United Health Foundation

9900 Bren Road East
Minnetonka MN 55343

June, 2005

Dear Colleague,

On behalf of United Health Foundation, it is my pleasure to provide you with the thirteenth edition of the BMJ Publishing Group's publication *Clinical Evidence Concise*. We remain committed to providing clinicians with each new update of this international source of the best available evidence for effective health care. It is our opinion that physicians should be supported in their best efforts to provide quality, safe and appropriate health care to their patients. From the many letters we receive from physicians across the nation, we know that *Clinical Evidence* is effective, not only in improving patient care, but also in enhancing patient-physician relationships and facilitating medical education.

As enthusiastic as we are about this thirteenth print version of *Clinical Evidence,* we are equally pleased to provide you with free access to the Internet version which is available at **www.clinicalevidence.com/uhf**. This website provides you with useful augmentations to the print version such as an efficient search tool, complete references, and monthly topic updates.

As a reader of *Clinical Evidence,* you demonstrate your commitment to the values of continuing professional development. On behalf of all of us at United Health Foundation, we thank you for your efforts to provide the best possible health care to all of your patients.

Sincerely,

William W. McGuire, M.D.
Chairman
United Health Foundation

D0366970

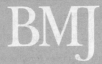

clinical
evidence

concise

The international source of the best available evidence for effective health care

13

SUMMER 2005

Editorial Office
BMJ Publishing Group, BMA House, Tavistock Square, London, WC1H 9JR, United Kingdom. Tel: +44 (0)20 7387 4499 • Fax: +44 (0)20 7383 6242 • www.bmjpg.com

Subscription prices for *Clinical Evidence*
Clinical Evidence and *Clinical Evidence Concise* are both published six monthly (June/December) by the BMJ Publishing Group. The annual subscription rates (for December, Issue 12 and June, Issue 13) are:

Concise edition
Personal: £95 • €140 • US$170
Institutional: £200 • €295 • US$365
Student/nurse: £42 • €62 • US$76

Full edition
Personal: £105 • €155 • US$190
Institutional: £220 • €325 • US$400
Student/nurse: £48 • €71 • US$87

There are special combined rates if you wish to purchase both editions.

All individual subscriptions (personal, student, nurse) include online access at no additional cost. Institutional subscriptions are for print editions only. Institutions may purchase online site licences separately. For information on site licences and individual electronic subscriptions please visit the subscription pages of our website www.clinicalevidence.com or email us at CEsubscriptions@bmjgroup.com (UK and ROW) or clinevid@pmds.com (Americas). You may also telephone us or fax us on the following numbers:

UK and ROW Tel: +44 (0)20 7383 6270 • Fax: +44 (0)20 7383 6402
Americas Tel: +1 800 373 2897/240 646 7000 • Fax: +1 240 646 7005

Bulk subscriptions for societies and organisations
The Publishers offer discounts for any society or organisation buying bulk quantities for their members/specific groups. Please contact Miranda Lonsdale, Sales Manager at mlonsdale@bmjgroup.com.

Rights and permission to reproduce
For information on translation rights, please contact Kate McPartlin at KMcPartlin@bmjgroup.com. To request permission to reprint all or part of any contribution in *Clinical Evidence* please contact Michelle McNeely at mmcneely@bmjgroup.com.

British Library Cataloguing in Publication Data. A catalogue record for this book is available from the British Library. ISSN 1475-9225, ISBN 0-9548965-4-8.

Printed by The Banta Book Group, Banta Harrisonburg, VA, USA.

Designed by Pete Wilder, The Designers Collective, London, UK.

Team and Advisors

Acknowledgements

The BMJ Publishing Group would like to thank United Health Foundation for its support.

The BMJ Publishing Group thanks the following people and organisations for their advice and support: The Cochrane Collaboration, and especially Iain Chalmers, Mike Clarke, Phil Alderson, and Carol Lefebvre; the National Health Service (NHS) Centre for Reviews and Dissemination, and especially Jos Kleijnen and Julie Glanville; the NHS, and especially Tom Mann, Ron Stamp, Ben Toth, Veronica Fraser, Muir Gray, and Nick Rosen; the British National Formulary, and especially Dinesh Mehta, Eric Connor, and John Martin; Martindale: The Complete Drug Reference, and especially Sean Sweetman; the Health Information Research Unit at McMaster University, and especially Brian Haynes and Ann McKibbon; the United Health Foundation (UHF), and especially Reed Tuckson and Yvette Krantz; Bazian Ltd, and especially Anna Donald and Vivek Muthu; Paul Dieppe, Tonya Fancher, and Richard Kravitz who are working with *Clinical Evidence* to explore ways of presenting evidence on the usefulness of diagnostic test; previous staff who have contributed to this issue; the clinicians, epidemiologists, and members of patient groups who have acted as contributors, advisors, and peer reviewers; and members of our user panels: Liz Hawthorne and colleagues at Didcot Health Centre; Murray Lough and colleagues at Airdrie Health Centre; Alex Potter and colleagues at Clydebank Health Centre; and Aimee Brame, Chris Clark, Gloria Daly, Hilary Durrant, Sarah Gwynne, James Harper, Diane Hickford, Sarosh Irani, Alison Kedward, Denise Knight, Sarah Lourenco, Michael Murphy, Ross Overshott, Deborah Rigby, and Catherine Tighe.

The BMJ Publishing Group values the ongoing support it has received from the global medical community for *Clinical Evidence*. We are grateful to the clinicians and patients who have taken part in focus groups, which are crucial to the development of *Clinical Evidence*. Finally, we would like to acknowledge the readers who have taken the time to send us their comments and suggestions.

The BMJ Publishing Group wishes to thank United Health Foundation for its efforts in providing educational funding which has allowed the wide dissemination of this valuable resource to millions of physicians and health professionals in the USA.

Contents

Welcome to Issue 13
A Guide to *Clinical Evidence Concise*

Some topics listed here are not printed in this issue but are available on the website while awaiting update (www.clinicalevidence.com).

Welcome to Issue 13

Welcome to Issue 13 of *Clinical Evidence,* the international source of the best available evidence on the effects of common clinical interventions. *Clinical Evidence* summarises the current state of knowledge and uncertainty about the prevention and treatment of clinical conditions, based on thorough searches and appraisal of the literature. It is neither a text book of medicine, nor a set of guidelines. It describes the best available evidence from systematic reviews, RCTs, and observational studies where appropriate, and if there is no good evidence it says so.

DEALING WITH UNCERTAINTY

Clinical Evidence and its sister product for patients, Best Treatments, aim to help people make informed decisions about which treatments to use. For clinicians and patients we wish to highlight treatments that work and for which the benefits outweigh the harms, especially those treatments that may currently be underused. We also wish to highlight treatments that do not work or for which the harms outweigh the benefits. Crucially, *Clinical Evidence* and Best Treatments can help people to distinguish between uncertainty due to gaps in the evidence or due to gaps in their own knowledge.

For the research community, *Clinical Evidence* and Best Treatments show where more research is needed—where there are currently no good RCTs or no RCTs that look at certain groups of people or important patient outcomes. We are pleased to be working closely with the James Lind Alliance, which is establishing partnerships between patients and clinicians to identify and prioritise current uncertainties about the effects of treatments. One important product of this initiative will be the free access Database of Uncertainties about the Effects of Treatments (DUET).

HOW MUCH DO WE KNOW?

So what can *Clinical Evidence* tell us about the state of our current knowledge? What proportion of commonly used treatments are supported by good evidence, what proportion should not be used or used only with caution, and how big are the gaps in our knowledge? Of the 2404 treatments covered in this issue, 360 (15%) are rated as beneficial, 538 (22%) likely to be beneficial, 180 (7%) as trade off between benefits and harms, 115 (5%) unlikely to be beneficial, 89 (4%) likely to be ineffective or harmful, and 1122 (47%), the largest proportion, as unknown effectiveness (see figure 1). Dividing treatments into categories is never easy. It always involves a degree of subjective judgement and is sometimes controversial. We do it because users tell us it is helpful, but judged by its own rules the categorisation is certainly of unknown effectiveness and may well have trade offs between benefits and harms. However, the figures above suggest that the research community has a large task ahead and that most decisions about treatments still rest on the individual judgements of clinicians and patients.

WHAT'S NEW

Clinical Evidence is continuously updated, with full literature searches on each topic every 12 months. Print copies containing the latest version of each topic are published every six months, and the website is refreshed, with new and updated content, every month. Before each topic is updated, we thoroughly review the structure of the topic, including the questions and the treatments covered, with the help of our expert authors and advisors in the field, to ensure maximum clinical relevance.

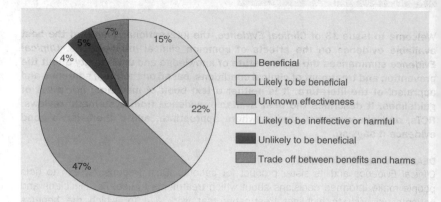

The content of *Clinical Evidence* Issue 13 is a snapshot of all content that was ready for publication in February 2005. Ten new topics have been added since Issue 12: Common cold, Angina (stable), Acne, Cervical cancer, Carbon monoxide poisoning, Non-Hodgkin's lymphoma, Glycaemic control in type 1 diabetes, End stage renal disease, Uncomplicated malaria and Kidney stones. In addition, 67 chapters have been updated, and by the time this reaches you more new and updated topics will have been posted on the website (www.clinicalevidence.com).

The regular updating of *Clinical Evidence* is now supplemented by BMJ Updates (www.bmjupdates.com), which provides readable summaries of the best and most relevant clinical research articles as they are published. You can ask the service to alert you to valid research in the areas that most interest you. BMJ Updates is a collaboration between the BMJ Publishing Group and McMaster University and can be accessed free via the *Clinical Evidence* website.

INTERNATIONAL REACH

Clinical Evidence has an international circulation, reaching more than a million clinicians worldwide in seven languages. In the USA, 500 000 clinicians receive copies of the concise edition thanks to the United Health Foundation. In the UK, the National Health Service distributes 50 000 copies of the concise edition to clinical staff in England, with free online access to everyone in England and Wales, and the BMA sends the concise edition to 10 500 UK medical students once a year. The governments of Norway and New Zealand now provide everyone in their countries with free online access, and thanks to the Italian Ministry of Health and the work of the Italian Cochrane Centre, 300 000 doctors in Italy receive a copy of the concise edition in Italian.

Clinical Evidence is available in other non-English language editions. The Spanish translation (published in collaboration with the Iberoamerican Cochrane Centre and Legis) now comes in all formats: full, concise and online. The full text is available in Japanese and Russian (seven broad speciality editions). The concise edition is also available in German and French.

Finally, *Clinical Evidence* continues to be available free online to people in developing countries as part of the HINARI initiative spearheaded by the World Health Organization and the BMJ Publishing Group. Details of those countries that qualify are available from the *Clinical Evidence* website (www.clinicalevidence.com).

FEEDBACK

Our web-site aims to encourage feedback, all of which we welcome. You can contact us at CEfeedback@bmjgroup.com, or use the Contact Us button on every page, or contact the editor on +44 (0)20 7383 6043. We are particularly interested to capture the clinical questions that first led you to use *Clinical Evidence* and to what extent your question was answered. If you have any comments on any of the material in *Clinical Evidence*, think that any important evidence has been missed, or have suggestions for new topics or questions please let us know.

Readers who would like to contribute either as authors or peer reviewers are also invited to send their CV to mmcneely@bmjgroup.com.

REFERENCES

1. *Clinical Evidence Conciso: La fonte delle migliori prove de efficacia per la pratica clínica.* Milan, Italy: Centro Cochrane Italiano/Editore Italiano/Editore Zadig, 2003.
2. *Evidencia Clinica.* Barcelona, Spain/Bogotá, Colombia: Asociacón Colaboración Cochrane Iberoamerican/Legis, 2004.
3. *Clinical Evidence (Japanese edition).* Tokyo, Japan: Nikkei Medical, 2004.
4. *Dokazatel'naya meditsina.* Moscow, Russia: Media Sphera Publishing Group, 2003.
5. *Kompendium evidenzbasierte Medizin.* Bern, Switzerland: Verlag Hans Huber, 2004.
6. *Décider pour traiter abrégé.* Meudon, France: RanD, 2004.

A guide to Clinical Evidence Concise

SUMMARY PAGE

Clinical Evidence Concise is an index of the summary information from each chapter in *Clinical Evidence* Issue 13. It contains evidence relating to hundreds of therapeutic or preventative interventions, derived from thousands of original studies, and presents it in around 600 pages. For each condition, interventions are categorised according to whether they have been found to be effective or not. The full evidence detail behind these summaries, including clinical questions, figures, tables, and appendices, are featured online at www.clinicalevidence.com, along with quantified, referenced, and up to date information about each condition. The full evidence is also available by subscription to our full text paper version.

Making summaries involves discarding detail, and users of *Clinical Evidence Concise* need to be aware of the limitations of the evidence that is presented. It is not possible to make global statements that are both useful and apply to every patient or clinical context that occur in practice. For example, when stating that we found evidence that a drug is beneficial, we mean that there is evidence that the drug has been shown to deliver more benefits than harms when assessed in at least one subgroup of people, using at least one outcome at a particular point in time. It does not mean that the drug will be effective in all people given that treatment or that other outcomes will be improved, or even that the same outcome will be improved at a different time after the treatment.

MEASURE OF TREATMENT EFFECTS

The dilemma is how to present summaries that are useful but not misleading. We have experimented with providing statements with no numerical information at all, with NNTs only, with a batch of absolute and relative risks, or with just the odds ratio. Each measure has its advantages and disadvantages, and not all are available from the included studies. Quantitative results may be misleading in the absence of discussion of their precision, reliability, and applicability. In *Clinical Evidence Concise*, we present non-numerical information only. Detailed quantitative results are presented online, where we are able to discuss their interpretation in more detail. Your suggestions on improvements are welcome.

USING *CLINICAL EVIDENCE CONCISE* ONLINE

Clinical Evidence Concise is intended to be used as a first point of call when trying to decide what the options for treatment might be. A detailed exploration of the evidence will require looking up the detail in the full print version, or on *Clinical Evidence* online. The electronic versions link, whenever possible, to abstracts of the original research in PubMed or published online versions. In this way, *Clinical Evidence* is also designed to act as a pointer, connecting the clinician rapidly to the relevant original evidence.

INDEX PAGE

Each topic online contains an index page listing interventions within their assigned categories of whether they have been found to be effective or not. Key messages summarising the evidence for each intervention are listed below the categorisation table. The full evidence detail supporting the categorisation, consisting of the question, a summary statement, benefits, harms, and a comment can be accessed by a hyperlink from the categorisation table. We would value your feedback on the presentation of interventions in future issues.

CATEGORISATION

We have developed these categories of effectiveness from one of the Cochrane Collaboration's first and most popular products, *A guide to effective care in pregnancy and childbirth*.[1] The categories are explained in the table below.

TABLE	**Categorisation of treatment effects in *Clinical Evidence***
Beneficial	Interventions for which effectiveness has been demonstrated by clear evidence from RCTs, and for which expectation of harms is small compared with the benefits.
Likely to be beneficial	Interventions for which effectiveness is less well established than for those listed under 'beneficial'.
Trade off between benefits and harms	Interventions for which clinicians and patients should weigh up the beneficial and harmful effects according to individual circumstances and priorities.
Unknown effectiveness	Interventions for which there are currently insufficient data or data of inadequate quality.
Unlikely to be beneficial	Interventions for which lack of effectiveness is less well established than for those listed under 'likely to be ineffective or harmful'.
Likely to be ineffective or harmful	Interventions for which ineffectiveness or harmfulness has been demonstrated by clear evidence.

Fitting interventions into these categories is not always straightforward. For one thing, the categories represent a mix of several hierarchies: the level of benefit (or harm), the level of evidence (RCT or observational data), and the level of certainty around the finding (represented by the confidence interval). Another problem is that much of the evidence that is most relevant to clinical decisions relates to comparisons between different interventions rather than to comparison with placebo or no intervention. Where necessary, we have indicated the comparisons. A third problem is that interventions may have been tested, or found to be effective, in only one group of people, such as those at high risk of an outcome. Again, we have indicated this where possible. But perhaps most difficult of all has been trying to maintain consistency across different topics. We are working on refining the criteria for putting interventions under each category.

REFERENCES

Full references to the individual studies cited in *Clinical Evidence Concise* are available online. References cited in the definition, incidence/prevalence, aetiology/risk factors, and prognosis sections are listed in the text but are available as hyperlinks from the equivalent section online.

TOPIC GLOSSARY

Topics may contain glossary listings; these are available in full online and can be accessed from the hyperlinks within the topic.

MAIN GLOSSARY

Words and terms that are used throughout *Clinical Evidence* are listed in the main glossary online.

TABLES AND FIGURES

The presence of figures and tables online are flagged up in a similar way to the glossary with the use of ⒻΦ for figures and ⓉΦ for tables.

FEEDBACK

The design of *Clinical Evidence Concise* will change progressively over the next few years. We will perform evaluation studies ourselves to measure the relevance of the material to the questions that are being asked in practice, the ease of use, and to check that the message extracted from the summary corresponds closely with that intended. If you have any comments, suggestions, or detect any errors, please let us know at CEfeedback@bmjgroup.com.

For more information on any of our products or processes, please visit our website at www.clinicalevidence.com.

REFERENCES

1. Enkin M, Keirse M, Renfrew M, et al. *A guide to effective care in pregnancy and childbirth*. Oxford: Oxford University Press, 1998.

Non-Hodgkin's lymphoma (diffuse large B cell lymphoma)

Search date February 2004

Ellen Roxane Copson

What are the effects of first line treatments for aggressive non-Hodgkin's lymphoma (diffuse large B cell lymphoma)? New

BENEFICIAL

CHOP 21* New

CHOP 21 is the standard treatment for aggressive non-Hodgkin's lymphoma (not including Burkitt's lymphoma) and placebo or no treatment controlled trials would be considered unethical. Six RCTs identified by two systematic reviews found that no alternative regimen (MACOP-B, m-BACOD, ProMACE-CytaBOM, or PACEBOM) was shown to be consistently superior to CHOP 21 in terms of overall survival. Toxicity was generally similar with the different regimens.

LIKELY TO BE BENEFICIAL

CHOP 14 New

We found one RCT comparing CHOP 21 with CHOP 14 in people aged 18–60 years with good prognosis aggressive lymphoma and a second RCT comparing CHOP 21 with CHOP 14 in people aged 61–75 years with aggressive lymphoma. The RCT in younger people found no significant difference between CHOP 14 and CHOP 21 in complete response rates or 5 year event free survival. However, overall 5 year survival was higher with CHOP 14. The RCT in older people found that CHOP 14 improved complete response rate, 5 year event free survival, and overall survival compared with CHOP 21. Toxicity was similar with CHOP 14 and CHOP 21 in both studies.

CHOP 21 plus rituximab (increased survival compared with CHOP 21 alone) New

One RCT found that in people aged 60–80 years with stage II–IV disease, CHOP 21 plus rituximab reduced events and death compared with CHOP 21 alone at 2 years.

Short schedule CHOP 21 plus adjuvant radiotherapy (increased survival compared with longer schedule CHOP 21 alone) New

One RCT found that short schedule CHOP 21 plus adjuvant radiotherapy improved 5 year progression free survival and overall survival compared with longer schedule CHOP 21 alone. Longer schedule CHOP 21 alone increased the risk of congestive heart failure, and slightly increased the risk of myelosuppression, although this increase was not significant.

What are the effects of treatments for relapsed aggressive non-Hodgkin's lymphoma (diffuse large B cell lymphoma)? New

LIKELY TO BE BENEFICIAL

Conventional dose salvage chemotherapy (consensus that treatment should be given but relative benefits of different regimens unclear)* New

We found no RCTs comparing different conventional dose salvage chemotherapy regimens (PACEBOM, ESHAP, RICE, IVAC) in people with relapsed aggressive non-Hodgkin's lymphoma. Consensus is that people with relapsed disease should be treated with salvage chemotherapy. One systematic review identified 22 phase II trials of various conventional dose salvage chemotherapy regimens. All regimens reported similar response rates and no single superior regimen could be identified.

High dose chemotherapy plus autologous transplant stem cell support (increased survival compared with conventional dose chemotherapy in people with chemosensitive disease) New

One systematic review identified one RCT comparing high dose chemotherapy plus autologous bone marrow transplantation with conventional dose chemotherapy in people with a chemosensitive relapse of aggressive non-Hodgkin's lymphoma. It found that high dose chemotherapy plus autologous bone marrow transplantation improved 5 year event free survival and overall survival compared with conventional chemotherapy. We found no RCTs in people in people with chemotherapy resistant disease.

*Based on consensus.

DEFINITION   Non-Hodgkin's lymphoma (NHL) consists of a complex group of cancers arising mainly from B lymphocytes (85% of cases) and occasionally from T lymphocytes. NHL usually develops in lymph nodes (nodal lymphoma) but can arise in other tissues almost anywhere in the body (extranodal lymphoma). NHL is categorised according to its appearance under the microscope (histology) and the extent of the disease (stage). **Histology:** Since 1966, four major different methods of classifying NHLs according to their histological appearance have been published (see table 1)❶;see table 2❶;see table 3❶;see table 4)❶. At present, the World Health Organization (WHO)[1] system is accepted as the gold standard of classification. The WHO system is based on the underlying principles of the REAL classification system.[2] Historically, NHLs have been divided into slow growing "low grade" lymphomas and fast growing "aggressive" lymphomas. This chapter deals only with the most common aggressive NHL – diffuse B cell lymphoma (WHO classification; see table 1❶). Interpretation of older studies is complicated by the fact that histological methods have changed and there is no direct correlation between lymphoma types in the WHO and other classification systems. Attempts to generalise results must therefore be treated with caution. We have however included some older studies referring to alternative classification methods if they included people with the following types of aggressive lymphomas, which overlap substantially with the WHO classification of interest: Working Formulation Classification – primarily intermediate grades (grades E–H; see table 2❶);[3] Kiel classification – centroblastic, Immunoblastic, and anaplastic (see table 3❶)[4] Rappaport classification – diffuse histiocytic, diffuse lymphocytic poorly differentiated, and diffuse mixed (lymphocytic and histiocytic; see table 4❶).[5] **Stage:** NHL has traditionally been staged according to extent of disease spread using the Ann Arbor system (see table 5❶).[6] The term "early disease" is used to describe disease that falls within Ann Arbor stage I or II while "advanced disease" refers to Ann Arbor stage III or IV disease. However, all people with bulky disease, usually defined as having a disease site larger ▶

Non-Hodgkin's lymphoma (diffuse large B cell lymphoma)

than 10 cm in diameter, are treated as having advanced disease regardless of their Ann Arbor staging. **Relapsed disease:** Relapsed disease refers to the recurrence of active disease in a person who had previously achieved a complete response to initial treatment for NHL. Most studies of treatments in relapsed disease require a minimum duration of complete response of 1 month before relapse.

INCIDENCE/ PREVALENCE
Non-Hodgkin's lymphoma occurs more commonly in males than females, and is increasing in incidence in the Western world by 4% a year. It is the seventh most common cancer in the UK with 9189 new cases per 100 000 population diagnosed in 2000 and causing 4654 deaths per 100 000 population in 2002.[7]

AETIOLOGY/ RISK FACTORS
The aetiology of most Non-Hodgkin's lymphomas (NHLs) is unknown. Incidence is higher in individuals who are immunosuppressed (congenital or acquired). Other risk factors include viral infection (human T cell leukaemia virus type-1, Epstein Barr virus, human immunodeficiency virus), bacterial infection (e.g. *Helicobacter pylori*), previous treatment with diphenylhydantoin or antineoplastic drugs, and exposure to pesticides or organic solvents.[8]

PROGNOSIS
Overall survival: Untreated aggressive Non-Hodgkin's lymphomas (NHLs) would generally result in death in a matter of months. High grade lymphomas, particularly diffuse large B cell lymphomas and Burkitt's lymphomas, have a high cure rate, with both initial and salvage chemotherapy.[9] The 5 year relative age standardised survival for people diagnosed with and treated for NHL between 2000 and 2001 was 55% for men and 56% for women.[7] **Relapse:** About 50% of people with NHL will be cured by initial treatment. Of the rest, about 30% will fail to respond to initial treatment (so called "chemotherapy refractory disease"), and about 20–30% will relapse. Most relapses occur within 2 years of completion of initial treatment. Up to 50% of these have chemosensitive disease; the remainder tend to have chemotherapy resistant disease. **Prognostic indicators:** Prognosis depends on histological type, stage, age, performance status, and lactate dehydrogenase levels. Prognosis varies substantially within each Ann Arbor stage, and further information regarding prognosis can be obtained from applying the International Prognostic Index (IPI).[8] The IPI model stratifies prognosis according to the presence or absence of five risk factors: age (< 60 years v > 60 years), serum lactate dehydrogenase (normal v elevated), performance status (0 or 1 v 2–4), Ann Arbor stage (I or II v III or IV), and number of extranodal sites involved (0 or 1 v 2–4). People with two or more high risk factors have a less than 50% chance of relapse free and overall survival at 5 years. IPI staging is currently the most important system used to define disease stage and treatment options. However, most studies identified by our search pre-date the IPI staging system.

Please refer to the Clinical Evidence website for full text and references.

Blood and lymph disorders

Sickle cell disease

Search date September 2003

Martin M Meremikwu

What are the effects of interventions to prevent sickle cell crisis and other acute complications in people with sickle cell disease?

BENEFICIAL

Penicillin prophylaxis in children under 5 years of age

One systematic review found that penicillin prophylaxis in children younger than 5 years reduced invasive pneumococcal infections and related deaths compared with no penicillin or placebo, irrespective of pneumococcal immunisation status.

LIKELY TO BE BENEFICIAL

Hydroxyurea

One RCT in adults identified by a systematic review found that hydroxyurea reduced the incidence of painful sickle cell crisis over a mean 21 months compared with placebo. Another RCT in children identified by a systematic review found that hydroxyurea reduced the duration of hospital stay compared with placebo. The RCT in adults also found that hydroxyurea reduced acute chest syndrome and the need for blood transfusion in people with sickle cell disease over a mean 21 months. It found no significant difference in stroke, hepatic sequestration, and mortality related to sickle cell disease between hydroxyurea and placebo, but it may have lacked power and fewer people taking hydroxyurea than taking placebo had these outcomes. Hydroxyurea has been associated with neutropenia, hair loss, skin rash, and gastrointestinal disturbances. We found no RCTs assessing the long term effects of hydroxyurea.

Piracetam

One RCT identified by a systematic review found that piracetam reduced the incidence of sickle cell crisis in children compared with placebo.

Zinc sulfate

One RCT identified by a systematic review found that zinc sulfate reduced the incidence of sickle cell crisis compared with placebo.

UNKNOWN EFFECTIVENESS

Malaria chemoprophylaxis

Falciparum malaria is believed to precipitate sickle cell crisis and to increase the risk of death in children with sickle cell anaemia, therefore regular chemoprophylaxis with anti-malarial drugs is advocated by consensus. However, one quasi randomised trial identified by a systematic review provided insufficient evidence to assess routine malaria chemoprophylaxis in people with sickle cell disease.

Pneumococcal vaccines

We found no RCTs evaluating the clinical benefits of pneumococcal vaccines in sickle cell disease. Three RCTs found that pneumococcal vaccines caused local reaction and fever but no severe adverse effects.

Avoidance of cold environment; limiting physical exercise

We found no RCTs or observational studies of sufficient quality evaluating these interventions in preventing sickle cell crisis and other life threatening complications.

What are the effects of interventions to treat pain in people with sickle cell crisis?

LIKELY TO BE BENEFICIAL

Controlled release oral morphine given after an initial intravenous bolus dose of morphine (as effective as repeated doses of intravenous morphine)

We found no RCTs comparing morphine versus placebo in people with sickle cell crisis. One RCT in children with painful crisis found that, after an intravenous loading dose of morphine at onset of treatment, controlled release oral morphine was as effective for reducing pain as intravenous morphine.

Patient controlled analgesia

Two small RCTs in adults with sickle cell crisis found no significant difference in pain between patient controlled analgesia using either meperidine or morphine and intermittent parenteral treatment. The incidence of adverse effects was also similar in both regimens.

TRADE OFF BETWEEN BENEFITS AND HARMS

Corticosteroid as adjunct to narcotic analgesics

One RCT found that adding high dose intravenous methylprednisolone to intravenous morphine reduced the duration of inpatient analgesia compared with placebo in people with acute, severe, painful sickle cell crisis. It found no significant difference between adding methylprednisolone and placebo in the proportion of people readmitted to hospital for recurrent pain within two weeks of stopping treatment, although more people taking methylprednisolone were readmitted. Another RCT found that adding dexamethasone to intravenous morphine reduced the number of doses and duration of intravenous analgesia compared with placebo in people with acute sickle cell chest syndrome. Some of the known adverse effects of corticosteroids are increased risk of infections, weight gain, hypertension, poor glucose metabolism, cataracts, and poor growth in children.

UNKNOWN EFFECTIVENESS

Acupuncture

We found no RCTs of acupuncture in people with sickle cell crisis.

Diflunisal

One RCT in adults with vaso-occlusive sickle cell crisis found no significant difference between adding diflunisal to intramuscular meperidine and adding placebo in pain or in dose of meperidine administered, but it is likely to have been underpowered to detect a clinically important difference.

Hydration

We found no RCTs on the effects of routinely giving extra fluids to treat people with sickle cell crisis.

Ketorolac

Four RCTs provided insufficient evidence to assess ketorolac in people with vaso-occlusive sickle cell crisis.

Oxygen

One RCT in children provided insufficient evidence to assess oxygen therapy in people with sickle cell crisis.

Aspirin; codeine; ibuprofen; paracetamol

We found no RCTs evaluating these analgesics in people with sickle cell crisis.

Sickle cell disease

DEFINITION

Sickle cell disease refers to a group of disorders caused by inheritance of a pair of abnormal haemoglobin genes, including the sickle cell gene. It is characterised by chronic haemolytic anaemia, dactylitis, and acute episodic clinical events called "crises".[1] Vaso-occlusive (painful) crisis is the most common and occurs when abnormal red cells clog small vessels causing tissue ischaemia. The others are hyper-haemolytic crisis (excessive haemolysis), acute chest syndrome, sequestration crisis, and aplastic crisis. A common variant of sickle cell disease, also characterised by haemolytic anaemia, occurs in people with one sickle and one thalassaemia gene. **Sickle cell trait** occurs in people with one sickle gene and one normal gene. People with sickle cell trait do not have any clinical manifestation of illness. This topic covers people with sickle cell disease with or without thalassaemia.

INCIDENCE/ PREVALENCE

Sickle cell disease is most common among people living in or originating from sub-Saharan Africa.[2] The disorder also affects people of Mediterranean, Caribbean, Middle Eastern, and Asian origin. The sickle cell gene is most common in areas where malaria is endemic: sickle cell trait affects about 10–30% of Africa's tropical populations.[3] Sickle cell disease affects an estimated 1–2% (120 000) of newborns in Africa annually. Approximately 178 babies (0.28 per 1000 conceptions) are affected by sickle cell disease in England annually.[4] About 60 000 people in the USA[4] and 10 000 in the UK suffer from the disease.[5]

AETIOLOGY/ RISK FACTORS

Sickle cell disease is inherited as an autosomal recessive disorder. For a baby to be affected, both parents must have the sickle cell gene. In parents with sickle cell trait, the risk of having of an affected baby is one in four for each pregnancy. Painful (vaso-occlusive) crisis is the most common and most distressing feature of the disease, and these episodes start in infancy and early childhood.[6] Factors that precipitate or modulate the occurrence of sickle cell crisis are not fully understood, but infections, hypoxia, dehydration, acidosis, stress (such as major surgery or childbirth), and cold are believed to play some role. In tropical Africa, malaria is the most common cause of anaemic and vaso-occlusive crisis.[3] High levels of fetal haemoglobin are known to ameliorate the severity and incidence of sickle cell crisis and other complications of the disease.

PROGNOSIS

People affected by sickle cell disease are predisposed to bacterial infections, especially to those caused by encapsulated organisms such as *Pneumococcus*, *Haemophilus influenzae*, *Meningococcus*, and *Salmonella* species. Severe bacterial infections such as pneumonia, meningitis, and septicaemia are common causes of morbidity and mortality, especially among young children.[7] About 10% of children with sickle cell anaemia may develop a stroke, and more than half of these may suffer recurrent strokes.[8] Abnormal features of cerebral blood vessels shown by transcranial Doppler scan predict a high risk of stroke in children with sickle cell disease.[9] Frequent episodes of crisis, infections, and organ damage reduce the quality of life of people with sickle cell disease. High rate of vaso-occlusive (painful) crisis is an index of clinical severity that correlates with early death. Life expectancy remains low, especially in communities with poor access to health services. In some parts of Africa, about 50% of children with sickle cell disease die before their first birthday.[3] The average life expectancy for men and women with sickle cell disease in the USA is about 42 and 48 years, respectively.[10] Frequent blood transfusions could increase the risk of immune reactions and infections, such as HIV and hepatitis B or C viruses, and Chagas' disease. The need for repeated blood transfusions in people with sickle cell disease predisposes them to the risk of iron overload.[11]

Please refer to the Clinical Evidence website for full text and references.

Search date October 2003

Nicolas Danchin, Edoardo De Benedetti, and Philip Urban

What treatments improve outcomes in acute myocardial infarction?

BENEFICIAL

Angiotensin converting enzyme inhibitors

One systematic review in people treated within 14 days of acute myocardial infarction has found that angiotensin converting enzyme inhibitors reduce mortality after 6 weeks compared with placebo. However, a non-systematic review found that angiotensin converting enzyme inhibitors increase persistent hypotension and renal dysfunction at 6 weeks compared with placebo.

Aspirin

One systematic review in people with acute myocardial infarction has found that aspirin reduces mortality, reinfarction, and stroke at 1 month compared with placebo.

β Blockers

Two reviews and one subsequent RCT found that β blockers reduced mortality compared with no β blockers. One RCT in people receiving thrombolytic treatment found that immediate treatment with metoprolol reduced rates of reinfarction and chest pain at 6 days compared with delayed treatment, but had no significant effect on mortality at 6 days or at 1 year.

Primary percutaneous transluminal coronary angioplasty versus thrombolysis (performed in specialist centres)

One systematic review found that primary percutaneous transluminal coronary angioplasty reduced a combined outcome of death, non-fatal reinfarction, and stroke compared with thrombolysis.

Thrombolysis

One non-systematic review in people with acute myocardial infarction and ST segment elevation or bundle branch block on their initial electrocardiogram found that prompt thrombolytic treatment (within 6 hours and perhaps up to 12 hours and longer after the onset of symptoms) reduced mortality compared with placebo. RCTs comparing different types of thrombolytic agents versus each other found no significant difference in mortality. One non-systematic review found that thrombolytic treatment increased the risk of stroke or major bleeding compared with control. The review also found that intracranial haemorrhage was more common in people of advanced age and low body weight, those with hypertension on admission, and those given tissue plasminogen activator rather than another thrombolytic agent. One non-systematic review found conflicting results for intracerebral haemorrhage with bolus treatment compared with infusion of thrombolytic agents. One systematic review found that thrombolysis was less effective at reducing a combined outcome of death, non-fatal reinfarction, and stroke compared with primary percutaneous transluminal coronary angioplasty.

LIKELY TO BE BENEFICIAL

Adding low molecular weight heparin (enoxaparin) to thrombolytics (reduces acute myocardial infarction rates)

One RCT found that adding enoxaparin (a low molecular weight heparin) to streptokinase reduced acute myocardial infarction rates compared with adding ▶

placebo in people with early evidence of a developing infarction. One systematic review identified five RCTs comparing enoxaparin (a low molecular weight heparin) plus thrombolytic treatment versus unfractionated heparin plus thrombolytic treatment. Two of the RCTs identified by the review found that enoxaparin plus thrombolytics reduced acute myocardial infarction rates compared with unfractionated heparin plus thrombolytics, while three RCTs found no significant difference between treatments. The review found no significant difference in mortality between enoxaparin and unfractionated heparin when added to thrombolytic treatment and no significant difference between added enoxaparin and added unfractionated heparin in the risk of intracranial or other major bleeding.

Nitrates (in the absence of thrombolysis)

One systematic review of the trials conducted in the prethrombolytic era found that nitrates reduced mortality in people with acute myocardial infarction compared with placebo.

TRADE OFF BETWEEN BENEFITS AND HARMS

Glycoprotein IIb/IIIa inhibitors

Two large RCTs found that combined treatment with half dose thrombolysis plus abciximab did not reduce mortality at 1 month in people with acute myocardial infarction compared with full dose thrombolysis, but found limited evidence that the combined treatment reduced non-fatal cardiovascular events. However, the RCTs found that combined treatment with abciximab increased bleeding complications, particularly extracranial haemorrhage. Three RCTs found conflicting evidence about the benefits of adding abciximab to primary coronary angioplasty or stenting in people with acute myocardial infarction, although all found that adding abciximab increased bleeding risk. One RCT found no difference in survival or morbidity outcomes between early or late tirofiban administration in people undergoing primary coronary angioplasty. It also found no difference in minor or major bleeding complications between early and late tirofiban administration, although the study may have been too small to detect clinically important differences.

UNLIKELY TO BE BENEFICIAL

Adding unfractionated heparin to thrombolytics

Two RCTs found no significant difference in mortality or acute myocardial infarction rates between unfractionated heparin plus thrombolytics and thrombolytics alone. One systematic review identified five RCTs comparing enoxaparin (a low molecular weight heparin) plus thrombolytic treatment versus unfractionated heparin plus thrombolytic treatment. Two of the RCTs identified by the review found that enoxaparin plus thrombolytics reduced acute myocardial infarction rates compared with unfractionated heparin plus thrombolytics, while three RCTs found no significant difference between treatments. The review found no significant difference in mortality between enoxaparin and unfractionated heparin when added to thrombolytic treatment and no significant difference between added enoxaparin and added unfractionated heparin in the risk of intracranial or other major bleeding.

Nitrates (in addition to thrombolysis)

Two RCTs in people with acute myocardial infarction (after thrombolysis was introduced) found no significant difference in mortality between nitrates and placebo.

LIKELY TO BE INEFFECTIVE OR HARMFUL

Calcium channel blockers

We found evidence that neither dihydropyridines nor verapamil reduce mortality compared with placebo. One RCT found limited evidence that, in people with left ventricular dysfunction, nifedipine given in the first few days after myocardial infarction may increase mortality compared with placebo.

Which treatments improve outcomes for cardiogenic shock after acute myocardial infarction?

BENEFICIAL

Early invasive cardiac revascularisation

One large RCT found that early invasive cardiac revascularisation reduced mortality after 6 and 12 months compared with medical treatment alone in people with cardiogenic shock within 48 hours of acute myocardial infarction. A second, smaller RCT found similar results, although the difference was not significant.

UNKNOWN EFFECTIVENESS

Intra-aortic balloon counterpulsation

An RCT presented only in abstract form found limited evidence of no significant difference in mortality at 6 months between intra-aortic balloon counterpulsation plus thrombolysis versus thrombolysis alone in people with cardiogenic shock.

Early cardiac surgery; positive inotropes; pulmonary artery catheterisation; vasodilators; ventricular assistance devices and cardiac transplantation

We found no evidence from RCTs about the effects of these interventions.

UNLIKELY TO BE BENEFICIAL

Thrombolysis

Subgroup analysis of one RCT found no significant difference in mortality after 21 days between thrombolysis and no thrombolysis in people with cardiogenic shock.

DEFINITION **Acute myocardial infarction (AMI):** The sudden occlusion of a coronary artery leading to myocardial cell death. **Cardiogenic shock:** Defined clinically as a poor cardiac output plus evidence of tissue hypoxia that is not improved by correcting reduced intravascular volume.[1] When a pulmonary artery catheter is used, cardiogenic shock may be defined as a cardiac index below 2.2 L/minute/m^2 despite an elevated pulmonary capillary wedge pressure ($\geq$ 15 mm Hg).[1–3]

INCIDENCE/ **AMI:** Acute myocardial infarction is one of the most common causes of
PREVALENCE mortality worldwide. In 1990, ischaemic heart disease was the world's leading cause of death, accounting for about 6.3 million deaths. The age standardised incidence varies among and within countries.[4] Each year, about 900 000 people in the USA experience AMI, about 225 000 of whom die. About half of these people die within 1 hour of symptoms and before reaching a hospital emergency room.[5] Event rates increase with age for both sexes and are higher in men than in women and in poorer than richer people at all ages. The incidence of death from AMI has fallen in many Western countries over the past 20 years. **Cardiogenic shock:** Cardiogenic shock occurs in about 7% of people admitted to hospital with AMI.[6] Of these, about half have established cardiogenic shock at the time of admission to hospital, and most of the others develop it during the first 24–48 hours after their admission.[7] ▶

Acute myocardial infarction

AETIOLOGY/ RISK FACTORS

AMI: The immediate mechanism of AMI is rupture or erosion of an atheromatous plaque causing thrombosis and occlusion of coronary arteries and myocardial cell death. Factors that may convert a stable plaque into an unstable plaque (the "active plaque") have yet to be fully elucidated. Shear stresses, inflammation, and autoimmunity have been proposed. The changing rates of coronary heart disease in different populations are only partly explained by changes in the standard risk factors for ischaemic heart disease (particularly a fall in blood pressure and smoking). **Cardiogenic shock:** Cardiogenic shock after AMI usually follows a reduction in functional ventricular myocardium, and is caused by left ventricular infarction (79% of people with cardiogenic shock) more often than by right ventricular infarction (3% of people with cardiogenic shock).[8] Cardiogenic shock after AMI may also be caused by cardiac structural defects, such as mitral valve regurgitation due to papillary muscle dysfunction (7% of people with cardiogenic shock), ventricular septal rupture (4% of people with cardiogenic shock), or cardiac tamponade after free cardiac wall rupture (1% of people with cardiogenic shock). Major risk factors for cardiogenic shock after AMI are previous myocardial infarction, diabetes mellitus, advanced age, hypotension, tachycardia or bradycardia, congestive heart failure with Killip class II–III, and low left ventricular ejection fraction (ejection fraction < 35%).[7,8]

PROGNOSIS

AMI: May lead to a host of mechanical and cardiac electrical complications, including death, ventricular dysfunction, congestive heart failure, fatal and non-fatal arrhythmias, valvular dysfunction, myocardial rupture, and cardiogenic shock. **Cardiogenic shock:** Mortality rates for people in hospital with cardiogenic shock after AMI vary between 50–80%.[2,3,6,7] Most deaths occur within 48 hours of the onset of shock **❺**. People surviving until discharge from hospital have a reasonable long term prognosis (88% survival at 1 year).[10]

Please refer to the Clinical Evidence website for full text and references.

What are effects of long term single drug treatment for stable angina? New

LIKELY TO BE BENEFICIAL

β Blockers* New

One small RCT found no significant difference between a β blocker (propranolol) and placebo in angina frequency or exercise duration after 6 months. However, this trial may have lacked power to detect a clinically important difference between groups. There is consensus that β blockers are effective for treating the symptoms of stable angina. RCTs found no significant difference between β blockers and calcium channel blockers in the frequency of angina attacks, exercise duration, mortality, or non-fatal cardiovascular events at 6 months to 3 years. However, these RCTs may have lacked power to detect clinically important differences between groups. One RCT also found no significant difference between β blockers and calcium channel blockers in quality of life.

Calcium channel blockers* New

One small RCT found no significant difference between bepridil and placebo in the frequency of angina attacks. It found that bepridil increased exercise duration compared with placebo at 6 months. There is consensus that calcium channel blockers are effective for treating the symptoms of stable angina. RCTs found no significant difference between calcium channel blockers and β blockers in the frequency of angina attacks, exercise duration, mortality, or non-fatal cardiovascular events at between 6 months and 3 years. However, these RCTs may have lacked power to detect clinically important differences between groups. One RCT also found no significant difference between calcium channel blockers and β blockers in quality of life. One RCT found no significant difference between amlodipine and isosorbide mononitrate in the frequency of angina attacks or in quality of life. It found that amlodipine increased exercise duration compared with isosorbide mononitrate at 6 months. The RCT found that peripheral oedema was more common with amlodipine than with isosorbide mononitrate, whereas headache was more common with isosorbide mononitrate.

Nitrates* New

We found no RCTs comparing long term single drug treatment with nitrates versus placebo for stable angina. However, there is consensus that nitrates are effective for treating the symptoms of stable angina. One RCT found no significant difference between amlodipine and isosorbide mononitrate in the frequency of angina attacks or in quality of life. It found that amlodipine increased exercise duration compared with isosorbide mononitrate at 6 months. The RCT found that peripheral oedema was more common with amlodipine than with isosorbide mononitrate, whereas headache was more common with isosorbide mononitrate.

Potassium channel openers* New

We found no RCTs on the effects of long term single drug treatment with potassium channel openers for stable angina. However, there is consensus that potassium channel openers are effective for treating the symptoms of stable angina.

*Based on consensus   ▶

Angina (stable)

DEFINITION Angina pectoris, often simply known as angina, is a clinical syndrome characterised by discomfort in the chest, shoulder, back, arm, or jaw.[1] Angina is usually caused by coronary artery atherosclerotic disease. Rarer causes include valvular heart disease, hypertrophic cardiomyopathy, uncontrolled hypertension, or vasospasm or endothelial dysfunction not related to atherosclerosis. The differential diagnosis of angina includes non-cardiac conditions affecting the chest wall, oesophagus, and lungs. Angina may be classified as stable or unstable. **Stable angina** is defined as regular or predictable angina symptoms that have been occurring for over 2 months. Symptoms are transient and are typically provoked by exertion, and alleviated by rest or nitroglycerin. Other precipitants include cold weather, eating, or emotional distress. This chapter deals specifically with stable angina caused by coronary artery atherosclerotic disease. **Unstable angina** is diagnosed if there is a rapid decline in exercise capacity or if there are episodes of pain at rest. This is usually associated with atherosclerotic plaque instability and, as myocardial infarction and death may ensue, should be treated as a medical emergency, usually requiring hospital admission.

INCIDENCE/ PREVALENCE The prevalence of stable angina remains unclear.[1,2] Epidemiological studies in the UK estimate that 6–16% of men and 3–10% of women aged 65–74 years have experienced angina.[3–5] Annually, about 1% of the population visits their general practitioner with symptoms of angina[4] and 23 000 people with new anginal symptoms present to their general practitioner each year in the UK.[6] These studies did not distinguish between stable and unstable angina.[3–6]

AETIOLOGY/ RISK FACTORS Stable angina resulting from coronary artery disease is characterised by focal atherosclerotic plaques in the intimal layer of the epicardial coronary artery. The plaques encroach on the coronary lumen and may limit blood flow to the myocardium, especially during periods of increased myocardial oxygen demand. The major risk factors that lead to the development of stable angina are similar to those that predispose to coronary heart disease. These risk factors include increasing age, male sex, overweight, hypertension, elevated serum cholesterol level, smoking, and relative physical inactivity.[7]

PROGNOSIS Stable angina is a marker of underlying coronary heart disease, which accounts for 1 in 4 deaths in the UK.[8] People with angina are 2–5 times more likely to develop other manifestations of coronary heart disease than people that do not have angina.[7,9] One population based study (7100 men aged 51–59 years at entry) found that people with angina had higher mortality than people with no history of coronary artery disease at baseline (16 year survival rate: 53% with angina v 72% without coronary artery disease v 34% with a history of myocardial infarction).[10] Clinical trials in people with stable angina have tended to recruit participants who were not felt to be in need of coronary revascularisation and in these people prognosis is better, with an annual mortality of 1–2% and annual rate of non-fatal myocardial infarction of 2–3%.[11–14] Features that indicate a poorer prognosis include: more severe symptoms, male sex,[15] abnormal resting electrocardiogram[16] (present in about 50% of people with angina[17]), previous myocardial infarction,[10,18] left ventricular dysfunction,[19] easily provoked or widespread coronary ischaemia on stress testing (present in about one third of people referred to hospital with stable angina), and significant stenosis of all three major coronary arteries or the left main coronary artery.[6,19] In addition, the standard coronary risk factors continue to exert a detrimental and additive effect on prognosis in people with stable angina.[9,20,21] Control of these risk factors is dealt with in the *Clinical Evidence* chapter on secondary prevention of ischaemic cardiac events, (Web only).

Please refer to the Clinical Evidence website for full text and references.

Search date October 2003

Gregory Y H Lip and Bethan Freestone

What are the effects of interventions to prevent embolism?

UNKNOWN EFFECTIVENESS

Antithrombotic treatment before cardioversion

We found no RCTs on use of aspirin, heparin, or warfarin as thromboprophylaxis before attempted cardioversion in acute atrial fibrillation.

What are the effects of interventions for conversion to sinus rhythm?

TRADE OFF BETWEEN BENEFITS AND HARMS

Flecainide

One RCT found that intravenous flecainide increased the proportion of people who reverted to sinus rhythm within 1 hour and in whom the sinus rhythm was maintained after 6 hours compared with placebo. Flecainide has been associated with serious adverse events such as severe hypotension and torsades de point. Two RCTs found that oral flecainide increased the proportion of people who reverted to sinus rhythm within 8 hours compared with intravenous amiodarone. We found insufficient evidence to draw any conclusions about comparisons between intravenous flecainide and intravenous amiodarone and between flecainide and quinidine. Three RCTs found no significant difference in rates of conversion to sinus rhythm between flecainide and propafenone. Flecainide and propafenone are not used in people with known or suspected ischaemic heart disease because they may cause arrhythmias.

Propafenone

One systematic review and subsequent RCTs have found that propafenone increased the proportion of people converting to sinus rhythm within 1–4 hours compared with placebo. One RCT in people with onset of atrial fibrillation of less than 48 hours found no significant difference between intravenous propafenone and amiodarone in the proportion of people who converted to sinus rhythm within 1 hour. Another RCT in people with onset of atrial fibrillation of less than 2 weeks found that a higher proportion of people converted to sinus rhythm with oral propafenone within 2.5 hours compared with amiodarone, but the difference did not remain significant at 24 hours. Three RCTs found insufficient evidence to compare rates of conversion to sinus rhythm between propafenone and flecqinide. Propafenone and flecainide are not used in people with known or suspected ischaemic heart disease.

UNKNOWN EFFECTIVENESS

Amiodarone

We found insufficient evidence from three RCTs about the effects of amiodarone as a single agent compared with placebo for conversion to sinus rhythm in people with acute atrial fibrillation in people who are haemodynamically stable. Four small RCTs found no significant difference in rate of conversion to sinus rhythm at 24–48 hours for amiodarone compared with digoxin, although the studies may have lacked power to exclude clinically important differences. One small RCT found that amiodarone increased rate of cardioversion compared with verapamil at 3 hours. One RCT in people with onset of atrial fibrillation of less than 48 hours found no ▶

Atrial fibrillation (acute)

significant difference between intravenous propafenone and amiodarone in conversion to sinus rhythm within 1 hour. Another RCT in people with onset of atrial fibrillation of less than 2 weeks found that a higher proportion of people converted to sinus rhythm with oral propafenone within 2.5 hours compared with amiodarone but the difference did not remain significant at 24 hours. Two RCTs found that intravenous amiodarone reduced the proportion of people who reverted to sinus rhythm within 8 hours compared with oral flecainide. We found insufficient evidence to draw any conclusion between intravenous flecainide compared with intravenous amiodarone. We found no RCTs comparing amiodarone with either DC cardioversion or diltiazem.

DC cardioversion

We found no RCTs of DC cardioversion in acute atrial fibrillation in people who are haemodynamically stable.

Quinidine

We found no RCTs of DC cardioversion that compared quinidine versus placebo. One small RCT in people with onset of atrial fibrillation of less than 48 hours found that quinidine plus digoxin increased the proportion of people converting to sinus rhythm within 12 hours compared with sotalol. We found insufficient evidence to draw any conclusions about comparisons between flecainide and quinidine.

Sotalol

We found no RCTs comparing sotalol versus placebo. One small RCT in people with onset of atrial fibrillation of less than 48 hours found that quinidine plus digoxin increased the proportion of people who converted to sinus rhythm within 12 hours compared with sotalol.

UNLIKELY TO BE BENEFICIAL

Digoxin

We found no placebo controlled RCTs limited to people with acute atrial fibrillation. Three RCTs in people with atrial fibrillation of up to 7 days' duration found no significant difference between digoxin and placebo in conversion to sinus rhythm. Four RCTs found no significant difference between amiodarone and digoxin in conversion to sinus rhythm at 24–48 hours, although these trials may have lacked power to detect clinically important differences.

What are the effects of interventions to control heart rate?

LIKELY TO BE BENEFICIAL

Digoxin

We found no placebo controlled RCTs limited to people with acute atrial fibrillation. Two RCTs found that compared with placebo, digoxin reduced ventricular rate after 30 minutes and after 2 hours in people with atrial fibrillation of up to 7 days' duration. One RCT found that compared with digoxin, intravenous diltiazem reduced heart rate within 5 minutes in people with acute atrial fibrillation and atrial flutter.

Diltiazem

One RCT in people with atrial fibrillation (of unspecified duration) or atrial flutter found that intravenous diltiazem reduced heart rate in people within 15 minutes compared with placebo. One RCT found that in people with acute atrial fibrillation and atrial flutter, intravenous diltiazem reduced heart rate within 5 minutes compared with intravenous digoxin. One RCT found no significant difference between intravenous verapamil and intravenous diltiazem in rate control or measures of systolic function in people with acute atrial fibrillation or atrial flutter, but verapamil caused hypotension in some people.

Timolol

We found no RCTs limited to people with acute atrial fibrillation. One small RCT in people with atrial fibrillation of unspecified duration found that intravenous timolol (a β blocker) reduced ventricular rate within 20 minutes compared with placebo.

Verapamil

Two RCTs found that intravenous verapamil reduced heart rate at 10 or 30 minutes compared with placebo in people with atrial fibrillation or atrial flutter. One RCT in people with atrial fibrillation or acute atrial flutter found no significant difference between intravenous verapamil and intravenous diltiazem in rate control or measures of systolic function, but verapamil caused hypotension in some people. The RCT found that amiodarone increased the rate of cardioversion compared with verapamil at 3 hours.

UNKNOWN EFFECTIVENESS

Amiodarone

We found no RCTs examining effects of amiodarone alone on heart rate in people with acute atrial fibrillation.

Sotalol

We found no RCTs comparing sotalol versus placebo.

DEFINITION **Acute atrial fibrillation** is rapid, irregular, and chaotic atrial activity of less than 48 hours' duration. It includes both the first symptomatic onset of chronic, or persistent, atrial fibrillation and episodes of paroxysmal atrial fibrillation. It is sometimes difficult to distinguish new onset of atrial fibrillation from long standing atrial fibrillation that was previously undiagnosed. Atrial fibrillation within 72 hours of onset is sometimes called recent onset atrial fibrillation. By contrast, **chronic atrial fibrillation** is more sustained and can be described as paroxysmal (with spontaneous termination and sinus rhythm between recurrences), persistent, or permanent atrial fibrillation. This review deals only with people with acute atrial fibrillation who are haemodynamically stable. The consensus is that people who are not haemodynamically stable should be treated with immediate DC cardiversion. We have excluded studies in people with atrial fibrillation arising during or soon after cardiac surgery.

INCIDENCE/ We found limited evidence of the incidence or prevalence of acute atrial
PREVALENCE fibrillation. Extrapolation from the Framingham study suggests an incidence in men of 3/1000 person years at age 55 years, rising to 38/1000 person years at 94 years.[1] In women, the incidence was 2/1000 person years at age 55 years and 32.5/1000 person years at 94 years. The prevalence of atrial fibrillation ranged from 0.5% for people aged 50–59 years to 9% in people aged 80–89 years. Among acute emergency medical admissions in the UK, 3–6% had atrial fibrillation, and about 40% were newly diagnosed.[2,3] Among acute hospital admissions in New Zealand, 10% (95% CI 9% to 12%) had documented atrial fibrillation.[4]

AETIOLOGY/ Common precipitants of acute atrial fibrillation are acute myocardial infarction
RISK FACTORS and the acute effects of alcohol. Age increases the risk of developing acute atrial fibrillation. Men are more likely to develop atrial fibrillation than women (38 years' follow up from the Framingham Study, RR after adjustment for age and known predisposing conditions 1.5).[5] Atrial fibrillation can occur in association with underlying disease (both cardiac and non-cardiac) or can arise in the absence of any other condition. Epidemiological surveys have found that risk factors for the development of acute atrial fibrillation include ischaemic ▶

Atrial fibrillation (acute)

heart disease, hypertension, heart failure, valve disease, diabetes, alcohol abuse, thyroid disorders, and disorders of the lung and pleura.[1] In a British survey of acute hospital admissions of patients with atrial fibrillation, a history of ischaemic heart disease was present in 33%, heart failure in 24%, hypertension in 26%, and rheumatic heart disease in 7%.[3] In some populations, the acute effects of alcohol explain a large proportion of the incidence of acute atrial fibrillation. Paroxysms of atrial fibrillation are more common in athletes.[6]

PROGNOSIS **Spontaneous reversion:** Observational studies and placebo arms of RCTs have found that more than 50% of people with acute atrial fibrillation revert spontaneously within 24–48 hours, especially if atrial fibrillation is associated with an identifiable precipitant such as alcohol or myocardial infarction. **Progression to chronic atrial fibrillation:** We found no evidence about the proportion of people with acute atrial fibrillation who develop more chronic forms of atrial fibrillation (e.g. paroxysmal, persistent, or permanent atrial fibrillation). **Mortality:** We found little evidence about the effects on mortality and morbidity of acute atrial fibrillation where no underlying cause is found. Acute atrial fibrillation during myocardial infarction is an independent predictor of both short term and long term mortality.[7] **Heart failure:** Onset of atrial fibrillation reduces cardiac output by 10–20% irrespective of the underlying ventricular rate[8,9] and can contribute to heart failure. People with acute atrial fibrillation who present with heart failure have worse prognoses. **Stroke:** Acute atrial fibrillation is associated with a risk of imminent stroke.[10–13] One case series used transoesophageal echocardiography in people who had developed acute atrial fibrillation within the preceding 48 hours; 15% had atrial thrombi.[14] An ischaemic stroke associated with atrial fibrillation is more likely to be fatal, have a recurrence, and leave a serious functional deficit among survivors than a stroke not associated with atrial fibrillation.[15]

Please refer to the Clinical Evidence website for full text and references.

Cardiovascular disorders

What are the effects of interventions aimed at changing people's behaviour?

BENEFICIAL

Advice from physicians and trained counsellors to quit smoking

Systematic reviews have found that simple, one off advice from a physician during a routine consultation increased the number of smokers quitting smoking and not relapsing for 1 year. One systematic review found that advice from trained counsellors also increased quit rates compared with minimal intervention.

Advice on a cholesterol lowering diet

Systematic reviews have found that advice on a cholesterol lowering diet (i.e. advice to lower total fat intake or increase the ratio of polyunsaturated : saturated fatty acid) leads to a small reduction in blood cholesterol concentrations in the long term (≥ 6 months).

Advice on reducing sodium intake to reduce blood pressure

One systematic review found that, compared with usual care, intensive interventions to reduce sodium intake provided small reductions in blood pressure, however effects on deaths and cardiovascular events are unclear.

Antidepressants (bupropion or nortriptyline) as part of a smoking cessation programme (but no evidence of benefit for selective serotonin reuptake inhibitors or moclobemide)

Systematic reviews have found that quit rates are increased by bupropion and nortriptyline given as part of a smoking cessation programme, but not by moclobemide or selective serotonin reuptake inhibitors.

Antismoking interventions in people at high risk of disease (evidence that counselling or bupropion are effective in this group)

Systematic reviews and four subsequent RCTs have found that antismoking advice improves smoking cessation in people at high risk of smoking related disease. We found no evidence that high intensity advice is more effective than low intensity advice in high risk people. One RCT found that bupropion increased cessation rates in smokers with cardiovascular disease.

Antismoking interventions for pregnant women

Two systematic reviews have found that antismoking interventions in pregnant women increased abstinence rates during pregnancy. One RCT found that nicotine patches did not significantly increase quit rates in pregnant women compared with placebo.

Exercise advice to women over 80 years of age

One RCT found that exercise advice delivered in the home by physiotherapists increased physical activity and reduced the risk of falling in women over 80 years.

Lifestyle interventions for sustained weight loss

Two large RCTs found that weight loss advice resulted in greater weight loss than no advice. One RCT found that cognitive behavioural therapy was more effective than usual care in promoting weight loss. Systematic reviews have found that using behavioural therapy to support advice on diet and exercise is probably more effective in achieving weight loss than diet advice alone. One systematic review ▶

Changing behaviour

found limited evidence that partial meal replacement plans reduced weight loss at 1 year compared with reduced calorie diet in people who completed the treatment.

Nicotine replacement for smoking cessation

One systematic review and one subsequent RCT have found that nicotine replacement is an effective additional component of cessation strategies in smokers who smoke at least 10 cigarettes daily. We found no evidence of any particular method of nicotine delivery having superior efficacy. We found limited evidence from five RCTs (follow up 2–8 years) that the benefit of nicotine replacement treatment on quit rates decreased with time.

LIKELY TO BE BENEFICIAL

Advice from nurses to quit smoking

One systematic review found limited evidence that advice from nurses to quit smoking increased quitting at 1 year compared with no advice.

Counselling sedentary people to increase physical activity

We found limited evidence from systematic reviews and subsequent RCTs that counselling sedentary people increased physical activity compared with no intervention. Limited evidence from RCTs suggests that consultation with an exercise specialist rather than or in addition to a physician may increase physical activity at 1 year. We found limited evidence that interventions delivered by new media can lead to short term changes in physical activity.

Lifestyle interventions to maintain weight loss

One systematic review and additional RCTs have found that most types of maintenance strategy result in smaller weight gains or greater weight losses compared with no contact. Strategies that involve personal contact with a therapist, family support, walking training programmes, or multiple interventions, or are weight focused, seem most effective.

Self help materials for people who want to stop smoking

One systematic review found that self help materials slightly improved smoking cessation compared with no intervention. It found that individually tailored materials were more effective than standard or stage based materials. One subsequent RCT found no significant difference in abstinence rates at 6 months between self help materials based on the stages of change model and standard self help literature.

Telephone advice to quit smoking

One systematic review found limited evidence that telephone counselling improved quit rates compared with interventions with no personal contact.

UNKNOWN EFFECTIVENESS

Lifestyle advice to prevent weight gain

One small RCT found that low intensity education plus a financial incentive increased weight loss compared with no treatment. A second RCT found no significant effect on prevention of weight gain from a postal newsletter with or without a linked financial incentive compared with no contact. One RCT found that lifestyle advice prevented weight gain in perimenopausal women compared with assessment alone. One small RCT comparing a nutrition course for female students with no nutrition course found no significant increase in weight from baseline in either group at 1 year.

Physical exercise to aid smoking cessation

One systematic review found limited evidence that exercise may increase smoking cessation.

Cardiovascular disorders

Training health professionals in promoting weight loss

One systematic review of poor quality RCTs provided insufficient evidence on the sustained effect of interventions to improve health professionals' management of obesity. One subsequent cluster RCT found limited evidence that training for primary care doctors in nutrition counselling plus a support programme reduced body weight of the people in their care over 1 year compared with usual care.

Training health professionals to give advice on smoking cessation (increases frequency of antismoking interventions, but may not improve effectiveness)

One systematic review found that training health professionals increased the frequency of antismoking interventions being offered. It found no good evidence that antismoking interventions are more effective if the health professionals delivering the interventions received training. One RCT found that a structured intervention delivered by trained community pharmacists increased smoking cessation rates compared with usual care delivered by untrained community pharmacists.

LIKELY TO BE INEFFECTIVE OR HARMFUL

Acupuncture for smoking cessation

One systematic review found no significant difference between acupuncture and control in smoking cessation rates at 1 year.

Anxiolytics for smoking cessation

One systematic review found no significant difference in quit rates between anxiolytics and control.

DEFINITION Cigarette smoking, diet, and level of physical activity are important in the aetiology of many chronic diseases. Individual change in behaviour has the potential to decrease the burden of chronic disease, particularly cardiovascular disease. This chapter focuses on the evidence that specific interventions lead to changed behaviour.

INCIDENCE/ PREVALENCE In the developed world, the decline in smoking has slowed and the prevalence of regular smoking is increasing in young people. A sedentary lifestyle is becoming increasingly common and the prevalence of obesity is increasing rapidly.

Please refer to the Clinical Evidence website for full text and references.

Heart failure

Search date February 2004

Robert McKelvie

What are the effects of non-drug treatments?

Exercise

One systematic review found that exercise training reduced death rates and hospital admissions compared with usual care.

Multidisciplinary interventions

One systematic review has found that multidisciplinary programmes reduced admissions to hospital compared with conventional care, but found no significant difference in mortality. The review found that telephone contact plus improved coordination of primary care had no significant effect on admission rate. Two RCTs included in the review found that home based support reduced cardiovascular events at 3–6 years compared with usual care. Subsequent RCTs found that education, nurse led support, and multidisciplinary programmes reduced death and hospital readmission and improved quality of life at 12 weeks to 1 year compared with usual care.

What are the effects of drug and invasive treatments?

Angiotensin converting enzyme inhibitors

Systematic reviews and RCTs found that angiotensin converting enzyme inhibitors reduced ischaemic events, mortality, and hospital admission for heart failure compared with placebo. Relative benefits were similar in different groups of people, but absolute benefits were greater in people with severe heart failure.

Angiotensin II receptor blockers

One systematic review and one subsequent RCT provided evidence that angiotensin II receptor blockers reduced mortality and admission for heart failure compared with placebo in people with New York Heart Association class II–IV heart failure, and were an effective alternative in people who were intolerant to angiotensin converting enzyme inhibitors. One systematic review found no significant difference between angiotensin II receptor blockers and angiotensin converting enzyme inhibitors in all cause mortality or hospital admission. One systematic review and one subsequent RCT found that angiotensin II receptor blockers plus angiotensin converting enzyme inhibitors reduced cardiovascular mortality and admission for heart failure compared with angiotensin converting enzyme inhibitors alone. Effects on all cause mortality remained uncertain.

β Blockers

Systematic reviews found strong evidence that adding a β blocker to an angiotensin converting enzyme inhibitor decreased mortality and hospital admission in symptomatic people with heart failure of any severity. Limited evidence from a subgroup analysis of one RCT found no significant effect on mortality in black people.

Digoxin (improves morbidity in people already receiving diuretics and angiotensin converting enzyme inhibitors)

One systematic review found that, in people in sinus rhythm with heart failure, digoxin reduced clinical worsening of heart failure compared with placebo. One ▶

large RCT in people already receiving diuretics and angiotensin converting enzyme inhibitors found that digoxin reduced the proportion of people admitted to hospital for worsening heart failure at 37 months compared with placebo, but found no significant difference between groups in mortality.

LIKELY TO BE BENEFICIAL

Eplerenone (in people with myocardial infarction complicated by left ventricular dysfunction and heart failure already on medical treatment)

One large RCT in people with recent myocardial infarction complicated by left ventricular dysfunction and clinical heart failure already on medical treatment (which could include angiotensin converting enzyme inhibitors, angiotensin receptor blockers, diuretics, β blockers, or coronary reperfusion therapy) found that adding eplerenone (an aldosterone receptor antagonist) reduced mortality compared with adding placebo.

Implantable cardiac defibrillators in people at high risk of arrhythmia

One RCT found good evidence that an implantable cardiac defibrillator reduced mortality in people with heart failure who had experienced a near fatal ventricular arrhythmia. Two RCTs found that implantable cardiac defibrillators reduced mortality compared with medical treatment in people with heart failure and at high risk of arrhythmia.

Spironolactone in people with severe heart failure

One large RCT in people with severe heart failure taking diuretics, angiotensin converting enzyme inhibitors, and digoxin found that adding spironolactone reduced mortality after 2 years compared with adding placebo.

UNKNOWN EFFECTIVENESS

Amiodarone

Systematic reviews found weak evidence that amiodarone may reduce mortality compared with placebo. However, we were not able to draw firm conclusions about the effects of amiodarone in people with heart failure.

Anticoagulation

A preliminary report from one RCT found no significant difference between warfarin and no antithrombotic treatment or between warfarin and aspirin in the combined outcome of death, myocardial infarction, and stroke after 27 months. However, the RCT may have lacked power to detect a clinically important difference.

Antiplatelet agents

A preliminary report from one RCT found no significant difference between aspirin and no antithrombotic treatment or between aspirin and warfarin in the combined outcome of death, myocardial infarction, and stroke after 27 months. However, the RCT may have lacked power to detect a clinically important difference.

UNLIKELY TO BE BENEFICIAL

Calcium channel blockers

One systematic review has found no significant difference in mortality between second generation dihydropyridine calcium channel blockers and placebo. RCTs comparing other calcium channel blockers versus placebo also found no evidence of benefit.

LIKELY TO BE INEFFECTIVE OR HARMFUL

Non-amiodarone antiarrhythmic drugs

Evidence extrapolated from one systematic review in people treated after a myocardial infarction suggested that other antiarrhythmic drugs (apart from β blockers) may have increased mortality in people with heart failure.

Positive inotropes (other than digoxin)

RCTs in people with heart failure found that positive inotropic drugs other than digoxin (ibopamine, milrinone, and vesnarinone) increased mortality over 6–11 months compared with placebo. One systematic review in people with heart failure found a non-significant increase in mortality with intravenous inotropic drugs that act through the adrenergic pathway compared with placebo or control, and insufficient data to determine whether symptoms improved. It suggested that their use may not be safe.

What are the effects of angiotensin converting enzyme inhibitors in people at high risk of heart failure?

BENEFICIAL

Angiotensin converting enzyme inhibitors in people with asymptomatic left ventricular dysfunction or other risk factors

RCTs in people with asymptomatic left ventricular systolic dysfunction and in people with other risk factors found that angiotensin converting enzyme inhibitors delayed the onset of symptomatic heart failure, reduced cardiovascular events, and improved long term survival compared with placebo.

What are the effects of treatments for diastolic heart failure?

LIKELY TO BE BENEFICIAL

Angiotensin II receptor blockers

One RCT found that candesartan, an angiotensin II receptor blocker, reduced the combined outcome of cardiovascular death or hospital admission for heart failure compared with placebo, although the difference was not significant. It found no significant difference in cardiovascular death between the two groups, but found that candesartan reduced hospital admission compared with placebo.

UNKNOWN EFFECTIVENESS

Other treatments

We found no RCTs examining effects of other treatments in people with diastolic heart failure.

DEFINITION   Heart failure occurs when abnormality of cardiac function causes failure of the heart to pump blood at a rate sufficient for metabolic requirements under normal filling pressure. It is characterised clinically by breathlessness, effort intolerance, fluid retention, and poor survival. It can be caused by systolic or diastolic dysfunction and is associated with neurohormonal changes.[1] Left ventricular systolic dysfunction (LVSD) is defined as a left ventricular ejection fraction below 0.40. It may be symptomatic or asymptomatic. Defining and diagnosing diastolic heart failure can be difficult. Recently proposed criteria include: (1) clinical evidence of heart failure; (2) normal or mildly abnormal left ventricular systolic function; and (3) evidence of abnormal left ventricular relaxation, filling, diastolic distensibility, or diastolic stiffness.[2] However, assessment of some of these criteria is not standardised.

INCIDENCE/ PREVALENCE Both the incidence and prevalence of heart failure increase with age. Studies of heart failure in the USA and Europe found that under 65 years of age the incidence is 1/1000 men a year and 0.4/1000 women a year. Over 65 years, incidence is 11/1000 men a year and 5/1000 women a year. Under 65 years the prevalence of heart failure is 1/1000 men and 1/1000 women; over 65 years the prevalence is 40/1000 men and 30/1000 women.[3] The prevalence of asymptomatic LVSD is 3% in the general population.[4-6] The mean age of people with asymptomatic LVSD is lower than that for symptomatic individuals. Both heart failure and asymptomatic LVSD are more common in men.[4-6] The prevalence of diastolic heart failure in the community is unknown. The prevalence of heart failure with preserved systolic function in people in hospital with clinical heart failure varies from 13–74%.[7,8] Fewer than 15% of people with heart failure under 65 years have normal systolic function, whereas the prevalence is about 40% in people over 65 years.[7]

AETIOLOGY/ RISK FACTORS Coronary artery disease is the most common cause of heart failure.[3] Other common causes include hypertension and idiopathic dilated congestive cardiomyopathy. After adjustment for hypertension, the presence of left ventricular hypertrophy remains a risk factor for the development of heart failure. Other risk factors include cigarette smoking, hyperlipidaemia, and diabetes mellitus.[4] The common causes of left ventricular diastolic dysfunction are coronary artery disease and systemic hypertension. Other causes are hypertrophic cardiomyopathy, restrictive or infiltrative cardiomyopathies, and valvular heart disease.[8]

PROGNOSIS The prognosis of heart failure is poor, with 5 year mortality ranging from 26–75%.[3] Up to 16% of people are readmitted with heart failure within 6 months of first admission. In the USA, heart failure is the leading cause of hospital admission among people over 65 years of age.[3] In people with heart failure, a new myocardial infarction increases the risk of death (RR 7.8, 95% CI 6.9 to 8.8). About a third of all deaths in people with heart failure are preceded by a major ischaemic event.[9] Sudden death, mainly caused by ventricular arrhythmia, is responsible for 25–50% of all deaths, and is the most common cause of death in people with heart failure.[10] The presence of asymptomatic LVSD increases an individual's risk of having a cardiovascular event. One large prevention trial found that for a 5% reduction in ejection fraction, the risk ratio for mortality was 1.20 (95% CI 1.13 to 1.29). For hospital admission for heart failure, the risk ratio was 1.28 (95% CI 1.18 to 1.38) and the risk ratio for heart failure was 1.20 (95% CI 1.13 to 1.26).[4] The annual mortality for people with diastolic heart failure varies in observational studies (1.3–17.5%).[7] Reasons for this variation include age, the presence of coronary artery disease, and variation in the partition value used to define abnormal ventricular systolic function. The annual mortality for left ventricular diastolic dysfunction is lower than that found in people with systolic dysfunction.[11]

Please refer to the Clinical Evidence website for full text and references.

Peripheral arterial disease

Search date December 2003

Paul Bachoo

What are the effects of treatments for people with chronic peripheral arterial disease?

BENEFICIAL

Antiplatelet treatment

Systematic reviews have found strong evidence that antiplatelet agents reduce major cardiovascular events over an average of about 2 years compared with control treatment. Systematic reviews have found that antiplatelet agents reduce the risk of arterial occlusion and revascularisation procedures compared with placebo or no treatment. The balance of benefits and harms is in favour of treatment for most people with symptomatic peripheral arterial disease, because as a group they are at much greater risk of cardiovascular events.

Exercise

Systematic reviews and subsequent RCTs in people with chronic stable claudication have found that regular exercise at least three times weekly for between 3 and 6 months improves total walking distance and maximal exercise time after 3–12 months compared with no exercise. One RCT found that a "stop smoking and keep walking" intervention increased the maximal walking distance compared with usual care at 12 months. One RCT found that vitamin E plus regular exercise increased walking duration compared with placebo at 6 months.

LIKELY TO BE BENEFICIAL

Bypass surgery (compared with thrombolysis in people with acute limb ischaemia)

One systematic review in people with acute limb ischaemia found that surgery reduced amputation rate and pain compared with thrombolysis, but found no significant difference in mortality after 1 year.

Percutaneous transluminal angioplasty (transient benefit only)

Two small RCTs in people with mild to moderate intermittent claudication found limited evidence that percutaneous angioplasty improved walking distance after 6 months compared with no angioplasty but found no significant difference after 2 or 6 years. Two small RCTs identified by a systematic review and four additional RCTs in people with femoro–popliteal or aorto-iliac artery stenoses found no significant difference between angioplasty alone and angioplasty plus stent placement in patency rates, occlusion rates, or clinical improvement. The RCTs may lack power to rule out an important clinical effect. One systematic review found that in people with chronic progressive peripheral arterial disease percutaneous transluminal angioplasty was less effective in improving patency compared with surgery after 12–24 months but found no significant difference after 4 years. The review found no difference in mortality after 12–24 months.

Smoking cessation*

RCTs of advice to stop smoking would be considered unethical. The consensus view is that smoking cessation improves symptoms in people with intermittent claudication. One systematic review of observational studies found inconclusive results from stopping smoking, both in terms of increasing absolute claudication distance and reducing the risk of symptom progression, compared with people who continue to smoke.

*Based on observational evidence and consensus.

TRADE OFF BETWEEN BENEFITS AND HARMS

Cilostazol

Six RCTs found that cilostazol improved claudication distance at 12 to 24 weeks compared with placebo. However, adverse effects of cilostazol were common in the RCTs, and included headache, diarrhoea, and palpitations. One RCT found limited evidence that cilostazol increased initial and absolute claudication distance compared with pentoxifylline.

UNKNOWN EFFECTIVENESS

Bypass surgery (compared with percutaneous transluminal angioplasty)

One systematic review found that surgery improved primary blood vessel patency after 12–24 months compared with percutaneous transluminal angioplasty, but found no significant difference after 4 years. The review found no significant difference in mortality after 12–24 months. Although the consensus view is that bypass surgery is the most effective treatment for people with debilitating symptomatic peripheral arterial disease, RCTs provided inadequate evidence on long term clinical outcomes to confirm this view.

Pentoxifylline

One systematic review and one subsequent RCT found insufficient evidence to compare pentoxifylline with placebo. One RCT found that pentoxifylline was less effective at improving initial and absolute claudication distance compared with cilostazol.

DEFINITION Peripheral arterial disease arises when there is significant narrowing of arteries distal to the arch of the aorta. Narrowing can arise from atheroma, arteritis, local thrombus formation, or embolisation from the heart or more central arteries. This topic includes treatment options for people with symptoms of reduced blood flow to the leg that are likely to arise from atheroma. These symptoms range from calf pain on exercise (intermittent claudication) to rest pain, skin ulceration, or symptoms of ischaemic necrosis (gangrene) in people with critical limb ischaemia.

INCIDENCE/ Peripheral arterial disease is more common in people aged over 50 years than
PREVALENCE in younger people, and is more common in men than women. The prevalence of peripheral arterial disease of the legs (assessed by non-invasive tests) is about 3% in people under the age of 60 years, but rises to over 20% in people over 75 years.[1] The overall annual incidence of intermittent claudication is 1.5–2.6/1000 men and 1.2–3.6/1000 women.[2]

AETIOLOGY/ Factors associated with the development of peripheral arterial disease include
RISK FACTORS age, gender, cigarette smoking, diabetes mellitus, hypertension, hyperlipidaemia, obesity, and physical inactivity. The strongest associations are with smoking (RR 2.0–4.0) and diabetes (RR 2.0–3.0).[3] Acute limb ischaemia may result from thrombosis arising within a peripheral artery or from embolic occlusion.

PROGNOSIS The symptoms of intermittent claudication can resolve spontaneously, remain stable over many years, or progress rapidly to critical limb ischaemia. About 15% of people with intermittent claudication eventually develop critical leg ischaemia, which endangers the viability of the limb. The annual incidence of critical limb ischaemia in Denmark and Italy in 1990 was 0.25–0.45/1000 people.[4,5] Coronary heart disease is the major cause of death in people with peripheral arterial disease of the legs. Over 5 years, about 20% of people with intermittent claudication have a non-fatal cardiovascular event (myocardial ▶

Peripheral arterial disease

infarction or stroke).[6] The mortality rate of people with peripheral arterial disease is two to three times higher than that of age and sex matched controls. Overall mortality after the diagnosis of peripheral arterial disease is about 30% after 5 years and 70% after 15 years.[6]

Please refer to the Clinical Evidence website for full text and references.

What are the effects of specialised care in people with stroke?

BENEFICIAL

Specialised care (specialist stroke rehabilitation)
One systematic review found that specialist stroke rehabilitation reduced death or dependency after a median follow up of 1 year compared with conventional (less specialised) care. Prospective observational data suggest that these findings may be reproducible in routine clinical settings. A second systematic review found no significant difference between care based on in-hospital care pathways and standard care in death or dependency rates. However, these results were based on one small RCT, which may have lacked power to detect clinically important effects. One small subsequent pilot study found no significant difference between intensive monitoring and usual stroke unit care in rates of poor outcome at 3 months but found that intensive monitoring reduced mortality.

What are the effects of medical treatment in acute ischaemic stroke?

BENEFICIAL

Aspirin
One systematic review in people with ischaemic stroke confirmed by computerised tomography scan found that aspirin taken within 48 hours of stroke onset reduced death or dependency at 6 months and increased the proportion of people making a complete recovery compared with placebo.

TRADE OFF BETWEEN BENEFITS AND HARMS

Thrombolysis (increases overall mortality and fatal haemorrhages but reduces dependency in survivors; beneficial effects on dependency do not extend to streptokinase)
One systematic review in people with confirmed ischaemic stroke found that thrombolysis reduced the risk of the composite outcome of death or dependency after 1–6 months compared with placebo. However, it increased the risk of death from intracranial haemorrhage measured in the first 7–10 days and risk of death after 1–6 months. The excess in deaths was offset by fewer people being alive but dependent 6 months after stroke onset, and the net effect was a reduction in people who were dead or dependent. Systematic reviews that undertook meta-analyses for specific thrombolytic agents found that benefits and harms of recombinant tissue plasminogen activator were similar to the overall results. However, streptokinase increased mortality compared with placebo, and this harm was not offset by reduced dependency in survivors. Results of the reviews may not extrapolate to people with the mildest or most severe strokes.

Immediate systemic anticoagulation
One systematic review comparing systemic anticoagulants (unfractionated heparin, low molecular weight heparin, heparinoids, oral anticoagulants, or specific thrombin inhibitors) with usual care without systemic anticoagulants found no significant difference in death or dependence after 3–6 months. One systematic review found no significant difference between anticoagulants (unfractionated and low molecular weight heparin) and aspirin in death or dependency at 3–6 months ▶

Stroke management

for all people with stroke or for the subset of people who also had atrial fibrillation. Systematic reviews provided evidence that systemic anticoagulation reduced the risk of symptomatic deep venous thrombosis in people with ischaemic stroke, but increased the risk of intracranial haemorrhage or extracranial haemorrhage.

UNLIKELY TO BE BENEFICIAL

Neuroprotective agents (calcium channel antagonists, γ-aminobutyric acid agonists, lubeluzole, glycine antagonists, tirilazad, N-methyl-D-aspartate antagonists)

RCTs found no evidence that calcium channel antagonists, lubeluzole, γ-aminobutyric acid agonists, tirilazad, glycine antagonists, or N-methyl-D-aspartate antagonists significantly improved clinical outcomes compared with placebo. One systematic review found that lubeluzole increased the risk of having Q-T prolongation to more than 450 milliseconds on electrocardiography compared with placebo.

LIKELY TO BE INEFFECTIVE OR HARMFUL

Acute reduction in blood pressure

One systematic review in people with acute stroke found insufficient evidence about the effects of lowering blood pressure compared with placebo on clinical outcomes. However, other studies found conflicting results. Two RCTs have suggested that people treated with antihypertensive agents may have a worse clinical outcome and increased mortality.

What are the effects of surgical treatment for intracerebral haematomas?

UNKNOWN EFFECTIVENESS

Evacuation

We found that the balance between benefits and harms has not been clearly established for the evacuation of supratentorial haematomas. We found no evidence from RCTs on the role of evacuation or ventricular shunting in people with infratentorial haematoma whose consciousness level is declining.

DEFINITION Stroke is characterised by rapidly developing clinical symptoms and signs of focal, and at times global, loss of cerebral function lasting more than 24 hours or leading to death, with no apparent cause other than that of vascular origin.[1] Ischaemic stroke is stroke caused by vascular insufficiency (such as cerebrovascular thromboembolism) rather than haemorrhage.

INCIDENCE/ PREVALENCE Stroke is the third most common cause of death in most developed countries.[2] It is a worldwide problem; about 4.5 million people die from stroke each year. Stroke can occur at any age, but half of all strokes occur in people over 70 years old.[3]

AETIOLOGY/ RISK FACTORS About 80% of all acute strokes are ischaemic, usually resulting from thrombotic or embolic occlusion of a cerebral artery.[4] The remainder are caused either by intracerebral or subarachnoid haemorrhage.

PROGNOSIS About 10% of all people with acute ischaemic strokes will die within 30 days of stroke onset.[5] Of those who survive the acute event, about 50% will experience some level of disability after 6 months.[6]

Please refer to the Clinical Evidence website for full text and references.

What are the effects of preventive interventions in people with prior stroke or transient ischaemic attack?

BENEFICIAL

Antiplatelet treatment

One systematic review found that prolonged antiplatelet treatment reduced the risk of serious vascular events including stroke in people with prior stroke or transient ischaemic attack compared with placebo or no antiplatelet treatment.

Blood pressure reduction

One systematic review and two subsequent large RCTs found that blood pressure lowering treatment reduced stroke and other major vascular events in people with a prior stroke or transient ischaemic attack, whether or not they were hypertensive. Two additional smaller RCTs in people with a prior stroke or transient ischaemic attack found no significant difference between atenolol and placebo in stroke, but these RCTs may have lacked power to detect clinically important differences.

Carotid endarterectomy in people with moderately severe (50–69%) symptomatic carotid artery stenosis

Evidence from a pooled analysis of individual patient data from three RCTs found that carotid endarterectomy reduced stroke and death compared with no endarterectomy in symptomatic people with 50–69% carotid stenosis.

Carotid endarterectomy in people with severe (> 70%) symptomatic carotid artery stenosis

Evidence from a pooled analysis of three RCTs found that carotid endarterectomy reduced stroke and death compared with no endarterectomy in symptomatic people with more than 70% carotid stenosis, although no benefit was found in people with near-occlusion. Benefit in symptomatic people with more than 70% stenosis was greater than in people with lower grade stenosis.

Cholesterol reduction

Systematic reviews of large RCTs found that statins reduced major vascular events, including stroke, compared with placebo in people with prior stroke or transient ischaemic attack. RCTs found no evidence that non-statin treatments reduced stroke compared with placebo or no treatment.

LIKELY TO BE BENEFICIAL

Carotid endarterectomy in people with asymptomatic but severe carotid artery stenosis

Two systematic reviews found that carotid endarterectomy reduced perioperative stroke, death, and subsequent ipsilateral stroke in people with asymptomatic but severe stenosis. However, because the risk of stroke without surgery in asymptomatic people is relatively low, the benefit from surgery is small.

Stroke prevention

UNKNOWN EFFECTIVENESS

Alternative antiplatelet regimens to aspirin (no evidence that any regimen more or less effective than aspirin alone)

Systematic reviews and subsequent RCTs found no good evidence that any antiplatelet regimen was superior to aspirin for long term secondary prevention of serious vascular events but found that clopidogrel was a safe and effective alternative to aspirin.

Carotid or vertebral percutaneous transluminal angioplasty

RCTs provided insufficient evidence about the effects of carotid or vertebral percutaneous transluminal angioplasty or stenting compared with medical treatment or carotid endarterectomy in people with a recent carotid or vertebral territory transient ischaemic attack or non-disabling ischaemic stroke who have severe stenosis of the ipsilateral carotid or vertebral artery.

Different blood pressure lowering regimens (no evidence that any regimen more or less effective than any other)

We found no RCTs comparing different blood pressure lowering regimens specifically among people with a prior stroke or transient ischaemic attack. Systematic reviews of RCTs in people with hypertension or vascular disease found little difference in stroke between regimens based on diuretics, angiotensin converting enzyme inhibitors, β blockers or calcium channel blockers. There was a direct relationship between the relative risk of stroke outcomes and the blood pressure reduction achieved.

UNLIKELY TO BE BENEFICIAL

Carotid endarterectomy in people with moderate (30–49%) symptomatic carotid artery stenosis

Evidence from a pooled analysis of individual patient data from three RCTs suggested that carotid endarterectomy was of no benefit in symptomatic people with 30–49% stenosis.

Carotid endarterectomy in people with symptomatic near-occlusion of the carotid artery

Three RCTs provided limited evidence that carotid endarterectomy increased the risk of stroke or death due to surgery in symptomatic people with near occlusion of the ipsilateral carotid artery.

High dose versus low dose aspirin (no additional benefit but may increase harms)

One systematic review and one subsequent RCT found that low dose aspirin (75–150 mg/day) was as effective as higher doses for preventing serious vascular events. It found insufficient evidence that doses lower than 75 mg daily were as effective. Systematic reviews found no evidence of an association between aspirin dose and risk of intracranial, major extracranial, or gastrointestinal haemorrhage. RCTs found that high dose aspirin (500–1500 mg/day) increased the risk of upper gastrointestinal upset compared with medium dose aspirin (75–325 mg/day).

LIKELY TO BE INEFFECTIVE OR HARMFUL

Anticoagulation in people in sinus rhythm

Systematic reviews found no significant difference between anticoagulation and placebo or antiplatelet treatment for preventing recurrent stroke after presumed ischaemic stroke in people in normal sinus rhythm. Anticoagulants increased the risk of fatal intracranial and extracranial haemorrhage compared with placebo. High intensity anticoagulation increased the risk of major bleeding compared with antiplatelet treatment.

Carotid endarterectomy in people with less than 30% symptomatic carotid artery stenosis

Evidence from a pooled analysis of individual patient data from three RCTs suggested that carotid endarterectomy increased the risk of stroke or death due to surgery in symptomatic people with less than 30% carotid stenosis.

What are the effects of preventive anticoagulant and antiplatelet treatment in people with atrial fibrillation and prior stroke or transient ischaemic attack?

BENEFICIAL

Oral anticoagulation

One systematic review found that adjusted dose warfarin reduced the risk of stroke compared with control in people with previous stroke or transient ischaemic attack. The best time to begin anticoagulation after an ischaemic stroke is unclear. One systematic review provided insufficient evidence to compare warfarin versus aspirin.

UNKNOWN EFFECTIVENESS

Aspirin

One sytematic review of one RCT found no significant diference between aspirin and placebo in stroke or death in people with previous stroke or transient ischaemic attack. One systematic review provided insufficient evidence to compare aspirin versus warfarin.

What are the effects of preventive anticoagulant and antiplatelet treatment in people with atrial fibrillation and without prior stroke or transient ischaemic attack?

LIKELY TO BE BENEFICIAL

Aspirin in people with contraindications to anticoagulants

One systematic review found that aspirin reduced the risk of stroke compared with placebo, but another review found no significant difference. These findings support the use of aspirin in people with atrial fibrillation and contraindications to anticoagulants.

Oral anticoagulation

One systematic review found that warfarin reduced fatal and non-fatal ischaemic stroke compared with placebo, provided there was a low risk of bleeding and careful monitoring. The people in the review had a mean age of 69 years. One overview in people less than 65 years old found no significant difference in the annual stroke rate between warfarin and placebo.

DEFINITION   Prevention in this context is the long term management of people with a prior stroke or transient ischaemic attack, and of people at high risk of stroke for other reasons such as atrial fibrillation. **Stroke:** See definition under stroke management, p 28. **Transient ischaemic attack:** This is similar to a mild ischaemic stroke except that symptoms last for less than 24 hours.[1]

Stroke prevention

INCIDENCE/ PREVALENCE See incidence/prevalence under stroke management, p 28.

AETIOLOGY/ RISK FACTORS See aetiology under stroke management, p 28. Risk factors for stroke include prior stroke or transient ischaemic attack, increasing age, hypertension, diabetes, cigarette smoking, and emboli associated with atrial fibrillation, artificial heart valves, or myocardial infarction. The relation with cholesterol is less clear. One overview of prospective studies among healthy middle aged people found no association between total cholesterol and overall stroke risk.[2] However, one review of prospective observational studies in eastern Asian people found that cholesterol was positively associated with ischaemic stroke but negatively associated with haemorrhagic stroke.[3]

PROGNOSIS People with a history of stroke or transient ischaemic attack are at high risk of all vascular events, such as myocardial infarction, but are at particular risk of subsequent stroke (about 10% in the first year and about 5% each year thereafter); see figure 1🅕, and figure 1 in secondary prevention of ischaemic cardiac events, (Web only).[4,5] People with intermittent atrial fibrillation treated with aspirin should be considered at similar risk of stroke, compared with people with sustained atrial fibrillation treated with aspirin (rate of ischaemic stroke/year: 3.2% with intermittent *v* 3.3% with sustained).[6]

Please refer to the Clinical Evidence website for full text and references.

Search date July 2003
David Fitzmaurice, FD Richard Hobbs, and Richard McManus

What are the effects of treatments for proximal deep vein thrombosis?

LIKELY TO BE BENEFICIAL

Low molecular weight heparin (reduced recurrence and reduced risk of major haemorrhage compared with unfractionated heparin)

Systematic reviews found that low molecular weight heparin reduced the incidence of recurrent thromboembolic disease in people with proximal deep vein thrombosis and decreased the risk of major haemorrhage over 3–6 months compared with unfractionated heparin. Two subsequent RCTs in people with proximal deep vein thrombosis receiving oral anticoagulation, some considered at high risk of pulmonary embolism, found no significant difference in pulmonary embolism or mortality at 12 days or recurrent venous thromboembolism over 2 years between adding low molecular weight heparin and adding unfractionated heparin. One of the RCTs also found no significant difference in rates of clinically important bleeding between low molecular weight heparin and unfractionated heparin. The reviews found no significant difference in thrombocytopenia between low molecular weight heparin and unfractionated heparin. One subsequent open label RCT found no significant difference in recurrent deep vein thrombosis at 2 years between low molecular weight heparin and unfractionated heparin.

Oral anticoagulation (vitamin K antagonists such as acenocoumarol, flutamide, warfarin)

We found no RCTs comparing vitamin K antagonists such as acenocoumarol, flutamide, and warfarin versus placebo in people with proximal deep vein thrombosis. One RCT found that fewer people had recurrence of proximal deep vein thrombosis within 6 months with acenocoumarol (nicoumalone) plus intravenous unfractionated heparin as initial treatment than with acenocoumarol alone; as a result, the trial was stopped. One systematic review found no significant difference between oral anticoagulation and long term low molecular weight heparin in recurrent thromboembolism, major haemorrhage, or mortality.

TRADE OFF BETWEEN BENEFITS AND HARMS

Prolonged duration of anticoagulation

Two systematic reviews and one large subsequent RCT found fewer deep vein thrombosis recurrences with up to 48 months compared with up to 24 weeks, duration of anticoagulation with vitamin K antagonists. Another systematic review and two additional open label RCTs found no significant difference in the risk of deep vein thrombosis recurrences between longer and shorter duration of anticoagulation, but their results were limited by the use of indirect comparisons and by lack of power. One review found limited evidence that prolonged compared with shorter anticoagulation increased major haemorrhage, but another review and one large subsequent RCT found no significant difference in major haemorrhage. The absolute risk of recurrent venous thromboembolism decreases with time, but the relative risk reduction with treatment remains constant. Harms of treatment, including major haemorrhage, continue during prolonged treatment. Individuals have different risk profiles, and it is likely that the optimal duration of anticoagulation will vary.

Thromboembolism

Venae cavae filters

One RCT in people with proximal deep vein thrombosis considered at high risk of pulmonary embolism, all receiving oral anticoagulation, found that venae cavae filters reduced rates of pulmonary embolism at 12 days compared with no filters. However, the difference in rates of pulmonary embolism was not significant at 2 years, and venae cavae filters increased rates of recurrent deep vein thrombosis at 2 years.

UNKNOWN EFFECTIVENESS

Abrupt discontinuation of oral anticoagulation

One RCT in people who had received warfarin for 3–6 months provided insufficient evidence to compare abrupt withdrawal of warfarin versus an additional month of warfarin at a fixed low dose of 1.25 mg daily.

Compression stockings

We found no RCTs of standard compression stockings for treating people with proximal deep vein thrombosis. One RCT found that made to measure knee length graduated compression stockings reduced post-thrombotic syndrome over 5–8 years compared with no stockings.

High intensity oral anticoagulation

One RCT found that bleeding rates with warfarin treatment were increased by higher international normalised ratio target ranges (international normalised ratio 3.0–4.5), but recurrence rates were not significantly different compared with a lower range (international normalised ratio 2.0–3.0).

Home treatment with short term low molecular weight heparin

One systematic review of weak RCTs found no significant difference in recurrence of thromboembolism between heparin treatment at home and in hospital.

Low molecular weight heparin versus oral anticoagulation (long term)

One systematic review found no significant difference between long term low molecular weight heparin and oral anticoagulation in recurrent thromboembolism, major haemorrhage, or mortality.

Once daily versus twice daily low molecular weight heparin

Systematic reviews found no significant difference between once and twice daily low molecular weight heparin in recurrent thromboembolism or mortality at 10 days or 3 months. However, the reviews may have been underpowered to detect a clinically important difference because of low rates of recurrent thromboembolism and mortality in the trials.

What are the effects of treatments for isolated calf vein thrombosis?

LIKELY TO BE BENEFICIAL

Warfarin (reduced rate of proximal extension compared with no treatment in people who had received initial heparin and wore compression stockings)

One RCT, in people who had received initial intravenous unfractionated heparin (international normalised ratio 2.5–4.2) and wore compression stockings, found that warfarin reduced rates of proximal extension compared with no further treatment.

UNKNOWN EFFECTIVENESS

Prolonged duration of anticoagulation

One open label RCT found no significant difference in recurrent thromboembolism or rates of major haemorrhage between 6 and 12 weeks of warfarin. The absolute risk of recurrent venous thromboembolism decreases with time, but the relative risk reduction with treatment remains constant. Harms of treatment, including major haemorrhage, continue during prolonged treatment. Individuals have different risk profiles and it is likely that the optimal duration of anticoagulation will vary.

What are the effects of treatments for pulmonary embolism?

TRADE OFF BETWEEN BENEFITS AND HARMS

Low molecular weight heparin (no clear evidence of a difference in mortality or new episodes of thromboembolism compared with unfractionated heparin, increased risk of major haemorrhage unclear)

One RCT in people with symptomatic pulmonary embolism who did not receive thrombolysis or embolectomy found no significant difference between low molecular weight heparin and unfractionated heparin in mortality or new episodes of thromboembolism. Another RCT in people with proximal deep vein thrombosis without clinical signs or symptoms of pulmonary embolism, but with high probability lung scan findings, found that low molecular weight heparin reduced the proportion of people with new episodes of venous thromboembolism compared with intravenous heparin. The RCTs found no significant difference in major haemorrhage between low molecular weight heparin and unfractionated heparin, but may have been underpowered to detect a clinically important difference.

Prolonged duration of anticoagulation

We found no direct evidence in people with pulmonary embolism about the optimum duration of anticoagulation. Evidence for duration of treatment has been extrapolated from RCTs in people with proximal deep vein thrombosis and any venous thromboembolism, which found that longer courses of anticoagulation reduced recurrence compared with shorter courses but may increase the risk of major haemorrhage.

Warfarin plus heparin

One small RCT in people with pulmonary embolism found that warfarin plus heparin reduced mortality at 1 year compared with no anticoagulation.

UNLIKELY TO BE BENEFICIAL

High intensity anticoagulation

We found no direct evidence in people with pulmonary embolism about the optimum intensity of anticoagulation. Evidence for intensity of treatment has been extrapolated from RCTs in people with proximal deep vein thrombosis and any venous thromboembolism, which found that bleeding rates were increased by higher international normalised ratio target ranges (international normalised ratio 3.0–4.5), but recurrence rates were not significantly different compared with a lower range (international normalised ratio 2.0–3.0).

Thrombolysis

Systematic reviews and one subsequent RCT found no significant difference in mortality between thrombolysis plus heparin and heparin alone, and found that thrombolysis may increase the incidence of intracranial haemorrhage. RCTs identified by a systematic review found no significant difference in mortality or recurrent pulmonary embolism among different thrombolytics.

Thromboembolism

What are the effects of computerised decision support on oral anticoagulation management?

Computerised decision support in oral anticoagulation

We found no RCTs comparing computerised decision support versus usual management of oral anticoagulation that used clinically important outcomes (major haemorrhage or death). One systematic review and four subsequent RCTs found that, compared with usual care, the use of computerised decision support in oral anticoagulation increased the time spent in the target international normalised range. Another subsequent RCT found no significant difference between computerised decision support and standard manual support in the time spent in the target international normalised ratio range.

DEFINITION
Venous thromboembolism is any thromboembolic event occurring within the venous system, including deep vein thrombosis and pulmonary embolism. **Deep vein thrombosis** is a radiologically confirmed partial or total thrombotic occlusion of the deep venous system of the legs sufficient to produce symptoms of pain or swelling. **Proximal deep vein thrombosis** affects the veins above the knee (popliteal, superficial femoral, common femoral, and iliac veins). **Isolated calf vein thrombosis** is confined to the deep veins of the calf and does not affect the veins above the knee. **Pulmonary embolism** is radiologically confirmed partial or total thromboembolic occlusion of pulmonary arteries, sufficient to cause symptoms of breathlessness, chest pain, or both. **Post-thrombotic syndrome** is oedema, ulceration, and impaired viability of the subcutaneous tissues of the leg occurring after deep vein thrombosis. **Recurrence** refers to symptomatic deterioration because of a further (radiologically confirmed) thrombosis, after a previously confirmed thromboembolic event, where there had been an initial, partial, or total symptomatic improvement. **Extension** refers to a radiologically confirmed new, constant, symptomatic intraluminal filling defect extending from an existing thrombosis.

INCIDENCE/ PREVALENCE
We found no reliable study of the incidence or prevalence of deep vein thrombosis or pulmonary embolism in the UK. A prospective Scandinavian study found an annual incidence of 1.6–1.8/1000 people in the general population.[1,2] One postmortem study estimated that 600 000 people develop pulmonary embolism each year in the USA, of whom 60 000 die as a result.[3]

AETIOLOGY/ RISK FACTORS
Risk factors for deep vein thrombosis include immobility, surgery (particularly orthopaedic), malignancy, smoking, pregnancy, older age, and inherited or acquired prothrombotic clotting disorders.[4] The oral contraceptive pill is associated with death due to venous thromboembolism (ARI with any combined oral contraception: 1–3/million women a year).[5] The principal cause of pulmonary embolism is a deep vein thrombosis.[4]

PROGNOSIS
The annual recurrence rate of symptomatic calf vein thrombosis in people without recent surgery is over 25%.[6,7] Proximal extension develops in 40–50% of people with symptomatic calf vein thrombosis.[8] Proximal deep vein thrombosis may cause fatal or non-fatal pulmonary embolism, recurrent venous thrombosis, and the post-thrombotic syndrome. One case series (462 people) published in 1946 found 5.8% mortality from pulmonary emboli in people in hospital with untreated deep vein thrombosis.[9] One non-systematic review of observational studies found that, in people after recent surgery who have an asymptomatic deep calf vein thrombosis, the rate of fatal pulmonary embolism ▶

was 13–15%.[10] The incidence of other complications without treatment is not known. The risk of recurrent venous thrombosis and complications is increased by thrombotic risk factors.[11]

Please refer to the Clinical Evidence website for full text and references.

Varicose veins

Search date March 2004

Paul Tisi

What are the effects of treatments in adults with varicose veins?

LIKELY TO BE BENEFICIAL

Surgery (more effective than injection sclerotherapy)

We found no RCTs comparing surgery versus no treatment or compression stockings. RCTs have found that surgery reduced varicose vein recurrence and incidence of new varicose veins at 1–10 years compared with injection sclerotherapy.

UNKNOWN EFFECTIVENESS

Compression stockings

One crossover RCT found no significant difference in symptoms between compression stockings for 4 weeks and no treatment in people with varicose veins. However, the study may have lacked power to detect clinically important effects. One systematic review found that, in pregnant women with varicose veins, sodium tetradecyl sulphate sclerotherapy improved symptoms and the cosmetic appearance of varicose veins compared with compression stockings after 6–24 months.

Injection sclerotherapy

One systematic review found no RCTs that compared injection sclerotherapy versus no treatment. One systematic review found that, in pregnant women with varicose veins, sodium tetradecyl sulphate sclerotherapy improved symptoms and the cosmetic appearance of varicose veins compared with compression stockings after 6–24 months. One RCT found no significant difference between polidocanol and sodium tetradecyl sulphate for improving the appearance of varicose veins at 16 weeks. One RCT reported a similar incidence of new varicose veins at 5 or 10 years with standard dose conventional sclerotherapy, high dose conventional sclerotherapy, and foam sclerotherapy. RCTs found that injection sclerotherapy was less effective at reducing varicose vein recurrence and incidence of new varicose veins at 1–10 years compared with surgery.

DEFINITION Although we found no consistent definition of varicose veins,[1] the term is commonly taken to mean veins that are distended and tortuous. Any vein may become varicose, but the term "varicose veins" conventionally applies to varices of the superficial leg veins. The condition is caused by poorly functioning valves within the lumen of the veins. Blood flows from the deep to the superficial venous systems through these incompetent valves, causing persistent superficial venous hypertension, which leads to varicosity of the superficial veins. Common sites of valvular incompetence include the saphenofemoral and saphenopopliteal junctions and perforating veins connecting the deep and superficial venous systems along the length of the leg. Sites of venous incompetence are determined by clinical examination, handheld Doppler, or duplex ultrasound. Symptoms of varicose veins include distress about cosmetic appearance, pain, itch, limb heaviness, and cramps. This review focuses on uncomplicated, symptomatic varicose veins. We have excluded treatments for chronic venous ulceration and other complications. We have also excluded studies that solely examine treatments for small, dilated veins in the skin of the leg, known as thread veins, spider veins, or superficial telangiectasia.

INCIDENCE/ PREVALENCE	One large US cohort study found the biannual incidence of varicose veins to be 2.6% in women and 2.0% in men.[2] Incidence was constant over the age of 40 years. The prevalence of varicose veins in Western populations has been estimated in one study to be about 25–30% among women and 10–20% in men.[3] A recent Scottish cohort study has, however, found a higher prevalence of varices of the saphenous trunks and their main branches in men than in women (40% men and 32% women).[4]
AETIOLOGY/ RISK FACTORS	One large case control study found that women with two or more pregnancies were at increased risk of varicose veins compared with women with fewer than two pregnancies (RR about 1.2–1.3 after adjustment for age, height, and weight).[2] It found that obesity was also a risk factor, although only among women (RR about 1.3). One narrative systematic review found insufficient evidence on the effects of other suggested risk factors, including genetic predisposition, prolonged sitting or standing, tight undergarments, low fibre diet, constipation, deep vein thrombosis, and smoking.[3]
PROGNOSIS	We found no reliable data on prognosis, nor on the frequency of complications, which include chronic inflammation of affected veins (phlebitis), venous ulceration, and rupture of varices.

Please refer to the Clinical Evidence website for full text and references.

Child health

Absence seizures in children

Search date September 2004

Ewa Posner

What are the effects of treatments for typical absence seizures in children?

TRADE OFF BETWEEN BENEFITS AND HARMS

Valproate*

We found one systematic review. It found no RCTs comparing valproate versus placebo. There is, however, consensus that valproate (sodium valproate or valproic acid) is beneficial, although it is associated with rare but serious adverse effects, including behavioural and cognitive abnormalities, liver necrosis, and pancreatitis. The review found three small RCTs comparing valproate versus ethosuximide. It found no significant difference between valproate and ethosuximide in clinical response (as determined by either electroencephalogram or telemetry recordings, or observer reports of seizure frequency). The review found no RCTs comparing valproate versus other anticonvulsants.

Ethosuximide*

We found one systematic review. It found no RCTs comparing ethosuximide versus placebo. There is, however, consensus that ethosuximide is beneficial, although it is associated with rare but serious adverse effects, including aplastic anaemia, skin reactions, and renal and hepatic impairment. The review found three small RCTs comparing ethosuximide versus valproate. It found no significant difference between ethosuximide and valproate in clinical response (as determined by either electroencephalogram or telemetry recordings, or observer reports of seizure frequency). The review found no RCTs comparing ethosuximide versus other anticonvulsants.

Lamotrigine

One RCT in children and adolescents who had previously benefited from lamotrigine found that lamotrigine increased the proportion of children who remained seizure free compared with placebo. However, lamotrigine was associated with serious skin reactions. We found no RCTs comparing lamotrigine versus other anticonvulsants.

UNKNOWN EFFECTIVENESS

Gabapentin

One RCT found no significant difference between gabapentin and placebo in the frequency of typical absence seizures. However, the study may have lacked power to detect clinically important effects.

*We found no RCT evidence comparing valproate or ethosuximide versus placebo but there is consensus belief that valproate and ethosuximide are beneficial in typical absence seizures.

DEFINITION   Absence seizures are sudden, frequent episodes of unconsciousness lasting a few seconds and are often accompanied by simple automatisms or clonic, atonic, or autonomic components. Typical absence seizures display a characteristic electroencephalogram showing regular symmetrical generalised spike and wave complexes with a frequency of 3 Hz and usually occur in children with normal development and intelligence. Typical absence seizures are often confused with complex partial seizures, especially in cases of prolonged seizure with automatisms. However, the abrupt ending of typical absence seizures, without a postictcal phase, is the most useful clinical ▶

feature in distinguishing the two types. Typical absence seizures should not be confused with atypical absence seizures, which differ markedly in electroencephalogram findings and ictal behaviour, and usually present with other seizure types in a child with a background of learning disability and severe epilepsy.[1] Typical absence seizures may be the sole seizure type experienced by a child. If this is the case and the child is of normal development and has no structural lesions, the child is said to have childhood absence epilepsy. Alternatively, typical absence seizures may coexist in children with other epileptic syndromes, such as juvenile myoclonic epilepsy or juvenile absence epilepsy, in which other seizure types are also present. This differentiation into typical versus atypical seizures is important, as the natural history and response to treatment varies in the two groups. Interventions for atypical absence seizures or for absence seizures secondary to structural lesions are not included in this chapter.

INCIDENCE/ PREVALENCE

About 10% of seizures in children with epilepsy are typical absence seizures.[1] Annual incidence has been estimated at 0.7–4.6/100 000 people in the general population and 6–8/100 000 in children aged 0–15 years. Prevalence is 5–50/100 000 people in the general population.[2] Age of onset ranges from 3–13 years, with a peak at 6–7 years.

AETIOLOGY/ RISK FACTORS

The cause of childhood absence epilepsy is presumed to be genetic. Seizures can be triggered by hyperventilation in susceptible children. Some anticonvulsants, such as phenytoin, carbamazepine, and vigabatrin are associated with an increased risk of absence seizures.

PROGNOSIS

In childhood absence epilepsy, in which typical absence seizures are the only type of seizures suffered by the child, seizures generally cease spontaneously by 12 years of age or sooner. Less than 10% of children develop infrequent generalised tonic clonic seizures and it is very rare for them to continue having absence seizures.[3] In other epileptic syndromes (in which absence seizures may coexist with other types of seizure) prognosis is varied, depending on the syndrome. Absence seizures have a significant impact on quality of life. The episode of unconsciousness may occur at any time, and usually without warning. Affected children need to take precautions to prevent injury during absences and refrain from activities that would put them at risk if seizures occurred (e.g. climbing heights, swimming unsupervised, or cycling on busy roads). Often, school staff members are the first to notice the recurrent episodes of absence seizures, and treatment is generally initiated because of the adverse impact on learning.

Please refer to the Clinical Evidence website for full text and references.

Acute otitis media in children

Search date February 2004

Paddy O'Neill and Tony Roberts

What are the effects of treatments?

LIKELY TO BE BENEFICIAL

Ibuprofen

One RCT in children aged 1–6 years receiving antibiotic treatment found that ibuprofen reduced earache as assessed by parental observation after 2 days compared with placebo.

Paracetamol

One RCT in children aged 1–6 years receiving antibiotic treatment found that paracetamol reduced earache as assessed by parental observation after 2 days compared with placebo.

TRADE OFF BETWEEN BENEFITS AND HARMS

Antibiotics (compared with placebo)

We found four systematic reviews comparing antibiotics versus placebo in acute otitis media. The reviews used different inclusion criteria and outcome measures. One review in children aged 4 months to 18 years found a reduction in symptoms with a range of antibiotics (cephalosporins, erythromycin, penicillins, trimethoprim–sulfamethoxazole [co-trimoxazole]) after 7–14 days of treatment compared with placebo. Another review in children younger than 2 years found no significant difference in clinical improvement after 7 days between antibiotics (penicillins, sulphonamides, amoxicillin/clavulanic acid [co-amoxiclav]) and placebo alone or placebo plus myringotomy. A third review in children aged 4 weeks to 18 years found that antibiotics (ampicillin, amoxicillin) reduced clinical failure rate within 2–7 days compared with placebo or observational treatment. The fourth review in children aged 6 months to 15 years found that, compared with placebo, the early use of antibiotics (erythromycin, penicillins) reduced the proportion of children still in pain 2–7 days after presentation, and reduced the risk of developing contralateral acute otitis media. This review also found that antibiotics increased the risk of vomiting, diarrhoea, or rashes.

Choice of antibiotic regimen

One systematic review in children aged 4 months to 18 years found no significant difference between a range of antibiotics in rate of treatment success at 7–14 days or of middle ear effusion at 30 days. Another systematic review in children aged 4 weeks to 18 years found no significant difference between antibiotics in clinical failure rates within 3–14 days. The second review also found that adverse effects, primarily gastrointestinal, were more common with cefixime than with amoxicillin or ampicillin, and were more common with amoxicillin/clavulanate (original formulation) than with azithromycin. Systematic reviews of placebo controlled RCTs have found that antibiotics increase the risk of vomiting, diarrhoea, and rashes.

Immediate compared with delayed antibiotic treatment

One RCT in children aged 6 months to 10 years found that immediate antibiotic treatment reduced the number of days of earache, ear discharge, and amount of daily paracetamol used after the first 24 hours of illness compared with delayed antibiotic treatment, but found no significant difference between groups in daily pain scores. It also found that immediate antibiotic treatment increased diarrhoea ▶

Child health

compared with delayed antibiotic treatment. Systematic reviews of placebo controlled RCTs have found that antibiotics increase the risk of vomiting, diarrhoea, and rashes.

Longer compared with short courses of antibiotics

One systematic review and two subsequent RCTs have found that 10 day courses of antibiotics reduce treatment failure, relapse, and reinfection at 8–19 days compared with 5 day courses, but found no significant difference between groups at 20–42 days. Systematic reviews of placebo controlled RCTs have found that antibiotics increase the risk of vomiting, diarrhoea, and rashes.

LIKELY TO BE INEFFECTIVE OR HARMFUL

Myringotomy

One RCT in infants aged 3 months to 1 year found higher rates of persistent infection and lower rates of otoscopic recovery in children treated with myringotomy plus placebo compared with children receiving antibiotic only. A second RCT in children aged 2–12 years found no significant difference between myringotomy only, amoxicillin only, and no treatment in reduction of pain at 24 hours or 7 days. A third RCT found higher rates of initial treatment failure (resolution of symptoms within 12 hours) with myringotomy plus placebo than with antibiotic only, for severe episodes of acute otitis media in children aged 2–12 years.

What are the effects of interventions to prevent recurrence?

LIKELY TO BE BENEFICIAL

Xylitol chewing gum or syrup

One RCT found that xylitol syrup or chewing gum reduced the proportion of children with at least one episode of acute otitis media compared with control. It found no significant difference between xylitol lozenges and control gum. It found that more children taking xylitol withdrew because of abdominal pain or other unspecified reasons compared with control.

TRADE OFF BETWEEN BENEFITS AND HARMS

Antibiotic prophylaxis (long term)

One systematic review in children and adults found that long term antibiotic prophylaxis reduced recurrence of acute otitis media compared with placebo. One subsequent RCT in children aged 3 months to 6 years found no significant difference between antibiotic prophylaxis and placebo in prevention of recurrence. A second subsequent RCT found that amoxicillin, but not sulfisoxazole reduced recurrence of acute otitis media within 6 months compared with placebo. The systematic review provided insufficient evidence on adverse effects of long term antibiotic prophylaxis, although one subsequent RCT reported that adverse effects included diarrhoea, vomiting, and thrombocytopenia. We found insufficient evidence on which antibiotic to use, for how long, and how many episodes of acute otitis media justify starting preventive treatment.

LIKELY TO BE INEFFECTIVE OR HARMFUL

Tympanostomy (ventilation tubes)

One small RCT found that tympanostomy tube insertion reduced the mean number of episodes of acute otitis media during the first 6 month period after treatment compared with myringotomy alone or no surgery, but not during the subsequent 18 months. It also found a non-significant trend toward more recurrent infections and ▶

Acute otitis media in children

worse hearing after tube extrusion in those treated with tympanostomy. It found more tympanosclerosis in ears that received ventilating tubes compared with those that received myringotomy alone or no surgery.

DEFINITION

Otitis media is an inflammation in the middle ear. Subcategories include acute otitis media (AOM), recurrent AOM, and chronic suppurative otitis media. AOM is the presence of middle ear effusion in conjunction with rapid onset of one or more signs or symptoms of inflammation of the middle ear. AOM presents with systemic and local signs, and has a rapid onset. The diagnosis is made on the basis of signs and symptoms, principally ear pain in the presence of a cloudy or bulging eardrum (and immobility of the eardrum if pneumatic otoscopy is performed). Erythema is a moderately useful sign for helping to establish the diagnosis. If the eardrum has a normal colour, then risk of AOM is low.[1] Uncomplicated AOM is limited to the middle ear cleft.[2] The persistence of an effusion beyond 3 months without signs of infection defines otitis media with effusion (also known as "glue ear"; see otitis media with effusion, p 136). Chronic suppurative otitis media is characterised by continuing inflammation in the middle ear causing discharge (otorrhoea) through a perforated tympanic membrane (see chronic suppurative otitis media, p 127).

INCIDENCE/ PREVALENCE

AOM is common and has a high morbidity and low mortality in otherwise healthy children. In the UK, about 30% of children under 3 years of age visit their general practitioner with AOM each year, and 97% receive antimicrobial treatment.[3] By 3 months of age, 10% of children have had an episode of AOM. It is the most common reason for outpatient antimicrobial treatment in the USA.[4]

AETIOLOGY/ RISK FACTORS

The most common bacterial causes for AOM in the USA and UK are *Streptococcus pneumoniae*, *Haemophilus influenzae*, and *Moraxella catarrhalis*.[3] Similar pathogens are found in Colombia.[5] The incidence of penicillin resistant *S pneumoniae* has risen, but rates differ between countries. The most important risk factors for AOM are young age and attendance at day care centres, such as nursery schools. Other risk factors include being white; male sex; a history of enlarged adenoids, tonsillitis, or asthma; multiple previous episodes; bottle feeding; a history of ear infections in parents or siblings; and use of a soother or pacifier. The evidence for an effect of environmental tobacco smoke is controversial.[3]

PROGNOSIS

Without antibiotic treatment AOM symptoms improve in 24 hours in about 60% of children, and in about 80% of children the condition resolves in about 3 days. Suppurative complications occur in about 0.12% of children if antibiotics are withheld.[6] Serious complications are rare in otherwise healthy children but include hearing loss, mastoiditis, meningitis, and recurrent attacks.[3] The World Health Organization estimates that each year 51 000 children under the age of 5 years die from complications of otitis media in developing countries.[7]

Please refer to the Clinical Evidence website for full text and references.

Asthma and other wheezing disorders in children

Search date June 2003

Duncan Keeley and Michael McKean

What are the effects of treatments for acute asthma in children?

BENEFICIAL

Oxygen*

An RCT comparing oxygen treatment with no oxygen treatment in acute severe asthma would be considered unethical. One prospective cohort study and clinical experience support the need for oxygen in acute asthma.

High dose inhaled corticosteroids

We found one systematic review that identified four RCTs comparing high dose inhaled with oral corticosteroids in children. Three RCTs found no significant difference in hospital admission with nebulised budesonide or dexamethasone compared with oral prednisolone in children with mild to moderate asthma. One RCT in children with moderate to severe asthma found that, compared with inhaled fluticasone, oral prednisolone reduced hospital admission and improved lung function at 4 hours. A subsequent RCT in children aged 4–16 years found that, compared with oral prednisolone, nebulised fluticasone improved lung function over 7 days. Another RCT in children aged 5–16 years admitted to hospital with severe asthma found no significant difference with nebulised budesonide compared with oral prednisolone in lung function at 24 hours or 24 days after admission.

Inhaled ipratropium bromide added to β_2 agonists (in emergency room)

One systematic review has found that, compared with β_2 agonist alone, multiple doses of inhaled ipratropium bromide plus an inhaled β_2 agonist (fenoterol or salbutamol) reduced hospital admissions and improved lung function in children aged 18 months to 17 years with severe asthma exacerbations. In children with mild to moderate asthma exacerbations, a single dose of inhaled ipratropium bromide plus a β_2 agonist (fenoterol, salbutamol, or terbutaline) compared with a β_2 agonist alone improved lung function for up to 2 hours, but did not reduce hospital admissions

Metered dose inhaler plus spacer devices for delivery of β_2 agonists (as effective as nebulisers)

One systematic review in children with acute but not life threatening asthma, who were old enough to use a spacer, has found no significant difference in hospital admission rates with a metered dose inhaler plus a spacer versus nebulisation for delivering β_2 agonists (fenoterol, salbutamol, or terbutaline) or β agonist (orciprenaline). Children using a metered dose inhaler with a spacer may have shorter stays in emergency departments, less hypoxia, and lower pulse rates compared with children receiving β_2 agonist by nebulisation.

Systemic corticosteroids

One systematic review has found that systemic corticosteroids increase the likelihood of early discharge and reduce the frequency of relapse within 1–3 months in children hospitalised with acute asthma.

*In the absence of RCT evidence, categorisation based on observational evidence and strong consensus belief that oxygen is beneficial.

Asthma and other wheezing disorders in children

Intravenous theophylline

One systematic review found that in children aged 1–19 years admitted to hospital with severe asthma, intravenous theophylline improved lung function and symptom scores 6–8 hours after treatment compared with placebo, but found no significant difference in number of bronchodilator treatments required or length of hospital stay. A subsequent RCT in children aged 1–17 years admitted to an intensive care unit with severe asthma found that, compared with controls, intravenous theophylline decreased the time to reach a clinical asthma score of 3 or less but found no significant difference in length of stay in the intensive care unit.

Inhaled ipratropium bromide added to salbutamol (after initial stabilisation)

One RCT in children admitted to hospital with initially stabilised severe asthma found no significant difference in clinical asthma scores during the first 36 hours with nebulised ipratropium bromide compared with placebo added to salbutamol (a β_2 agonist) and corticosteroid (hydrocortisone or prednisone).

What are the effects of single agent prophylaxis in childhood asthma?

Inhaled corticosteroids

One systematic review has found that, compared with placebo, prophylactic inhaled corticosteroids improve symptoms and lung function in children with asthma. Several RCTs have found that inhaled corticosteroids slightly reduce growth rate compared with placebo, although studies with long term follow up suggest attainment of normal adult height. Inhaled corticosteroids have been associated with rare reports of adrenal suppression. One RCT in children aged 6–16 years found no significant difference in improvement of asthma symptoms with inhaled beclometasone compared with theophylline, but found less use of bronchodilators and oral corticosteroids with inhaled beclometasone. Small RCTs have found inhaled corticosteroids to be more effective than sodium cromoglicate in improving symptoms and lung function. RCTs in children aged 5–16 years have found that, compared with inhaled long acting β_2 agonists (salmeterol) or inhaled nedocromil, inhaled corticosteroids (beclometasone, budesonide, or fluticasone) improve symptoms and lung function in children with asthma. RCTs in children aged 5–16 years have found that inhaled corticosteroids (beclometasone, budesonide, or fluticasone) versus inhaled long acting β_2 agonists (salmeterol) or inhaled nedocromil improve symptoms and lung function in children with asthma.

Inhaled nedocromil

Two RCTs in children aged 6–12 years found that, compared with placebo, inhaled nedocromil reduces asthma symptom scores, asthma severity, and bronchodilator use, and improves lung function. One large RCT in children aged 5–12 years with mild to moderate asthma found no significant difference between nedocromil and budesonide or placebo in lung function, hospital admission rate, or the symptom score on diary cards, but found that budesonide was superior to nedocromil, and that nedocromil was superior to placebo in several measures of asthma symptoms and morbidity.

Oral montelukast

One RCT in children aged 6–14 years found that, compared with placebo, oral montelukast (a leukotriene receptor antagonist) increased from baseline the mean morning forced expiratory volume in 1 second and reduced the total daily β_2 agonist use, but found no significant difference in daytime asthma symptom score or in nocturnal awakenings with asthma. Another RCT in children aged 2–5 years found that, compared with placebo, oral montelukast improved average daytime symptom scores and reduced the need for rescue oral steroid courses, but found no significant difference in average overnight asthma symptom scores. We found no RCTs directly comparing oral montelukast with inhaled corticosteroids.

TRADE OFF BETWEEN BENEFITS AND HARMS

Inhaled salmeterol

Two RCTs in children aged 4–14 years found that, compared with placebo, inhaled salmeterol improved lung function but found conflicting evidence about reduced use of salbutamol. One RCT comparing inhaled salmeterol with beclometasone found that salmeterol was associated with a significant deterioration in bronchial reactivity.

Oral theophylline

One small RCT in children aged 6–15 years found that, compared with placebo, oral theophylline increased mean morning peak expiratory flow rate and reduced the mean number of acute night time attacks and doses of bronchodilator used. Another RCT in children aged 6–16 years found no significant difference in improvement of asthma symptoms with oral theophylline compared with inhaled beclometasone, but found greater use of bronchodilators and oral corticosteroids with theophylline over 1 year. Theophylline has serious adverse effects (cardiac arrhythmia, convulsions) if therapeutic blood concentrations are exceeded.

UNKNOWN EFFECTIVENESS

Inhaled sodium cromoglicate

One systematic review found insufficient evidence for prophylactic treatment with sodium cromoglicate in children aged less than 1 year to 18 years. Several small comparative RCTs found sodium cromoglicate to be less effective than inhaled corticosteroids in improving symptoms and lung function.

What are the effects of additional prophylactic treatments in childhood asthma inadequately controlled by standard dose inhaled corticosteroids?

UNKNOWN EFFECTIVENESS

Increased dose of inhaled beclometasone

One RCT in children aged 6–16 years taking inhaled beclometasone (a corticosteroid) comparing the addition of a second dose of inhaled beclometasone with placebo found no significant difference in lung function, symptom scores, exacerbation rates, or bronchial reactivity but found a reduction in growth velocity at 1 year.

Inhaled salmeterol

One RCT in children aged 6–16 years found that addition of salmeterol (a long acting β_2 agonist) increased peak expiratory flow rates in the first few months of treatment but found no increase after 1 year. A second short term RCT in children aged 4–16 years also found increased morning peak expiratory flow rates and more symptom free days at 3 months with addition of salmeterol.

Asthma and other wheezing disorders in children

Oral montelukast

One crossover RCT in children aged 6–14 years with persistent asthma who had been taking inhaled budesonide for at least 6 weeks found that, compared with addition of placebo, oral montelukast (a leukotriene receptor antagonist) improved lung function and decreased the proportion of days with asthma exacerbations over 4 weeks. These differences were statistically significant but modest in clinical terms.

Oral theophylline

One small RCT found that addition of theophylline, compared with placebo, to previous treatment increased the proportion of symptom free days and reduced the use of additional orciprenaline (a β agonist) and additional corticosteroid (beclometasone or prednisolone) over 4 weeks. We found insufficient evidence to weigh these short term benefits and possible long term harms.

What are the effects of treatments for acute wheezing in infants?

LIKELY TO BE BENEFICIAL

Addition of ipratropium bromide to fenoterol

One RCT identified by a systematic review in infants aged 3–24 months found that addition of ipratropium bromide to fenoterol (a long acting β_2 agonist) compared with fenoterol alone reduced the proportion of infants receiving further treatment 45 minutes after initial treatment.

Inhaled salbutamol

One RCT in infants aged 3 months to 2 years found that, compared with placebo, nebulised salbutamol (a short acting β_2 agonist) improved respiratory rate but found no significant difference in hospital admission. Another RCT that included infants aged less than 18 months to 36 months found no significant difference in change from baseline in clinical symptom scores with nebulised salbutamol versus placebo.

Short acting β_2 agonists delivered by metered dose inhaler/spacer versus nebuliser

Two RCTs in children aged up to 5 years found no significant difference in hospital admissions with delivery of salbutamol through a metered dose inhaler plus spacer compared with nebulised salbutamol. Another RCT in infants aged 1–24 months found no significant difference in improvement of symptoms with delivery of terbutaline through a metered dose inhaler plus spacer compared with nebulised terbutaline. Nebulised β_2 agonists may cause tachycardia, tremor, and hypokalaemia.

UNKNOWN EFFECTIVENESS

High dose inhaled corticosteroids

One systematic review found that high dose inhaled corticosteroids compared with placebo reduced the requirement for oral corticosteroids, but the difference was not statistically significant. The review also found a clear preference for the inhaled corticosteroids by the children's parents over placebo. The clinical importance of these results is unclear.

Inhaled ipratropium bromide

We found no RCTs comparing inhaled ipratropium bromide compared with placebo for treating acute wheeze.

◄ **Oral prednisolone**
One small RCT found no significant difference in daily symptom scores with oral prednisolone (a corticosteroid) versus placebo.

What are the effects of prophylaxis in wheezing infants?

LIKELY TO BE BENEFICIAL

Oral salbutamol
One RCT identified by a systematic review in infants aged 3–14 months found that oral salbutamol (a short acting β_2 agonist) compared with placebo reduced treatment failures.

TRADE OFF BETWEEN BENEFITS AND HARMS

Higher dose inhaled budesonide
One RCT in infants aged 6–30 months found that higher prophylactic doses of inhaled budesonide (a corticosteroid) compared with placebo reduced symptoms and the proportion of children with acute wheezing episodes during a 12 week period but found no significant reduction in the proportion of wheezing episodes per infant. Another RCT in infants aged 11–36 months found that higher prophylactic doses of inhaled budesonide significantly reduced the proportion of days requiring oral prednisolone, and symptoms of wheezing and sleep disturbance, but found no significant improvement for cough. Higher doses of inhaled corticosteroids have the potential for adverse effects.

UNKNOWN EFFECTIVENESS

Inhaled ipratropium bromide
One small RCT identified by a systematic review found no significant difference in relief of symptoms with nebulised ipratropium bromide compared with placebo. The study may have lacked power to exclude a clinically important difference between treatments.

Inhaled salbutamol
Two RCTs identified by a systematic review in infants aged up to 2 years found no significant improvement in symptoms with inhaled salbutamol (a short acting β_2 agonist) compared with placebo.

Lower dose inhaled budesonide
Three RCTs found no clear evidence of effectiveness with lower prophylactic doses of inhaled budesonide (a corticosteroid) in children aged 1 week to 6 years with recurrent wheeze.

UNLIKELY TO BE BENEFICIAL

Addition of inhaled beclometasone to salbutamol
One RCT found no significant improvement in symptoms with addition of inhaled beclometasone compared with placebo to inhaled salbutamol.

DEFINITION   Differentiation between asthma and non-asthmatic viral associated wheeze may be difficult; persisting symptoms and signs between acute attacks are suggestive of asthma, as are a personal or family history of atopic conditions such as eczema and hay fever. **Childhood asthma** is characterised by chronic or recurrent cough and wheeze. The diagnosis is confirmed by demonstrating reversible airway obstruction, preferably on several occasions over time, in children old enough to perform peak flow measurements or spirometry. Diagnosing asthma in children requires exclusion of other causes of recurrent respiratory symptoms. Acute asthma is a term used to describe a ▶

severe exacerbation of asthma symptoms accompanied by tachycardia and tachypnoea. The aim of prophylactic treatments in asthma is to minimise persistent symptoms and prevent acute exacerbations. **Wheezing in infants** is characterised by a high pitched purring or whistling sound produced mainly on the out breath and is commonly associated with an acute viral infection such as bronchiolitis (see bronchiolitis in children, p 53) or asthma. These are not easy to distinguish clinically.

INCIDENCE/ PREVALENCE

Childhood asthma: Surveys have found an increase in the proportion of children diagnosed with asthma. The increase is higher than can be explained by an increased readiness to diagnose asthma. One questionnaire study from Aberdeen, Scotland, surveyed 2510 children aged 8–13 years in 1964 and 3403 children in 1989. Over the 25 years, the diagnosis of asthma rose from 4% to 10%.[1] The increase in prevalence of childhood asthma from the 1960s to 1980s was accompanied by an increase in hospitals admissions over the same period. In England and Wales this was a sixfold increase.[2] **Wheezing in infants** is common and seems to be increasing, although the magnitude of any increase is not clear. One Scottish cross-sectional study (2510 children aged 8–13 years in 1964 and 3403 children in 1989) found that the prevalence of wheeze rose from 10% in 1964 to 20% in 1989, and episodes of shortness of breath rose from 5% to 10% over the same period.[1] Difficulties in defining clear groups (phenotypes) and the transient nature of the symptoms, which often resolve spontaneously, have confounded many studies.

AETIOLOGY/ RISK FACTORS

Childhood asthma: Asthma is more common in children with a personal or family history of atopy, increased severity and frequency of wheezing episodes and presence of variable airway obstruction or bronchial hyperresponsiveness. Precipitating factors for symptoms and acute episodes include infection, house dust mites, allergens from pet animals, exposure to tobacco smoke, and anxiety. **Wheezing in infants:** Most wheezing episodes in infancy are precipitated by viral respiratory infections.

PROGNOSIS

Childhood asthma: A British longitudinal study of children born in 1970 found that 29% of 5 year olds wheezing in the past year were still wheezing at the age of 10 years.[3] Another study followed a group of children in Melbourne, Australia from the age of 7 years (in 1964) into adulthood. The study found that a large proportion (73%) of 14 year olds with infrequent symptoms had few or no symptoms by the age of 28 years, whereas two thirds of those 14 year olds with frequent wheezing still had recurrent attacks at the age of 28 years.[4] **Wheezing in infants:** One cohort study (826 infants followed from birth to 6 years) suggests that there may be at least three different prognostic categories for wheezing in infants: "persistant wheezers" (14% of total, with risk factors for atopic asthma such as elevated immunoglobulin E levels and a maternal history of asthma), who initially suffered wheeze during viral infections, and in whom the wheezing persisted into school age; "transient wheezers" (20% of total, with reduced lung function as infants but no early markers of atopy), who also suffered wheeze during viral infections but stopped wheezing after the first 3 years of life; and "late onset wheezers" (15% of total), who did not wheeze when aged under 3 years but had developed wheeze by school age.[5] Another retrospective cohort study found that 14% of children with one attack and 23% of children with four or more attacks in the first year of life had experienced at least one wheezing illness in the past year at age 10 years.[3] Administering inhaled treatments to young children can be difficult. Inconsistencies in results could reflect the effects of the differences in the drugs used, delivery devices used, dosages used, and the differences in the pattern of wheezing illnesses and treatment responses among young children.

Please refer to the Clinical Evidence website for full text and references.

Attention deficit hyperactivity disorder in children

Search date May 2004

Deborah Pritchard

What are the effects of treatments for attention deficit hyperactivity disorder in children?

LIKELY TO BE BENEFICIAL

Atomoxetine *New*

Four RCTs found that atomoxetine reduced symptoms of attention deficit hyperactivity disorder compared with placebo after up to 9 weeks of treatment. The RCTs found that atomoxetine decreased appetite and increased nausea, vomiting, asthenia, dyspepsia, infection, and pruritus compared with placebo.

Dexamfetamine sulphate

Two systematic reviews and one subsequent RCT found limited evidence that dexamfetamine improved some behavioural outcomes compared with placebo. One systematic review found insufficient evidence to compare the effects of dexamfetamine versus methylphenidate. One RCT found limited evidence that, in children already taking dexamfetamine or methylphenidate, adding clonidine reduced conduct symptoms of ADHD compared with added placebo after 6 weeks.

Methylphenidate

One systematic review and subsequent RCTs found that methylphenidate reduced core symptoms of attention deficit hyperactivity disorder in the short term compared with placebo, but disturbed sleep and appetite. The review found insufficient to compare the effects of methylphenidate versus dexamfetamine or tricyclic antidepressants. The review also found limited evidence that methylphenidate versus psychological/behavioural treatment improved symptoms in the medium term, but the clinical importance of these findings is unclear. One small RCT provided insufficient evidence to compare clonidine alone; methylphenidate alone, and the combination. A second RCT found limited evidence that, in children already taking dexamfetamine or methylphenidate, added clonidine reduced conduct symptoms of ADHD compared with added placebo after 6 weeks.

Methylphenidate plus psychological/behavioural treatment

One systematic review found inconsistent results for combination treatments (methylphenidate plus psychological/behavioural treatment) compared with placebo in children with attention deficit hyperactivity disorder. A second systematic review found that combination treatments improved attention deficit hyperactivity disorder symptoms compared with psychological/behavioural treatments alone. It also suggested that combined medication management plus intensive behavioural treatment was better than medication management alone.

UNKNOWN EFFECTIVENESS

Clonidine

Limited evidence from one systematic review suggested that clonidine reduced core attention deficit hyperactivity disorder symptoms compared with placebo, but the clinical importance of these findings is unclear. One small RCT provided insufficient evidence to compare clonidine alone; methylphenidate alone, and the combination. A second RCT found limited evidence that, in children already taking dexamfetamine or methylphenidate, added clonidine reduced conduct symptoms of ADHD compared with added placebo after 6 weeks.

Attention deficit hyperactivity disorder in children

Psychological/behavioural treatment

One systematic review of two small RCTs provided insufficient evidence to assess the effects of psychological/behavioural treatment compared with standard care. One large subsequent RCT found no significant difference between psychological/behavioural treatment and standard care in behaviour rating scales.

DEFINITION
Attention deficit hyperactivity disorder (ADHD) is "a persistent pattern of inattention and hyperactivity and impulsivity that is more frequent and severe than is typically observed in people at a comparable level of development" (DSM-IV).[1] Inattention, hyperactivity, and impulsivity are commonly known as the core symptoms of ADHD. Symptoms must be present for at least 6 months, observed before the age of 7 years, and "clinically important impairment in social, academic, or occupational functioning" must be evident in more than one setting. The symptoms must not be better explained by another disorder, such as an anxiety disorder, mood disorder, psychosis, or autistic disorder.[1] The World Health Organization's *International statistical classification of diseases and related health problems* (ICD-10)[2] uses the term "hyperkinetic disorder" for a more restricted diagnosis. It differs from the DSM-IV classification[3] as all three problems of attention, hyperactivity, and impulsiveness must be present, more stringent criteria for "pervasiveness" across situations must be met, and the presence of another disorder is an exclusion criterion. The evidence presented in this topic largely relates to children aged 5 years and above. There is a paucity of evidence of efficacy and safety of treatments in pre-school children.

INCIDENCE/ PREVALENCE
Prevalence estimates of ADHD vary according to the diagnostic criteria used and the population sampled. DSM-IV prevalence estimates among school children range from 3–5%,[1] but other estimates vary from 1.7–16.0%.[4,5] No objective test exists to confirm the diagnosis of ADHD, which remains a clinical diagnosis. Other conditions frequently co-exist with ADHD. Oppositional defiant disorder is present in 35% (95% CI 27% to 44%) of children with ADHD, conduct disorder in 26% (95% CI 13% to 41%), anxiety disorder in 26% (95% CI 18% to 35%), and depressive disorder in 18% (95% CI 11% to 27%).[6]

AETIOLOGY/ RISK FACTORS
The underlying causes of ADHD are not known.[6] There is limited evidence that it has a genetic component.[7–9] Risk factors also include psychosocial factors.[10] There is increased risk in boys compared with girls, with ratios varying from 3 : 1[6] to 4 : 1.[3]

PROGNOSIS
More than 70% of hyperactive children may continue to meet criteria for ADHD in adolescence, and up to 65% of adolescents may continue to meet criteria for ADHD in adulthood.[5] Changes in diagnostic criteria cause difficulty with interpretation of the few outcome studies. One cohort of boys followed up for an average of 16 years found a ninefold increase in antisocial personality disorder and a fourfold increase in substance misuse disorder.[7]

Please refer to the Clinical Evidence website for full text and references.

What are the effects of preventive interventions?

BENEFICIAL

Respiratory syncytial virus immunoglobulins or palivizumab (monoclonal antibody) in children at high risk

One systematic review has found that, in children born prematurely, in children with bronchopulmonary dysplasia, and in children with a combination of risk factors, prophylactic respiratory syncytial virus immunoglobulin or palivizumab (monoclonal antibody) reduces admission rates to hospital and intensive care units compared with placebo or no prophylaxis. Treatment duration varied between 4 and 6 months.

UNKNOWN EFFECTIVENESS

Nursing interventions (cohort segregation, handwashing, gowns, masks, gloves, and goggles) in children admitted to hospital

We found no RCTs about the effects of these interventions to prevent spread of bronchiolitis to other children.

What are the effects of treatments?

UNKNOWN EFFECTIVENESS

Bronchodilators (inhaled salbutamol, inhaled adrenaline [epinephrine])

Systematic reviews have found that inhaled bronchodilators improve overall clinical scores in the short term (up to 24 hours after treatment) compared with placebo in children treated in hospital, emergency departments, and outpatient clinics. They found no significant difference in admission rates between bronchodilators and placebo and no clinically important improvement in oxygen saturation. Subsequent RCTs found no evidence that nebulised adrenaline improved short term outcomes during the first 4 days of illness in infants, the rate of hospital admission, the duration of hospital stay, or the time to resolution of illness compared with 0.9% sodium chloride. Four RCTs provided insufficient evidence of a difference between nebulised adrenaline and nebulised salbutamol in clinical severity, rate of hospital admission or duration of admission.

Corticosteroids

RCTs provided limited and inconclusive evidence on the effects of corticosteroids compared with placebo.

Respiratory syncytial virus immunoglobulins, pooled immunoglobulins, or palivizumab (monoclonal antibody)

One systematic review has found that, in children born prematurely, in children with bronchopulmonary dysplasia, and in children with a combination of risk factors, prophylactic respiratory syncytial virus immunoglobulin or palivizumab (monoclonal antibody) reduces admission rates to hospital and intensive care units compared with placebo or no prophylaxis. Treatment duration varied between 4 and 6 months.

Ribavirin

One systematic review found no significant difference between ribavirin and placebo in mortality, risk of respiratory deterioration, or duration of hospital stay in ▶

children admitted to hospital with respiratory syncytial virus bronchiolitis. It found limited evidence that ribavirin reduced the duration of mechanical ventilation. Two subsequent RCTs found no significant difference between ribavirin and placebo in duration of hospital stay or admission rate because of lower respiratory tract symptoms during the first year after the acute episode, or in the frequency of recurrent wheezing illness over 1 year of follow up.

DEFINITION Bronchiolitis is a virally induced acute bronchiolar inflammation that is associated with signs and symptoms of airway obstruction. Diagnosis is based on clinical findings. Clinical manifestations include fever, rhinitis (inflammation of the nasal mucosa), tachypnoea (rapid breathing), expiratory wheezing, cough, rales, use of accessory muscles, apnoea (absence of breathing), dyspnoea (difficulty in breathing), alar flaring (flaring of the nostrils), and retractions (indrawing of the intercostal soft tissues on inspiration). Disease severity of bronchiolitis may be classified clinically as mild, moderate, or severe.

INCIDENCE/ PREVALENCE Bronchiolitis is the most common lower respiratory tract infection in infants, occurring in a seasonal pattern with highest incidence in the winter in temperate climates,[1] and in the rainy season in warmer countries. Each year in the USA about 21% of infants have lower respiratory tract disease and 6–10/1000 infants are admitted to hospital for bronchiolitis (1–2% of children < 12 months of age).[2] The peak rate of admission occurs in infants aged 2–6 months.[3]

AETIOLOGY/ RISK FACTORS Respiratory syncytial virus is responsible for bronchiolitis in 70% of cases. This figure reaches 80–100% in the winter months. However, in early spring, parainfluenza virus type 3 is often responsible.[1]

PROGNOSIS **Morbidity and mortality:** Disease severity is related to the size of the infant, and to the proximity and frequency of contact with infective infants. Children at increased risk of morbidity and mortality are those with congenital heart disease, chronic lung disease, history of premature birth, hypoxia, and age less than 6 weeks.[4] Other factors associated with a prolonged or complicated hospital stay include a history of apnoea or respiratory arrest, pulmonary consolidation seen on a chest radiograph, and (in North America) people of Native American or Inuit race.[5] The risk of death within 2 weeks is high for children with congenital heart disease (3.4%) or chronic lung disease (3.5%) as compared with other groups combined (0.1%).[4] Rates of admission to intensive care units (range 31–36%) and need for mechanical ventilation (range 11–19%) are similar among all high risk groups. [4] The percentage of these children needing oxygen supplementation is also high (range 63–80%).[4] In contrast, rates of intensive care unit admission (15%) and ventilation (8%) in children who do not have high risk characteristics are markedly lower.[6] **Long term prognosis:** Information on long term prognosis varies among studies. One small prospective study of two matched cohorts (25 children with bronchiolitis; 25 children without) found no evidence that bronchiolitis requiring outpatient treatment is associated with an increased risk of asthma in the long term.[7] Possible confounding factors include variation in illness severity, smoke exposure, and being in overcrowded environments.[8] We found one prospective study in 50 randomly selected infants admitted with bronchiolitis, followed up by questionnaires for 5 years and a visit in the fifth year. It found a doubling of asthma incidence compared with the general population, although there was large (30%) loss to follow up and no matched control group.[9]

Please refer to the Clinical Evidence website for full text and references.

Search date February 2004

Kate Ackerman and David Creery

What are the effects of treatments for non-submersion out of hospital cardiorespiratory arrest?

Bag–mask ventilation

We found no RCTs. One non-randomised controlled trial found no significant difference in survival or neurological outcome between endotracheal intubation and bag–mask ventilation in children with non-submersion cardiorespiratory arrest requiring airway management in the community.

Bystander cardiopulmonary resuscitation

It is widely accepted that cardiopulmonary resuscitation and ventilation should be undertaken in children who have arrested. Placebo controlled trials would be considered unethical. One systematic review of observational studies has found that children whose arrest was witnessed and who received bystander cardiopulmonary resuscitation were more likely to survive to hospital discharge compared with no bystander cardiopulmonary resuscitation. We found no RCTs on the effects of training parents to perform cardiopulmonary resuscitation.

Intubation

We found no RCTs. One controlled trial found no significant difference in survival or neurological outcome between endotracheal intubation and bag–mask ventilation in children with non-submersion cardiorespiratory arrest.

Airway management and ventilation; direct current cardiac shock (for ventricular fibrillation or pulseless ventricular tachycardia); intravenous adrenaline (epinephrine) at standard dose

Although we found no direct evidence to support their use, widespread consensus based on indirect evidence and extrapolation from adult data holds that these interventions should be universally applied to children who have arrested. Placebo controlled trials would be considered unethical.

Intravenous adrenaline at high dose; intravenous sodium bicarbonate; intravenous calcium; training parents to perform cardiopulmonary resuscitation

We found no RCTs or prospective observational studies on the effects of these interventions in children who have arrested in the community.

DEFINITION The chapter deals with non-submersion, out of hospital cardiorespiratory arrest in children, which is defined as a state of pulselessness and apnoea occurring outside of a medical facility and not caused by submersion in water.[1]

INCIDENCE/ PREVALENCE We found 12 studies (3 prospective, 9 retrospective) reporting the incidence of non-submersion out of hospital cardiorespiratory arrest in children (see table 1❶).[2–13] Eleven studies reported the incidence in both adults and children, and eight reported the incidence in children.[2–9,11–13] Incidence in the general population ranged from 2.2–5.7/100 000 people a year (mean 3.1, 95% CI 2.1 to 4.1). Incidence in children ranged from 6.9–18.0/ 100 000 children a year (mean 10.6, 95% CI 7.1 to 14.1).[8] One prospective ▶

study (300 children) found that about 50% of out of hospital cardiorespiratory arrests occurred in children under 12 months, and about two thirds occurred in children under 18 months.[11]

AETIOLOGY/ RISK FACTORS We found 26 studies reporting the causes of non-submersion pulseless arrests in a total of 1574 children. The commonest causes were undetermined (as in sudden infant death syndrome) (39%), trauma (18%), chronic disease (7%), and pneumonia (4%).[1,3–12,14–20]

PROGNOSIS We found no observational studies that investigated non-submersion arrests alone. We found 27 studies (5 prospective, 22 retrospective; total of 1754 children) that reported out of hospital arrest.[1–12,14–28] The overall survival rate following out of hospital arrest was 5% (87 children). Nineteen of these studies (1140 children) found that of the 48 surviving children, 12 (25%) had no or mild neurological disability and 36 (75%) had moderate or severe neurological disability. We found one systematic review (search date 1997), which reported outcomes after cardiopulmonary resuscitation for both in hospital and out of hospital arrests in children of any cause, including submersion.[29] Studies were excluded if they did not report survival. The review found evidence from prospective and retrospective observational studies that out of hospital arrest of any cause in children carries a poorer prognosis than arrest within hospital (132/1568 [8%] children survived to hospital discharge after out of hospital arrest v 129/544 [24%] children after in hospital arrests). About half of the survivors were involved in studies that reported neurological outcome. Of these, survival with "good neurological outcome" (i.e. normal or mild neurological deficit) was higher in children who arrested in hospital compared with those who arrested elsewhere (60/77 [78%] surviving children in hospital v 28/68 [41%] elsewhere).[29]

Please refer to the Clinical Evidence website for full text and references.

Search date August 2003

Gregory Rubin

What are the effects of treatments?

TRADE OFF BETWEEN BENEFITS AND HARMS

Cisapride with or without magnesium oxide

Two RCTs in people aged 2–18 years found that cisapride improved stool frequency and symptoms of constipation after 8–12 weeks of treatment in an outpatient setting compared with placebo. One RCT in children aged 1–7 years with chronic constipation found that combined treatment with cisapride and magnesium oxide significantly improved stool frequency after 3–4 weeks of treatment in an outpatient setting compared with magnesium oxide alone. We found no evidence from primary care settings. Use of cisapride has been restricted in some countries because of adverse cardiac effects.

UNKNOWN EFFECTIVENESS

Biofeedback training

One systematic review found no significant difference between biofeedback plus conventional treatment and conventional treatment alone in persisting defecation disorders at 12 months.

Increased dietary fibre

We found no systematic review or RCTs in children on the effects of increasing dietary fibre.

Osmotic laxatives

We found no RCTs that compared osmotic laxatives versus placebo in children. Two small RCTs found no significant difference in stool frequency or consistency between lactulose and lactitol after 2–4 weeks in children aged 8 months to 16 years. One of the RCTs found that lactulose increased abdominal pain and flatulence compared with lactitol. A third RCT in non-breastfed constipated infants found no difference between different strengths of lactulose.

Stimulant laxatives

One systematic review found no reliable RCTs comparing stimulant laxatives versus placebo or other treatments.

DEFINITION **Constipation** is characterised by infrequent bowel evacuations; hard, small faeces; or difficult or painful defecation. The frequency of bowel evacuation varies from person to person.[1] According to the Rome II diagnostic criteria for childhood defecation disorders, functional constipation can be defined as "either having hard or pellet-like stools for the majority of stools or firm stools two or less times per week in the absence of structural, endocrine or metabolic diseases".[2] Some studies reported in this chapter used other diagnostic criteria.[3] **Encopresis** is defined as involuntary bowel movements in inappropriate places at least once a month for 3 months or more, in children aged 4 years and older.[4]

INCIDENCE/ PREVALENCE Constipation with or without encopresis is common in children. It accounts for 3% of consultations to paediatric outpatient clinics and 25% of paediatric gastroenterology consultations in the USA.[5] Encopresis has been reported in 2% of children at school entry. The peak incidence is at 2–4 years of age.

AETIOLOGY/ RISK FACTORS No cause is discovered in 90–95% of children with constipation. Low fibre intake and a family history of constipation may be associated factors.[6] Psychosocial factors are often suspected, although most children with constipation are ▶

developmentally normal.[5] Chronic constipation can lead to progressive faecal retention, distension of the rectum, and loss of sensory and motor function. Organic causes for constipation are uncommon, but include Hirschsprung's disease (1/5000 births; male to female ratio of 4 : 1; constipation invariably present from birth), cystic fibrosis, anorectal physiological abnormalities, anal fissures, constipating drugs, dehydrating metabolic conditions, and other forms of malabsorption.[5] This chapter aims to cover children in whom no underlying cause is identified.

PROGNOSIS Childhood constipation can be difficult to treat and often requires prolonged support, explanation, and medical treatment. In one long term follow up study of children presenting under the age of 5 years, 50% recovered within 1 year and 65–70% recovered within 2 years; the remainder required laxatives for daily bowel movements or continued to soil for several years.[5] It is not known what proportion continue to have problems into adult life, although adults presenting with megarectum or megacolon often have a history of bowel problems from childhood.

Please refer to the Clinical Evidence website for full text and references.

Topic search November 2003

David Johnson

What are the effects of treatments in mild croup?

BENEFICIAL

Dexamethasone (oral single dose)

One RCT found that, compared with placebo, a single oral dose of dexamethasone (0.15 mg/kg) reduced the proportion of children treated for mild croup seeking additional medical attention for ongoing croup symptoms within 7–10 days. We found no RCTs evaluating single versus multiple doses of dexamethasone, or other corticosteroids in children with mild croup.

UNKNOWN EFFECTIVENESS

Decongestants (oral)

We found no systematic review, RCTs, or prospective cohort studies on oral decongestant in children with mild croup.

Humidification

We found no systematic review, RCTs, or any observational studies evaluating the effects of humidification in children with mild croup.

UNLIKELY TO BE BENEFICIAL

Antibiotics

We found no systematic review, RCTs, or prospective cohort studies evaluating any type of antibiotic in children with mild croup. However, there is widespread consensus that antibiotics do not shorten the clinical course of a disease that is predominantly viral in origin.

What are the effects of treatments in moderate to severe croup?

BENEFICIAL

Adrenaline (epinephrine) (nebulised)

Three RCTs found that, compared with placebo, nebulised racemic adrenaline (epinephrine) 2.25% improved croup score within 30 minutes after starting treatment. One of these RCTs found that, by 2 hours, the treatment effect of adrenaline (epinephrine) had largely disappeared. None of the RCTs reported adverse effects suggesting myocardial insufficiency, nor any evidence suggesting that treatment increases cardiac demand (for example, following treatment, the heart rate did not rise). However, we found one well documented case report of a previously normal child with severe croup who sustained a small myocardial infarction after being treated with three adrenaline (epinephrine) nebulisations within 1 hour. One small RCT found no significant difference between nebulised racemic adrenaline (epinephrine) and heliox (helium–oxygen mixture) in overall mean change in croup scores over 4 hours in children already treated with humidified oxygen and intramuscular dexamethasone 0.6 mg/kg.

Budesonide (nebulised) (compared with placebo)

One systematic review found that, compared with placebo, nebulised budesonide improved croup score at 6, 12, and 24 hours and reduced the need for adrenaline (epinephrine) treatment in children with moderate to severe croup. One RCT found ▶

that, compared with placebo, nebulised budesonide, 2 mg administered every 12 hours, improved the time to a two point improvement in children's croup score.

Dexamethasone (compared with placebo)

One systematic review found that, compared with placebo, dexamethasone improved croup score at 6, 12, and 24 hours and reduced the need for adrenaline (epinephrine) treatment in children with moderate to severe croup. One subsequent RCT found that, compared with placebo, a single oral dose of dexamethasone 0.6 mg/kg reduced the proportion of children seeking additional medical attention for ongoing croup symptoms within 7 days.

LIKELY TO BE BENEFICIAL

Dexamethasone, oral (compared with nebulised budesonide)

One RCT found no significant difference between oral dexamethasone 0.6 mg/kg and nebulised budesonide 2 mg in the proportion of children treated with adrenaline (epinephrine) or admitted to hospital after 1 week. Another RCT found no significant difference between oral dexamethasone 0.6 mg/kg and nebulised budesonide 2 mg in the proportion of children treated with adrenaline (epinephrine) after 1 hour or admitted to hospital at 24 hours. This RCT also found that, compared with placebo, both oral dexamethasone and nebulised budesonide reduced hospital admission at 24 hours. Although oral dexamethasone and nebulised budesonide appear to be equivalent, it is preferable to use oral dexamethasone because nebulisation usually causes prolonged agitation and crying, which worsens the child's respiratory distress, and it takes on average 15 minutes to deliver nebulised budesonide compared with 1–2 minutes with oral dexamethasone.

Dexamethasone, intramuscular (compared with nebulised budesonide for croup scores)

One RCT found that, compared with nebulised budesonide, intramuscular dexamethasone 0.6 mg/kg improved croup scores at 5 hours but found no significant difference in hospital admission. In this RCT, those children randomised to receive budesonide did not receive a placebo intramuscular injection, but had an elastic bandage placed on their thigh to aid in masking. Therefore it is possible that masking may not have been maintained, potentially biasing the study's result.

Oxygen

We found no systematic review, RCTs, or any analytical observational studies evaluating the effects of oxygen in children with moderate to severe croup. An RCT of oxygen versus no oxygen in children with severe croup would be considered unethical. There is widespread consensus that oxygen is beneficial in children with severe respiratory distress. Given the lack of harm and the compelling logic for administering oxygen in children with severe respiratory distress, oxygen will continue to be administered to these children. One RCT found no significant difference in mean change from baseline in croup score with heliox (helium 70%, oxygen 30%) compared with oxygen 30% alone, but was too small to detect reliably a clinically important difference.

UNKNOWN EFFECTIVENESS

L-adrenaline (epinephrine) compared with racemic adrenaline (epinephrine)

One small RCT reported no significant difference in overall improvement in croup scores between L-adrenaline (epinephrine) (1 : 1000, 5 mL) and racemic adrenaline (epinephrine) (2.25%, 5 mL).

β₂ agonists, short-acting (nebulised)

We found no systematic review, RCTs, or observational studies evaluating the effects of nebulised short acting β_2 agonists in children with moderate to severe croup. Although there is neither empirical evidence showing benefit nor a clear theoretical reason for using nebulised short acting β_2 agonists, in some communities, a significant proportion of children with croup are treated with nebulised short acting β_2 agonists.

Decongestants (oral)

We found no systematic review, RCTs, or prospective cohort studies evaluating the effects of any oral decongestant in children with moderate to severe croup.

Dexamethasone (different doses and routes of administration)

One RCT found no significant difference between single oral dexamethasone doses of 0.6 mg/kg and 0.3 mg/kg or between 0.3 mg/kg and 0.15 mg/kg for the need for adrenaline (epinephrine) after 1 hour, remaining in the short stay unit at 24 hours, or returning for care for croup symptoms following discharge. A systematic review (including studies using several different corticosteroids other than dexamethasone) found that the higher the dose administered, the greater the difference in the proportion of children reported to be improved between the corticosteroid and placebo groups. Two RCTs found no significant difference between intramuscular and oral dexamethasone 0.6 mg/kg for resolution of symptoms, unscheduled return for medical care, or after reassessment with further treatment with corticosteroid, adrenaline (epinephrine), and/or hospital admission. In both RCTs, children randomised to receive oral dexamethasone did not receive a placebo intramuscular injection, but had an elastic bandage placed on their thigh to aid in masking. Therefore, it is possible that masking may not have been maintained, potentially biasing the studies results.

Dexamethasone (oral) plus budesonide (nebulised)

One RCT found no significant difference in mean change from baseline in croup score within 4 hours between nebulised budesonide 2 mg added to oral dexamethasone 0.6 mg/kg and oral dexamethasone 0.6 mg/kg alone.

Heliox (helium–oxygen mixture)

One RCT found no significant difference in mean change from baseline in croup score with heliox (helium 70%, oxygen 30%) compared with oxygen 30% alone, both delivered by humidification for 20 minutes. However, this RCT, was too small to detect reliably a clinically important difference. Another RCT found no significant difference between nebulised racemic adrenaline (epinephrine) and heliox (helium–oxygen mixture) in overall mean change in croup scores over 4 hours in children already treated with humidified oxygen and intramuscular dexamethasone 0.6 mg/kg.

Humidification

One RCT found no significant difference between humidification and controls in mean change in croup scores at 2 hours in children who had already received a single oral dose of dexamethasone 0.6 mg/kg. In this RCT, humidification was delivered by a corrugated tube held to the child's face by a parent. Another RCT found no significant difference in improvement in croup scores at 12 hours between placing children with croup in a high humidity atmosphere (87–95%) in a humidified tent, and room air. One small case series of children with croup reported scalds from hot humidified air.

Croup

Nebulised adrenaline (epinephrine) alone compared with intermittent positive pressure breathing

One crossover RCT in 14 children aged 4 months to 5 years admitted to hospital with minimum inspiratory stridor at rest found no significant difference in overall improvement in croup scores between nebulised adrenaline (epinephrine) plus intermittent positive pressure breathing at 15–17 cm pressure and nebulised adrenaline (epinephrine) alone.

UNLIKELY TO BE BENEFICIAL

Antibiotics

We found no systematic reviews, RCTs, or prospective cohort studies that examined the benefit of any type of antibiotics in children with croup. However, there is strong consensus belief that antibiotics do not shorten the clinical course of a disease that is predominantly viral in origin. This statement does not apply if bacterial tracheitis is suspected.

What are the effects of treatments in children with impending respiratory failure in severe croup?

BENEFICIAL

Adrenaline (epinephrine) (nebulised)

We found no systematic review or RCTs evaluating the effects of adrenaline (epinephrine) in children with impending respiratory failure in severe croup. An RCT of adrenaline (epinephrine) versus no adrenaline (epinephrine) would be considered unethical. One cohort study in children with acute upper airway obstruction found that nebulised L adrenaline (epinephrine) improved mean croup score and reduced carbon dioxide levels. Another cohort study found that nebulised racemic adrenaline (epinephrine) reduced both stridor and paradoxical breathing.

Corticosteroids

One systematic review found that, compared with placebo, treatment with corticosteroids significantly reduced the rate of endotracheal intubation. One RCT in intubated children showed that, compared with placebo, treatment with prednisolone (1 mg/kg via nasogastric tube every 12 hours until 24 hours after extubation) significantly reduced the duration of intubation and the need for reintubation.

LIKELY TO BE BENEFICIAL

Oxygen

We found no systematic review, RCTs, or any analytical observational studies evaluating the effects of oxygen in children with impending respiratory failure in severe croup. An RCT of oxygen versus no oxygen in children with severe croup would be considered unethical. There is widespread consensus that oxygen is beneficial in children with severe respiratory distress.

UNKNOWN EFFECTIVENESS

Heliox (helium–oxygen mixture)

We found no systematic review, RCTs, or any analytical observational studies evaluating the effects of heliox (helium–oxygen mixture) in children with impending respiratory failure in severe croup.

▶

Antibiotics

We found no systematic reviews, RCTs, or prospective cohort studies that examined the benefit of any type of antibiotics in children with croup. However, there is strong consensus belief that antibiotics do not shorten the clinical course of a disease that is predominantly viral in origin. This statement does not apply if bacterial tracheitis is suspected.

Sedatives

We found no systematic review or RCTs evaluating the effects of sedatives in children with impending respiratory failure in severe croup. One prospective cohort study showed that children with severe croup who were treated with sedatives had decreased croup scores but no decrease in transcutaneous carbon dioxide pressure. This suggests that sedatives decrease respiratory effort without improving ventilation.

DEFINITION Croup is characterised by the abrupt onset, most commonly at night, of a barking cough, inspiratory stridor, hoarseness, and respiratory distress due to upper airway obstruction. Croup symptoms are often preceded by symptoms of upper respiratory tract infection-like symptoms. The most important diagnoses to differentiate from croup include bacterial tracheitis, epiglottitis, and the inhalation of a foreign body. Some investigators distinguish subtypes of croup;[1-3] the subtypes most commonly distinguished are acute laryngotracheitis and spasmodic croup. Children with acute laryngotracheitis have an antecedent upper respiratory tract infection, are usually febrile, and are thought to have more persistent symptoms. Children with spasmodic croup do not have an antecedent upper respiratory tract infection, are afebrile, have recurrent croup, and are thought to have more transient symptoms. However, there is little empirical evidence justifying the view that spasmodic croup responds differently from acute laryngotracheitis. **Population:** For this review, we have included children up to the age of 12 years with croup; no attempt has been made to exclude spasmodic croup. We could not find definitions of clinical severity that are either widely accepted or rigorously derived. For this review, we have elected to use definitions derived by a committee consisting of a range of specialists and sub-specialists during the development of a clinical practise guideline from Alberta Medical Association (Canada).[4] The definitions of severity have been correlated with the Westley croup score,[5] since it is the most widely used clinical score, and its validity and reliability have been well demonstrated).[6,7] The Westley croup score is the most widely used clinical score, and its validity and reliability have been well-demonstrated.[6,7] **Mild croup:** Occasional barking cough, none to limited stridor at rest, and none to mild suprasternal and/or intercostal indrawing (retractions of the skin of the chest wall), corresponding to a Westley croup score of 0–2. **Moderate croup:** Frequent barking cough, easily audible stridor at rest, and suprasternal and sternal wall retraction at rest, but no or little distress or agitation, corresponding to a Westley croup score of 3–5. **Severe croup:** Frequent barking cough, prominent inspiratory and — occasionally — expiratory stridor, marked sternal wall retractions, decreased air entry on auscultation, and significant distress and agitation, corresponding to a Westley croup score of 6–11. **Impending respiratory failure:** Barking cough (often not prominent), audible stridor at rest (occasionally can be hard to hear), sternal wall retractions (may not be marked), usually lethargic or decreased level of consciousness, and often dusky complexion without supplemental oxygen, corresponding to a Westley croup score of > 11. When ▶

having severe respiratory distress, a young child's compliant chest wall "caves in" during inspiration, causing unsynchronised chest and abdominal wall expansion (paradoxical breathing). Approximately 85% of children attending general emergency departments, by this classification scheme, have mild croup, and less than 1% have severe croup (unpublished prospective data obtained from 21 Alberta general emergency departments).

INCIDENCE/ PREVALENCE Croup has an average annual incidence of 3% and accounts for 5% of emergent admissions to hospital in children under 6 years of age in North America (unpublished population based data from Calgary Health Region, Alberta, Canada, 1996–2000).[8] One retrospective Belgian study found that 16% of 5–8 year old children had suffered from croup at least once during their life, and 5% had experienced recurrent croup (3 or more episodes).[9] We are not aware of epidemiological studies establishing the incidence of croup in other parts of the world.

AETIOLOGY/ RISK FACTORS Croup occurs most commonly in children between 6 months and 3 years of age, but can also occur in children as young as 3 months and as old as 12–15 years of age.[8] Croup is extremely rare in adults.[10] Croup occurs predominantly in late autumn, but can occur during any season, including summer.[8] Croup is caused by a variety of viral agents and, occasionally, by *Mycoplasma pneumoniae*.[8] Parainfluenza accounts for 75% of all cases, with the commonest type being parainfluenza type 1. The remaining proportion of cases are largely accounted for by respiratory syncytial virus, metapneumovirus, influenza A and B, adenovirus, and mycoplasma.[8,11–13] Viral invasion of the laryngeal mucosa leads to inflammation, hyperaemia, and oedema.[1] This leads to narrowing of the subglottic region. Children compensate for this narrowing by breathing more quickly and deeply. In children with more severe illness, as the narrowing progresses, their increased effort at breathing becomes counterproductive, airflow through the upper airway becomes turbulent (stridor), their compliant chest wall begins to cave in during inspiration, resulting in paradoxical breathing, and consequently the child becomes fatigued. With these events — if untreated — the child becomes hypoxic and hypercapnoeic, which eventually results in respiratory failure and arrest.[14,15]

PROGNOSIS Croup symptoms resolve in the majority of children within 48 hours.[16] However, a small percentage of children with croup have symptoms that persist for up to 1 week.[16] Hospitalisation rates vary significantly between communities but, on average, less than 5% of all children with croup are admitted to hospital.[17–20] Of those admitted to hospital, only 1–3% are intubated.[21–24] Mortality is low; in one 10-year study, less than 0.5% of intubated children died.[22] Uncommon complications of croup include pneumonia, pulmonary oedema, and bacterial tracheitis.[25–27]

Please refer to the Clinical Evidence website for full text and references.

Search date January 2004

Philip Hazell

In the light of emerging evidence and consensus on harms data on some of the pharmacological treatments included in this review since the time of writing, and the current FDA sponsored meta-analysis of safety data, this chapter will be undergoing review in its next updated version. These data relate to increased risks of suicide and self harm with some pharmacological agents. In the interim, practitioners should be guided by the recommendations and warnings issued by their national drug regulatory authorities with respect to the prescribing of antidepressants to juveniles.

What are the effects of treatments?

BENEFICIAL

Cognitive behavioural therapy (in children and adolescents with mild to moderate depression)

One systematic review in children and adolescents with mild to moderate depression found that cognitive behavioural therapy improved symptoms compared with non-specific support.

LIKELY TO BE BENEFICIAL

Interpersonal therapy (in adolescents with mild to moderate depression)

Two RCTs found that interpersonal therapy increased recovery rate after 12 weeks in adolescents with mild to moderate depression compared with clinical monitoring or waiting list control.

TRADE OFF BETWEEN BENEFITS AND HARMS

Selective serotonin reuptake inhibitors

Three RCTs provided limited evidence that fluoxetine improved symptoms of depression compared with placebo. One RCT found that, in adolescents with major depression, paroxetine improved response rate after 8 weeks compared with placebo. Another RCT in people with major depression (aged 12–20 years) found no significant difference in effects on improvement rates between paroxetine and clomipramine, although it may have lacked power to detect clinically important effects. Pooled analysis of two RCTs found that, in children and adolescents with major depression, sertraline improved depressive symptoms compared with placebo, but this improvement was clinically small. We found no RCTs on other selective serotonin reuptake inhibitors. RCTs found that adverse effects such as dizziness, sleepiness, headache, tremor, and gastrointestinal symptoms are common with selective serotonin reuptake inhibitors, although adverse effect profiles vary among different drugs in the class. Selective serotonin reuptake inhibitors are frequently associated with dizziness, light-headedness, drowsiness, poor concentration, nausea, headache, and fatigue if treatment is reduced or stopped. On the basis of unpublished data, regulatory authorities in both the UK and the USA have recommended that paroxetine should not be prescribed for people under 18 years of age.

Depression in children and adolescents

UNKNOWN EFFECTIVENESS

Cognitive behavioural therapy (in adolescents with major depression or dysthymia with depressed parents)

One RCT in depressed adolescents with major depression or dysthymia with depressed parents found no significant difference in recovery from depression between cognitive behavioural therapy plus usual care and usual care alone over 2 years.

Electroconvulsive therapy

We found no RCTs on electroconvulsive therapy in children and adolescents with depression.

Family therapy

We found insufficient evidence in children and adolescents about the effects of family therapy.

Intravenous clomipramine (in adolescents)

One small RCT found that, in non-suicidal adolescents, intravenous clomipramine improved depression scores at 6 days compared with placebo. However, the trial was too small and brief for us to draw reliable conclusions.

Lithium

One small RCT in children with depression and a family history of bipolar affective disorder found no significant difference between lithium and placebo in global assessment or depression scores after 6 weeks. However, the study may have lacked power to detect clinically important effects.

Monoamine oxidase inhibitors

One small RCT provided insufficient evidence to compare the reversible monoamine oxidase inhibitor, moclobemide, versus placebo in children aged 9–15 years with major depression, some of whom had a comorbid disorder. We found no RCTs on non-reversible monoamine oxidase inhibitors in children or adolescents.

Specific psychological treatments other than cognitive behavioural therapy

We found insufficient evidence in children and adolescents about the effects of specific psychological treatments other than cognitive behavioural therapy.

St John's Wort (Hypericum perforatum)

We found no RCTs on St John's Wort (Hypericum perforatum) in children or adolescents with depression.

Venlafaxine

One small RCT in children and adolescents with major depression receiving psychotherapy found no significant difference between venlafaxine and placebo in improvement of depressive symptoms after 6 weeks. However, the study may have lacked power to detect clinically important effects.

UNLIKELY TO BE BENEFICIAL

Tricyclic antidepressants (in adolescents)

One systematic review in adolescents and children found no significant difference in depression scores between oral tricyclic antidepressants (amitriptyline, desipramine, imipramine, nortriptyline) and placebo after 4–10 weeks. However, subgroup analyses found that oral tricyclic antidepressants improved symptoms compared with placebo in adolescents but not children. There was no significant difference in rates of remission. The review also found that oral tricyclic antide-pressants were associated with adverse effects. One RCT found no significant difference in improvement rates between oral clomipramine and paroxetine after 8 weeks.

LIKELY TO BE INEFFECTIVE OR HARMFUL

Tricyclic antidepressants (in children)

Subgroup analyses in one systematic review found no significant difference between oral tricyclic antidepressants (amitriptyline, desipramine, imipramine, nortriptyline) and placebo in children with depression. The review also found that oral tricyclic antidepressants were associated with adverse effects.

DEFINITION Compared with adult depression (see depressive disorders, p 291), depres-sion in children (6–12 years) and adolescents (13–18 years) may have a more insidious onset, may be characterised more by irritability than sadness, and occurs more often in association with other conditions such as anxiety, conduct disorder, hyperkinesis, and learning problems.[1] The term "major depression" is used to distinguish discrete episodes of depression from mild, chronic (1 year or longer) low mood, or irritability, which is known as "dysthymia".[1] The severity of depression may be defined by the level of impairment and the presence or absence of psychomotor changes and somatic symptoms (see depressive disorders, p 291). In some studies, severity of depression is defined according to cut-off scores on depression rating scales. A manic episode is defined by abnormally and persistently elevated, expansive, or irritable mood. Additional symptoms may include grandiosity, decreased need for sleep, pressured speech, flight of ideas, distractibility, psychomotor agitation, and impaired judgement.[2]

INCIDENCE/ Estimates of prevalence of depression among children and adolescents in the
PREVALENCE community range from 2–6%.[3,4] Prevalence tends to increase with age, with a sharp rise at around the onset of puberty. Pre-adolescent boys and girls are affected equally by the condition, but in adolescents, depression is more common among girls than boys.[5]

AETIOLOGY/ The aetiology is uncertain, but may include genetic vulnerability,[6] childhood
RISK FACTORS events, and current psychosocial adversity.[1]

PROGNOSIS In children and adolescents, the recurrence rate after a first depressive episode is 40%.[7] Young people experiencing a moderate to severe depressive episode may be more likely than adults to have a manic episode within the following few years.[1,8] Trials of treatments for child and adolescent depression have found high rates of response to placebo (as much as two thirds of people in some inpatient studies) suggesting that episodes of depression may be self limiting in many cases.[9] A third of young people who experience a depressive episode will make a suicide attempt at some stage, and 3–4% will die from suicide.[1]

Please refer to the Clinical Evidence website for full text and references.

Gastroenteritis in children

Search date August 2004

Jacqueline Dalby-Payne and Elizabeth Elliott

What are the effects of treatments for acute gastroenteritis?

BENEFICIAL

Oral rehydration solutions (as effective as iv fluids)

One systematic review and two additional RCTs in children with mild to moderate dehydration in developed countries found no significant difference between oral rehydration solutions and intravenous fluids in duration of diarrhoea, time spent in hospital, or weight gain at discharge. One small RCT in children with mild to moderate dehydration managed in the emergency department found that oral rehydration reduced length of stay in the department. However, it did not significantly reduce rate of hospital admission compared with intravenous fluids. One RCT in children with severe dehydration in a developing country found that oral rehydration solutions reduced the duration of diarrhoea and increased weight gain at discharge, and were associated with fewer adverse effects compared with intravenous fluids.

LIKELY TO BE BENEFICIAL

Lactose-free feeds (reduces duration of diarrhoea)

One systematic review and three of five subsequent RCTs found limited evidence that lactose-free feeds reduced the duration of diarrhoea in children with mild to severe dehydration compared with feeds containing lactose. The remaining two subsequent RCTs found no significant difference between lactose-free and lactose containing feeds in diarrhoea duration.

Loperamide (reduces duration of diarrhoea, but adverse effects unclear)

Two RCTs found that, in children with mild to moderate dehydration, loperamide reduces the duration of diarrhoea compared with placebo. Another RCT found no significant difference between loperamide and placebo in the duration of diarrhoea. We found insufficient evidence to assess the risk of adverse effects.

Nasogastric rehydration (as effective as iv fluids)

Two RCTs conducted in the USA compared nasogastric with intravenous rehydration fluids and found different results. One small RCT, in children with moderate dehydration, found limited evidence that nasogastric rehydration fluids reduced the duration of diarrhoea and length of hospital stay compared with intravenous fluids. The second, larger RCT found no significant difference in stool output between nasogastric and intravenous fluids. However, it found a greater percentage weight gain with intravenous fluids. It found that more attempts at reinsertion were required for intravenous catheters compared with nasogastric catheters.

UNKNOWN EFFECTIVENESS

Clear fluids (other than oral rehydration solutions)

We found no systematic review or RCTs comparing "clear fluids" (water, carbonated drinks, and translucent fruit juices) versus oral rehydration solutions for treatment of acute gastroenteritis.

DEFINITION   Acute gastroenteritis is caused by infection of the gastrointestinal tract, commonly caused by a virus. It is characterised by rapid onset of diarrhoea with or without vomiting, nausea, fever, and abdominal pain.[1] In children, the symptoms and signs can be non-specific.[2] Diarrhoea is defined as the frequent passage of unformed liquid stools.[3] Regardless of the cause, the mainstay of management of acute gastroenteritis is provision of adequate fluids to prevent and treat dehydration. In this chapter we examine the benefits and harms of different treatments irrespective of cause.

INCIDENCE/   Worldwide, about 3–5 billion cases of acute gastroenteritis occur in children
PREVALENCE   under 5 years of age each year.[4] In the UK, acute gastroenteritis accounts for 204/1000 general practitioner consultations in children under 5 years of age.[5] Gastroenteritis leads to hospital admission in 7/1000 children under 5 years of age a year in the UK[5] and 13/1000 in the USA.[6] In Australia, gastroenteritis accounts for 6% of all hospital admissions in children under 15 years of age.[7]

AETIOLOGY/   In developed countries, acute gastroenteritis is predominantly caused by
RISK FACTORS   viruses (87%), of which rotavirus is most common;[8-11] bacteria cause most of the remaining cases, predominantly Campylobacter, Salmonella, Shigella, and Escherichia coli. In developing countries, bacterial pathogens are more frequent, although rotavirus is also a major cause of gastroenteritis.

PROGNOSIS   Acute gastroenteritis is usually self limiting but if untreated can result in morbidity and mortality secondary to water and electrolyte losses. Acute diarrhoea causes 4 million deaths a year in children under 5 years of age in Asia (excluding China), Africa, and Latin America, and over 80% of deaths occur in children under 2 years of age.[12] Although death is uncommon in developed countries, dehydration secondary to gastroenteritis is a significant cause of morbidity and need for hospital admission.[6,7,13]

Please refer to the Clinical Evidence website for full text and references.

Gastro-oesophageal reflux in children

Search date September 2003

Yadlapalli Kumar and Rajini Sarvananthan

What are the effects of treatments?

LIKELY TO BE BENEFICIAL

Feed thickeners in infants

One systematic review of feed thickeners found no RCTs in newborn infants. One RCT in infants aged 14–120 days found that a pre-thickened infant formula reduces regurgitation, choking and gagging, and coughing within a week without causing constipation. One small RCT in infants aged 1–6 weeks found no significant difference between carob flour and placebo thickening after 1 week, although the study may have lacked power to detect a clinically important difference.

Sodium alginate

Two RCTs in infants and in children under 2 years found that sodium alginate reduced the frequency of regurgitation at 8–14 days compared with placebo. A third small RCT of children under 17 years of age comparing sodium alginate with metoclopramide and with placebo found no significant difference between treatments.

UNKNOWN EFFECTIVENESS

Domperidone

One small RCT provided insufficient evidence about the effects of domperidone in children with gastro-oesophageal reflux.

H$_2$ antagonists

Two small RCTs provided insufficient evidence about the effects of H$_2$ antagonists in children with gastro-oesophagael reflux. Neither RCT reported clinically meaningful results.

Metoclopramide

We found insufficient evidence from three small RCTs about the clinical effects of metoclopramide compared with placebo or other treatments.

Proton pump inhibitors

We found no RCTs of proton pump inhibitors for gastro-oesophageal reflux in children.

Surgery

We found no RCTs of surgery for gastro-oesophageal reflux in children.

TRADE OFF BETWEEN BENEFITS AND HARMS

Positioning (left lateral or prone) in infants

Three crossover RCTs in children aged under 6 months found limited evidence that prone or left lateral positioning improved oesophageal pH variables compared with supine positioning. Both prone and left lateral positions may be associated with a higher risk of sudden infant death syndrome compared with supine positioning.

LIKELY TO BE INEFFECTIVE OR HARMFUL

Cisapride

One systematic review found no significant difference between cisapride and placebo in the proportion of children with improved symptoms at the end of ▶

treatment. Cisapride has been withdrawn or restricted in several countries because of an association with life-threatening heart rhythm abnormalities.

DEFINITION Gastro-oesophageal reflux disease is the passive transfer of gastric contents into the oesophagus due to transient or chronic relaxation of the lower oesophageal sphincter.[1] A survey of 69 children (median age 16 months) with gastro-oesophageal reflux disease attending a tertiary referral centre found that presenting symptoms were recurrent vomiting (72%), epigastric and abdominal pain (36%), feeding difficulties (29%), failure to thrive (28%), and irritability (19%).[2] However, results may not be generalisable to younger children or children presenting in primary care, who make up the majority of cases. Over 90% of children with gastro-oesophageal reflux disease have vomiting before 6 weeks of age.[1]

INCIDENCE/ PREVALENCE Gastro-oesophageal regurgitation is considered a problem if it is frequent, persistent, and is associated with other symptoms such as increased crying, discomfort with regurgitation, and frequent back arching.[1,3] A cross-sectional survey of parents of 948 infants attending 19 primary care paediatric practices found that regurgitation of at least one episode a day was reported in 51% of infants aged 0–3 months. "Problematic" regurgitation occurred in significantly fewer infants (14% v 51%; P < 0.001).[3] Peak regurgitation reported as "problematic" was reported in 23% of infants aged 6 months.[3]

AETIOLOGY/ RISK FACTORS Risk factors for gastro-oesophageal reflux disease include immaturity of the lower oesophageal sphincter, chronic relaxation of the sphincter, increased abdominal pressure, gastric distension, hiatus hernia, and oesophageal dysmotility.[1] Premature infants and children with severe neurodevelopmental problems or congenital oesophageal anomalies are particularly at risk.[1]

PROGNOSIS Regurgitation is considered benign, and most cases resolve spontaneously by 12–18 months of age.[4] In a cross-sectional survey of 948 parents, the peak age for reporting four or more episodes of regurgitation was at 5 months of age (23%), which decreased to 7% at 7 months (P < 0.001). One cohort study found that those infants with frequent spilling in the first 2 years of life (90 days or more in the first 2 years) were more likely to have symptoms of gastro-oesophageal reflux at 9 years of age than those with no spilling (RR 2.3, 95% CI 1.3 to 4.0).[5] The prevalence of "problematic" regurgitation also reduced from 23% in infants aged 6 months to 3.25% in infants aged 10–12 months.[3] Rare complications of gastro-oesophageal reflux disease include oesophagitis with haematemesis and anaemia, respiratory problems (such as cough, apnoea, and recurrent wheeze), and failure to thrive.[1] A small comparative study (40 children) suggested that, when compared with healthy children, infants with gastro-oesophageal reflux disease had slower development of feeding skills and had problems affecting behaviour, swallowing, food intake, and mother–child interaction.[6]

Please refer to the Clinical Evidence website for full text and references.

Infantile colic

Child health

Search date September 2004

Teresa Kilgour and Sally Wade

What are the effects of treatments for infantile colic?

LIKELY TO BE BENEFICIAL

Whey hydrolysate milk

One small RCT found limited evidence that replacing cows' milk formula with whey hydrolysate formula reduced crying recorded in a parental diary.

TRADE OFF BETWEEN BENEFITS AND HARMS

Dicycloverine (dicyclomine)

Two systematic reviews of RCTs of variable quality found limited evidence that dicycloverine reduced crying in infants with colic compared with placebo. RCTs found that dicycloverine increased drowsiness, constipation, and loose stools compared with placebo, but the difference did not reach significance. Case reports of harms in infants have included breathing difficulties, seizures, syncope, asphyxia, muscular hypotonia, and coma.

UNKNOWN EFFECTIVENESS

Advice to reduce stimulation

One RCT found limited evidence that advice to reduce stimulation (by not patting, lifting, or jiggling the baby, or by reducing auditory stimulation) reduced crying after 7 days in infants under 12 weeks compared with an empathetic interview giving no advice. However, we were unable to draw reliable conclusions from this small study.

Car ride simulation

One RCT found no significant difference between car ride simulation plus reassurance; counselling mothers about specific management techniques (responding to crying with gentle soothing motion, avoiding over stimulation, using a pacifier, and prophylactic carrying) plus reassurance; and reassurance alone, in terms of maternal anxiety or hours of infant crying over 2 weeks.

Casein hydrolysate milk

Two RCTs found insufficient evidence about the effects of replacing cows' milk formula with casein hydrolysate hypoallergenic formula. Another small RCT found that substituting soya or cows' milk with casein hydroysate formula was less effective at reducing the duration and extent of crying with focused counselling.

Cranial osteopathy

We found no RCTs on the effects of cranial osteopathy in infants with colic.

Focused counselling

One RCT found no significant difference between counselling mothers about specific management techniques (responding to crying with gentle soothing motion, avoiding over stimulation, using a pacifier, and prophylactic carrying) plus reassurance; car ride simulation plus reassurance; and reassurance alone, in terms of maternal anxiety or hours of infant crying over 2 weeks. Another small RCT found that counselling decreased the duration and extent of crying compared with substitution of soya or cows' milk with casein hydrolysate formula.

Herbal tea

One small RCT found that herbal tea (containing extracts of camomile, vervain, licorice, fennel, and balm mint in a sucrose solution) improved symptoms of colic rated by parents at 7 days compared with sucrose solution alone. However, we were unable to draw reliable conclusions from this small study.

Infant massage

One RCT found no significant difference between massage and a crib vibrator for colic related crying or parental rating of symptoms of infantile colic, but it may have lacked power to detect a clinically important difference.

Low lactose milk

Four small crossover RCTs provided insufficient evidence on the effects of low lactose milk in infants with colic.

Soya based infant feeds

One small RCT found that soya based infant feeds reduced the duration of crying in infants with colic compared with standard cows' milk formula. However, we were unable to draw reliable conclusions from this small study.

Spinal manipulation

Two RCTs found insufficient evidence about the effects of spinal manipulation.

Sucrose solution

One small crossover RCT found limited evidence that sucrose solution improved symptoms of colic as rated by parents after 12 days compared with placebo. However, we were unable to draw reliable conclusions from this small study.

UNLIKELY TO BE BENEFICIAL

Advice to increase carrying

One RCT found no significant difference in daily crying time between advice to carry the infant, even when not crying, for at least an additional 3 hours a day and general advice (to carry, check baby's nappy, feed, offer pacifier, place baby near mother, or use background stimulation such as music).

Simethicone (activated dimeticone)

One RCT found no significant difference between simethicone and placebo in colic rated by carers. Another RCT found no significant difference between simethicone and placebo in improvement as rated by parental interview, 24 hour diary, or behavioural observation. Another poor quality RCT found that simethicone reduced the number of crying attacks on days 4–7 of treatment compared with placebo. One RCT found insufficient evidence to compare simethicone with spinal manipulation.

DEFINITION
Infantile colic is defined as excessive crying in an otherwise healthy baby. The crying typically starts in the first few weeks of life and ends by 4–5 months. Excessive crying is defined as crying that lasts at least 3 hours a day, for 3 days a week, for at least 3 weeks.[1] Due to the natural course of infantile colic, it can be difficult to interpret trials which do not include a placebo or have no treatment group for comparison.

INCIDENCE/ PREVALENCE
Infantile colic causes one out of six families (17%) to consult a health professional. One systematic review of 15 community based studies found a wide variation in prevalence, which depended on study design and method of recording.[2] Two prospective studies identified by the review yielded prevalence rates of 5% and 19%.[2] One RCT (89 breast and formula fed infants) found that, at 2 weeks of age, the prevalence of crying more than 3 hours a day was 43% among formula fed infants and 16% among breast fed infants. The prevalence at 6 weeks was 12% (formula fed) and 31% (breast fed).[3] ▶

AETIOLOGY/
RISK FACTORS
The cause is unclear and, despite its name, infantile colic may not have an abdominal cause. It may reflect part of the normal distribution of infantile crying. Other possible explanations are painful intestinal contractions, lactose intolerance, gas, or parental misinterpretation of normal crying.[1]

PROGNOSIS
Infantile colic improves with time. One study found that 29% of infants aged 1–3 months cried for more than 3 hours a day, but by 4–6 months of age the prevalence had fallen to 7–11%.[4]

Please refer to the Clinical Evidence website for full text and references.

Nitu Sengupta, Helen Bedford, David Elliman, and Robert Booy

What are the effects of measles vaccination?

BENEFICIAL

Monovalent measles vaccine or combined MMR vaccine (reduced incidence of measles and child mortality compared with placebo or no vaccine)

We found no RCTs comparing the clinical effects of combined measles, mumps, and rubella (MMR) versus no vaccine or placebo. One large RCT, one quasi randomised trial, one large retrospective cohort study, and several observational studies found that monovalent vaccine reduced the incidence of measles. Mass population cohort studies and other observational studies also consistently found important reductions in child mortality after measles vaccination. Observational studies found that measles vaccination programmes were followed by a reduction in the incidence of subacute sclerosing panencephalitis. Several features of measles infection occur or are suspected to occur after the vaccine, but we found no studies comparing rates of occurrence between people with naturally acquired measles and those who have been vaccinated. Severe complications are rare with measles immunisation. One non-systematic review found that, compared with placebo, measles vaccination increased the incidence of fever and febrile seizures, although febrile seizures are rare and do not progress into afebrile seizures. Observational studies found that aseptic meningitis, a rare complication, increased after mass vaccination with the L-Z and Urabe strains of MMR, but no increased incidence has been reported with Jeryl Lynn, Hoshino, or Rubini strains. Observational studies found that both measles vaccination and naturally acquired measles increased the incidence of idiopathic thrombocytopenic purpura. Observational studies found no association between the incidence of asthma in healthy children and MMR vaccination. They also found no significant change in the incidence of Guillain–Barré syndrome, autism, diabetes, or inflammatory bowel disease as a result of measles vaccination. Anaphylaxis has been reported after vaccination with MMR, but this is extremely rare.

UNKNOWN EFFECTIVENESS

Comparative effects of combined MMR and monovalent measles vaccine

We found no RCTs comparing the clinical effects of MMR versus monovalent vaccines in children. Seroconversion rates are similar with both vaccines.

DEFINITION Measles is an infectious disease caused by a ribonucleic acid paramyxovirus. The illness is characterised by an incubation period of 6–19 days (median 13 days);[1] a prodromal period of 2–4 days with upper respiratory tract symptoms; conjunctivitis, Koplik's spots on mucosal membranes, and high fever; followed by a widespread maculopapular rash that persists, with fever, for 5–6 days.

INCIDENCE/ PREVALENCE Incidence varies according to vaccination coverage. Worldwide, there are an estimated 30 million cases of measles each year,[2] but the incidence is only 0–10/100 000 people in countries with widespread vaccination programmes such as the USA, UK, Mexico, India, China, Brazil, and Australia.[3] In the USA, before licensing of effective vaccines, more than 90% of people were infected by the age of 15 years. After licensing in 1963, incidence fell by about 98%.[4] The mean annual incidence in Finland was 366/100 000 in 1970,[5] but declined to about zero by the late 1990s.[6] Similarly, the annual incidence ▶

Measles: prevention

declined to almost zero in Chile, the English speaking Caribbean, and Cuba during the 1990s when vaccination programmes were introduced.[7,8]

AETIOLOGY/ RISK FACTORS Measles is highly contagious and spreads through airborne droplets. As with most other infectious diseases, risk factors include overcrowding and low herd immunity. Newborn babies have a lower risk of measles than do older infants, owing to protective maternal antibodies, although in recent US outbreaks maternal antibody protection was lower than expected.[4] Antibody levels are lower in babies born to immunised mothers compared with offspring of naturally infected mothers.[9,10]

PROGNOSIS The World Health Organization estimated that measles caused 777 000 deaths and 27.5 million disability adjusted life years in 2000.[11] **Disease in healthy people:** In developed countries, most prognostic data come from the pre-vaccination era and from subsequent outbreaks in non-vaccinated populations. The overall rate of complications in the UK was 6.7% before the introduction of measles vaccination. Encephalitis affected 1.2/1000 diseased people, and respiratory complications in 38/1000 diseased people.[12] Other complications before the introduction of the vaccine included seizures, with or without fever, affecting 5/1000 people with measles.[13] Idiopathic thrombocytopenic purpura has been reported, but the frequency is not known. Subacute sclerosing panencephalitis (SSPE) is an inevitably fatal, progressive degenerative disorder of the central nervous system with a mean onset 7–10 years after measles infection. It is more common when measles occurs under the age of 1 year (18/100 000 in children < 1 year of age v 4/100 000 overall), as identified by a passive reporting system set up in England and Wales to monitor the incidence of SSPE.[14] Between 1989–1991 in the USA, measles resurgence among young children (< 5 years) who had not been immunised led to 55 622 cases, with more than 11 000 hospital admissions and 166 deaths.[15–17] Measles complications include diarrhoea (9%), pneumonia (6%), and acute encephalitis (about 0.14%).[17] Measles during pregnancy results in higher risk of premature labour[18] but no proven increase in congenital anomalies.[19] **Disease in malnourished or immunocompromised people:** In malnourished people, particularly those with vitamin A deficiency, measles case fatality can be as high as 25%. Immunocompromised people have a higher morbidity and mortality. Children younger than 5 years, and adults older than 20 years, have a higher risk of severe complications and death.[15,20] In the period 1974–1984, four UK centres reported that 15/51 (29%) deaths in children in their first remission from leukaemia resulted from measles.[21] Another report reviewing cases from the same four UK centres between 1973 and 1986 found that five out of 17 cases of measles in children with malignancies proved fatal.[22] At least 5 out of 36 (14%) measles associated deaths in 1991 in the USA were in HIV infected persons.[15] Worldwide, measles is a major cause of blindness, and causes 5% of deaths in young children (< 5 years).[23]

Please refer to the Clinical Evidence website for full text and references.

Nick Barnes, Guy Millman, and Elizabeth James

What are the effects of treatments for acute attacks of migraine headache in children?

UNKNOWN EFFECTIVENESS

$5HT_1$ antagonists (e.g. Triptans)
Two RCTs provided insufficient evidence that nasal sumatriptan reduced symptoms of migraine, but found that sumatriptan increased taste disturbance compared with placebo. One RCT found no significant difference in pain relief between oral rizatriptan and placebo.

Antiemetics
We found no RCTs of antiemetics in children with migraine headache.

Codeine phosphate
We found no RCTs.

Non-steroidal anti-inflammatory drugs
We found no reliable RCTs assessing the effects of non-steroidal anti-inflammatory drugs in children and adolescents with migraine headache.

Paracetamol
We found no RCTs of sufficient quality addressing the effects of paracetamol (acetaminophen) in children or adolescents with migraine headache.

What are the effects of prophylaxis for migraine in children?

LIKELY TO BE BENEFICIAL

Stress management
One small RCT provided limited evidence that a stress management programme improved headache severity and frequency compared with no stress management at 1 month.

UNKNOWN EFFECTIVENESS

Dietary manipulation
We found no RCTs of sufficient quality in children and adolescents with migraine headache.

Pizotifen
We found no RCTs of sufficient quality.

Progressive muscle relaxation
We found no RCTs of sufficient quality examining effects of progressive muscle relaxation in children with migraine headache.

Thermal biofeedback
We found no RCTs of sufficient quality examining effects of thermal biofeedback in children with migraine headache.

▶

Child health

Migraine headache in children

β blockers

One RCT found that propranolol increased perception of benefit compared with placebo. However, one RCT found no significant difference in migraine episodes and another RCT found that propranolol increased headache duration compared with placebo.

DEFINITION   Migraine is defined by the International Headache Society (IHS) as a recurrent headache that occurs with or without aura and lasts 2–48 hours.[1] It is usually unilateral in nature, pulsating in quality, of moderate or severe intensity, and is aggravated by routine physical activity. Nausea, vomiting, photophobia, and phonophobia are common accompanying symptoms. This topic focuses on children younger than 18 years. Diagnostic criteria for children are broader than criteria for adults, allowing for a broader range of duration and a broader localisation of the pain).[2] Diagnosis is difficult in young children, because the condition is defined by subjective symptoms. Studies that do not explicitly use criteria that are congruent with IHS diagnostic criteria (or revised IHS criteria in children < 15 years of age) have been excluded from this topic.

INCIDENCE/   Migraine occurs in 3–10% of children,[3–7] and currently affects 50/1000
PREVALENCE   school age children in the UK and an estimated 7.8 million children in the European Union.[8] Studies in developed countries suggest that migraine is the most common diagnosis among children presenting with headache to a medical practitioner. It is rarely diagnosed in children under 2 years of age because of the symptom based definition, but increases steadily with age thereafter.[1,9,10] It affects boys and girls similarly before puberty, but after puberty girls are more likely to suffer from migraine.[4,6,10] See incidence/ prevalence of migraine headache, p 369.

AETIOLOGY/   The cause of migraine headaches is unknown. We found few reliable data
RISK FACTORS identifying risk factors or measuring their effects in children. Suggested risk factors include stress, foods, menses, and exercise in genetically predisposed children and adolescents.[10,11]

PROGNOSIS   We found no reliable data about prognosis of childhood migraine headache diagnosed by IHS criteria. It has been suggested that more than half the children will have spontaneous remission after puberty.[10] It is believed that migraine that develops during adolescence tends to continue in adult life, although attacks tend to be less frequent and severe in later life.[12] We found one longitudinal study from Sweden (73 children with "pronounced" migraine and mean age onset 6 years) with over 40 years follow up, which predated the IHS criteria for migraine headache.[13] It found that migraine headaches had ceased before the age of 25 years in 23% of people. However, by the age of 50 years, more than 50% of people continued to have migraine headaches. We found no prospective data examining long term risks in children with migraine.

Please refer to the Clinical Evidence website for full text and references.

What are the effects of treatments for unconjugated hyperbilirubinaemia in term and preterm infants?

BENEFICIAL

Exchange transfusion

We found no RCTs on the effects of exchange transfusion versus no treatment or versus phototherapy. There is general consensus that exchange transfusion is effective in reducing serum bilirubin levels and in preventing neuro-developmental sequelae. In most of the RCTs comparing other interventions, exchange transfusion was used successfully to reduce serum bilirubin levels when those interventions failed to control the rise of serum bilirubin.

Phototherapy

Two RCTs found that both conventional phototherapy and fibreoptic phototherapy reduced neonatal jaundice more effectively than no treatment. One systematic review (which included quasi-randomised as well as randomised controlled trials) and one subsequent RCT found that conventional phototherapy was more effective than fibreoptic phototherapy, although subgroup analysis in the systematic review found no significant difference between groups in preterm infants. No trials included in the review evaluated the impact of either phototherapy method on parent–infant bonding. One RCT found a greater effect with double conventional compared with single conventional phototherapy, whilst another RCT found no significant difference between double fibreoptic and single conventional phototherapy. One systematic review (which included quasi-randomised as well as randomised controlled trials) found no significant difference between fibreoptic plus conventional and conventional phototherapy alone in additional phototherapy, exchange transfusion, or percentage change in bilirubin after 24 hours, although it noted a trend favouring the fibreoptic plus conventional group. Most trials did not report kernicterus as an outcome. We found insufficient evidence on the adverse effects of phototherapy.

UNKNOWN EFFECTIVENESS

Albumin infusion

We found no RCTs on the effects of albumin infusion versus no treatment or versus other treatment.

Home versus hospital phototherapy

We found no RCTs on the effects of home phototherapy versus no treatment or versus hospital phototherapy.

DEFINITION   Neonatal jaundice refers to the yellow colouration of the skin and sclera of newborn babies that results from hyperbilirubinaemia.

INCIDENCE/   Jaundice is the most common condition requiring medical attention in
PREVALENCE   newborn babies. About 50% of term and 80% of preterm babies develop jaundice in the first week of life.[1] Jaundice is also a common cause of readmission to hospital after early discharge of newborn babies.[2] Jaundice usually appears 2–4 days after birth and disappears 1–2 weeks later, usually without the need for treatment.

▶

Neonatal jaundice

AETIOLOGY/ RISK FACTORS In most infants with jaundice, there is no underlying disease and the jaundice is termed physiological. Physiological jaundice occurs when there is accumulation of unconjugated bilirubin in the skin and mucous membranes. It typically presents on the second or third day of life and results from the increased production of bilirubin (due to increased circulating red cell mass and a shortened red cell lifespan) and the decreased excretion of bilirubin (due to low concentrations of the hepatocyte binding protein, low activity of glucuronyl transferase, and increased enterohepatic circulation) that normally occur in newborn babies. In some infants, unconjugated hyperbilirubinaemia may be associated with breast feeding (breast milk jaundice), and this typically occurs after the third day of life. Although the exact cause of breast milk jaundice is not clear, it is generally believed to be due to an unidentified factor in breast milk. Non-physiological causes include blood group incompatibility (Rhesus or ABO problems), other causes of haemolysis, sepsis, bruising, and metabolic disorders. Gilbert's and Crigler-Najjar syndromes are rare causes of neonatal jaundice.

PROGNOSIS In the newborn baby, unconjugated bilirubin can penetrate the blood–brain barrier and is potentially neurotoxic. Unconjugated hyperbilirubinaemia can, therefore, result in neuro-developmental sequelae including the development of kernicterus. Kernicterus is brain damage arising from the deposition of bilirubin in brain tissue. However, the exact level of bilirubin that is neurotoxic is unclear, and kernicterus at autopsy has been reported in infants in the absence of markedly elevated levels of bilirubin.[3] Recent reports suggest a resurgence of kernicterus in countries in which this complication had virtually disappeared.[4] This has been attributed mainly to early discharge of newborns from hospital.

Please refer to the Clinical Evidence website for full text and references.

Search date February 2003

Natalie Lyth and Sara Bosson

What are the effects of interventions?

BENEFICIAL

Enuresis alarm plus dry-bed training (as effective as enuresis alarm alone)

One systematic review has found limited evidence that a higher proportion of children achieve 14 consecutive dry nights with alarm plus dry bed training than with no treatment. A second systematic review found no significant difference between alarm plus dry bed training and alarm alone for achieving 14 consecutive dry nights.

Desmopressin (in short term)

One systematic review has found that desmopressin reduces bedwetting by at least one night per week and increases the chance of attaining initial success (14 consecutive dry nights) compared with placebo. The review found insufficient evidence comparing either intranasal versus oral administration of desmopressin or desmopressin versus tricyclic drugs. There was some evidence that higher doses of desmopressin were more likely to reduce the number of wet nights during treatment compared with lower doses. The review found no difference between desmopressin and enuresis alarms in the number of children achieving initial success, although one RCT found that, after 3 months of treatment, enuresis alarms were better than desmopressin at reducing the number of wet nights per week.

Dry bed training (in short term)

One systematic review has found that a greater proportion of children achieved 14 consecutive dry nights with dry bed training than with no treatment.

Enuresis alarm (in short and long term)

One systematic review has found that enuresis alarms increase initial success rates compared with no treatment, and that 31–61% of children using alarms were still dry at 3 months. We found limited evidence from one small RCT that dry bed training reduced bedwetting compared with an enuresis alarm after initial treatment and after 6 months. One systematic review found no significant difference between alarm plus dry bed training and alarm alone for achieving 14 consecutive dry nights. One systematic review found that desmopressin plus alarm was better at reducing the number of wet nights per week during treatment compared with alarm alone or alarm plus placebo, although there was no significant difference in the rate of initial success.

LIKELY TO BE BENEFICIAL

Laser acupuncture (as effective as desmopressin in one RCT)

One RCT found no difference between laser acupuncture and intranasal desmopressin in the number of wet nights in children aged over 5 years.

Standard home alarm clock (in short term)

One RCT found that a higher proportion of children achieved 14 consecutive dry nights with standard home alarm clock than with waking after 3 hours' sleep. ▶

Child health

Nocturnal enuresis in children

◄

UNKNOWN EFFECTIVENESS

Dry bed training (in long term)

One systematic review has found no significant long term difference in the proportion of dry nights between dry bed training and no treatment. However, one small RCT showed some long-term advantages of dry bed training.

Standard home alarm clock (in long term)

One RCT found no significant difference in the proportion of dry nights achieved at 3 months between standard home alarm clock and waking after 3 hours' sleep.

Ultrasound

We found no RCTs. One small controlled trial in children aged 6–14 years found that ultrasound increased the proportion of dry nights for up to 12 months compared with control.

UNLIKELY TO BE BENEFICIAL

Adding desmopressin to an alarm (in long term)

One systematic review found that desmopressin plus alarm was better at reducing the number of wet nights per week during treatment compared with alarm alone or alarm plus placebo, although there was no significant difference in the rate of initial success.

TRADE OFF BETWEEN BENEFITS AND HARMS

Tricyclic drugs (imipramine, desipramine)

One systematic review has found that tricyclic drugs (imipramine, desipramine) increase the chance of attaining 14 consecutive dry nights compared with placebo, although tricyclic drugs increased adverse effects such as anorexia, anxiety reaction, constipation, depression, diarrhoea, dizziness, drowsiness, dry mouth, headache, irritability, lethargy, sleep disturbance, upset stomach, and vomiting compared with placebo. We found no good studies comparing tricyclic drugs versus desmopressin. The review found no significant difference between imipramine and an enuresis alarm during the treatment period, but it found limited evidence that an alarm reduced bedwetting after the treatment had stopped compared with imipramine.

DEFINITION
Nocturnal enuresis is the involuntary discharge of urine at night in the absence of congenital or acquired defects of the central nervous system or urinary tract in a child aged 5 years or older.[1] Disorders that have bedwetting as a symptom (termed "nocturnal incontinence") can be excluded by a thorough history, examination, and urinalysis. "Monosymptomatic" nocturnal enuresis is characterised by night time symptoms only and accounts for 85% of cases. Nocturnal enuresis is defined as primary if the child has not been dry for a period of more than 6 months, and secondary if such a period of dryness preceded the onset of wetting.

INCIDENCE/ PREVALENCE
Between 15% and 20% of 5 year olds, 7% of 7 year olds, 5% of 10 year olds, 2–3% of 12–14 year olds, and 1–2% of people aged 15 years and over wet the bed twice a week on average.[2]

AETIOLOGY/ RISK FACTORS
Nocturnal enuresis is associated with several factors, including small functional bladder capacity, nocturnal polyuria, and arousal dysfunction. Linkage studies have identified associated genetic loci on chromosomes 8q, 12q, 13q, and 22q11.[3–6]

PROGRESS Nocturnal enuresis has widely differing outcomes, from spontaneous resolution to complete resistance to all current treatments. About 1% of adults remain enuretic. Without treatment, about 15% of children with enuresis become dry each year.[7] We found no RCTs on the best age at which to start treatment in children with nocturnal enuresis. Anecdotal experience suggests that reassurance is sufficient below the age of 7 years. Behavioural treatments, such as alarms, require motivation and commitment from the child and a parent. Anecdotal experience suggests that children under the age of 7 years may not exhibit the commitment needed.

Please refer to the Clinical Evidence website for full text and references.

Nosebleeds in children

Search date February 2004

Gerald McGarry

What are the effects of treatments for recurrent idiopathic epistaxis in children?

LIKELY TO BE BENEFICIAL

Antiseptic cream versus no treatment

One RCT found that chlorhexidine/neomycin cream reduced nosebleeds compared with no treatment at 8 weeks.

UNKNOWN EFFECTIVENESS

Antiseptic cream versus cautery

One small RCT found no significant difference in nosebleeds between chlorhexidine/neomycin cream and silver nitrate cautery at 8 weeks. However, the study may have lacked power to detect clinically important differences between treatments. Some children found the smell and taste of the antiseptic cream unpleasant. All children found cautery painful, despite the use of local anaesthesia.

Cautery plus antiseptic cream

One small RCT found insufficient evidence about the effects of silver nitrate cautery plus chlorhexidine/neomycin cream compared with chlorhexidine/neomycin cream alone.

Cautery versus no treatment

We found no RCTs about the effects of this intervention.

DEFINITION	Recurrent idiopathic epistaxis is recurrent, self limiting, nasal bleeding for which no specific cause is identified. There is no consensus on the frequency or severity of recurrences.
INCIDENCE/ PREVALENCE	A cross sectional study of 1218 children (aged 11–14 years) found that 9% had frequent episodes of epistaxis.[1] It is likely that only the most severe episodes are considered for treatment.
AETIOLOGY/ RISK FACTORS	In children, most epistaxis occurs from the anterior part of the septum in the region of Little's area.[2] Initiating factors include local inflammation, mucosal drying, and local trauma (including nose picking).[2] Epistaxis caused by other specific local (e.g. tumours) or systemic factors (e.g. clotting disorders) is not considered here.
PROGNOSIS	Recurrent epistaxis is less common in adolescents over 14 years and many children "grow out" of this problem.

Please refer to the Clinical Evidence website for full text and references.

Perinatal asphyxia 85

Search date June 2004

William McGuire

What are the effects of interventions in term or near term newborns with perinatal asphyxia?

UNKNOWN EFFECTIVENESS

Antioxidants

One systematic review found insufficient evidence from two small RCTs about the effects of antioxidants in infants with perinatal asphyxia.

Calcium channel blockers

We found no RCTs on the effects of calcium channel blockers in infants with asphyxia.

Corticosteroids

We found no RCTs on the effects of corticosteroids in infants with perinatal asphyxia.

Fluid restriction

We found no RCTs on the effects of fluid restriction in infants with perinatal asphyxia.

Hyperventilation

We found no RCTs on the effects of hyperventilation in infants with perinatal asphyxia.

Magnesium sulphate

We found no RCTs on the effects of magnesium sulphate in infants with asphyxia.

Mannitol

One small RCT provided insufficient evidence on the effects of mannitol in infants with asphyxia.

Opiate antagonists

One small RCT identified by a systematic review did not report on the effects of opiate antagonists, mortality or neurodevelopmental outcomes in infants with perinatal asphyxia.

UNLIKELY TO BE BENEFICIAL

Prophylactic anticonvulsants

One systematic review of three small, methodologically flawed RCTs found no significant difference in mortality or neurodevelopmental outcomes between barbiturates and no drug treatment in term infants with perinatal asphyxia.

DEFINITION   The clinical diagnosis of perinatal asphyxia is based on several criteria, the two main ones being: evidence of cardiorespiratory and neurological depression, defined as an Apgar score of less than 7 at 5 minutes after birth; and evidence of acute hypoxic compromise with acidaemia, defined as an arterial blood pH of less than 7 or base excess greater than 12 mmol/L.[1] In many settings, especially in resource poor countries, it may be impossible to assess fetal or neonatal acidaemia. Signs of "hypoxic-ischaemic" encephalopathy (neonatal encephalopathy) or other organ dysfunction can also be part of the clinical picture. In the immediate postpartum period when resuscitation is being undertaken, it may not be possible to determine whether the neurological and ▶

Perinatal asphyxia

cardiorespiratory depression is secondary to hypoxia-ischaemia, or to another condition such as feto-maternal infection or metabolic disease. However, these features often take time to develop and are therefore not useful in deciding the immediate management of infants with suspected perinatal asphyxia. In addition, neonatal encephalopathy may have a variety of causes which may be unrelated to an hypoxia-ischaemic event.[2–4]

INCIDENCE/ PREVALENCE Estimates of the incidence of perinatal asphyxia vary depending on the definitions used. In resource rich countries the incidence of severe perinatal asphyxia (causing death or severe neurological impairment) is about 1/1000 live births.[5,6] In resource poor countries, perinatal asphyxia is probably much more common. Data from hospital based studies in such settings suggest an incidence of 5–10/1000 live births.[7–9] This probably represents an underestimate of the true community incidence of perinatal asphyxia in resource poor countries.

AETIOLOGY/ RISK FACTORS Perinatal asphyxia may occur *in utero*, during labour and delivery, or in the immediate postnatal period. There are numerous causes, including placental abruption, cord compression, transplacental anaesthetic or narcotic administration, intrauterine pneumonia, severe meconium aspiration, congenital cardiac or pulmonary anomalies, and birth trauma. Postnatal asphyxia can be caused by an obstructed airway, maternal opiates which can cause respiratory depression, or congenital sepsis.

PROGNOSIS Worldwide, perinatal asphyxia is a major cause of death and of acquired brain damage in newborn infants.[9] The prognosis depends on the severity of the asphyxia. Only a minority of infants with severe encephalopathy after perinatal asphyxia survive without handicap.[5] However, there are limited population based data on long term outcomes after perinatal asphyxia, such as cerebral palsy, developmental delay, visual and hearing impairment, and learning and behavioural problems. After an asphyxial event, there may be an opportunity to intervene to minimise brain damage. The first phase of brain damage, early cell death, results from primary exhaustion of the cellular energy stores. Early cell death can occur within minutes. Immediate resuscitation to restore oxygen supply and blood circulation aims to limit the extent of this damage. A secondary phase of neuronal injury may occur several hours after the initial insult. The mechanisms believed to be important in this process include oxygen free radical production, intracellular calcium entry, and apoptosis. Treatments during the post-resuscitation phase aim to block these processes thereby limiting secondary cell damage and minimising the extent of any brain damage.

Please refer to the Clinical Evidence website for full text and references.

Search date May 2003

Deborah Pritchard

What are the effects of interventions to reduce pain related distress during heel puncture?

LIKELY TO BE BENEFICIAL

Holding (skin to skin) versus swaddling in term infants

RCTs found that holding reduced crying during heel puncture compared with swaddling in term infants.

Oral glucose

RCTs found that oral glucose reduced pain responses (particularly the duration of crying) in preterm and term infants compared with water or no treatment.

Oral sucrose

Systematic reviews and additional RCTs found good evidence in preterm infants and limited evidence in term infants that oral sucrose reduced pain responses (particularly the duration of crying) compared with water or no treatment. One RCT found that sucrose did not appear to increase the benefit of holding. Three RCTs in term infants found that sucrose plus pacifier was more effective than pacifier alone, although one RCT in preterm infants found no significant difference in pain score between a pacifier dipped in sucrose and pacifier alone. One RCT found insufficient evidence about the effects of oral sucrose compared with lidocaine–prilocaine emulsion in term infants undergoing heel puncture.

Other sweeteners

RCTs have found that other sweeteners (hydrogenated glucose or an artificial sweetener, 10 parts cyclamate and 1 part saccharin) reduce pain scores and the percentage of time spent crying in term infants compared with water.

Pacifiers

RCTs in term and preterm infants have found that pacifiers given before heel puncture reduce pain responses compared with no treatment.

Positioning (tucking arms and legs) in preterm infants

One RCT found limited evidence that pain responses were reduced by tucking the arms and legs into a mid-line flexed position during heel puncture.

Rocking

We found limited evidence that rocking reduces pain related stress compared with placebo.

UNKNOWN EFFECTIVENESS

Multiple doses of sweet solution

One small RCT found no significant difference with multiple versus single doses of sucrose in pain scores for heel puncture.

Swaddling

One small RCT found no significant difference in pain responses from swaddling compared with no swaddling.

▶

Reducing pain during blood sampling in infants

UNLIKELY TO BE BENEFICIAL

Breast milk or breast feeding

RCTs found no evidence that breast milk or breast feeding during heel puncture reduced pain responses or crying in neonates compared with water.

Prone position

One RCT found no significant difference in pain score between prone position and either side or supine position during heel puncture.

Topical anaesthetics

Systematic reviews and additional RCTs found no evidence of reduced pain responses, particularly crying, following heel puncture with topical anaesthetic (lidocaine, lidocaine–prilocaine emulsion, or tetracaine [amethocaine]) compared with placebo.

Warming

Two RCTs in term infants found no benefit of warming before heel puncture.

What are the effects of interventions to reduce pain related distress during venepuncture?

LIKELY TO BE BENEFICIAL

Breast feeding

One RCT found that breast feeding during venepuncture reduced pain responses compared with oral water or being held. The RCT found no significant difference in pain response between breast feeding and oral glucose.

Oral glucose

RCTs have found that oral glucose reduces pain responses (particularly the duration of crying) in term and preterm infants compared with water or no treatment. One RCT found no significant difference in pain scores between sucrose and glucose.

Oral sucrose

RCTs have found that oral sucrose reduces pain responses (particularly the duration of crying) in term and preterm infants compared with water or no treatment. One RCT found no significant difference in pain between sucrose and glucose.

Pacifiers

One RCT found that pacifiers reduced pain responses compared with water or no treatment in term infants undergoing venepuncture.

Topical anaesthetics

Four RCTs found limited evidence that lidocaine–prilocaine emulsion reduced pain responses to venepuncture compared with placebo. Two RCTs found that tetracaine (amethocaine) gel reduced pain and crying during venepuncture compared with placebo.

UNKNOWN EFFECTIVENESS

Other sweeteners

We found no RCTs of other sweeteners for venepuncture.

DEFINITION Methods of sampling blood in infants include heel puncture, venepuncture, and arterial puncture. Heel puncture involves lancing of the lateral aspect of the infant's heel, squeezing the heel, and collecting the pooled capillary blood. Venepuncture involves aspirating blood through a needle from a peripheral vein. Arterial blood sampling is not discussed in this review. RCTs in this review were performed in a hospital care setting and the evidence relates to preterm and ill infants who have multiple blood tests, rather than infants undergoing heel puncture tests for routine screening. The results therefore cannot be applied to routine screening heel puncture tests in healthy infants.

INCIDENCE/ PREVALENCE Almost every infant in the developed world undergoes heel puncture to screen for metabolic disorders (e.g. phenylketonuria). Many infants have repeated heel punctures or venepunctures to monitor blood glucose or haemoglobin. Preterm or ill neonates may undergo 1–21 heel punctures or venepunctures per day.[1–3] These punctures are likely to be painful. Heel punctures comprise 61–87% and venepunctures comprise 8–13% of the invasive procedures performed on ill infants. Analgesics are rarely given specifically for blood sampling procedures, but 5–19% of infants receive analgesia for other indications.[2,3] In one study, comfort measures were provided during 63% of venepunctures and 75% of heel punctures.[3]

AETIOLOGY/ RISK FACTORS Blood sampling in infants can be difficult to perform, particularly in preterm or ill infants. Young infants may have increased sensitivity and more prolonged responses to pain than older age groups.[4] Factors that may affect the infant's pain responses include postconceptional age, previous pain experience, and procedural technique.

PROGNOSIS Pain caused by blood sampling is associated with acute behavioural and physiological deterioration.[4] Experience of pain during heel puncture seems to heighten pain responses during subsequent blood sampling.[5] Other adverse effects of blood sampling include bleeding, bruising, haematoma, and infection.

Please refer to the Clinical Evidence website for full text and references.

Sudden infant death syndrome

Search date July 2004

David Creery and Angelo Mikrogianakis

What are the effects of interventions to reduce the risk of sudden infant death syndrome?

BENEFICIAL

Advice to avoid prone sleeping

One non-systematic review and 12 observational studies found that eight campaigns encouraging non-prone positioning and seven campaigns involving, among other recommendations, advice to encourage non-prone sleeping positions were followed by a reduced incidence of sudden infant death syndrome.

LIKELY TO BE BENEFICIAL

Advice to avoid tobacco smoke exposure*

One non-systematic review and four observational studies found limited evidence that campaigns to reduce several risk factors for sudden infant death, which included tobacco smoke exposure, were followed by a reduced incidence of sudden infant death syndrome. One observational study found that smoking was associated with an increased risk of sudden infant death.

UNKNOWN EFFECTIVENESS

Advice to avoid bed sharing*

One observational study found that a campaign to reduce several risk factors for sudden infant death, which included advice to avoid bed sharing, was followed by a reduced incidence of sudden infant death syndrome. However, it is not clear whether effects were specifically due to the advice to avoid bed sharing.

Advice to avoid over heating or over wrapping*

One non-systematic review and one observational study found limited evidence that campaigns to reduce several risk factors for sudden infant death, which included over wrapping and over heating, were followed by a reduced incidence of sudden infant death syndrome. However, it is not clear whether effects were specifically due to the advice to avoid over wrapping or over heating.

Advice to avoid soft sleeping surfaces*

We found no evidence on the effects of advice to avoid soft sleeping surfaces in the prevention of sudden infant death syndrome.

Advice to breastfeed*

One non-systematic review and three observational studies found that campaigns to reduce several risk factors for sudden infant death, which included advice to breastfeed, were followed by a reduced incidence of sudden infant death syndrome. However, it is not clear whether effects were specifically due to the advice to breastfeed.

Advice to promote soother use*

One systematic review found insufficient evidence on soother use in the prevention of sudden infant death syndrome.

*Observational evidence only; RCTs unlikely to be conducted.

DEFINITION Sudden infant death syndrome (SIDS) is the sudden death of an infant aged under 1 year that remains unexplained after review of the clinical history, examination of the scene of death, and postmortem.

INCIDENCE/ PREVALENCE The incidence of SIDS has varied over time and among nations (incidence per 1000 live births of SIDS in 1996: The Netherlands 0.3, Japan 0.4, Canada 0.5, England and Wales 0.7, USA 0.8, and Australia 0.9).[1]

AETIOLOGY/ RISK FACTORS By definition, the cause of SIDS is not known. Observational studies have found an association between SIDS and several risk factors, including prone sleeping position,[2,3] prenatal or postnatal exposure to tobacco smoke,[4] soft sleeping surfaces,[5,6] hyperthermia/over wrapping (see tables A, B, and C on web extra),[7,8] bed sharing (particularly with mothers who smoke),[9,10] lack of breastfeeding,[11,12] and lack of soother use.[7,13] The incidence of SIDS is increased in the siblings of that infant.[14,15]

PROGNOSIS Prognosis is not applicable.

Please refer to the Clinical Evidence website for full text and references.

Urinary tract infection in children

Search date January 2004

James Larcombe

What are the effects of treatment of acute urinary tract infection in children?

Antibiotics (more effective than placebo)*

There is consensus that antibiotics are likely to be beneficial compared with placebo. Placebo controlled trials of antibiotics for symptomatic acute urinary tract infection in children are considered unethical.

Oral antibiotics (as effective as initial intravenous antibiotics in children without severe vesicoureteric reflux or renal scarring)

One RCT identified by a systematic review found no significant difference between oral cephalosporins alone and a regimen of 3 days of intravenous cephalosporins plus continued oral cephalosporins in duration of fever, reinfection rate, renal scarring, or extent of scarring in children aged 2 years or younger with a first confirmed urinary tract infection. The RCT found weak evidence that in children with grades III–IV reflux, initial intravenous treatment plus oral treatment may reduce renal scarring compared with oral treatment alone at 6 months.

Immediate empirical antibiotic treatment (unclear benefit compared with delayed treatment based on microscopy and culture)

We found no RCTs comparing early empirical treatment with delayed treatment based on the results of microscopy or culture in acute urinary tract infection in children. Retrospective analysis of one RCT found no significant difference in risk of renal scarring between cephalosporin treatment within 24 hours compared with 24 hours after the onset of fever in children under 2 years of age with urinary tract infections.

Longer (7–14 days) courses of initial intravenous antibiotics (no more effective than shorter [3–4 days] courses of intravenous antibiotics in children with acute pyelonephritis)

One systematic review found no significant difference between long (7–14 days) and short (3–4 days) courses of initial intravenous antibiotics in persistence of bacteriuria after treatment, recurrent urinary tract infection at 6–12 months, or renal scarring at 3–6 months in children with acute pyelonephritis.

Longer (7–14 days) courses of oral antibiotics (no more effective than shorter [2–4 days] courses for non-recurrent lower urinary tract infections in the absence of renal tract abnormality)

One systematic review found no significant difference between longer courses (7–14 days) and shorter courses (2–4 days) of the same oral antibiotic in cure rate at 7 days after treatment in children with no history of renal tract abnormality and judged not to have acute pyelonephritis. Another systematic review found no significant difference between 7–14 day courses and 3 day courses of any antibiotic in cure rate. However, longer courses may be associated with more adverse effects.

▶

◀ **LIKELY TO BE INEFFECTIVE OR HARMFUL**

Prolonged delay in treatment (> 4 days)
We found no RCTs. Five retrospective studies found that medium to long term delays (4 days to 7 years) in treatment may be associated with an increased risk of renal scarring.

Single dose of oral antibiotics (less effective than longer course [7–10 days])
One systematic review found that single dose oral amoxicillin decreased cure rate at 3–30 days compared with a longer (10 days) course of oral amoxicillin. Another systematic review found that single day or single dose regimens increased treatment failure compared with 7–14 day courses of any antibiotic.

What are the effects of interventions to prevent recurrence?

LIKELY TO BE BENEFICIAL

Immunotherapy
One RCT in children with recurrent urinary tract infection found that adding pidotimod (an immunotherapeutic agent) to antibiotic treatment reduced recurrence compared with adding placebo.

Prophylactic antibiotics
One systematic review found limited evidence that prophylactic antibiotics (co-trimoxazole, nitrofurantoin, given for 10 weeks to 12 months) reduced urinary tract infection recurrence in children compared with placebo or no treatment. One RCT found that nitrofurantoin reduced recurrence of urinary tract infection over 6 months compared with trimethoprim. However, more children discontinued treatment with nitrofurantoin because of adverse effects. We found no RCTs evaluating the optimum duration of prophylactic antibiotics.

UNKNOWN EFFECTIVENESS

Surgical correction of moderate to severe vesicoureteric reflux (grades III–IV) with bilateral nephropathy
One small RCT found a non-significantly greater decline in glomerular filtration rate over 10 years with medical treatment compared with surgery in children with moderate to severe bilateral vesicoureteric reflux and bilateral nephropathy.

UNLIKELY TO BE BENEFICIAL

Surgical correction of minor functional anomalies
We found no RCTs. One observational study suggested that children with minor anomalies do not develop renal scarring and therefore may not benefit from surgery.

Surgical correction of moderate to severe vesicoureteric reflux with adequate glomerular filtration rate (similar benefits to medical management)
One systematic review found no significant difference between surgical and medical management (prophylactic antibiotic treatment) in urinary tract infections or their complications from after 1–5 years in children with moderate to severe vesicoureteric reflux, although surgery abolished reflux. One subsequent RCT, reporting 10 years' follow-up, found that new renal scars rarely occurred with either management strategy after 5 years.

*Based on consensus. Placebo controlled RCTs would be considered unethical. ▷

Urinary tract infection in children

DEFINITION Urinary tract infection (UTI) is defined by the presence of a pure growth of more than 10^5 colony forming units of bacteria per millilitre of urine. Lower counts of bacteria may be clinically important, especially in boys and in specimens obtained by urinary catheter. Any growth of typical urinary pathogens is considered clinically important if obtained by suprapubic aspiration. In practice, three age ranges are usually considered on the basis of differential risk and different approaches to management: children under 1 year; young children (1 4, 5, or 7 years, depending on the information source); and older children (up to 12–16 years). Recurrent UTI is defined as a further infection by a new organism. Relapsing UTI is defined as a further infection with the same organism.

INCIDENCE/ PREVALENCE Boys are more susceptible before the age of 3 months; thereafter the incidence is substantially higher in girls. Estimates of the true incidence of UTI depend on rates of diagnosis and investigation. At least 8% of girls and 2% of boys will have a UTI in childhood.[1]

AETIOLOGY/ RISK FACTORS The normal urinary tract is sterile. Contamination by bowel flora may result in urinary infection if a virulent organism is involved or if the child is immunosuppressed. In neonates, infection may originate from other sources. *Escherichia coli* accounts for about 75% of all pathogens. *Proteus* is more common in boys (about 30% of infections). Obstructive anomalies are found in 0–4% and vesicoureteric reflux in 8–40% of children being investigated for their first UTI.[2] One meta-analysis of 12 cohort studies (537 children admitted to hospital for UTI, 1062 kidneys) found that 36% of all kidneys had some scarring on DMSA scintigraphy and that 59% of children with vesicoureteric reflux on micturating cystourethography had at least one scarred kidney (pooled positive likelihood ratio 1.96, 95% CI 1.51 to 2.54; pooled negative likelihood ratio 0.71, 95% CI 0.58 to 0.85). There was evidence of heterogeneity in likelihood ratios among studies. The authors concluded that vesicoureteric reflux is a weak predictor of renal damage in children admitted to hospital.[3] Thus, although vesicoureteric reflux is a major risk factor for adverse outcome, other factors, some of which have not yet been identified, are also important. Vesicoureteric reflux itself runs in families: in one review article, the incidence of reflux in siblings ranged from 26% (a cohort of asymptomatic siblings) to 86% (siblings with a history of urinary tract infection) compared with a rate of less than 1% in the normal population.[4] Although some gene variants appear to be more common in children who suffer renal damage, no clear link has yet been established between specific genes and an adverse outcome.[5] Local or systemic immune problems are also likely to be factors in the development of urinary tract infection.

PROGNOSIS After first infection, about 50% of girls have a further infection in the first year and 75% within 2 years.[6] We found no figures for boys, but a review suggests that recurrences are common under 1 year of age, but rare subsequently.[7] Renal scarring occurs in 5–15% of children within 1–2 years of their first UTI, although 32–70% of these scars are noted at the time of initial assessment.[2] The incidence of renal scarring rises with each episode of infection in childhood.[8] Retrospective analysis of an RCT comparing oral versus intravenous antibiotics found that new renal scarring after a first UTI was more common in children with vesicoureteric reflux than in children without reflux (logistic regression model; AR of scarring: 16/107 [15%] with reflux v 10/165 [6%] without reflux; RR 2.47, 95% CI 1.17 to 5.24).[9] A study (287 children with severe vesicoureteric reflux treated either medically or surgically for any UTI) evaluated the risk of renal scarring with serial DMSA scintigraphy over 5 years. It found that younger children (aged < 2 years) were at greater risk of renal scarring than older children regardless of treatment for the infection (AR for deterioration in DMSA scan over 5 years: 21/86 [24%] for younger children v 27/201 [13%] for older children; RR 1.82, 95% CI 1.09 to 3.03).[10] One prospective study found that children of all ages who presented with symptoms of pyelonephritis were likely to have renal abnormalities (abnormal initial scans in 34/65 [52%] children).[11] Another prospective study found that the highest rates of renal scarring after pyelonephritis occurred between 1–5 years of age.[12] A further prospective study by the same team found that children aged over 1 year had more abnormalities on DMSA scans at 3 months after an episode of pyelonephritis (54/129 [42%] older children v 22/91 [24%] younger children; RR 1.73, 95% CI 1.14 to 2.63).[13] They noted conflicting results in previous literature on this subject.[14] They also found that girls were more likely than boys to develop scarring on DMSA scan at 3 months after an episode of pyelonephritis (67/171 [39%] girls v 9/49 [18%] boys; RR 2.13, 95% CI 1.15 to 3.96).[13] Renal scarring is associated with future complications: poor renal growth, recurrent adult pyelonephritis, impaired glomerular function, early hypertension, and end stage renal failure.[14–17] A combination of recurrent UTI, severe vesicoureteric reflux, and the presence of renal scarring at first presentation is associated with the worst prognosis. One prospective observational study assessed the persistence of scarring on DMSA scans in children with a first UTI.[18] Grading of scars was as follows: mild (< 25% of kidney affected), moderate (25–50% of kidney), and severe (> 50% of kidney). The study found that vesicoureteric reflux was associated with more persistent scarring at 6 months (in children with severe scarring on initial scan: 7/8 [88%] with reflux had a persisting lesion v 1/7 [14%] without reflux; RR 6.13, 95% CI 0.98 to 38.00; in children with mild to moderate scarring on initial scan: 3/8 [38%] with reflux had a persisting lesion v 5/31 [16%] without reflux; RR 2.70, 95% CI 0.81 to 9.10).[18] The study also found that vesicoureteric reflux was associated with a higher risk of pyelonephritis on the initial scan (RR for pyelonephritis with reflux v without reflux 1.62, 95% CI 1.14 to 2.31).

Please refer to the Clinical Evidence website for full text and references.

Anal fissure (chronic)

Search date January 2004

Marion Jonas and John Scholefield

What are the effects of treatments for chronic anal fissure?

BENEFICIAL

Internal anal sphincterotomy

One systematic review found that internal anal sphincterotomy improved fissure healing compared with topical glyceryl trinitrate after 6 weeks to 2 years. One systematic review found that internal anal sphincterotomy reduced fissure persistence compared with botulinum A toxin-haemagglutinin complex at 12 months. One systematic review found no significant difference between internal anal sphincterotomy and anal stretch in persistence of fissures, and found that both procedures healed 70–95% of fissures. However, it found that anal stretch increased rates of flatus incontinence compared with internal anal sphincterotomy. One systematic review found no significant difference between open and closed internal anal sphincterotomy in persistence of fissures. One small RCT found no significant difference between internal anal sphincterotomy and anal advancement flap in patient satisfaction or fissure healing.

LIKELY TO BE BENEFICIAL

Anal advancement flap (as effective as internal anal sphincterotomy based on 1 small RCT)

One small RCT found no significant difference between lateral internal anal sphincterotomy and anal advancement flap in patient satisfaction or fissure healing.

Topical glyceral trinitrate

One systematic review and one subsequent RCT found limited evidence from heterogeneous RCTs that topical glyceryl trinitrate reduced persistence of fissures compared with placebo. Results were difficult to interpret because of differing durations and doses of treatments. Consensus opinion regards glyceryl trinitrate as an effective first line treatment for chronic anal fissure. One systematic review found that internal anal sphincterotomy improved fissure healing compared with topical glyceryl trinitrate after 6 weeks to 2 years. One systematic review found no significant difference in fissure persistence between topical glyceryl trinitrate ointment and botulinum A toxin-hc injection after 2 months. Two RCTs found no significant difference between glyceryl trinitrate ointment and a glyceryl trinitrate patch in fissure healing after 8–12 weeks. Two RCTs found no significant difference between topical glyceryl trinitrate and topical diltiazem in fissure healing at 8 weeks.

TRADE OFF BETWEEN BENEFITS AND HARMS

Anal stretch (as effective as internal anal sphincterotomy but higher rates of flatus incontinence)

One systematic review found no significant difference between internal anal sphincterotomy and anal stretch in persistence of fissures. It found that both procedures healed 70–95% of fissures. Anal stretch increased rates of flatus incontinence compared with internal anal sphincterotomy.

UNKNOWN EFFECTIVENESS

Botulinum A toxin-haemagglutinin complex

One systematic review found no significant difference in fissure persistence between botulinum A toxin haemagglutinin and placebo or topical glyceryl nitrate at 2 months. One systematic review and one additional RCT found no significant difference between high and low dose botulinum A toxin-haemagglutinin complex after 2–3 months. One systematic review found that botulinum A toxin-haemagglutinin complex significantly increased fissure persistence compared with anal sphincterotomy at 12 months.

Botulinum A toxin-haemagglutinin complex plus nitrates

We found no RCTs comparing botulinum A toxin-haemagglutinin complex plus nitrates versus placebo. One small RCT found that botulinum A toxin-haemagglutinin complex plus topical isosorbide dinitrate three times daily increased fissure healing at 6 weeks compared with botulinum A toxin-haemagglutinin complex alone. It found no significant difference at 8 or 12 weeks.

Diltiazem

We found no placebo controlled RCTs. Two RCTs found no significant difference between topical diltiazem and topical glyceryl trinitrate in fissure healing at 8 weeks. One small RCT identified by a systematic review found no significant difference in fissure persistence after 8 weeks between oral diltiazem and topical diltiazem but that adverse events were more common with oral diltiazem.

Indoramin

One RCT found no significant difference between oral indoramin and placebo in fissure healing after 6 weeks, but it may have been too small to detect a clinically important difference.

DEFINITION   Anal fissure is a split or tear in the lining of the distal anal canal. It is a painful condition often associated with fresh blood loss from the anus and perianal itching. **Acute anal fissures** have sharply demarcated, fresh mucosal edges, often with granulation tissue at the base. The majority of acute fissures will heal spontaneously, or with increased oral fluid and dietary fibre intake as well as laxatives where there is a history of constipation. Fissures persisting for longer than 6 weeks are generally defined as chronic. **Chronic anal fissures** have margins that are indurated, with less granulation tissue; the muscle fibres of the internal anal sphincter may be seen at the base. These require intervention in order to heal.

INCIDENCE/   Anal fissures are common in all age groups, but we found no reliable evidence
PREVALENCE   about incidence.

AETIOLOGY/   Low intake of dietary fibre may be a risk factor for the development of acute anal
RISK FACTORS   fissure.[1] People with anal fissure often have raised resting anal canal pressures with anal spasm.[2,3] Men and women are equally affected by anal fissure, and up to 11% of women develop anal fissure after childbirth.[4]

PROGNOSIS   Placebo controlled studies found that 70–90% of untreated "chronic" fissures did not heal during the study.[5,6]

Please refer to the Clinical Evidence website for full text and references.

Appendicitis

Search date October 2003

John Simpson and William Speake

What are the effects of treatments?

BENEFICIAL

Adjuvant antibiotics

One systematic review and one subsequent RCT in children and adults with simple or complicated appendicitis undergoing appendicectomy have found that prophylactic antibiotics reduce wound infections and intra-abdominal abscesses compared with no antibiotics. Subgroup analysis from the systematic review has found that antibiotics reduce the number of wound infections in children with complicated appendicitis compared with no antibiotics. However, subgroup analysis from the systematic review found no significant difference in the number of wound infections between antibiotics and no antibiotics in children with simple appendicitis. One subsequent RCT in children with simple appendicitis found no significant difference with antibiotic prophylaxis compared with no antibiotic prophylaxis in wound infections, but the RCT may have been too small to exclude a clinically important difference.

LIKELY TO BE BENEFICIAL

Laparoscopic surgery versus open surgery (in children)

One systematic review has found that, in children, laparoscopic surgery reduced the number of wound infections and the length of hospital stay compared with open surgery, but found no significant difference in postoperative pain, time to mobilisation, or proportion of intra-abdominal abscesses.

TRADE OFF BETWEEN BENEFITS AND HARMS

Antibiotics versus surgery

One small RCT in adults with suspected appendicitis found that conservative treatment with antibiotics reduced pain and morphine consumption for the first 10 days compared with appendicectomy. However, the RCT found that 35% of people treated with antibiotics were readmitted within 1 year with acute appendicitis and subsequently had an appendicectomy.

Laparoscopic surgery versus open surgery (in adults)

One systematic review and one subsequent RCT have found that laparoscopic surgery in adults reduces wound infections, postoperative pain, duration of hospital stay, and time taken to return to work compared with open surgery. However, the systematic review found that laparoscopic surgery increased postoperative intra-abdominal abscesses compared with open surgery.

UNKNOWN EFFECTIVENESS

Open surgery versus no treatment

We found no RCTs comparing open surgery with no surgery.

Stump inversion at open appendicectomy

One RCT found no significant difference between stump inversion and simple ligation in wound infection, length of hospital stay, or intra-abdominal abscesses. Another RCT found that stump inversion increased wound infections compared with simple ligation, but found no significant difference between groups for intra-abdominal abscesses or length of hospital stay.

▶

DEFINITION Acute appendicitis is acute inflammation of the vermiform appendix.

INCIDENCE/ PREVALENCE The incidence of acute appendicitis is falling, although the reason for this is unclear. The reported lifetime risk of appendicitis in the USA is 8.7% in men and 6.7% in women,[1] and there are about 60 000 cases reported annually in England and Wales. Appendicitis is the most common surgical emergency requiring operation.

AETIOLOGY/ RISK FACTORS The cause of appendicitis is uncertain, although various theories exist. Most relate to luminal obstruction, which prevents escape of secretions and inevitably leads to a rise in intraluminal pressure within the appendix. This can lead to subsequent mucosal ischaemia, and the stasis provides an ideal environment for bacterial overgrowth. Potential causes of the obstruction are faecoliths, often because of constipation, lymphoid hyperplasia, or caecal carcinoma.[2]

PROGNOSIS The prognosis of untreated appendicitis is unknown, although spontaneous resolution has been reported in at least 1/13 (8%) episodes.[3] The recurrence of appendicitis after conservative management,[3,4] and recurrent abdominal symptoms in certain people,[5] suggests that chronic appendicitis and recurrent acute or subacute appendicitis may also exist.[6] The standard treatment for acute appendicitis is appendicectomy. RCTs comparing treatment with no treatment would be regarded as unethical. The mortality from acute appendicitis is less than 0.3%, rising to 1.7% after perforation.[7] The most common complication of appendicectomy is wound infection, occurring in between 5 and 33% of cases.[8] Intra-abdominal abscess formation occurs less frequently in 2% of appendicectomies.[9] A perforated appendix in childhood does not appear to have subsequent negative consequences on female fertility.[10]

Please refer to the Clinical Evidence website for full text and references.

Cholecystitis (acute)

Search date December 2003

Julie Margenthaler, Douglas Schuerer, and Robb Whinney

What are the effects of treatments for acute cholecystitis?

BENEFICIAL

Early cholecystectomy

Four RCTs found that operation before the scheduled date because of recurrent or worsening symptoms was necessary in 13–19% of people receiving delayed cholecystectomy (open or laparoscopic cholecystectomy after 6–8 weeks). The RCTs found no significant difference between early (within 72 hours) and delayed cholecystectomy (open or laparoscopic) in intraoperative or postoperative complications, but found that early cholecystectomy reduced hospital stay. Two RCTs found that early laparoscopic cholecystectomy increased duration of operation compared with delayed laparoscopic cholecystectomy but reduced use of analgesics. The RCTs found no significant difference between early and delayed laparoscopic cholecystectomy in the rate of conversion to open cholecystectomy.

Laparoscopic cholecystectomy

One RCT found that observation alone had a failure rate after 8 years of 30%, but found no difference in the rate of gallstone related complications (recurrent cholecystitis, pancreatitis, intractable pain) or emergency admissions for pain compared with cholecystectomy (open or laparoscopic). Three RCTs found that laparoscopic cholecystectomy reduced hospital stay, and found limited evidence that it reduced duration of surgery and intraoperative/postoperative complications compared with open cholecystectomy. One RCT found no difference between conventional laparoscopic cholecystectomy and minilaparoscopic cholecystectomy in use of analgesics, hospital stay, and rates of conversion to open cholecystectomy. Duration of surgery was marginally shorter with conventional laparoscopic cholecystectomy.

Minilaparoscopic cholecystectomy

One RCT found no difference between minilaparoscopic and conventional laparoscopic cholecystectomy in use of analgesics, hospital stay, and rates of conversion to open cholecystectomy. Duration of surgery was marginally longer with minilaparoscopic cholecystectomy.

TRADE OFF BETWEEN BENEFITS AND HARMS

Open cholecystectomy

One RCT found that observation alone had a failure rate after 8 years of 30%, but found no difference in the rate of gallstone related complications (recurrent cholecystitis, pancreatitis, intractable pain) or emergency admissions for pain compared with cholecystectomy (open or laparoscopic). Three RCTs found that open cholecystectomy increased hospital stay and found limited evidence that it increased duration of surgery and intraoperative/postoperative complications compared with laparoscopic cholecystectomy.

Observation alone

One RCT found that observation alone had a failure rate after 8 years of 30%, but found no difference in the rate of gallstone related complications (recurrent cholecystitis, pancreatitis, intractable pain) or emergency admissions for pain compared with cholecystectomy (open or laparoscopic).

▶

◀ **DEFINITION**   **Acute cholecystitis** results from obstruction of the cystic duct usually by a gallstone followed by distension and subsequent chemical or bacterial inflammation of the gallbladder. People with acute cholecystitis usually have unremitting right upper quadrant pain, anorexia, nausea, vomiting, and fever. About 95% of people with acute cholecystitis have gallstones (calculous cholecystitis) and 5% lack gallstones (acalculous cholecystitis).[1] Severe acute cholecystitis may lead to necrosis of the gallbladder wall known as gangrenous cholecystitis. This review does not include people with acute cholangitis, which is a severe complication of gallstone disease and generally a result of bacterial infection.

INCIDENCE/   The incidence of acute cholecystitis among people with gallstones is
PREVALENCE   unknown. Twenty per cent of people admitted to hospital for biliary tract disease have acute cholecystitis.[1] The number of cholecystectomies carried out for acute cholecystitis has increased from the mid 1980s to the early 1990s, especially in elderly people.[2] Acute calculous cholecystitis is three times more common in women than men up to the age of 50 years, and about 1.5 times more common in women than men thereafter.[1]

AETIOLOGY/   Acute calculous cholecystitis seems to be caused by obstruction of the cystic
RISK FACTORS   duct by a gallstone or local mucosal erosion and inflammation caused by a stone, but cystic duct ligation alone does not produce acute cholecystitis in animal studies. The role of bacteria in the pathogenesis of acute cholecystitis is not clear; positive cultures of bile or gallbladder wall are found in 50–75% of cases.[3,4] The cause of acute acalculous cholecystitis is uncertain and may be multifactorial, including increased susceptibility to bacterial colonisation of static gallbladder bile.[1]

PROGNOSIS   Complications of acute cholecystitis include perforation of the gallbladder, pericholecystic abscess, and fistula caused by gallbladder wall ischaemia and infection. In the USA, the overall mortality from untreated complications is about 20%.[5]

Please refer to the Clinical Evidence website for full text and references.

Colonic diverticular disease

Search date February 2004

John Simpson and Robin Spiller

What are the effects of treatments for uncomplicated diverticular disease?

LIKELY TO BE BENEFICIAL

Rifaximin (plus dietary fibre supplementation v dietary fibre supplementation alone)

Two RCTs in people with uncomplicated diverticular disease found that rifaximin plus dietary fibre supplementation improved symptoms compared with dietary fibre supplementation alone after 12 months of treatment.

UNKNOWN EFFECTIVENESS

Bran and ispaghula husk

One small RCT in people with uncomplicated diverticular disease found no significant difference between bran or ispaghula husk and placebo in symptom relief after 16 weeks.

Elective surgery

We found no RCTs of elective open or laparoscopic colonic resection in people with uncomplicated diverticular disease.

Lactulose

One small RCT in people with uncomplicated diverticular disease found no significant difference between lactulose and a high fibre diet in self rated improvement after 12 weeks.

Methylcellulose

One small RCT in people with uncomplicated diverticular disease found no significant difference between methylcellulose and placebo in mean symptom scores at 3 months.

What are the effects of treatments to prevent complications of diverticular disease?

UNKNOWN EFFECTIVENESS

Increased fibre intake

We found no RCTs examining complication rates after advice to consume a high fibre diet or of dietary fibre supplementation.

Mesalazine (after an attack of acute diverticulitis)

One methodologically flawed RCT provided insufficient evidence about effects of mesalazine compared with no treatment in people previously treated for an episode of acute diverticulitis.

▶

What are the effects of treatments for acute diverticulitis?

UNKNOWN EFFECTIVENESS

Medical treatment

We found no RCTs comparing medical treatment versus placebo in people with acute diverticulitis. One small RCT found no significant difference between intravenous cefoxitin and intravenous gentamicin plus intravenous clindamycin in rates of clinical cure. Observational studies in people with acute diverticulitis have found low mortality with medical treatment, but found that recurrence rates may be high.

Surgery (for diverticulitis complicated by generalised peritonitis)

We found no RCTs comparing surgery versus no surgery or versus medical treatment. One RCT found no significant difference in mortality between acute resection and transverse colostomy of the sigmoid colon. A second RCT found no significant difference in mortality between primary and secondary sigmoid colonic resection, but found that primary resection reduced rates of postoperative peritonitis and emergency reoperation. We found no RCTs comparing open versus laparoscopic surgery.

DEFINITION   Colonic diverticula are mucosal out pouchings through the large bowel wall. They are often accompanied by structural changes (elastosis of the taenia coli, muscular thickening, and mucosal folding). They are usually multiple and occur most frequently in the sigmoid colon. If diverticula are associated with symptoms, then this is termed diverticular disease. If asymptomatic, then the condition is known as diverticulosis.

INCIDENCE/   In the UK the incidence of diverticulosis increases with age; about 5% of
PREVALENCE   people are affected in their fifth decade of life and about 50% by their ninth decade.[1] Diverticulosis is common in developed countries, although there is a lower prevalence of diverticulosis in Western vegetarians consuming a diet high in roughage.[2] Diverticulosis is almost unknown in rural Africa and Asia.[3]

AETIOLOGY/   There is an association between low fibre diets and diverticulosis of the colon.[3]
RISK FACTORS   Prospective observational studies have found that both physical activity and a high fibre diet are associated with a lower risk of developing diverticular disease.[4,5] Case control studies have found an association between perforated diverticular disease and non-steroidal anti-inflammatory drugs, corticosteroids, and opiate analgesics, whereas calcium antagonists have a protective effect.[6-9] People in Japan, Singapore, and Thailand develop diverticula that affect mainly the right side of the colon.[10]

PROGNOSIS   Symptoms will develop in 10–25% of people with diverticula at some point in their lives.[1] It is unclear why some people develop symptoms and some do not. Even after successful medical treatment of acute diverticulitis almost two thirds of people suffer recurrent pain in the lower abdomen.[11] Recurrent diverticulitis is observed in 7–42% of people with diverticular disease, and after recovery from the initial attack the calculated yearly risk of suffering a further episode is 3%.[12] About half of recurrences occur within 1 year of the initial episode and 90% occur within 5 years.[13] Complications of diverticular disease (perforation, obstruction, haemorrhage, and fistula formation) are each seen in about 5% of people with colonic diverticula when followed up for 10–30 years.[14] In the UK the incidence of perforation is 4 cases per 100,000 people per year, leading to approximately 2000 cases annually.[15] Intra-abdominal abscess formation is also a recognised complication.

Please refer to the Clinical Evidence website for full text and references.

Constipation in adults

Search date December 2003

Frank Frizelle and Murray Barclay

What are the effects of lifestyle advice in adults with idiopathic chronic constipation?

UNKNOWN EFFECTIVENESS

Lifestyle advice

We found no RCTs of lifestyle advice in adults with idiopathic chronic constipation.

What are the effects of bulking agents in adults with idiopathic chronic constipation?

LIKELY TO BE BENEFICIAL

Ispaghula husk (psyllium)

One RCT identified by a systematic review found that ispaghula husk increased the frequency of bowel movements and improved overall symptoms compared with placebo after 2 weeks. We found limited evidence from two RCTs that ispaghula husk improved symptoms compared with lactulose at 4 weeks. One RCT provided insufficient evidence to compare ispagula husk versus macrogol 3350. One RCT found no clinically important difference between ispaghula husk and docusate in frequency of bowel movements, stool consistency, straining, or pain after 2 weeks.

UNKNOWN EFFECTIVENESS

Bran

We found no RCTs of sufficient quality comparing bran versus placebo in adults with idiopathic chronic constipation.

What are the effects of stool softeners in adults with idiopathic chronic constipation?

UNKNOWN EFFECTIVENESS

Paraffin; seed oils/arachis oil

We found no RCTs in adults with idiopathic chronic constipation.

What are the effects of osmotic laxatives in adults with idiopathic chronic constipation?

BENEFICIAL

Macrogols

Three RCTs identified by a systematic review and one small additional RCT found that macrogols (polyethylene glycols) improved symptoms after 2–20 weeks compared with placebo. One RCT found insufficient evidence to compare macrogol 3350 versus ispaghula husk. One systematic review and one subsequent RCT found that macrogols improved global satisfaction and severity of constipation at 4 weeks compared with lactulose.

▶

Lactulose
We found limited evidence from two RCTs that lactulose improved symptoms compared with placebo. We found limited evidence from two RCTs that lactulose was less effective in improving symptoms at 4 weeks than ispaghula husk. Three RCTs identified by systematic reviews compared lactulose versus lactitol and found different results. Two RCTs found no significant difference in effectiveness at 2–4 weeks and one RCT found that lactulose was less effective than lactitol in increasing bowel movement frequency at 2 weeks. One RCT identified by a systematic review and one subsequent RCT found that lactulose was less effective than macrogols in improving global satisfaction and severity of constipation at 4 weeks.

Lactitol
One small crossover RCT identified by a systematic review found that lactitol increased the frequency of bowel movements compared with placebo after 4 weeks. Three RCTs identified by systematic reviews compared lactitol versus lactulose and found different results. Two RCTs found no significant difference in frequency of bowel movements at 2–4 weeks and one RCT found that lactitol increased frequency of bowel movements at 2 weeks compared with lactulose.

Magnesium salts; phosphate enemas; sodium citrate enemas
We found no RCTs in adults with idiopathic chronic constipation.

What are the effects of stimulant laxatives in adults with idiopathic chronic constipation?

Dantron
We found no RCTs of dantron in adults with idiopathic chronic constipation. Animal studies have suggested that dantron may be carcinogenic. Its use is, therefore, recommended only in people who are terminally ill.

Docusate
One systematic review identified no RCTs of sufficient quality comparing docusate versus placebo. One RCT identified by a systematic review found no clinically important difference between docusate and ispaghula husk in frequency of bowel movements, stool consistency, straining, or pain after 2 weeks.

Bisacodyl; glycerol/glycerin suppositories; picosulphate (picosulfate); senna
We found no RCTs in adults with idiopathic chronic constipation.

DEFINITION   Bowel habits and perception of bowel habit vary widely within and among populations, making constipation difficult to define strictly. The Rome II criteria is a standardised tool that diagnoses chronic constipation on the basis of two or more of the following symptoms for at least 12 weeks in the preceding year: straining at defecation on at least a quarter of occasions; stools that are lumpy/hard on at least a quarter of occasions; sensation of incomplete evacuation on at least a quarter of occasions; and three or fewer bowel movements a week.[1] In practice, however, diagnostic criteria are less rigid and are in part dependent on perception of normal bowel habit. Typically, chronic constipation might be diagnosed when a person has bowel actions twice a week or less, for two consecutive weeks, especially in the presence of features such as straining at stool, abdominal discomfort, and sensation of ▶

incomplete evacuation. In this chapter, we have included all RCTs that stated that all participants had chronic constipation, whether or not this diagnosis was made according to strict Rome II criteria. Where the definitions of constipation in the RCTs differ markedly from those presented here, we have made this difference explicit. In this chapter, we deal with chronic constipation that is not caused by a specific underlying disease (sometimes known as idiopathic constipation) in adults aged over 18 years. We have excluded studies in pregnant women and in people with constipation associated with underlying specific organic diseases such as autonomic neuropathy, spinal cord injury, bowel obstruction, and paralytic ileus.

INCIDENCE/ PREVALENCE Twelve million general practitioner prescriptions were written for laxatives in England in 2001.[2] Prevalence data are limited by small samples and problems with definition. One UK survey of 731 women found that 8.2% had constipation meeting Rome II criteria, and 8.5% defined themselves as being constipated.[3] A larger survey (1892 adults) found that 39% of men and 52% of women reported straining at stool on more than a quarter of occasions.[4] Prevalence rises in the elderly. Several surveys from around the world suggest that in a community setting, prevalence among the elderly is about 20%.[4–7]

AETIOLOGY/ RISK FACTORS One systematic review found that factors associated with increased risk of constipation included low fibre diet, low fluid intake, reduced mobility, and consumption of drugs such as opioids and anticholinergic antidepressants.[8]

PROGNOSIS Untreated constipation may lead to faecal impaction, particularly in elderly and confused people.[9] Constipation has been suggested as a risk factor for haemorrhoids and colorectal cancer, but evidence of causality is lacking.[9]

Please refer to the Clinical Evidence website for full text and references.

Search date July 2003

Paul Moayyedi, Brendan Delaney, and David Foreman

What are the effects of initial treatment of gastro-oesophageal reflux disease (GORD) associated with oesophagitis?

BENEFICIAL

H₂ receptor antagonists

One systematic review has found that H_2 receptor antagonists reduce the risk of persisting oesophagitis compared with placebo, but are not as effective as proton pump inhibitors.

Proton pump inhibitors

One systematic review, one additional RCT, and one subsequent RCT found that proton pump inhibitors increase healing compared with placebo or H_2 receptor antagonists. One systematic review found that esomeprazole 40 mg daily increased healing at 4 weeks compared with omeprazole 20 mg daily. RCTs have found no significant differences in clinical benefit among other proton pump inhibitors.

UNKNOWN EFFECTIVENESS

Antacids/alginates

Two RCTs provided limited evidence that antacids reduced symptom scores at 4–8 weeks compared with placebo, but neither found a significant difference in endoscopic healing. We found limited evidence on the effects of antacids compared with H_2 receptor antagonists. The first RCT found no significant difference between antacids compared with cimetidine in endoscopic healing at 8 weeks. The second RCT found that antacids were less effective for heartburn symptoms compared with ranitidine at 12 weeks.

Lifestyle advice

Small RCTs provided insufficient evidence on the effects of raising the head of the bed or weight loss for the treatment of reflux oesophagitis. We found no RCTs on the effects of reducing coffee intake, stopping smoking, reducing alcohol intake, or reducing fatty food intake.

LIKELY TO BE INEFFECTIVE OR HARMFUL

Motility stimulants

One RCT found that cisapride increased endoscopic healing compared with placebo at 12 weeks. The use of cisapride has been restricted in some countries because of concerns about heart rhythm abnormalities. We found no RCTs of domperidone or metoclopramide.

What are the effects of maintenance treatment of GORD associated with oesophagitis?

BENEFICIAL

Proton pump inhibitors

RCTs have found that proton pump inhibitors reduce relapse in people with healed reflux oesophagitis compared with placebo or H_2 receptor antagonist at 6–18 months. One systematic review has found that standard dose lansoprazole ▶

Gastro-oesophageal reflux disease

(30 mg/day) was as effective as omeprazole (20 mg/day) for maintaining healing at 12 months. However, the systematic review and one subsequent RCT provided evidence that lower dose lansoprazole (15 mg/day) was less effective than higher dose lansoprazole (30 mg/day), omeprazole, or esomeprazole for maintaining healing for up to 12 months.

TRADE OFF BETWEEN BENEFITS AND HARMS

Laparoscopic surgery

One systematic review found no fully published RCTs comparing laparoscopic surgery versus medical treatment for maintenance of remission. Two RCTs found no significant difference between open and laparoscopic fundoplication for remission at 3 months to 2 years. One RCT found that laparoscopic treatment was associated with surgical complications, although the rate was lower than with open surgery.

Open surgery

RCTs have found that open Nissen fundoplication compared with medical treatment improved the endoscopic grade of oesophagitis in people with chronic gastro-oesophageal reflux disease and oesophagitis at between 3 and 38 months. However, longer term follow up from one of these RCTs found no significant difference in endoscopic appearance between surgery and medical treatment at 10 years. Two RCTs found no significant difference between open and laparoscopic fundoplication for remission at 3 months to 2 years. One RCT found that mortality was higher with open surgery than with medical treatment. One RCT found that complication rates were higher with open than with laparoscopic surgery.

UNKNOWN EFFECTIVENESS

Antacids/alginates

We found no RCTs on the effects of antacids/alginates on the long term management of reflux oesophagitis.

H$_2$ receptor antagonists

One RCT found no significant difference between ranitidine and placebo for relapse of oesophagitis at 6 months in people with previously healed reflux oesophagitis. RCTs have found that H$_2$ receptor antagonists are less effective than proton pump inhibitors for maintaining remission up to 12 months.

Lifestyle advice

We found no RCTs on the effects of lifestyle advice on the long term management of reflux oesophagitis.

LIKELY TO BE INEFFECTIVE OR HARMFUL

Motility stimulants

Three RCTs have found that cisapride compared with placebo improved maintenance of healing at 6–12 months. Two further RCTs found no evidence of a difference, but they might have lacked power to detect a clinically significant effect. The use of cisapride has been restricted in some countries because of concerns about effects on heart rhythms. We found no RCTs comparing other prokinetic drugs with placebo or each other in people with gastro-oesophageal reflux disease and oesophagitis.

DEFINITION   Gastro-oesophageal reflux disease (GORD) is defined as reflux of gastroduodenal contents into the oesophagus, causing symptoms that are sufficient to interfere with quality of life.[1] People with GORD often have symptoms of heartburn and acid regurgitation.[2] GORD can be classified according to the results of upper gastrointestinal endoscopy. Currently the most validated ►

method is the Los Angeles classification, where an endoscopy showing mucosal breaks in the distal oesophagus indicate the presence of oesophagitis, which is graded in severity from grade A (mucosal breaks of < 5 mm in the oesophagus) to grade D (circumferential breaks in the oesophageal mucosa).[1,3] Alternatively, severity may be graded according to the Savary–Miller classification (grade I: linear, non-confluent erosions, to grade IV: severe ulceration or stricture).

INCIDENCE/ PREVALENCE Surveys from Europe and the USA suggest that 20–25% of the population have symptoms of GORD, and 7% have heartburn daily.[4,5] In primary care settings, about 25–40% of people with GORD have oesophagitis on endoscopy, but most have endoscopy negative reflux disease.[3]

AETIOLOGY/ RISK FACTORS We found no evidence of clear predictive factors for GORD. Obesity is reported to be a risk factor for GORD but epidemiological data are conflicting.[6,7] Smoking and alcohol are also thought to predispose to GORD, but observational data are limited.[7,8] It has been suggested that some foods, such as coffee, mints, dietary fat, onions, citrus fruits, or tomatoes, may predispose to GORD.[9] However, we found insufficient data on the role of these factors. We found limited evidence that drugs that relax the lower oesophageal sphincter, such as calcium channel blockers, may promote GORD.[10] Twin studies suggest that there may be a genetic predisposition to GORD.[8]

PROGNOSIS GORD is a chronic condition, with about 80% of people relapsing once medication is discontinued.[11] Many people therefore require long term medical treatment or surgery. Endoscopy negative reflux disease remains stable, with a minority of people developing oesophagitis over time.[12] However, people with severe oesophagitis may develop complications such as oesophageal stricture and Barrett's oesophagus.[1]

Please refer to the Clinical Evidence website for full text and references.

Helicobacter pylori infection

Search date October 2004

Brendan Delaney, Paul Moayyedi, and David Forman

What are the effects of H pylori eradication treatment in people with a proven duodenal ulcer?

BENEFICIAL

H pylori eradication for healing and preventing recurrence of duodenal ulcer

> One systematic review found that *H pylori* eradication treatment increased duodenal ulcer healing compared with no treatment, and that *H pylori* eradication treatment plus 1 month of antisecretory drug treatment increased duodenal ulcer healing compared with antisecretory drugs alone for 1 month. It also found that eradication treatment reduced recurrence compared with no treatment, although there was no significant difference in recurrence between eradication treatment plus antisecretory drug treatment for 1 month compared with ongoing antisecretory maintenance treatment alone in people with healed duodenal ulcers. One systematic review found that *H pylori* eradication treatment reduced the risk of bleeding compared with ulcer healing treatment alone, or compared with ulcer treatment plus subsequent antisecretory maintenance treatment in people with duodenal or gastric ulcer.

What are the effects of H pylori eradication treatment for people with a proven gastric ulcer?

BENEFICIAL

H pylori eradication for preventing recurrence of gastric ulcer

> One systematic review found no significant difference in healing between *H pylori* eradication treatment plus antisecretory drugs and antisecretory drugs alone. It found that *H pylori* eradication treatment reduced recurrence compared with no treatment. One systematic review found that *H pylori* eradication treatment reduced the risk of bleeding compared with ulcer healing treatment alone, or compared with ulcer treatment plus subsequent antisecretory maintenance treatment in people with duodenal or gastric ulcer.

What are the effects of H pylori eradication treatment in people with non-steroidal anti-inflammatory drug (NSAID) related peptic ulcers?

UNKNOWN EFFECTIVENESS

H pylori eradication for healing of NSAID related peptic ulcers

> One RCT found no significant difference between *H pylori* eradication and antisecretory treatment alone in healing of peptic ulcer in people who were taking NSAIDs and had bleeding peptic ulcers.

◄ **What are the effects of H pylori eradication treatment for preventing non-steroidal anti-inflammatory drug (NSAID) related peptic ulcers in people with previous ulcers or dyspepsia?**

UNKNOWN EFFECTIVENESS

H pylori eradication for prevention of NSAID related peptic ulcers in people with previous ulcers or dyspepsia

One RCT found that, in people with *H pylori* infection and taking non-steroidal anti-inflammatory drugs who had previous ulcers or dyspepsia, *H pylori* eradication treatment reduced the risk of developing new peptic ulcers compared with omeprazole at 6 months. Another RCT found that, in people with *H pylori* infection and with a previous bleeding ulcer, *H pylori* eradication was less effective than maintenance treatment with omeprazole in preventing a recurrent bleeding peptic ulcer in people taking naproxen, but there was no significant difference between treatments in people taking low dose aspirin.

What are the effects of H pylori eradication treatment for preventing non-steroidal anti-inflammatory drug (NSAID) related peptic ulcers in people without previous ulcers?

LIKELY TO BE BENEFICIAL

H pylori eradication for the prevention of non-steroidal anti-inflammatory drug (NSAID) related peptic ulcers in people without previous ulcers (more effective than placebo and as effective as antisecretory treatment)

One RCT found that *H pylori* eradication treatment reduced the risk of non-steroidal anti-inflammatory drug (NSAID) related peptic ulcers compared with no treatment in people without previous ulcers. Another RCT found that *H pylori* eradication reduced the risk of NSAID related peptic ulcers compared with placebo, but was not significantly different from antisecretory treatment alone.

What are the effects of H pylori eradication treatment in people with proved gastro-oesophageal reflux disease?

UNLIKELY TO BE BENEFICIAL

H pylori eradication in H pylori positive people with gastro-oesophageal reflux disease

Two RCTs in *H pylori* positive people with gastro-oesophageal reflux disease found no significant difference between *H pylori* eradication treatment and placebo in symptoms over 2 years.

What are the effects of H pylori eradication treatment in people with B cell lymphoma of the stomach?

UNKNOWN EFFECTIVENESS

H pylori eradication for gastric B cell lymphoma

We found no RCTs of *H pylori* eradication treatment in people with B cell gastric lymphoma. Observational studies provided limited evidence that 60–93% of ▶

Helicobacter pylori infection

people with localised, low grade B cell lymphoma experience tumour regression in response to *H pylori* eradication treatment, possibly avoiding, or delaying, the need for radical surgery, radiotherapy, or chemotherapy.

What are the effects of H pylori eradication treatment on the risk of developing gastric cancer?

UNKNOWN EFFECTIVENESS

H pylori eradication for prevention of gastric cancer (adenocarcinoma)

One RCT in people positive for *H pylori* found no significant difference in the risk of gastric cancer between eradication treatment and placebo at 7.5 years. In people with gastric atrophy or intestinal metaplasia, one RCT found that *H pylori* eradication increased the regression of high risk lesions compared with no eradication. However, the RCT did not assess the effects of eradication treatment on development of gastric cancer. We found consistent evidence from observational studies of an association between *H pylori* infection and increased risk of distal gastric adenocarcinoma.

What are the effects of H pylori eradication treatment in people with proved non-ulcer dyspepsia?

BENEFICIAL

H pylori eradication for non-ulcer dyspepsia

One systematic review in people with non-ulcer dyspepsia found that *H pylori* eradication reduced dyspeptic symptoms at 3–12 months compared with placebo.

What are the effects of H pylori eradication treatment in people with uninvestigated dyspepsia?

BENEFICIAL

H pylori eradication in people with uninvestigated dyspepsia (more effective than placebo and as effective as endoscopy based management)*

One RCT in people with *H pylori* found that *H pylori* eradication increased relief from dyspeptic symptoms at 1 year compared with placebo. One systematic review and one subsequent RCT in people at low risk of gastrointestinal malignancy found no significant difference in dyspepsia between *H pylori* testing plus eradication compared with management based on initial endoscopy after 1 year. However, delaying endoscopy is not safe in people at increased risk of gastrointestinal malignancy.

Do eradication treatments differ in their effects?

LIKELY TO BE BENEFICIAL

Quadruple regimen (as effective as triple regimen)

Two RCTs found that quadruple treatments were as effective as triple treatments for eradication of *H pylori* in people with or without a history of duodenal ulcer.

◀ **Three day quadruple regimen (as effective as 1 week triple regimen but with fewer adverse effects)**

One RCT comparing a 3 day quadruple regimen versus a 1 week triple regimen found no significant difference in *H pylori* eradication at 6 weeks. However, it found that people taking the 3 day quadruple regimen experienced fewer days of adverse effects.

Triple regimen (more effective than dual regimen)

We found no systematic review or RCTs of the effects of triple regimens compared with dual regimens on dyspeptic symptom scores, proportion of individuals with symptoms, quality of life, or mortality. One systematic review found that triple regimens eradicated *H pylori* from more people than dual regimens.

Two week triple regimen (more effective than 1 week triple regimen)

One systematic review found that 14 days of treatment with proton pump inhibitor based triple regimens increased *H pylori* eradication rates compared with 7 days of treatment with the same regimen.

UNKNOWN EFFECTIVENESS

Different triple regimens (relative effects on clinical outcomes unclear)

We found no systematic review or RCTs of the effects of different triple regimens on dyspeptic symptom scores, proportion of individuals with symptoms, quality of life, or mortality. One systematic review found that increasing the clarithromycin dose in a triple regimen containing amoxicillin increased *H pylori* eradication. However, increasing the clarithromycin dose in a triple regimen containing metronidazole had no significant additional effect on *H pylori* eradication. Another systematic review found that a triple regimen of metronidazole plus clarithromycin plus ranitidine bismuth increased eradication at 5–7 days compared with a triple regimen containing amoxicillin plus clarithromycin plus ranitidine bismuth.

*Endoscopy should not be delayed in people at risk of malignancy.

DEFINITION   *Helicobacter pylori* is a Gram negative flagellated spiral bacterium found in the stomach. Infection with *H pylori* is predominantly acquired in childhood. *H pylori* infection is not associated with a specific type of dyspeptic symptom. The organism is associated with lifelong chronic gastritis and may cause other gastroduodenal disorders.[1] *H pylori* can be identified indirectly by serology or by the C13 urea breath test. The urea breath test is more accurate than serology, with a sensitivity and specificity greater than 95%, and indicates active infection, whereas serology may lack specificity and cannot be used reliably as a test of active infection. Thus, the urea breath test is the test of choice where prevalence, and hence predictive value of serology may be low, or where a "test of cure" is required. In some areas stool antigen tests, which have a similar performance to the urea breath test are now available. This chapter focuses on *H pylori* positive people throughout.

INCIDENCE/ PREVALENCE   In the developed world, *H pylori* prevalence rates vary with year of birth and social class. Prevalence in many developed countries tends to be much higher (50–80%) in individuals born before 1950 compared with prevalence (< 20%) in individuals born more recently.[2] In many developing countries, the infection has a high prevalence (80–95%) irrespective of the period of birth.[3] Adult prevalence is believed to represent the persistence of a historically higher rate of infection acquired in childhood, rather than increasing acquisition of infection during life.

AETIOLOGY/ RISK FACTORS   Overcrowded conditions associated with childhood poverty lead to increased transmission and higher prevalence rates. Adult reinfection rates are low — less than 1% a year.[3]

Helicobacter pylori infection

◄ **PROGNOSIS** *H pylori* infection is believed to be causally related to the development of duodenal and gastric ulceration, B cell gastric lymphoma, and distal gastric cancer. About 15% of people infected with *H pylori* will develop a peptic ulcer, and 1% of people will develop gastric cancer during their lifetime.[4] One systematic review of observational studies (search date 2000, 16 studies, 1625 people)[5] found that the frequency of peptic ulcer disease in people taking non-steroidal anti-inflammatory drugs (NSAIDs) was greater in those who were *H pylori* positive than in those who were *H pylori* negative (peptic ulcer: 341/817 [41.7%] in *H pylori* positive NSAID users v 209/808 [25.9%] in *H pylori* negative NSAID users, OR 2.12, 95% CI 1.68 to 2.67).

Please refer to the Clinical Evidence website for full text and references.

Sanjay Purkayastha, Thanos Athanasiou, Paris Tekkis, Ara Darzi

What are the effects of elective treatment for primary unilateral inguinal hernia?

BENEFICIAL

Open mesh repair (reduced recurrence compared with open suture repair, with no increase in surgical complications)

We found no systematic review, RCTs, or cohort studies of sufficient quality comparing open mesh repair versus expectant management. One systematic review found that open mesh repair reduced inguinal hernia recurrence and slightly reduced the length of hospital stay compared with open suture repair. The review and one subsequent RCT found no significant difference in surgical complications between open mesh and open suture repair. One systematic review and three subsequent RCTs found that open mesh repair increased the overall recovery time compared with totally extraperitoneal (TEP) laparoscopic repair and found limited evidence that open mesh repair slightly increased hospital stay and postoperative pain. They found no significant difference between open mesh repair and TEP laparoscopic repair in either recurrence or most postoperative complications, although the systematic review and one RCT found limited evidence that open mesh repair increased postoperative haematoma compared with TEP laparoscopic repair. One systematic review found that open mesh repair increased postoperative pain at 3 months and time to return to usual activities compared with transabdominal preperitoneal (TAPP) laparoscopic repair. It found insufficient evidence to compare the effects of open mesh repair versus TAPP laparoscopic repair on recurrence rates. One subsequent RCT found that open mesh repair increased postoperative pain and length of hospital stay compared with TAPP laparoscopic repair. Adverse effects of open mesh repair and TAPP laparoscopic repair were similar, although the review found that open mesh repair decreased the risk of seroma and increased postoperative numbness and superficial infection compared with TAPP laparoscopic repair.

Totally extraperitoneal (TEP) laparoscopic repair (reduced pain and time to return to usual activities compared with open repair)

We found no systematic review, RCTs, or cohort studies of sufficient quality comparing totally extraperitoneal (TEP) laparoscopic repair versus expectant management. One systematic review and three subsequent RCTs found that TEP laparoscopic repair decreased the overall recovery time compared with open mesh repair and found limited evidence that TEP laparoscopic repair slightly reduced hospital stay and postoperative pain compared with open mesh repair. They found no significant difference between open mesh repair and TEP laparoscopic repair in either recurrence or most postoperative complications, although the systematic review and one RCT found limited evidence that TEP laparoscopic repair reduced postoperative haematoma compared with open mesh repair. One systematic review found that TEP laparoscopic repair reduced pain after 3 months and reduced length of hospital stay slightly compared with open suture repair, but found no significant difference in risk of recurrence or time to return to normal activities. One subsequent RCT found no significant difference between TEP laparoscopic repair and open suture repair in recurrence, length of hospital stay, or groin pain. Adverse effects were similar for TEP laparoscopic and open suture repair, although the review found that TEP laparoscopic repair increased the risk of seroma but decreased the risk of infection compared with open suture repair.

Inguinal hernia

Transabdominal preperitoneal (TAPP) laparoscopic repair (reduced pain and time to return to usual activities compared with open mesh repair)

We found no systematic review, RCTs, or cohort studies of sufficient quality comparing transabdominal preperitoneal (TAPP) laparoscopic repair versus expectant management. One systematic review found that TAPP laparoscopic repair reduced postoperative pain at 3 months, and time to return to usual activities compared with open mesh repair. It found insufficient evidence to compare effects of TAPP laparoscopic repair versus open mesh repair on recurrence rates. One subsequent RCT found that TAPP laparoscopic repair reduced postoperative pain and length of hospital stay compared with open mesh repair. Adverse effects of open mesh repair and TAPP laparoscopic repair were similar, although TAPP laparoscopic repair increased the risk of seroma and decreased postoperative numbness and superficial infection compared with open mesh repair. One systematic review and subsequent RCTs found that TAPP laparoscopic repair decreased postoperative pain and time to return to usual activities compared with open suture repair. The systematic review found limited evidence that TAPP laparoscopic repair reduced recurrence compared with open suture repair, although two subsequent RCTs found no significant difference. Adverse effects of TAPP laparoscopic repair and open suture repair were similar.

LIKELY TO BE BENEFICIAL

Open suture repair (conventional, well established surgical technique but less effective for improving clinically important outcomes than open mesh repair, TEP laparoscopic repair or TAPP laparoscopic repair)*

Clinical experience and consensus opinion suggest that surgery is effective for primary unilateral inguinal hernia. Open suture repair is a well established surgical technique. However, we found no systematic review, RCTs, or cohort studies of sufficient quality comparing open suture repair versus expectant management. One systematic review found that open suture repair was less effective at reducing inguinal hernia recurrence than open mesh repair and that it increased length of hospital stay. The review and one subsequent RCT found no significant difference in surgical complications between open suture repair and open mesh repair. One systematic review found that open suture repair increased pain after 3 months and increased length of hospital stay slightly compared with totally extraperitoneal (TEP) laparoscopic repair, but found no significant difference in risk of recurrence or time to return to normal activities, whereas one subsequent RCT found no significant difference between TEP laparoscopic repair and open suture repair in recurrence, length of hospital stay, or groin pain. Adverse effects were similar for TEP laparoscopic repair and open suture repair, although the review found that open suture repair decreased the risk of seroma but increased the risk of infection compared with TEP laparoscopic repair. One systematic review and subsequent RCTs found that open suture repair increased postoperative pain, and time to return to usual activities compared with transabdominal preperitoneal (TAPP) laparoscopic repair. The systematic review found limited evidence that open suture repair was less effective at reducing recurrence compared with TAPP laparoscopic repair, although two subsequent RCTs found no significant difference. Adverse effects of open suture repair and TAPP laparoscopic repair were similar.

UNKNOWN EFFECTIVENESS

Expectant management

We found no systematic review, RCTs, or cohort studies of sufficient quality of expectant management in people with unilateral inguinal hernia.

◄ *What are the effects of elective treatment for primary bilateral inguinal hernia?*

LIKELY TO BE BENEFICIAL

Open mesh repair (may reduce length of hospital stay compared with open suture repair)

We found no systematic review, RCTs, or cohort studies of sufficient quality comparing open mesh repair versus expectant management in people with bilateral inguinal hernia. One systematic review found limited evidence that open mesh repair reduced length of hospital stay compared with open suture repair but found insufficient evidence to compare other clinical effects. One systematic review found limited evidence that open mesh repair increased the time taken to return to normal activities and postoperative superficial infection compared with transabdominal preperitoneal laparoscopic repair. It found insufficient evidence to compare other clinical effects and insufficient evidence to compare clinical effects of open mesh repair versus totally extraperitoneal laparoscopic repair.

Open suture repair (conventional, well established surgical technique but may be less effective in improving clinically important outcomes than open mesh repair or TAPP laparoscopic repair)*

Clinical experience and consensus opinion suggest that surgical intervention is an effective treatment for bilateral inguinal hernia. Open suture repair is a well established surgical technique. However, we found no systematic review, RCTs, or cohort studies of sufficient quality comparing open suture repair versus expectant management in people with bilateral inguinal hernia. One systematic review found limited evidence that open suture repair increased length of hospital stay compared with open mesh repair but found insufficient evidence to compare other clinical effects. One systematic review found limited evidence that open suture repair increased the time taken to return to normal activities compared with transabdominal preperitoneal laparoscopic repair. It found insufficient evidence to compare other clinical effects, and found insufficient evidence to compare clinical effects of open suture repairs versus totally extraperitoneal laparoscopic repair.

Transabdominal preperitoneal (TAPP) laparoscopic repair (may reduce time to return to normal activities compared with open repair)

We found no systematic review, RCTs, or cohort studies of sufficient quality comparing transabdominal preperitoneal (TAPP) laparoscopic repair versus expectant management in people with bilateral inguinal hernia. One systematic review found limited evidence that TAPP laparoscopic repair reduced the time taken to return to normal activities compared with open suture repair or open mesh repair, and that TAPP laparoscopic repair reduced postoperative superficial infection compared with open mesh repair. It found insufficient evidence to compare other clinical effects.

UNKNOWN EFFECTIVENESS

Expectant management

We found no systematic review, RCTs, or cohort studies of sufficient quality of expectant management in people with bilateral inguinal hernia.

Inguinal hernia

Totally extraperitoneal (TEP) laparoscopic repair

We found no systematic review, RCTs, or cohort studies of sufficient quality comparing totally extraperitoneal laparoscopic (TEP) repair versus expectant management in people with bilateral inguinal hernia. One systematic review found insufficient evidence to compare clinical effects of TEP laparoscopic repair versus open suture and open mesh repairs.

What are the effects of elective treatment for recurrent inguinal hernia?

BENEFICIAL

Open mesh repair (slightly reduced length of hospital stay compared with open suture repair; other effects uncertain)

We found no systematic review, RCTs, or cohort studies of sufficient quality comparing open mesh repair versus expectant management. One systematic review found limited evidence that open mesh repair slightly reduced length of hospital stay compared with open suture repair in people with recurrent inguinal hernia. However, the review found insufficient evidence to compare effects on pain, time to return to usual activities, further recurrence, or other complications of surgery. One systematic review found limited evidence that open mesh repair increased the time taken to return to normal activities compared with transabdominal preperitoneal and totally extraperitoneal laparoscopic repair techniques, but it found insufficient evidence to compare other clinical effects.

LIKELY TO BE BENEFICIAL

Open suture repair (conventional, well established surgical technique but may be less effective in improving clinically important outcomes than open mesh repair or TAPP laparoscopic repair)*

Clinical experience and consensus opinion suggest that surgery is an effective treatment for recurrent inguinal hernia. Open suture repair is a well established surgical technique. However, we found no systematic review, RCTs, or cohort studies of sufficient quality comparing open suture repair versus expectant management. One systematic review found limited evidence that open suture repair slightly increased length of hospital stay compared with open mesh repair in people with recurrent inguinal hernia but found insufficient evidence to compare effects on pain, time to return to usual activities, further recurrence, or other complications of surgery. One systematic review found limited evidence that open suture repair increased the time taken to return to normal activities compared with transabdominal preperitoneal laparoscopic repair. It found insufficient evidence to compare other clinical effects and insufficient data to compare benefits of open suture repair versus totally extraperitoneal laparoscopic repair.

Totally extraperitoneal (TEP) laparoscopic repair (may reduce time to return to normal activities compared with open mesh repair; other effects uncertain)

We found no systematic review, RCTs, or cohort studies of sufficient quality comparing totally extraperitoneal laparoscopic (TEP) repair versus expectant management in people with recurrent inguinal hernia. One systematic review found limited evidence that TEP laparoscopic repair reduced the time taken to return to normal activities compared with open mesh repair. However, it found insufficient evidence to compare other clinical effects and insufficient data to compare the effects of TEP laparoscopic repair versus open suture repair.

◀ **Transabdominal preperitoneal (TAPP) laparoscopic repair (may reduce time to return to normal activities compared with open repair; other effects uncertain)**

We found no systematic review, RCTs, or cohort studies of sufficient quality comparing transabdominal preperitoneal laparoscopic repair versus expectant management. One systematic review found limited evidence that transabdominal preperitoneal laparoscopic repair reduced the time taken to return to normal activities compared with open suture repair and open mesh repair in people with recurrent inguinal hernia but found insufficient evidence to compare other clinical effects.

UNKNOWN EFFECTIVENESS

Expectant management

We found no systematic review, RCTs, or cohort studies of sufficient quality of expectant management in people with recurrent inguinal hernia.

*Based on clinical experience and consensus.

DEFINITION   Inguinal hernia is an out-pouching of peritoneum, with or without its contents, which occurs through the muscles of the anterior abdominal wall at the level of the inguinal canal, in the groin. It almost always occurs in men, because of the inherent weakness of the abdominal wall where the spermatic cord passes through the inguinal canal. A portion of bowel may become caught in the peritoneal pouch, and present as a lump in the groin. The hernia may extend into the scrotum, and can cause discomfort or ache. Primary hernias relate to the first presentation of a hernia and are distinct from recurrent hernias. A hernia is described as reducible if it occurs intermittently (e.g. on straining or standing) and can be pushed back into the abdominal cavity and is irreducible if it remains permanently outside the abdominal cavity. Inguinal hernia is usually a long standing condition and diagnosis is made clinically, on the basis of these typical symptoms and signs. The condition may occur in one groin (unilateral hernia) or both groins simultaneously (bilateral hernia), and may recur after treatment (recurrent hernia). Occasionally, hernia may present acutely because of complications (see prognosis below). In this chapter we deal only with non-acute, uncomplicated inguinal hernias in adults. Clinical experience and consensus opinion suggest that surgical intervention is an effective treatment for inguinal hernia. However, surgery is associated with complications (see outcomes below), therefore, much of this chapter examines the relative effectiveness and safety of different surgical techniques. Inguinal hernias are frequently classified as direct or indirect, depending on whether the hernia sac bulges directly through the posterior wall of the inguinal canal (direct hernia), or rather passes through the internal inguinal ring alongside the spermatic cord, and follows the course of the inguinal canal (indirect hernia). However, none of the studies that we identified distinguished between these two types of inguinal hernia. Identified studies gave little detail about the severity of hernia among included participants. In general, studies explicitly excluded people with irreducible or complicated hernia, large hernia (extending into the scrotum), or serious co-morbidity, and those at high surgical risk (e.g. because of coagulation disorders).

INCIDENCE/   We found one nationally mandated guideline, which reported that 105 000
PREVALENCE   people (about 0.2% of people) develop an inguinal hernia each year in England and Wales.[1] Inguinal hernia is usually repaired surgically in resource rich countries. Surgical audit data therefore provide reasonable estimates of incidence, and support estimates of this order of magnitude. National statistical survey data from England reported that about 70 000 inguinal hernia repairs were undertaken in public health care settings in England in 2002–2003.[2] Similarly, in the USA estimates based on cross-sectional data ▶

suggest that about 700 000 inguinal hernia repairs were undertaken in 1993.[3] A national survey of general practices covering about 1% of the population of England and Wales in 1991–1992 found that about 95% of people presenting to primary care settings with inguinal hernia were male.[4] It found that the incidence rose from about 11/10 000 person-years in men aged 16–24 years to about 200/10 000 person-years in men aged 75 years or above.

AETIOLOGY/ RISK FACTORS Age and male sex are risk factors (see incidence/prevalence above). Chronic cough and manual labour involving heavy lifting are conventionally regarded as risk factors because they lead to high intra-abdominal pressure. Obesity has also been suggested to be a risk factor. However, we found no reliable data to quantify these risks.

PROGNOSIS We found few reliable data on untreated prognosis. Strangulation, intestinal obstruction, and infarction are the most important acute complications of untreated hernia and are potentially life threatening. National statistics from England found that 5% of primary inguinal hernia repairs were undertaken as emergencies (presumably because of acute complications) in 1998–1999.[2] Older age, longer duration of hernia, and longer duration of irreducibility are thought to be risk factors for acute complication,[5] although we found no reliable data to quantify these effects.

Please refer to the Clinical Evidence website for full text and references.

What are the effects of treatments in people with irritable bowel syndrome?

LIKELY TO BE BENEFICIAL

Antidepressants (amitriptyline, clomipramine, desipramine, doxepin, mianserin, trimipramine)

One systematic review found limited evidence from low to moderate quality RCTs that antidepressants (amitriptyline, clomipramine, desipramine, doxepin, mianserin, trimipramine) reduced symptoms of irritable bowel syndrome compared with placebo in the short term. It was not clear whether the effects on irritable bowel syndrome were independent of the effects on psychological symptoms.

Smooth muscle relaxants (cimetropium bromide, hyoscine butyl bromide, mebeverine hydrochloride, otilonium bromide, pinaverium bromide, trimebutine)

One systematic review found limited evidence that smooth muscle relaxants (cimetropium bromide, hyoscine butyl bromide, mebeverine hydrochloride, otilonium bromide, pinaverium bromide, trimebutine) improved symptoms compared with placebo. One subsequent RCT found no significant difference between alverine and placebo in improvement in abdominal pain, although the study may have lacked power to detect a clinically important effect. One RCT identified by a systematic review found that mebeverine was less effective for symptoms than alosetron in women with diarrhoea predominant irritable bowel syndrome, although there are concerns that alosetron may be associated with ischaemic colitis.

TRADE OFF BETWEEN BENEFITS AND HARMS

$5HT_4$ receptor agonists (tegaserod)

One systematic review found that in women with constipation predominant irritable bowel syndrome, tegaserod improved symptoms compared with placebo. It found insufficient evidence about the effects of tegaserod in men. One subsequent RCT found that in adults with irritable bowel syndrome and without diarrhoea, tegaserod improved symptoms compared with placebo. The systematic review and the RCT found that tegaserod increased diarrhoea compared with placebo.

Alosetron

One systematic review found that alosetron (a $5HT_3$ receptor antagonist) improved symptoms in women with diarrhoea predominant irritable bowel syndrome compared with placebo or mebeverine. However, alosetron is associated with adverse effects, particularly constipation, and has been restricted in some countries because of concerns that it may be associated with ischaemic colitis. The systematic review provided insufficient evidence about the effects of alosetron in men.

UNKNOWN EFFECTIVENESS

$5HT_3$ receptor antagonists other than alosetron

We found no RCTs examining $5HT_3$ receptor antagonists other than alosetron. ▶

Irritable bowel syndrome

Digestive system disorders

Fibre supplementation

One systematic review found limited evidence that fibre supplementation improved symptoms of irritable bowel syndrome and irritable bowel syndrome related constipation.

DEFINITION Irritable bowel syndrome (IBS) is a chronic non-inflammatory condition characterised by abdominal pain, altered bowel habit (diarrhoea or constipation), and abdominal bloating, but with no identifiable structural or biochemical disorder. Symptom based criteria, such as the Manning criteria (see table 1❶),[1] the Rome I criteria (see table 2❶),[2] and the Rome II criteria (see table 3❶),[3] aid diagnosis but their main use is in defining populations in clinical trials. The Rome criteria also subcategorise IBS according to predominant symptoms (diarrhoea, constipation, or alternating between diarrhoea and constipation). In practice, the division between constipation predominant and diarrhoea predominant IBS may not be clear-cut in all people. Restriction of trial entry to a subcategory of IBS limits the generalisability of study results.

INCIDENCE/ PREVALENCE Estimates of incidence and prevalence vary depending on the diagnostic criteria used to define IBS. One cross-sectional postal survey (4476 people aged 20–69 years) in Teeside, UK, defined IBS as recurrent abdominal pain on more than six occasions during the previous year plus two or more of the Manning criteria (see table 1❶).[4] It estimated prevalence in the UK to be 16.7% (95% CI 15.4% to 18.0%) overall, with a prevalence of 22.8% (95% CI 20.8% to 24.8%) among women and 10.5% (95% CI 8.9% to 12.1%) among men.[4] A cross-sectional postal survey (4500 people aged > 17 years) in Australia found prevalences of IBS of 13.6% (95% CI 12.3% to 14.8%) using the Manning criteria (see table 1❶), 6.9% (95% CI 6.0% to 7.8%) using the Rome I criteria (see table 2❶), and 4.4% (95% CI 3.5% to 5.1%) using the Rome II criteria (see table 3❶).[5]

AETIOLOGY/ RISK FACTORS The pathophysiology of IBS is not certain. Studies on the aetiology of IBS have been descriptive or retrospective, and are of limited reliability. Suggested aetiological factors include: abnormal gastrointestinal motor function,[6–8] enhanced visceral perception,[9–11] psychosocial factors such as a history of childhood abuse,[12] genetic predisposition,[13–15] and a history of enteric mucosal inflammation.[16,17] We found no reliable prospective data to measure these associations.

PROGNOSIS A retrospective study reviewed the medical records of people with IBS (112 people aged 20–64 years when diagnosed with IBS at the Mayo Clinic, USA, in 1961–1963). IBS was defined as the presence of abdominal pain associated with either disturbed defecation or abdominal distension and the absence of organic bowel disease.[18] Over a 32 year period, death rates were similar among people with IBS compared with age and gender matched controls. One postal survey (4432 adults aged 20–69 years) found that people with IBS are significantly more likely to have had a cholecystectomy than controls (OR 1.9, 95% CI 1.2 to 3.2).[4] A paper reporting on the same survey population (2238 women aged 20–69 years) found that women with IBS were significantly more likely to have had a hysterectomy than controls (OR 1.6, 95% CI 1.1 to 2.2).[19] We found no reliable estimates of the duration of IBS if left untreated.

Please refer to the Clinical Evidence website for full text and references.

What are the effects of surgical treatments in people with pancreatic cancer that is considered suitable for complete tumour resection?

UNKNOWN EFFECTIVENESS

Pancreaticoduodenectomy (Whipple's procedure)

We found no RCTs comparing pancreaticoduodenectomy (Whipple's procedure) with non-surgical treatment in people with resectable pancreatic cancer, although such studies may be considered unethical. Observational data provide limited evidence that surgery may reduce mortality compared with non-surgical treatment, although results may be confounded by differences in disease stage. Small RCTs found no significant difference in quality of life or survival at 5 years between pancreaticoduodenectomy and pylorus preserving pancreaticoduodenectomy.

Pylorus preserving pancreaticoduodenectomy (compared with Whipple's procedure)

Small RCTs found no significant difference between pylorus preserving surgery and classical pancreaticoduodenectomy (Whipple's procedure) for overall quality of life at 1 year or survival at 5 years in people with resectable tumours. However, the studies may have lacked power to exclude clinically important differences for these outcomes.

What are effects of adjuvant treatments in people with completely resected pancreatic cancer?

TRADE OFF BETWEEN BENEFITS AND HARMS

Systemic fluorouracil based chemotherapy

One RCT has found that adjuvant fluorouracil based chemotherapy improves median survival compared with no adjuvant chemotherapy in people with resected pancreatic cancer. This RCT and a second RCT found no significant difference in 5 year survival between adjuvant chemotherapy with fluorouracil based chemotherapy and no chemotherapy but the RCTs may have lacked power to detect a clinically important effect. The second RCT found that adjuvant fluorouracil based chemotherapy increased $\geq$ Grade 2 leukopenia, anorexia, and nausea or emesis compared with no chemotherapy. A third RCT did not compare chemotherapy alone with no chemotherapy directly.

UNKNOWN EFFECTIVENESS

Systemic gemcitabine based chemotherapy

One systematic review found insufficient evidence about effects of adjuvant gemcitabine compared with no adjuvant chemotherapy in people with resected pancreatic cancer.

DEFINITION   In this chapter, the term "pancreatic cancer" refers to primary adenocarcinoma of the pancreas. Other pancreatic malignancies, such as carcinoid tumour, are not considered. Symptoms of pancreatic cancer include pain, jaundice, nausea, weight loss, loss of appetite, and symptoms of gastrointestinal obstruction and diabetes. Pancreatic cancer is staged from I to IV according to disease spread. Stage I disease is limited to the pancreas, ▶

Pancreatic cancer

duodenum, bile duct, or peri-pancreatic tissues, with no distant metastases or regional lymph node involvement. Stages II–IV describe disease that has spread more extensively or become metastatic. A pancreatic tumour is considered resectable if there is a possibility that surgery could remove all cancerous tissue completely. Early stage tumours in the tail or body of the pancreas are more likely to be resectable than the more common, later stage cancers in the head of the pancreas. Other factors that influence resectability include proximity of the tumour to major blood vessels and perceived peri-operative risk.

INCIDENCE/ PREVALENCE Pancreatic cancer is the eighth most common cancer in the UK with an annual incidence in England and Wales of about 12/100 000.[1] It is the fourth most common cause of cancer death in higher income countries, responsible for about 30 000 deaths each year in the USA.[2] Prevalence is similar in men and women, with 5–10% presenting with resectable disease.[3]

AETIOLOGY/ RISK FACTORS Pancreatic cancer is more likely in people who smoke and have high alcohol intake. Dietary factors, such as lack of fruit and vegetables, are also reported risk factors.[4] One meta-analysis of observational studies found that people with diabetes mellitus of more than 5 years' duration are more likely to develop pancreatic cancer compared with the general population.[5] However, estimates of the magnitude of increased risk vary. Additional risk factors include pancreatitis and, in some cases, a family history.[1]

PROGNOSIS Prognosis is poor. One year survival is about 12%, with 5 year survival ranging from less than 1% in those with advanced cancer at presentation to 5% in those with early stage cancer at presentation.[1,6]

Please refer to the Clinical Evidence website for full text and references.

What are the effects of radical versus conservative surgical resection?

LIKELY TO BE BENEFICIAL

Complete tumour resection*

RCTs of complete tumour resection are unlikely to be conducted. Observational studies and multivariate analysis of RCTs have found a strong association between survival and complete resection of the primary tumour.

*Observational evidence only; RCTs unlikely to be conducted.

Subtotal gastrectomy for resectable distal tumours (as effective as total gastrectomy)

Two RCTs in people with primary tumours in the distal stomach found no significant difference in 5 year survival or postoperative mortality between total and subtotal gastrectomy.

UNKNOWN EFFECTIVENESS

Radical versus conservative lymphadenectomy

Two large RCTs found no significant difference in 5 year survival rates between radical and conservative lymphadenectomy. However, confounding factors may have affected reliability of results, and we found conflicting data from subgroup analyses of prospective cohort studies.

LIKELY TO BE INEFFECTIVE OR HARMFUL

Removal of adjacent organs

One RCT found no significant difference between radical gastrectomy plus splenectomy and radical gastrectomy alone in 5 year survival rates or postoperative mortality. The RCT found that radical gastrectomy plus splenectomy significantly increased the number of postoperative infections compared with radical gastrectomy alone. Retrospective analyses of observational studies and RCTs in people with stomach cancer found that removal of additional organs (spleen and distal pancreas) increased morbidity and mortality compared with no organ removal.

What are the effects of adjuvant chemotherapy?

LIKELY TO BE BENEFICIAL

Adjuvant chemotherapy

One large systematic review and two subsequent RCTs found that adjuvant chemotherapy increased survival compared with surgery alone. Two subsequent RCTs found no significant difference between adjuvant chemotherapy and surgery alone in 5 year survival.

DEFINITION   Stomach cancer is usually an adenocarcinoma arising in the stomach and includes tumours arising at or just below the gastro-oesophageal junction (type II and III junctional tumours). Tumours are staged according to degree of invasion and spread (see table 1❶). Only non-metastatic stomach cancers are considered in this chapter.

⯈

Stomach cancer

INCIDENCE/ PREVALENCE
The incidence of stomach cancer varies among countries and by gender (incidence per 100 000 population a year in Japanese men is about 80, Japanese women 30, British men 18, British women 10, white American men 11, white American women 7).[1] Incidence has declined dramatically in North America, Australia, and New Zealand since 1930, but the decline in Europe has been slower.[2] In the USA, stomach cancer remains relatively common among particular ethnic groups, especially Japanese–Americans and some Hispanic groups. The incidence of cancer of the proximal stomach and gastro-oesophageal junction is rising rapidly in many European populations and in North America.[3,4] The reasons for this are poorly understood.

AETIOLOGY/ RISK FACTORS
Distal stomach cancer is strongly associated with lifelong infection with *Helicobacter pylori* and poor dietary intake of antioxidant vitamins (A, C, and E).[5,6] In Western Europe and North America, distal stomach cancer is associated with relative socioeconomic deprivation. Proximal stomach cancer is strongly associated with smoking (OR about 4),[7] and is probably associated with gastro-oesophageal reflux, obesity, high fat intake, and medium to high socioeconomic status.

PROGNOSIS
Invasive stomach cancer (stages T2–T4) is fatal without surgery. Mean survival without treatment is less than 6 months from diagnosis.[8,9] Intramucosal or submucosal cancer (stage T1) may progress slowly to invasive cancer over several years.[10] In the USA, over 50% of people recently diagnosed with stomach cancer have regional lymph node metastasis or involvement of adjacent organs. The prognosis after macroscopically and microscopically complete resection (R0) is related strongly to disease stage, particularly penetration of the serosa (stage T3) and lymph node involvement. Five year survival rates range from over 90% in intramucosal cancer to about 20% in people with stage T3N2 disease (see table 1❶). In Japan, the 5 year survival rate for people with advanced disease is reported to be about 50%, but the explanation for the difference remains unclear. Comparisons between Japanese and Western practice are confounded by factors such as age, fitness, and disease stage, as well as by tumour location, because many Western series include gastro-oesophageal junction adenocarcinoma, which is associated with a much lower survival rate after surgery.

Please refer to the Clinical Evidence website for full text and references.

What are the effects of treatments in adults?

LIKELY TO BE BENEFICIAL

Topical antibiotics

We found no RCTs with long term follow up. Two RCTs found limited evidence that topical quinolone antibiotics improved otoscopic appearances compared with placebo in adults with chronic suppurative otitis media. Six RCTs found no clear evidence of clinically important differences among topical antibiotics in adults. One systematic review found that topical antibiotics were more effective than systemic antibiotics for reducing otoscopic features of chronic suppurative otitis media. One RCT found no significant difference between topical ceftizoxime plus systemic ceftizoxime and systemic ceftizoxime alone. One RCT found no significant difference between preoperative topical antibiotics and no preoperative treatment in people undergoing tympanoplasty. Short term topical antibiotics have been associated with few adverse events in RCTs. Uncontrolled case studies have reported vestibular ototoxicity after topical non-quinolone antibiotics.

UNKNOWN EFFECTIVENESS

Ear cleansing (aural toilet)

We found no RCTs comparing ear cleansing versus no treatment.

Systemic antibiotics

We found insufficient evidence about the effects of systemic antibiotics compared with placebo, no treatment, each other, or topical antiseptics. One systematic review found that systemic antibiotics were less effective than topical antibiotics in reducing otoscopic features of chronic suppurative otitis media. Two RCTs found no significant difference between systemic plus topical antibiotics and topical antibiotics alone, although a third RCT found that topical quinolone was more effective than oral plus topical non-quinolones. We found no evidence about long term treatment.

Topical antibiotics plus topical steroids

One systematic review found insufficient evidence from three RCTs about effects on symptoms of topical antibiotics plus topical steroids compared with placebo or topical steroids alone.

Topical antiseptics

We found no systematic reviews and no RCTs comparing topical antiseptics versus placebo or no treatment. One RCT in adults found no significant difference between topical antiseptics plus ear cleansing under microscopic control and either topical or oral antibiotics. One RCT found no significant difference in resolution of ear discharge between topical povidone–iodine and topical quinolone. The RCTs were too small to establish or exclude a clinically important effect from topical antiseptics in adults.

Topical steroids

We found no RCTs comparing topical steroids versus placebo or no treatment.

Tympanoplasty with or without mastoidectomy

We found no RCTs comparing tympanoplasty with or without mastoidectomy versus no surgery for chronic suppurative otitis media without cholesteatoma. ▶

Chronic suppurative otitis media

What are the effects of treatments in children?

UNKNOWN EFFECTIVENESS

Ear cleansing

One systematic review found insufficient evidence from two RCTs to compare a simple form of ear cleansing versus no ear cleansing in children with chronic suppurative otitis media.

Systemic antibiotics

RCTs found insufficient evidence about the effects of systemic antibiotics in children with chronic suppurative otitis media.

Topical antibiotics

We found no systematic reviews and no RCTs comparing topical antibiotics versus placebo in children. One RCT with a high drop-out rate found that topical ciprofloxacin increased the proportion of children with no discharge at 10–21 days compared with a combination of framycetin, gramicidin, and dexamethasone eardrops.

Topical antibiotics plus topical steroids

Small RCTs found insufficient evidence to compare topical antibiotics plus topical steroids versus cleansing only or topical antiseptics. One RCT with a high drop-out rate found that topical ciprofloxacin increased the proportion of children with no discharge at 10–21 days compared with a combination of framycetin, gramicidin, and dexamethasone eardrops.

Topical antiseptics

Two RCTs found no significant reduction in otorrhoea between topical antiseptics and control after 2 weeks. One RCT found no significant difference in otorrhoea between topical antiseptics and topical antibiotic plus steroid. However, the RCTs were too small to exclude a clinically important effect.

Topical steroids

We found no RCTs comparing topical steroids versus placebo or no treatment in children.

Tympanoplasty with or without mastoidectomy

We found no RCTs comparing tympanoplasty with or without mastoidectomy versus no surgery for chronic suppurative otitis media without cholesteatoma.

DEFINITION Chronic suppurative otitis media is persistent inflammation of the middle ear or mastoid cavity. Synonyms include "chronic otitis media (without effusion)", chronic mastoiditis, and chronic tympanomastoiditis. Chronic suppurative otitis media is characterised by recurrent or persistent ear discharge (otorrhoea) over 2–6 weeks through a perforation of the tympanic membrane. Typical findings also include thickened granular middle ear mucosa, mucosal polyps, and cholesteatoma within the middle ear. Chronic suppurative otitis media is differentiated from chronic otitis media with effusion, in which there is an intact tympanic membrane with fluid in the middle ear but no active infection. Chronic suppurative otitis media does not include chronic perforations of the eardrum that are dry, or only occasionally discharge, and have no signs of active infection.

INCIDENCE/ The worldwide prevalence of chronic suppurative otitis media is 65–330
PREVALENCE million people. Between 39–200 million (60%) suffer from clinically significant hearing impairment. Otitis media was estimated to have caused 28 000 deaths and loss of over 2 million Disability Adjusted Life Years in 2000,[1] 94% of which were in developing countries. Most of these deaths were probably ▶

due to chronic suppurative otitis media because acute otitis media is a self limiting infection. Estimates of prevalence are shown in table A on web extra.[2-32]

AETIOLOGY/ RISK FACTORS Chronic suppurative otitis media is assumed to be a complication of acute otitis media, but the risk factors for chronic suppurative otitis media are not clear. Frequent upper respiratory tract infections and poor socioeconomic conditions (overcrowded housing,[33] hygiene, and nutrition) may be related to the development of chronic suppurative otitis media.[34,35] Improvement of housing, hygiene, and nutrition in Maori children was associated with a halving of the prevalence of chronic suppurative otitis media between 1978 and 1987.[36] See also acute otitis media in children, p 42.

PROGNOSIS Most children with chronic suppurative otitis media have mild to moderate hearing impairment (about 26–60 dB increase in hearing thresholds) based on surveys among children in Africa, Brazil,[37] India,[38] and Sierra Leone,[39] and among the general population in Thailand.[40] In many developing countries, chronic suppurative otitis media represents the most frequent cause of moderate hearing loss (40–60 dB).[41] Persistent hearing loss during the first 2 years of life may increase learning disabilities and poor scholastic performance.[42] Spread of infection may lead to life threatening complications such as intracranial infections and acute mastoiditis.[43] The frequency of serious complications fell from 20% in 1938 to 2.5% in 1948 and is currently estimated to be about 0.24% in Thailand and 1.8% in Africa. This is believed to be associated with increased use of antibiotic treatment, tympanoplasty, and mastoidectomy.[44-46] Cholesteatoma is another serious complication that has been found in a variable proportion of people with chronic suppurative otitis media (range 0–60%).[47 50] In the West, the incidence of cholesteatoma is low (in 1993 in Finland the age standardised incidence of cholesteatoma was eight new cases per 100 000 population/year).[51]

Please refer to the Clinical Evidence website for full text and references.

Ear wax

Search date December 2003

George Browning

What are the effects of methods to remove symptomatic ear wax?

TRADE OFF BETWEEN BENEFITS AND HARMS

Ear syringing

There is consensus that ear syringing is effective, but we found no RCTs comparing ear syringing versus no treatment or versus other treatment. RCTs provided insufficient evidence to assess syringing after the use of wax softeners. Reported complications of ear syringing include otitis externa, perforation of the ear drum, damage to the skin of the external canal, tinnitus, pain, and vertigo.

UNKNOWN EFFECTIVENESS

Manual removal (other than ear syringing)

We found no RCTs about mechanical methods of removing ear wax other than syringing, although many practitioners consider these to be standard treatments.

Wax softeners

Two RCTs provided inconclusive evidence about the effects of wax softeners compared with no treatment, saline, or placebo (sterile water). The first RCT in elderly people with impacted wax found that a proprietary wax softening agent containing arachis oil/chlorobutanol/*p*-dichlorobenzene reduced the proportion of ears requiring syringing compared with no treatment, but found no significant difference between the proprietary wax softening agent and saline/sterile water. It also found no significant difference between sodium bicarbonate and either no treatment or saline/sterile water in the proportion of ears requiring syringing. Another RCT in children found no significant difference in the proportion of ears requiring syringing between either docusate sodium or triethanolamine and saline. RCTs found no consistent evidence that any one type of wax softener was superior to the others. RCTs also provided insufficient evidence to assess wax softeners prior to syringing.

DEFINITION	Ear wax is normal and becomes a problem only if it produces deafness, pain, or other aural symptoms. Ear wax may also need to be removed if it prevents inspection of the ear drum. The term "impacted wax" is used in different ways, and can merely imply the coexistence of wax obscuring the ear drum with symptoms in that ear.[1]
INCIDENCE/ PREVALENCE	We found four surveys of the prevalence of impacted wax.[2–5] The studies were carried out in a variety of populations and used a variety of definitions of impacted wax; prevalence ranged from 7–35%. It is unclear how these figures relate to prevalence in the general population.
AETIOLOGY/ RISK FACTORS	Factors that prevent the normal extrusion of wax from the ear canal (e.g. wearing a hearing aid, using cotton buds to clean ears) increase the chance of ear wax accumulating.
PROGNOSIS	Most ear wax emerges from the external canal spontaneously; one RCT that included a no treatment group found that 32% of ears with impacted wax showed spontaneous resolution after 5 days.[1] Without impaction or adherence to the drum, there is likely to be minimal, if any, hearing loss.

Please refer to the Clinical Evidence website for full text and references.

What are the effects of treatments for acute attacks?

Anticholinergics; benzodiazepines; betahistine

We found no RCTs on the effects of these interventions in treating acute attacks of Menière's disease.

What are the effects of interventions to prevent attacks and delay disease progression?

Betahistine (for vertigo or tinnitus)

Seven RCTs provided insufficient evidence to compare betahistine versus placebo in terms of their effects on the frequency and severity of attacks of vertigo, tinnitus, and aural fullness. Two small RCTs in people with definite or possible Menière's disease found no significant difference in tinnitus between betahistine and trimetazidine. One of these RCTs found that trimetazidine reduced the intensity of vertigo compared with betahistine, but the other RCT found no significant difference in vertigo intensity between trimetazidine and betahistine.

Diuretics

One small crossover RCT provided insufficient evidence about the effects of triamterene plus hydrochlorothiazide on hearing, vertigo, or tinnitus. We found no evidence on their effects on disease progression.

Trimetazidine

We found no RCTs comparing trimetazidine versus placebo in Menière's disease. Two small RCTs in people with definite or possible Menière's disease found no significant difference in tinnitus between betahistine and trimetazidine. One of these RCTs found that trimetazidine reduced the intensity vertigo compared with betahistine, but the other RCT found no significant difference in vertigo intensity between trimetazidine and betahistine. We found no evidence on the effects of trimetazidine on disease progression.

Aminoglycosides; dietary modification; psychological support; vestibular rehabilitation

We found no RCTs on the effects of these interventions in preventing attacks of Menière's disease or delaying disease progression.

Betahistine (for hearing loss)

Four RCTs in people with possible Menière's disease found no significant difference between betahistine and placebo in change in hearing assessed by pure tone audiograms. Two small RCTs in people with definite or possible Menière's disease found no significant difference in hearing between betahistine and trimetazidine. ▶

Menière's disease

Lithium

Two small crossover RCTs in people with possible Menière's disease provided insufficient evidence to compare lithium versus placebo in terms of their effects on vertigo, tinnitus, aural fullness, or hearing, although they found that lithium was associated with tremor, thirst, and polyuria in some people.

DEFINITION Menière's disease is characterised by recurrent episodes of spontaneous rotational vertigo, sensorineural hearing loss, tinnitus, and a feeling of fullness or pressure in the ear. It may be unilateral or bilateral. Acute episodes can occur in clusters of about 6–11 a year, although remission may last several months.[1] The diagnosis is made clinically.[2] It is important to distinguish Menière's disease from other types of vertigo that might occur independently with hearing loss and tinnitus, and respond differently to treatment (e.g. benign positional vertigo, acute labyrinthitis). Strict diagnostic criteria help to identify the condition. In this chapter we applied the classification of the American Academy of Otolaryngology — Head and Neck Surgery to assess the diagnostic rigour used in RCTs (see table 1 ❶).[3–5]

INCIDENCE/ PREVALENCE Menière's disease is most common between 40–60 years of age, although younger people may be affected.[6,7] In Europe, the incidence is about 50–200/100 000 a year. A survey of general practitioner records of 27 365 people in the UK found an incidence of 43 affected people in a 1 year period (157/100 000).[8] Diagnostic criteria were not defined in this survey. A survey of over 8 million people in Sweden found an incidence of 46/100 000 a year with diagnosis strictly based on the triad of vertigo, hearing loss, and tinnitus.[9] From smaller studies, the incidence appears lower in Uganda[10] and higher in Japan (350/100 000, based on a national survey of hospital attendances during a single week).[7]

AETIOLOGY/ RISK FACTORS Menière's disease is associated with endolymphatic hydrops (raised endolymph pressure in the membranous labyrinth of the inner ear),[11] but a causal relationship remains unproven.[12] Specific disorders associated with hydrops (such as temporal bone fracture, syphilis, hypothyroidism, Cogan's syndrome, and Mondini dysplasia) can produce symptoms similar to those of Menière's disease.

PROGNOSIS Menière's disease is progressive but fluctuates unpredictably. It is difficult to distinguish natural resolution from the effects of treatment. Significant improvement in vertigo is usually seen in the placebo arm of RCTs.[13,14] Acute attacks of vertigo often increase in frequency during the first few years after presentation and then decrease in frequency in association with sustained deterioration in hearing.[6] In most people, vertiginous episodes eventually cease completely.[15] In one 20 year cohort study in 34 people, 28 (82%) people had at least moderate hearing loss (mean pure tone hearing loss > 50 dB)[1] and 16 (47%) developed bilateral disease. Symptoms other than hearing loss improve in 60–80% of people irrespective of treatment.[16]

Please refer to the Clinical Evidence website for full text and references.

Search date March 2004

Simon Janvrin

What are the effects of preventive interventions?

LIKELY TO BE BENEFICIAL

Oral decongestants in adults

One RCT in adult passengers with a history of ear pain during air travel found limited evidence that oral pseudoephedrine decreased symptoms of barotrauma during air travel compared with placebo. One other RCT in adult passengers with a history of ear pain during air travel found limited evidence that oral pseudoephedrine decreased ear pain and hearing loss compared with placebo.

UNKNOWN EFFECTIVENESS

Oral decongestants in children

One small RCT in children up to the age of 6 years found no significant difference between oral pseudoephedrine and placebo in ear pain at take off or landing.

Topical nasal decongestants

One small RCT in adults with a history of ear pain during air travel found no significant difference with oxymetazoline nasal spray and placebo in symptoms of barotrauma.

DEFINITION The effects of air travel on the middle ear can include ear drum pain, vertigo, hearing loss, and ear drum perforation.

INCIDENCE/ PREVALENCE The prevalence of symptoms depends on the altitude, type of aircraft, and characteristics of the passengers. One point prevalence study found that 20% of adult and 40% of child passengers had negative pressure in the middle ear after flight, and that 10% of adults and 22% of children had auroscopic evidence of damage to the ear drum.[1] We found no data on the incidence of perforation, which seems to be extremely rare in commercial passengers.

AETIOLOGY/ RISK FACTORS During aircraft descent, the pressure in the middle ear drops relative to that in the ear canal. A narrow, inflamed, or poorly functioning Eustachian tube impedes the necessary influx of air. As the pressure difference between the middle and outer ear increases, the ear drum is pulled inward.

PROGNOSIS In most people, symptoms resolve spontaneously. Experience in military aviation shows that most ear drum perforations will heal spontaneously.[2]

Please refer to the Clinical Evidence website for full text and references.

Otitis externa

Search date March 2004

Daniel Hajioff

What are the effects of empirical treatment?

Topical aluminium acetate drops (as effective as topical anti-infective agents)

We found no RCTs that compared topical aluminium acetate versus placebo. One RCT in people with acute diffuse otitis externa found no significant difference between aluminium acetate drops and topical polymyxin–neomycin–hydrocortisone drops in time to clinical cure or clinical cure rate at 4 weeks.

Topical anti-infective agents (antibiotics or antifungals with or without steroids)

One RCT found that methylprednisolone–neomycin drops improved symptoms and signs compared with placebo at 28 days. Two RCTs found no significant difference in cure rate between topical quinolones and other topical anti-infective agents. One RCT found that triamcinolone–neomycin drops improved resolution rates compared with hydrocortisone–neomycin–polymyxin B drops. Two RCTs found limited evidence that neomycin–dexamethasone–acetic acid spray improved clinical cure compared with topical anti-infective drops that did not contain acetic acid. We found no RCTs on the effects of topical anti-infective agents versus oral antibiotics. One RCT found limited evidence of no significant difference between topical anti-infective ointment plus oral co-trimoxazole and topical anti-infective ointment alone in symptom severity, symptom duration, and cure rate. One RCT in people with acute diffuse otitis externa found no significant difference between topical polymyxin-neomycin-hydrocortisone drops and aluminium acetate drops in time to clinical cure or cure rate at 4 weeks.

Topical steroids

One RCT in people with mild or moderate, acute or chronic otitis externa found that topical budesonide improved symptoms and signs compared with placebo. We found no RCTs of topical steroids compared with topical anti-infective agents. One RCT found no significant difference in symptom scores between low potency steroid (topical hydrocortisone) and high potency steroid (topical hydrocortisone butyrate) after 1 week.

Oral antibiotics

We found no RCTs of oral antibiotics compared with placebo or topical anti-infective agents. One RCT found limited evidence of no significant difference between oral co-trimoxazole plus topical anti-infective ointment and topical anti-infective ointment alone in symptom severity, symptom duration, and cure rate.

Specialist aural toilet

We found no RCTs that compared specialist aural toilet versus no aural toilet. One RCT found no significant difference between an ear wick plus anti-infective drops versus ribbon gauze impregnated with anti-infective ointment in resolution rates after 4 weeks.

◄ **Topical acetic acid (insufficient evidence to demonstrate effectiveness compared with placebo)**

We found no RCTs comparing topical acetic acid versus placebo. One RCT in adults with acute diffuse otitis externa found that topical steroids plus antibiotics and topical acetic acid plus steroids reduced the duration of symptoms, increased overall cure rates, and reduced recurrence compared with acetic acid alone.

UNLIKELY TO BE BENEFICIAL

Oral antibiotics plus topical anti-infective agents (no better than topical anti-infective agents alone)

One RCT found limited evidence of no significant difference between oral co-trimoxazole plus topical anti-infective ointment and topical anti-infective ointment alone in symptom severity, symptom duration, and cure rate.

DEFINITION   Otitis externa is inflammation, often with infection, of the external ear canal. This inflammation is usually generalised throughout the ear canal, so it is often referred to as "diffuse otitis externa". The present topic excludes localised inflammations such as furuncles. Otitis externa has acute (< 6 weeks), chronic (> 3 months), and necrotising (malignant) forms. Acute otitis externa may present as a single episode, or recur. It causes severe pain with aural discharge and associated hearing loss.[1] If the ear canal is visible, it appears red and inflamed. Chronic otitis externa may result in canal stenosis with associated hearing loss, for which it may be difficult to fit hearing aids. Necrotising otitis externa is defined by destruction of the temporal bone, usually in people with diabetes or in people who are immunocompromised, and can be life threatening.[2] In this chapter, we look at empirical treatment of acute and chronic otitis externa only.

INCIDENCE/ PREVALENCE   Otitis externa is common in all parts of the world. The incidence is not known precisely, but 10% of people are thought to have been affected at some time.[3] The condition affects children but is more common in adults. It accounts for a large proportion of the workload of otolaryngology departments, but milder cases are often managed in primary care.[3]

AETIOLOGY/ RISK FACTORS   Otitis externa may be associated with local or generalised eczema of the ear canal. It is more common in swimmers, in humid environments, in people with an absence of ear wax or narrow external ear canals, in hearing aid users, and after mechanical trauma.[4]

PROGNOSIS   We found few reliable data. Many cases of otitis externa resolve spontaneously over several weeks or months. Acute episodes have a tendency to recur, although the risk of recurrence is unknown. Experience suggests that chronic inflammation affects a small proportion of people after a single episode of acute otitis externa, and may rarely lead to canal stenosis.[1]

Please refer to the Clinical Evidence website for full text and references.

Otitis media with effusion

Search date March 2004

Ian Williamson

What are the effects of preventive interventions?

UNKNOWN EFFECTIVENESS

Modifying risk factors to prevent otitis media with effusion

We found no RCTs on the effects of interventions aimed at modifying risk factors, such as passive smoking and bottle feeding, in preventing otitis media with effusion.

What are the effects of pharmacological, mechanical, and surgical treatments?

LIKELY TO BE BENEFICIAL

Autoinflation (with purpose-manufactured nasal balloon)

One systematic review found that autoinflation with a purpose-manufactured nasal balloon significantly improved effusion compared with no treatment. Some children may find autoinflation difficult. We found no evidence on other methods of autoinflation.

Ventilation tubes plus adenoidectomy/adenotonsillectomy

We found one systematic review, which found that ventilation tubes and adenoidectomy alone or in combination were equally effective and reduced mean hearing impairment by less than 12 decibels. The clinical significance of this hearing improvement was variable. One RCT from the review, which subsequently reported outcomes after 5 years, found that ventilation tubes plus adenoidectomy/ adenotonsillectomy was more effective than adenoidectomy/adenotonsillectomy or ventilation tubes alone; all of these surgical interventions were more effective than no treatment in reducing duration of otitis media with effusion. Two subsequent RCTs found different effects on language development with ventilation tubes compared with watchful waiting. A third subsequent RCT found that early insertion of ventilation tubes reduced behavioural problems at 9 months compared with watchful waiting.

UNKNOWN EFFECTIVENESS

Corticosteroids (intranasal)

One small RCT found no significant difference between intranasal corticosteroids alone compared with placebo for resolution of effusion. A second small RCT found limited evidence that intranasal corticosteroids plus antibiotics improved symptoms compared with antibiotics alone.

Adenoidectomy alone; adenotonsillectomy alone; autoinflation (with other devices); tonsillectomy; ventilation tubes alone

We found insufficient evidence on the effects of these interventions.

UNLIKELY TO BE BENEFICIAL

Antibiotics (oral)

One systematic review found limited evidence that antibiotics improved short term outcomes compared with placebo or no treatment. However, a second systematic review of higher quality and incorporating six RCTs from the first review found no significant difference between antibiotics and placebo. A third systematic review ▶

found limited evidence from four RCTs that antibiotics plus oral corticosteroids improved resolution rates compared with antibiotics alone. Another small RCT in the same review found limited evidence that intranasal corticosteroids plus antibiotics improved symptoms compared with antibiotics alone. Adverse effects with antibiotics (mainly nausea, vomiting, and diarrhoea) were reported in 2–32% of children.

Mucolytics

One systematic review found no significant difference between 1–3 month courses of carbocisteine or carbocisteine lysine and placebo or no treatment in resolution of effusion. Three small RCTs of bromhexine versus placebo found inconclusive results.

LIKELY TO BE INEFFECTIVE OR HARMFUL

Antihistamines plus oral decongestants

One systematic review found no significant difference between antihistamines plus oral decongestants compared with placebo in clearance of effusion after 4 weeks.

Corticosteroids (oral)

One systematic review found no significant difference between oral corticosteroids and placebo in clearance of effusion after 2 weeks. It found limited evidence that oral corticosteroids plus antibiotics improved resolution rates compared with antibiotics alone.

DEFINITION Otitis media with effusion (OME), or "glue ear", is serous or mucoid but not mucopurulent fluid in the middle ear. Children usually present with hearing loss and speech problems. In contrast to those with acute otitis media (see acute otitis media in children, p 42), children with OME do not suffer from acute ear pain, fever, or malaise. Hearing loss is usually mild and often identified when parents express concern regarding their child's behaviour, performance at school, or language development.

INCIDENCE/ PREVALENCE OME is commonly seen in paediatric practice and accounts for 25–35% of all cases of otitis media.[1] One study in the UK found that, at any time, 5% of children aged 5 years had persistent (at least 3 months) bilateral hearing loss associated with OME.[2] The prevalence declines considerably beyond 6 years of age.[3] About 50–80% of children aged 4 years have been affected by OME some time in the past.[3,4] One study estimated that, between the ages of 2 months and 2 years, 91.1% of young children will have one episode of middle ear effusion, and 52.2% will have bilateral involvement.[5] OME is the most common reason for referral for surgery in children in the UK. The number of consultations for otitis media increased by 150% between 1975 and 1990. Middle ear effusions also occur infrequently in adults after upper respiratory tract infection or after air travel, and may persist for weeks or months after an episode of acute otitis media.[6] OME is estimated to account for 25–35% of all cases of otitis media.

AETIOLOGY/ RISK FACTORS Contributory factors include upper respiratory tract infection and narrow upper respiratory airways.[6,7] Case control studies have identified risk factors, including age 6 years or younger at first onset, day care centre attendance, large number of siblings, low socioeconomic group, frequent upper respiratory tract infection, bottle feeding, and household smoking.[3,6] These factors may be associated with about twice the risk of developing OME.[7]

PROGNOSIS Data from one prospective study of children aged 2–4 years showed that 50% of OME cases resolved within three months and 95% within a year.[8] In 5% of preschool children, OME (identified by tympanometric screening) persists for at least 1 year.[8,9] One cohort study of 3 year olds found that 65% of OME cases cleared within three months.[9] Most children aged 6 years or older will not have ▶

Otitis media with effusion

further problems.[2] The disease is ultimately self limiting in most cases.[2,5,10] However, one large cohort study (534 children) found that middle ear disease increased reported hearing difficulty at 5 years of age (OR 1.44, 95% CI 1.18 to 1.76) and was associated with delayed language development in children up to 10 years of age.[11] Hearing loss is the most common complication of OME. Most children with OME have fluctuating or persistent hearing deficits with mild to moderate degrees of hearing loss, averaging 27 decibels. The type of hearing loss is usually conductive, but may be sensorineural, or both. The sensorineural type is usually permanent.[12] Tympanic membrane perforation, tympanosclerosis, otorrhoea, and cholesteatoma occur more frequently among children with OME than those without OME. These conditions are especially common among children with OME who have had myringotomy with ventilation tube placement.[13]

Please refer to the Clinical Evidence website for full text and references.

Search date September 2003

Aziz Sheikh, Sukhmeet Singh Panesar, and Sangeeta Dhami

What are the effects of treatments on quality of life?

BENEFICIAL

Oral fexofenadine
Of all the oral antihistamines, only fexofenadine has been shown in RCTs to improve quality of life as well as rhinitis symptoms compared with placebo.

LIKELY TO BE BENEFICIAL

Oral leukotriene receptor antagonists
One systematic review provides good evidence that montelukast improves quality of life compared with placebo.

Oral leukotriene receptor antagonists plus oral antihistamines
One systematic review has found that montelukast plus loratadine improves quality of life compared with placebo. However, it found no evidence that combined treatment was any more effective than loratadine or montelukast alone.

UNKNOWN EFFECTIVENESS

Intranasal antihistamines; intranasal ipratropium bromide; oral decongestants; oral decongestants plus oral antihistamines; other oral antihistamines
We found no RCTs evaluating the effects of these interventions on quality of life.

What are the effects of treatments on rhinitis symptoms?

BENEFICIAL

Oral antihistamines
Numerous RCTs have found that oral antihistamines (acrivastine, azatadine, brompheniramine, cetirizine, ebastine, loratadine, desloratadine, or mizolastine) improve rhinitis symptoms compared with placebo. Drowsiness, sedation, and somnolence were the most commonly reported adverse effects.

Oral pseudoephedrine plus oral antihistamines
RCTs have found that pseudoephedrine plus oral antihistamines (fexofenadine, acrivastine, cetirizine, terfenadine, triprolidine, loratadine, or azatadine) improve overall symptoms of seasonal allergic rhinitis compared with pseudoephedrine or oral antihistamine or placebo alone. The most common adverse effects reported with combination treatment were headache and insomnia.

LIKELY TO BE BENEFICIAL

Intranasal levocabastine
RCTs found that intranasal levocabastine improved symptoms of seasonal allergic rhinitis compared with placebo.

Oral leukotriene receptor antagonists
One systematic review provided good evidence that montelukast improved nasal symptoms compared with placebo. One RCT provided inconclusive evidence about effects of pranlukast compared with placebo.

▶

Seasonal allergic rhinitis

Oral leukotriene receptor antagonists plus oral antihistamines

One systematic review has found that montelukast plus loratadine improves nasal symptoms compared with placebo. However, it found no evidence that combined treatment was any more effective than loratadine or montelukast alone.

TRADE OFF BETWEEN BENEFITS AND HARMS

Oral astemizole

RCTs have found that astemizole improves rhinitis symptoms compared with placebo but astemizole has been associated with prolongation of the QTc interval, and may induce ventricular arrhythmias.

Oral terfenadine

RCTs have found conflicting results about the effectiveness of terfenadine compared with placebo on rhinitis symptoms. Terfenadine is associated with risk of fatal cardiac toxicity if used in conjunction with macrolide antibiotics, oral antifungal agents, or grapefruit juice.

UNKNOWN EFFECTIVENESS

Intranasal azelastine

RCTs have found conflicting results about effectiveness of intranasal azelastine compared with placebo on symptoms of seasonal allergic rhinitis. Two small RCTs found no significant difference in nasal symptoms between intranasal antihistamines (azelastine, levocabastine) and oral antihistamines (cetirizine, terfenadine).

Intranasal ipratropium bromide

We found no systematic review or published RCTs.

DEFINITION
Seasonal allergic rhinitis is a symptom complex that may affect several organ systems. Symptoms will typically consist of seasonal sneezing, nasal itching, nasal blockage, and watery nasal discharge.[1] Eye symptoms (red eyes, itchy eyes, and tearing) are common. Other symptoms may include peak seasonal coughing, wheezing, and shortness of breath, oral allergy syndrome (manifesting as an itchy swollen oropharynx on eating stoned fruits), and systemic symptoms such as tiredness, fever, a pressure sensation in the head, and itchiness. Confirming the presence of pollen hypersensitivity using objective allergy tests such as skin prick tests, detection of serum specific IgE, and nasal provocation challenge testing may improve diagnostic accuracy.

INCIDENCE/ PREVALENCE
Seasonal allergic rhinitis is found throughout the world. Epidemiological evidence suggests that there is considerable geographical variation in its prevalence. Prevalence is highest in socioeconomically developed countries, where the condition may affect as much as 25% of the population.[2–4] Prevalence and severity are increasing. It is thought that improved living standards and reduced risk of childhood infections may lead to immune deviation of T helper cells in early life, which may increase susceptibility to seasonal allergic rhinitis (the so called "hygiene hypothesis").[5,6] Although people of all ages may be affected, the peak age of onset is adolescence.[7]

AETIOLOGY/ RISK FACTORS
The symptoms of seasonal allergic rhinitis are caused by an IgE mediated type 1 hypersensitivity reaction to grass, tree, or weed pollen. Allergy to other seasonal aeroallergens such as fungal spores may also provoke symptoms. Typically, symptoms become worse during the relevant pollen season and in the open, when pollen exposure is increased. Risk factors include a personal or family history of atopy or other allergic disorders, male sex, birth order (increased risk being seen in first born), and small family size.[8,9]

PROGNOSIS Seasonal allergic rhinitis may impair quality of life, interfering with work, sleep, and recreational activities.[10] Other allergic problems such as asthma and eczema frequently coexist, adding to the impact of rhinitis.[11]

Please refer to the Clinical Evidence website for full text and references.

Sinusitis (acute)

Search date August 2004

Kim Ah-See

What are the effects of treatments in people with clinically diagnosed acute sinusitis?

UNKNOWN EFFECTIVENESS

Antibiotics

Three RCTs found no good evidence that amoxicillin, with or without clavulanate, reduced or cured symptoms compared with placebo in people with clinically diagnosed acute sinusitis, who had not had radiological or bacteriological confirmation of disease. Two RCTs found that amoxicillin, with or without clavulanate, increased diarrhoea compared with placebo. We found no RCTs examining effects of other antibiotics (co-trimoxazole, cephalosporins, azithromycin, and erythromycin) compared with placebo or each other.

Antihistamines

We found no RCTs examining clinical effects of antihistamines in people with clinically diagnosed acute sinusitis.

Decongestants

We found no RCTs examining clinical effects of topical or systemic decongestants in people with clinically diagnosed acute sinusitis.

Topical steroids

We found no RCTs examining clinical effects of topical steroids in people with clinically diagnosed acute sinusitis.

What are the effects of antibiotics in people with radiologically or bacteriologically confirmed acute sinusitis?

LIKELY TO BE BENEFICIAL

Cephalosporins and macrolides (fewer adverse effects than amoxicillin or amoxicillin–clavulanate)

We found no RCTs comparing cephalosporins or macrolides with placebo. One systematic review and two subsequent RCTs in people with radiologically or bacteriologically confirmed acute sinusitis found no significant difference in clinical resolution between amoxicillin or amoxicillin–clavulanate and cephalosporins or macrolides. However, cephalosporins and macrolides caused fewer adverse effects than amoxicillin and amoxicillin–clavulanate. One RCT found no significant difference in clinical improvement or clinical cure between cefaclor (a cephalosporin) and azithromycin (a macrolide).

TRADE OFF BETWEEN BENEFITS AND HARMS

Amoxicillin and amoxicillin–clavulanate (more adverse effects than cephalosporins or macrolides)

One systematic review identified two RCTs in people with radiologically or bacteriologically confirmed acute maxillary sinusitis, which found that amoxicillin improved early clinical cure rate compared with placebo, but was associated with more frequent adverse effects, mainly gastrointestinal. One systematic review and two subsequent RCTs in people with radiologically or bacteriologically confirmed acute sinusitis found no significant difference in clinical resolution between ▶

amoxicillin or amoxicillin–clavulanate and cephalosporins or macrolides. However, amoxicillin and amoxicillin–clavulanate caused more adverse effects.

UNKNOWN EFFECTIVENESS

Antihistamines
We found no RCTs examining the effects of antihistamines in people with radiologically or bacteriologically confirmed acute sinusitis.

Decongestants
We found no RCTs examining the effects of decongestants in people with radiologically or bacteriologically confirmed acute sinusitis.

Different dosages of antibiotics
One RCT in people with radiologically or bacteriologically confirmed acute sinusitis found no significant difference in clinical resolution rates or adverse events between two and three daily doses of cefaclor. We found no RCTs of other antibiotics comparing different dosage regimens.

Topical steroids
We found no RCTs examining the effects of topical steroids in people with radiologically or bacteriologically confirmed acute sinusitis.

UNLIKELY TO BE BENEFICIAL

Long course antibiotic regimens (no more effective than short course regimens, and more adverse effects)
RCTs in people with confirmed acute sinusitis found no significant difference in clinical resolution rates between 6–10 day courses and 3–5 day courses of azithromycin, telithromycin, co-trimoxazole or cefuroxime (a cephalosporin) up to 3 weeks after treatment. RCTs found similar rates of adverse effects and diarrhoea between longer and shorter courses of azithromycin and telithromycin. One RCT found that adverse effects, which were mainly gastrointestinal, were more frequent with a longer course of cefuroxime than with a shorter course of cefuroxime.

DEFINITION Acute sinusitis is defined pathologically, by transient inflammation of the mucosal lining of the paranasal sinuses lasting less than 4 weeks. Clinically, it is characterised by nasal congestion, rhinorrhoea, facial pain, hyposmia, sneezing, and, if more severe, additional malaise and fever. The diagnosis is usually made clinically (on the basis of history and examination, but without radiological or bacteriological investigation). Clinically diagnosed acute sinusitis is less likely to be caused by bacterial infection than is acute sinusitis confirmed by radiological or bacteriological investigation.[1] In this chapter, we have excluded studies in children, in people with symptoms for more than 4 weeks (chronic sinusitis), and in people with symptoms after facial trauma. We have made it clear in each section whether we are dealing with clinically diagnosed acute sinusitis or acute sinusitis that has been confirmed by bacteriological or radiological investigation, because the effects of treatment may be different in these groups.

INCIDENCE/ PREVALENCE Each year in Europe, 1–5% of adults are diagnosed with acute sinusitis by their general practitioner.[2] Extrapolated to the British population, this is estimated to cause 6 million restricted working days a year.[3,4] Most people with acute sinusitis are assessed and treated in a primary care setting. The prevalence varies according to whether diagnosis is made on clinical grounds or on the basis of radiological or bacteriological investigation.

AETIOLOGY/ RISK FACTORS One systematic review (search date 1998) reported that about 50% of people with a clinical diagnosis of acute sinusitis have bacterial sinus infection.[1] The usual pathogens in acute bacterial sinusitis are *Streptococcus pneumoniae* ▶

Sinusitis (acute)

and *Haemophilus influenzae*, with occasional infection with *Moraxella catarrhalis*. Preceding viral upper respiratory tract infection is often the trigger for acute bacterial sinusitis,[5] with about 0.5% of common colds becoming complicated by the development of acute sinusitis.[6]

PROGNOSIS One meta-analysis of RCTs found that up to two thirds of people with acute sinusitis had spontaneous resolution of symptoms without active treatment.[7] One non-systematic review reported that people with acute sinusitis are at risk of chronic sinusitis and irreversible damage to the normal mucociliary mucosal surface.[8] One further non-systematic review reported rare life-threatening complications such as orbital cellulitis and meningitis after acute sinusitis.[9] However, we found no reliable data to measure these risks.

Please refer to the Clinical Evidence website for full text and references.

Search date February 2004

Angus Waddell

What are the effects of treatments for chronic tinnitus?

TRADE OFF BETWEEN BENEFITS AND HARMS

Tricyclic antidepressants

One systematic review of one RCT in people with depression and chronic tinnitus found that tricyclic antidepressants (nortriptyline) improved tinnitus related disability and symptoms of depression at 6 weeks, but found no significant difference in self reported tinnitus severity compared with placebo. One small RCT in people with tinnitus but without depression found that a greater proportion of people rated themselves as improved with tricyclic antidepressants (amitriptyline) compared with placebo at 6 weeks. Tricyclic antidepressants are associated with adverse effects such as dry mouth, blurred vision, and constipation.

UNKNOWN EFFECTIVENESS

Benzodiazepines (alprazolam)

One systematic review found limited evidence from one RCT that alprazolam, a benzodiazepine, improved self reported tinnitus severity after 12 weeks. Benzodiazepines can have adverse effects that may outweigh potential benefits.

Psychotherapy

One systematic review found insufficient evidence about the effects of cognitive behavioural treatment, relaxation therapy, education, or biofeedback compared with other or no treatment in people with chronic tinnitus.

Acupuncture; baclofen; cinnarizine; electromagnetic stimulation; ginkgo biloba; hyperbaric oxygen; hypnosis; lamotrigine; low power laser; nicotinamide; tinnitus masking devices; zinc

We found insufficient evidence about the effects of these interventions.

LIKELY TO BE INEFFECTIVE OR HARMFUL

Carbamazepine

One systematic review of one RCT found no significant difference between carbamazepine and placebo in tinnitus severity at 30 days. Treatment with carbamazepine was associated with an increased risk of dizziness, nausea, and headaches.

DEFINITION   Tinnitus is defined as the perception of sound, which does not arise from the external environment, from within the body (e.g. vascular sounds), or from auditory hallucinations related to mental illness. This review is concerned with tinnitus, where tinnitus is the only, or the predominant, symptom in an affected person.

INCIDENCE/ PREVALENCE   Up to 18% of the general population in industrialised countries are mildly affected by chronic tinnitus, and 0.5% report tinnitus having a severe effect on their ability to lead a normal life.[1]

AETIOLOGY/ RISK FACTORS   Tinnitus may occur as an isolated idiopathic symptom or in association with any type of hearing loss. Tinnitus may be a particular feature of presbycusis, noise induced hearing loss, Menière's disease (see Menière's disease, p 131), or the presence of an acoustic neuroma. In people with toxicity from aspirin or quinine, tinnitus can occur while hearing thresholds remain normal. Tinnitus is ▶

also associated with depression, although it may be unclear whether the tinnitus is a manifestation of the depressive illness or a factor contributing to its development.[2]

PROGNOSIS   Tinnitus may have an insidious onset, with a long delay before clinical presentation. It may persist for many years or decades, particularly when associated with a sensorineural hearing loss. In Menière's disease, both the presence and intensity of tinnitus can fluctuate. Tinnitus may cause disruption of sleep patterns, an inability to concentrate, and depression.[3]

Please refer to the Clinical Evidence website for full text and references.

What are the effects of tonsillectomy in children and adults with severe tonsillitis?

TRADE OFF BETWEEN BENEFITS AND HARMS

Tonsillectomy compared with antibiotics in children

Two systematic reviews that included the same two RCTs in children found insufficient evidence to compare surgical versus medical treatment. One subsequent RCT in less severely affected children found that surgery reduced the frequency of throat infection compared with medical treatment over 3 years. It suggested that the modest benefit may be outweighed by the morbidity associated with the surgery in populations with a low incidence of tonsillitis.

UNKNOWN EFFECTIVENESS

Tonsillectomy compared with antibiotics in adults

We found no RCTs evaluating tonsillectomy in adults.

DEFINITION Tonsillitis is infection of the parenchyma of the palatine tonsils. The definition of severe recurrent tonsillitis is arbitrary, but recent criteria have defined tonsillitis as five or more episodes of true tonsillitis a year, symptoms for at least a year, and episodes that are disabling and prevent normal functioning.[1] The definition does not include tonsillitis due to infectious mononucleosis, which usually occurs as a single episode. However, acute tonsillitis in this situation may be followed by recurrent tonsillitis in some people. Tonsillitis may occur in isolation or as part of a generalised pharyngitis. The clinical distinction between tonsillitis and pharyngitis is unclear in the literature and the condition is often referred to simply as "acute sore throat". A sore throat lasting for 24–48 hours as part of the prodrome of minor upper respiratory tract infection is excluded from this definition. **Diagnosis** of acute tonsillitis is primarily clinical, with the main interest being in whether the illness is viral or bacterial, this being of relevance if antibiotics are being considered. Studies have attempted to distinguish viral from bacterial sore throat on clinical grounds, but the results are conflicting, suggesting a lack of reliable diagnostic criteria. Investigations to assist with this distinction include throat swabs and serological tests, including the rapid antigen test and the antistreptolysin O titre. Rapid antigen testing is convenient and popular in North America but has doubtful sensitivity (61–95%), at least when measured against throat swab results, although specificity is higher (88–100%).

INCIDENCE/ PREVALENCE Recurrent sore throat has an incidence in general practice in the UK of 100 per 1000 population a year.[2] Acute tonsillitis is more common in childhood.

AETIOLOGY/ RISK FACTORS Common bacterial pathogens include β haemolytic and other streptococci. Bacteria are cultured only from a minority of people with tonsillitis. The role of viruses is uncertain. In tonsillitis associated with infectious mononucleosis, the most common infective agent is the Epstein–Barr virus (present in 50% of children and 90% of adults with the condition). Cytomegalovirus infection may also result in the clinical picture of infectious mononucleosis, and the differential diagnosis also includes toxoplasmosis, HIV, hepatitis A, and rubella.[3]

PROGNOSIS We found no good data on the natural history of tonsillitis or recurrent sore throat in children or adults. People in RCTs randomised to medical treatment (courses of antibiotics as required) have shown a tendency towards improvement over time.[4,5] Recurrent severe tonsillitis results in considerable morbidity, ▶

Tonsillitis

including time lost from school or work. The most common complication of acute tonsillitis is peritonsillar abscess, but we found no good evidence on its incidence. Rheumatic fever and acute glomerulonephritis are recognised complications of acute tonsillitis associated with group A β haemolytic streptococci. These diseases are rare in developed countries, but do occasionally occur. They are still a common problem in certain populations, notably Australian Aboriginals, and may be effectively prevented in closed communities by the use of penicillin. A systematic review found no evidence that aggressive antibiotic treatment of acute sore throat in the developed world was useful in the prevention of these diseases.[6]

Please refer to the Clinical Evidence website for full text and references.

What are the effects of treatments in people with type 1 diabetes and early nephropathy?

BENEFICIAL

Angiotensin converting enzyme (ACE) inhibitors (progression to late nephropathy)

One systematic review found that, compared with placebo or controls, ACE inhibitors (captopril, lisinopril, enalapril, perindopril, and ramipril) reduced progression to macroalbuminuria and increased regression to normoalbuminuria in normotensive people with type 1 diabetes and microalbuminuria. We found no systematic review or RCTs comparing effects of ACE inhibitors versus placebo in people with type 1 diabetes and early nephropathy for the outcomes mortality (all cause), incidence of end stage renal disease, or incidence of cardiovascular events (stroke, heart failure, myocardial infarction).

Glycaemic control (progression to late nephropathy)

One systematic review found that, compared with conventional control, intensive glycaemic control reduced progression of nephropathy in people with type 1 diabetes and either normal albumin excretion or microalbuminuria. The review found no significant difference between intensive glycaemic control and conventional control in the incidence of severe hypoglycaemia, but found higher incidence of diabetic ketoacidosis in people treated with continuous subcutaneous insulin infusion compared with conventional multiple injection treatment. We found no systematic review or RCT evaluating effects of glycaemic control in people with type 1 diabetes and early nephropathy for the outcomes of mortality, or incidence of cardiovascular events (stroke, heart failure, myocardial infarction).

UNKNOWN EFFECTIVENESS

Angiotensin II receptor antagonists

We found no systematic review or RCTs comparing effects of angiotensin II receptor antagonists versus placebo in people with type 1 diabetes and early nephropathy for outcomes of interest. Long term placebo controlled RCTs would not be ethical because of the established benefits of ACE inhibitors and similarity between these two drug classes. We found no RCTs comparing angiotensin II receptor antagonists versus ACE inhibitors in people with type 1 diabetes and early nephropathy.

Lipid lowering

We found no systematic review or RCTs on lipid lowering in people with type 1 diabetes and early nephropathy for the outcomes of progression to late nephropathy, mortality (all cause), incidence of end stage renal disease, or incidence of cardiovascular events (stroke, heart failure, myocardial infarction).

Protein restriction

We found no systematic review or RCTs comparing effects of low protein diet versus usual diet in people with type 1 diabetes and early nephropathy for the outcomes of progression to late nephropathy, mortality (all cause), incidence of end stage renal disease, or incidence of cardiovascular events (stroke, heart failure, myocardial infarction).

Diabetic nephropathy

Tight control of blood pressure

We found no systematic review or RCTs comparing tight control of blood pressure versus conventional control in people with type 1 diabetes and early nephropathy for the outcomes of progression to late nephropathy, mortality (all cause), incidence of end stage renal disease, or incidence of cardiovascular events (stroke, heart failure, myocardial infarction).

What are the effects of treatments in people with type 1 diabetes and late nephropathy?

BENEFICIAL

Captopril

One RCT in people with type 1 diabetes and late nephropathy found that, compared with placebo, captopril (an ACE inhibitor) reduced the combined outcome of renal transplant, end stage renal disease, or death over 3 years. We found no systematic review or RCTs comparing effects of captopril versus placebo in people with type 1 diabetes and late nephropathy for the outcome of incidence of cardiovascular events (stroke, heart failure, myocardial infarction) or on effects of other ACE inhibitors for the outcomes of interest.

UNKNOWN EFFECTIVENESS

Angiotensin II receptor antagonists

We found no systematic review or RCTs comparing effects of angiotensin II receptor antagonists versus placebo in people with type 1 diabetes and late nephropathy for outcomes of mortality (all cause), incidence of end stage renal disease, or incidence of cardiovascular events (stroke, heart failure, myocardial infarction). Long term placebo controlled RCTs would not be ethical because of the established benefits of ACE inhibitors and similarity between these two drug classes. We found no RCTs comparing angiotensin II receptor antagonists with ACE inhibitors in people with type 1 diabetes and late nephropathy.

Glycaemic control

We found no systematic review or RCTs comparing intensive glycaemic control with conventional glycaemic control in people with type 1 diabetes and late nephropathy for the outcomes of mortality (all cause), incidence of end stage renal disease, or incidence of cardiovascular events (stroke, heart failure, myocardial infarction).

Lipid lowering

We found no systematic review or RCTs evaluating effects of lipid lowering in people with type 1 diabetes and late nephropathy for the outcomes of mortality, incidence of end stage renal disease, or incidence of cardiovascular events (stroke, heart failure, myocardial infarction).

Protein restriction

One small RCT found that, compared with usual protein intake, a low protein diet significantly reduced the cumulative incidence of end stage renal disease or death over 4 years in people with type 1 diabetes and late nephropathy. This RCT was small, and neither participants nor study investigators could be blinded to the randomisation owing to the nature of the intervention. We found no systematic review or RCTs comparing effects of low protein diet versus usual diet in people with type 1 diabetes and late nephropathy for the outcome of incidence of cardiovascular events (stroke, heart failure, myocardial infarction).

◀ **Tight control of blood pressure**

We found no systematic review or RCT evaluating effects of tight blood pressure control versus conventional control in people with type 1 diabetes and late nephropathy for the outcomes of mortality, incidence of end stage renal disease, or incidence of cardiovascular events (stroke, heart failure, myocardial infarction).

What are the effects of treatments in people with type 2 diabetes and early nephropathy?

BENEFICIAL

ACE inhibitors

One RCT found that, compared with placebo, enalapril significantly reduced progression to late nephropathy. One RCT comparing ramipril versus placebo with subgroup analysis in people with diabetes and early nephropathy found that ramipril reduced the combined outcome of myocardial infarction, stroke, or cardiovascular death. One systematic review in people with diabetes and nephropathy, which did not stratify the results by the type of diabetes, found that, compared with placebo, ACE inhibitors significantly reduced progression to late nephropathy in people with diabetes and microalbuminuria over 3 years. We found no systematic review or RCTs comparing ACE inhibitors versus placebo in people with type 2 diabetes and early nephropathy for the outcomes of mortality (all cause), incidence of end stage renal disease, or incidence of cardiovascular events (stroke, heart failure, myocardial infarction).

Irbesartan (progression to late nephropathy)

One RCT in people with type 2 diabetes, hypertension, and microalbuminuria found that, compared with placebo, an angiotensin II receptor antagonist irbesartan 300 mg reduced progression from early to late nephropathy over 2 years, but found no significant decrease with irbesartan 150 mg. We found no systematic review or RCTs comparing angiotensin II receptor antagonists versus placebo in people with type 2 diabetes and early nephropathy for the outcomes of mortality (all cause), incidence of end stage renal disease, or incidence of cardiovascular events (stroke, heart failure, myocardial infarction).

Tight control of blood pressure (progression to late nephropathy)

One RCT found that, in people with type 2 diabetes, early nephropathy, and baseline blood pressure within the normal range, a lower diastolic blood pressure target (10 mm Hg below baseline) significantly reduced progression from microalbuminuria to overt albuminuria over 5 years compared with a moderate diastolic blood pressure target (80–89 mm Hg). We found no systematic review or RCTs on tight blood pressure control in people with type 2 diabetes and early nephropathy for the outcomes of progression to late nephropathy, mortality (all cause), incidence of end stage renal disease, or incidence of cardiovascular events (stroke, heart failure, myocardial infarction).

UNKNOWN EFFECTIVENESS

Glycaemic control

We found no systematic review or RCTs evaluating effects of glycaemic control in people with type 2 diabetes and early nephropathy for the outcomes of progression to late nephropathy, mortality, incidence of end stage renal disease, or incidence of cardiovascular events (stroke, heart failure, myocardial infarction). ▶

Diabetic nephropathy

Lipid lowering

We found no systematic review or RCTs on lipid lowering in people with type 2 diabetes and early nephropathy for the outcomes of progression to late nephropathy, mortality (all cause), incidence of end stage renal disease, or incidence of cardiovascular events (stroke, heart failure, myocardial infarction).

Protein restriction

We found no systematic review or RCTs on protein restriction in people with type 2 diabetes and early nephropathy for the outcomes of progression to late nephropathy, mortality (all cause), incidence of end stage renal disease, or incidence of cardiovascular events (stroke, heart failure, myocardial infarction).

What are the effects of treatments in people with type 2 diabetes and late nephropathy?

BENEFICIAL

Losartan (progression to end stage renal disease)

We found two RCTs comparing angiotensin II receptor antagonists versus placebo for the outcomes of progression to end stage renal disease, cardiovascular events, and all cause mortality. One RCT in people with type 2 diabetes and late nephropathy found that, compared with placebo, losartan reduced progression to end stage renal disease over 3.4 years but found no significant difference in fatal or non-fatal cardiovascular events or death from any cause. Another RCT in people with type 2 diabetes and late nephropathy found no significant difference between irbesartan and placebo in progression to end stage renal disease or death from any cause over 2.6 years. It also found that irbesartan significantly reduced the incidence of congestive heart failure compared with placebo, but no significant difference for a composite cardiovascular outcome, cardiovascular death, myocardial infarction, cerebrovascular accident, or cardiac revascularisation. In both RCTs, angiotensin II receptor antagonist was discontinued if hyperkalemia occurred.

UNKNOWN EFFECTIVENESS

ACE inhibitors

We found no systematic review or RCTs comparing ACE inhibitors versus placebo in people with type 2 diabetes and late nephropathy for the outcomes of mortality (all cause), incidence of end stage renal disease, or incidence of cardiovascular events (stroke, heart failure, myocardial infarction).

Glycaemic control

We found no systematic review or RCTs on glycaemic control in people with type 2 diabetes and late nephropathy for the outcomes of mortality (all cause), incidence of end stage renal disease, or incidence of cardiovascular events (stroke, heart failure, myocardial infarction).

Lipid lowering

We found no systematic review or RCTs on lipid lowering in people with type 2 diabetes and late nephropathy for the outcomes of mortality (all cause), incidence of end stage renal disease, or incidence of cardiovascular events (stroke, heart failure, myocardial infarction).

◀ **Protein restriction**

We found no systematic review or RCTs on protein restriction in people with type 2 diabetes and late nephropathy for the outcomes of mortality (all cause), incidence of end stage renal disease, or incidence of cardiovascular events (stroke, heart failure, myocardial infarction).

Tight control of blood pressure

We found no systematic review or RCTs on tight blood pressure control in people with type 2 diabetes and late nephropathy for the outcomes of mortality (all cause), incidence of end stage renal disease, or incidence of cardiovascular events (stroke, heart failure, myocardial infarction).

DEFINITION
Diabetic nephropathy is a clinical syndrome characterised by albuminuria on at least two occasions that are separated by 3–6 months, in people with diabetes. Diabetic nephropathy is usually accompanied by hypertension, progressive rise in proteinuria, and decline in renal function. In type 1 diabetes, five stages have been proposed. Of these stages, stages 1 and 2 are equivalent to pre-clinical nephropathy and are detected only by imaging or biopsy. Stage 3 is synonymous with early nephropathy, the clinical term used in this chapter. Stage 4 nephropathy is also known clinically as late nephropathy, and this term will be used for the remainder of this chapter. Stage 5 represents the progression to end stage renal disease. **Population:** For the purpose of this review, we have included people with diabetes and both early nephropathy, synonymous with microalbuminuria, usually defined by albuminuria level of 30–300 mg/day (or albumin/creatinine ratio of 30–300 mg/g [3.4–34 mg/mmol]), and late nephropathy, synonymous with macroalbuminuria, characterised by albuminuria > 300 mg/day (or albumin/creatinine ratio > 300 mg/g [34 mg/mmol]). The treatment of people with diabetes and end stage renal disease is not covered in this chapter.

INCIDENCE/ PREVALENCE
In 1997, the worldwide prevalence of diabetes was 124 million and is expected to increase to 221 million in 2010.[1] In the UK, 1.4 million people had been diagnosed with diabetes in 1998, and estimates suggest 1 million more have diabetes, but have not yet been diagnosed.[2] After 20 years of diabetes, the cumulative risk of proteinuria is 27% in type 2 and 28% in type 1.[3] In both type 1 and type 2 diabetes, the overall prevalence of microalbuminuria and macroalbuminuria is about 30–35%.[4] In addition, the incidence of diabetic nephropathy is increasing, in part due to the growing epidemic of type 2 diabetes and increased life expectancies; for example, in the USA, the incidence has increased by 150% in the past decade.[5]

AETIOLOGY/ RISK FACTORS
Duration of diabetes, older age, male gender, smoking status, and poor glycaemic control have all been found to be risk factors in the development of nephropathy.[6,7] In addition, certain ethnic groups seem to be at greater risk for developing diabetic nephropathy. Microalbuminuria is less pathognomonic among type 2 diabetics, because hypertension, which commonly complicates type 2 diabetes, can also cause microalbuminuria. Hypertension can also cause renal insufficiency, so the time to development of renal insufficiency can be shorter in type 2 diabetes than in type 1. For people who have an atypical course, renal biopsy may be advisable. In addition, there are some differences in the progression of type 1 and type 2 diabetic nephropathy. In type 2 diabetics, albuminuria is more often present at diagnosis. Hypertension is also more common in type 2 diabetic nephropathy. Finally, microalbuminuria is less predictive of late nephropathy in type 2 diabetics compared with type 1.[8]

PROGNOSIS
People with microalbuminuria are at increased risk for progression to macroalbuminuria and end stage renal disease. The course of renal function is similar between type 1 and type 2 diabetes. The natural history of diabetic nephropathy is better defined in type 1 than type 2 diabetes. In type 2 diabetes, the course can be more difficult to predict, primarily because the date of onset ▶

of diabetes is less commonly known and comorbid conditions can contribute to renal disease. Without specific interventions, about 80% of people with type 1 diabetes and 20–40% of people with type 2 diabetes with microalbuminuria will progress to macroalbuminuria.[9] Diabetic nephropathy is associated with poor outcomes. Diabetic nephropathy is the most common cause of end stage renal disease in the UK, accounting for 20% of all cases[10] whereas, in the USA, diabetes accounts for 48% of all new cases of end stage renal disease.[11] People with type 1 diabetes and proteinuria have been found to have a 40-fold greater risk of mortality than people without proteinuria.[12] The prognostic significance of proteinuria is less extreme in type 2 diabetes, although people with proteinuria do have a four-fold risk of death compared with people without proteinuria.[13] In addition, increased cardiovascular risk has been associated with albuminuria in people with diabetes.[14] African Americans, Native Americans, and Mexican Americans have a much higher risk of developing end stage renal disease in the setting of diabetes compared with white people.[9,15] In the USA, African American people with diabetes progress to end stage renal disease at a significantly more rapid rate than white people with diabetes.[16] In England, the rates for initiating treatment for end stage renal disease are 4.2 and 3.7 times higher for African Caribbeans and Indo Asians compared with white people.[17] The Pima tribe of Native Americans, located in southwestern USA, have much higher rates of diabetic nephropathy compared with white people, and also progress to end stage renal disease at a faster rate.[18]

Please refer to the Clinical Evidence website for full text and references.

What are the effects of preventive interventions?

LIKELY TO BE BENEFICIAL

Screening and referral to foot care clinics

One RCT found that a diabetes screening and protection programme (involving referral to a foot clinic if high risk features were present) reduced the risk of major amputation compared with usual care after 2 years.

UNKNOWN EFFECTIVENESS

Education

One systematic review found insufficient evidence about the effects of patient education for preventing foot ulcers, serious foot lesions, or amputation.

Therapeutic footwear

In people with diabetes and previous diabetic foot ulcer, one RCT found no significant difference in rates of foot ulceration between therapeutic footwear and usual footwear.

What are the effects of treatments?

BENEFICIAL

Pressure off-loading with non-removable cast

RCTs found that pressure off-loading with total contact casting or non-removable fibreglass casts improved healing of non-infected diabetic foot ulcers compared with traditional dressing changes, removable cast walkers or half shoes, or specialised cloth shoes.

LIKELY TO BE BENEFICIAL

Human skin equivalent

One RCT found that human skin equivalent increased ulcer healing rates compared with saline moistened gauze in people with chronic neuropathic non-infected foot ulcers.

Systemic hyperbaric oxygen (for infected ulcers)

One RCT identified by a systematic review found that systemic hyperbaric oxygen plus usual care reduced amputation rates at 10 weeks compared with usual care alone in people with severely infected diabetic foot ulcers, but one small RCT found no significant difference between treatments in major amputation rates. The second RCT but may have been too small to detect a clinically important difference.

Topical growth factors

One systematic review found that topical growth factors increased healing rates compared with placebo in people with non-infected diabetic foot ulcers.

UNKNOWN EFFECTIVENESS

Cultured human dermis

One systematic review found insufficient evidence of the effects of cultured human dermis on ulcer healing in people with non-infected diabetic foot ulcers.

Foot ulcers and amputations in diabetes

◄ **Pressure off-loading with felted foam versus pressure relief half shoe**

One RCT found no significant difference in time to ulcer healing between a pressure off-loading felted foam dressing and a pressure relief half shoe.

Systemic hyperbaric oxygen (for non-infected, non-ischaemic ulcers)

One small RCT found no significant difference between hyperbaric oxygen plus usual care and usual care alone in ulcer healing at 4 weeks in people with non-infected, neuropathic, non-ischaemic ulcers.

DEFINITION Diabetic foot ulceration is full thickness penetration of the dermis of the foot in a person with diabetes. Ulcer severity is often classified using the Wagner system. Grade 1 ulcers are superficial ulcers involving the full skin thickness but no underlying tissues. Grade 2 ulcers are deeper, penetrating down to ligaments and muscle, but not involving bone or abscess formation. Grade 3 ulcers are deep ulcers with cellulitis or abscess formation, often complicated with osteomyelitis. Ulcers with localised gangrene are classified as Grade 4 and those with extensive gangrene involving the entire foot are classified as Grade 5.

INCIDENCE/ PREVALENCE Studies conducted in Australia, Finland, the UK, and the USA have reported the annual incidence of foot ulcers among people with diabetes as 2.5–10.7%, and the annual incidence of amputation as 0.25–1.8%.[1–10]

AETIOLOGY/ RISK FACTORS Long term risk factors for foot ulcers and amputation include duration of diabetes, poor glycaemic control, microvascular complications (retinopathy, nephropathy, and neuropathy) and peripheral vascular disease. The strongest predictors of foot complications are altered foot sensation, foot deformities, and previous foot ulcer or amputation.[1–10]

PROGNOSIS People with diabetes are at risk of foot ulcers, infections, and vascular insufficiency. Amputation is indicated if these are severe or do not improve with conservative treatment. As well as affecting quality of life, these complications account for a large proportion of the healthcare costs of diabetes. For people with healed diabetic foot ulcers, the 5 year cumulative rate of ulcer recurrence is 66% and of amputation is 12%.[11]

Please refer to the Clinical Evidence website for full text and references.

Search date September 2003

Amaryllis Campbell

What are the effects of interventions in adolescents with type 1 diabetes? New

LIKELY TO BE BENEFICIAL

Educational interventions (compared with controls) New

We found no systematic review or RCTs evaluating a specific type of education or using HbA1c as the only method for measuring glycated haemoglobin. One systematic review found that, compared with controls, different educational and psychosocial interventions in adolescents with type 1 diabetes produced a small improvement in quality of life and glycated haemoglobin (measured using a variety of methods). However, most of the RCTs in the review were small studies, most of the interventions lacked any theoretical basis, and many of the outcome measures were not validated or standardised. We found no systematic review or RCTs evaluating the effects of education in adolescents with type 1 diabetes on the incidence of hypoglycaemia, diabetic ketoacidosis, neuropsychological impairment, weight gain, or fluid retention.

UNKNOWN EFFECTIVENESS

Different frequencies of insulin administration New

We found no systematic review or RCTs specifically evaluating the effects of frequency of insulin administration in adolescents with type 1 diabetes for the outcomes of rate of rise of glycated haemoglobin (measured as HbA1c), quality of life, incidence of and mortality from hypoglycaemia or diabetic ketoacidosis, weight gain, fluid retention, neuropsychological impairment, or all cause mortality.

Different frequencies of self blood glucose monitoring New

We found no systematic review or RCTs specifically evaluating the effects of frequency of self blood glucose monitoring in adolescents with type 1 diabetes for the outcomes of rate of rise of glycated haemoglobin (measured as HbA1c), quality of life, incidence of and mortality from hypoglycaemia or diabetic ketoacidosis, weight gain, fluid retention, neuropsychological impairment, or all cause mortality.

Intensive treatment programmes (compared with conventional treatment programmes) New

We found no systematic review or RCTs specifically in adolescents comparing intensive treatment programmes with conventional treatment programmes for the outcomes of rate of rise of glycated haemoglobin (measured as HbA1c), quality of life, incidence of and mortality from hypoglycaemia or diabetic ketoacidosis, weight gain, fluid retention, neuropsychological impairment, or all cause mortality.

What are the effects of interventions in adults with type 1 diabetes? New

TRADE OFF BETWEEN BENEFITS AND HARMS

Intensive treatment programmes (compared with conventional treatment programmes) New

One RCT identified by a systematic review and two RCTs found that, compared with conventional treatment programmes, intensive treatment programmes reduced ▶

Glycaemic control in diabetes: type 1

glycated haemoglobin levels at follow up varying from 1 to 10 years. The two RCTs reported different findings on quality of life measures and hypoglycaemia. One RCT found no significant difference between intensive and conventional treatment programmes in diabetes related quality of life but found an increase in incidence of severe hypoglycaemia with intensive treatment programmes. The other RCT found that, compared with conventional treatment, intensive treatment improved diabetes dependent quality of life but found no significant difference in the perceived frequency of hypoglycaemia. One systematic review found that compared with conventional treatment, intensive treatment increased hypoglycaemia, diabetic ketoacidosis (when the treatment programme involved the use of insulin pumps), and mortality associated with acute complications of intensive treatment but found no significant difference in all cause mortality.

Continuous subcutaneous insulin infusion (compared with multiple daily subcutaneous insulin injections) New

One crossover RCT found that, compared with multiple daily subcutaneous injections of a quick acting insulin analogue insulin aspart, delivery of insulin aspart by continuous subcutaneous infusion improved glycated haemoglobin levels (measured as HbA1c) and quality of life scores at 16 weeks in people with type 1 diabetes and longstanding poor glycaemic control. This RCT found more episodes of mild hypoglycaemia per patient week with continuous subcutaneous infusion but found no significant difference in incidence of severe hypoglycaemia at 16 weeks. Another RCT found no significant difference at 9 months between continuous subcutaneous infusion of insulin lispro and multiple daily injections of insulin lispro in glycated haemoglobin (measured as HbA1c), quality of life scores, or hypoglycaemia in people with type 1 diabetes previously receiving two or more insulin injections a day. The potential disadvantages of continuous subcutaneous insulin infusion include the risk of diabetic ketoacidosis owing to disconnection or malfunction of the pump and infection.

UNKNOWN EFFECTIVENESS

Different frequencies of self blood glucose monitoring New

We found no systematic review or RCTs specifically evaluating the effects of frequency of self blood glucose monitoring in adults with type 1 diabetes for the outcomes of rate of rise of glycated haemoglobin (measured as HbA1c), quality of life, incidence of and mortality from hypoglycaemia or diabetic ketoacidosis, weight gain, fluid retention, neuropsychological impairment, or all cause mortality.

Educational interventions (compared with controls) New

One RCT identified by a systematic review found no significant difference in glycated haemoglobin (measured as HbA1c) levels at 18 months between education in self monitoring of blood glucose, self management education, or usual care but was incompletely reported and may have lacked power to detect clinically important differences. We found no systematic review or RCTs specifically comparing the effects of group versus individual educational interventions or secondary care versus primary care educational interventions in adults with type 1 diabetes for the outcomes of interest. Given the nature of type 1 diabetes and the central importance of self management of the condition, all individuals with type 1 diabetes will have received some education at diagnosis; most studies of the effects of education will therefore be examining the impact of subsequent educational interventions. It may be difficult to separate out the effects of individual components of what typically will be a complex package of care, including elements of education, self management training, psychological support, and optimisation of insulin regimes. ►

DEFINITION

The term diabetes mellitus encompasses a group of disorders characterised by chronic hyperglycaemia with disturbances of carbohydrate, fat, and protein metabolism resulting from defects of insulin secretion, insulin action, or both. The World Health Organization definition now recognises diabetes as a progressive disorder of glucose metabolism in which individuals may move between normoglycaemia, impaired glucose tolerance, or impaired fasting glycaemia and frank hyperglycaemia. Type 1 diabetes occurs when the pancreas produces too little insulin or no insulin at all, because of destruction of the pancreatic islet β cells, usually attributable to an autoimmune process. Markers of autoimmune destruction (autoantibodies to islet cells, autoantibodies to insulin, or autoantibodies to both islet cells and insulin, and to glutamic acid decarboxylase) can be found in 85–90% of individuals with type 1 diabetes when fasting diabetic hyperglycaemia is first detected.[1] The definition of type 1 diabetes also includes individuals with β cell destruction who are prone to ketoacidosis but for which no specific cause can be found. However it excludes those forms of β cell destruction for which a specific cause can be found (e.g. cystic fibrosis, pancreatitis, cancer of the pancreas).[2] Type 2 diabetes results from defects in both insulin secretion and insulin action. The risk of type 2 diabetes increases with age and lack of physical activity, and occurs more frequently in individuals with obesity, hypertension, and dyslipidaemia (the metabolic syndrome). It occurs more frequently in women with previous gestational diabetes. There is also evidence of a familial predisposition. Type 2 diabetes is not covered in this chapter. **Diagnosis:** In the presence of symptoms (such as thirst, passing increased volumes of urine, blurring of vision, and weight loss) diabetes may be diagnosed on the basis of a single random elevated plasma glucose (≥ 11.1 mmol/L). In the absence of symptoms the diagnosis should be based on at least one additional blood glucose result in the diabetic range, either from a random sample, or fasting (plasma blood glucose ≥ 7.0 mmol/L) or from the oral glucose tolerance test (plasma blood glucose ≥ 11.1 mmol/L 2 hours after a 75 g glucose load).[2] **Population:** For the purpose of this chapter, we have included adolescents and adults with type 1 diabetes, but excluded pregnant women and people who are acutely unwell for example after surgery or myocardial infarction.

INCIDENCE/ PREVALENCE

It is estimated that slightly more than 218 000 people develop type 1 diabetes worldwide annually, of whom about 40% are children. The incidence varies considerably between populations, with 60 000 new cases occurring annually in Europe, 45 000 new cases in the South East Asian region, 36 000 new cases in North America, and the lowest number of new cases, 6,900 annually, in the African region.[3] There seems to be a worldwide increase in the incidence of type 1 diabetes in both high and low incidence populations.[4] The prevalence of type 1 diabetes is currently estimated as 5.3 million people worldwide, and also varies between populations, reflecting both the variation in incidence rates and differing population structures and mortality.[3]

AETIOLOGY/ RISK FACTORS

Two main aetiological forms of type 1 diabetes are recognised. Autoimmune diabetes mellitus results from autoimmune mediated destruction of the β cells of the pancreas. The rate of destruction varies, but all individuals with this form of diabetes eventually become dependent on insulin for survival. Peak incidence of autoimmune diabetes is during childhood and adolescence but it may occur at any age. There is a genetic predisposition and people with this type of diabetes may have other autoimmune disorders.[5] Certain viruses have been associated with β cell destruction, including rubella, Coxsackie B, and cytomegalovirus. Other environmental factors are probably also contributory, but these are poorly defined and understood. Idiopathic diabetes (in which the cause is unidentified) is more common in individuals of African and Asian origin.[2]

Glycaemic control in diabetes: type 1

PROGNOSIS   Untreated, most people with type 1 diabetes, particularly those with autoimmune diabetes mellitus, will experience increasing blood glucose levels, progressing to ketoacidosis or non-ketotic hyperosmolar states resulting in coma and death. The course of idiopathic diabetes may be more varied with some people experiencing permanent lack of insulin and a tendency to ketoacidosis, although in others the requirement for insulin treatment may fluctuate.[2] However most people with type 1 diabetes require insulin for survival, and are described as insulin dependent. The long term effects of diabetes include retinopathy, nephropathy, and neuropathy. Individuals with diabetes mellitus are also at increased risk of cardiovascular, cerebrovascular, and peripheral vascular disease. Good glycaemic control can reduce the risk of developing diabetic complications.[6]

Please refer to the Clinical Evidence website for full text and references.

Endocrine disorders

What are the effects of drug treatments in adults with obesity?

TRADE OFF BETWEEN BENEFITS AND HARMS

Sibutramine alone

Systematic reviews and subsequent RCTs found that, in people having dietary interventions with or without exercise, sibutramine promoted modest weight loss at 8 weeks, 6 months, and 1 year compared with placebo in obese adults, in both those who did and who did not have diabetes, hypertension, hyperlipidaemia, or binge eating disorder. RCTs in obese adults who had lost weight by taking sibutramine found limited evidence that sibutramine was more effective than placebo for weight maintenance. Other RCTs found that weight regain occurred when sibutramine was discontinued. One RCT found that sibutramine achieved greater weight loss than orlistat or metformin. RCTs provided insufficient evidence to compare sibutramine versus other agents. Sibutramine was temporarily suspended from the market in Italy for use in obesity because of concerns about severe adverse reactions, including arrhythmias, hypertension, and two deaths resulting from cardiac arrest. Two RCTs found no significant difference in the incidence of valvular heart disease between sibutramine and placebo, although these trials may have lacked power to detect a clinically important difference.

Phentermine

One systematic review found that, in people having lifestyle interventions, phentermine promoted modest weight loss compared with placebo in obese adults. RCTs identified by the review provided insufficient evidence to compare phentermine versus other agents. We found insufficient evidence on weight regain and long term safety with phentermine. A European Commission review concluded that a link between phentermine and heart and lung problems could not be excluded.

Mazindol

One systematic review found that, in people having lifestyle interventions, mazindol promoted modest weight loss compared with placebo in obese adults. The review provided insufficient evidence to compare mazindol versus other agents. We found one case report of pulmonary hypertension diagnosed 1 year after stopping treatment with mazindol. We found one case series of mazindol in people with stable cardiac disease that reported cardiac events such as atrial fibrillation and syncope. We found insufficient evidence on weight regain and long term safety.

Diethylpropion

One systematic review found that, in people having lifestyle interventions, diethylpropion promoted modest weight loss compared with placebo in obese adults. The review provided insufficient evidence to compare diethylpropion versus other agents. We found two case reports describing pulmonary hypertension and psychosis with diethylpropion. We found insufficient evidence on weight regain and long term safety. A European Commission review concluded that a link between diethylpropion and heart and lung problems could not be excluded.

Fluoxetine

One systematic review found that, in people having lifestyle interventions, fluoxetine promoted modest weight loss compared with placebo in obese adults. We ▶

found insufficient evidence on weight regain and long term safety of fluoxetine in obesity. One systematic review of antidepressant treatment found an association between selective serotonin reuptake inhibitors such as fluoxetine and uncommon but serious adverse events, including bradycardia, bleeding, granulocytopenia, seizures, hyponatraemia, hepatotoxicity, serotonin syndrome, and extrapyramidal effects.

Orlistat

Systematic reviews and subsequent RCTs found that, in people on a low calorie diet, orlistat modestly increased weight loss at 6–12 months compared with placebo in obese adults, in both those who did and who did not have diabetes, hyperlipidaemia, and hypertension. One RCT in obese people with hypercholesterolaemia found that orlistat plus fluvastatin increased weight loss compared with orlistat or fluvastatin alone. Another RCT found that orlistat was less effective than sibutramine in achieving weight loss. Adverse effects such as oily spotting from the rectum, flatulence, and faecal urgency occurred in a high proportion of people taking orlistat. We found insufficient evidence on weight regain and long term safety.

UNKNOWN EFFECTIVENESS

Sibutramine plus orlistat (insufficient evidence to compare with sibutramine alone)

One RCT provided insufficient evidence to compare sibutramine plus orlistat versus sibutramine alone.

What are the effects of bariatric surgery in adults with morbid obesity?

LIKELY TO BE BENEFICIAL

Gastric bypass (increased weight loss compared with gastroplasty or gastric banding)

RCTs provided moderate evidence that gastric bypass promoted greater weight loss than either gastroplasty or gastric banding. Five RCTs identified by a systematic review found that gastric bypass increased weight loss compared with horizontal gastroplasty. Two RCTs identified by the review found that gastric bypass increased weight loss at 1–3 years compared with vertical banded gastroplasty but another two RCTs found no significant difference between the procedures. One small RCT identified by the review found limited evidence of greater weight loss with gastric bypass than with gastric banding or vertical banded gastroplasty. Another small RCT identified by the review found that gastric bypass increased the proportion of people with 50% weight loss at 18 months compared with vertical banded gastroplasty or gastrogastrostomy. Perioperative mortalities were similar for these procedures. Postoperative complications were common and varied by type of procedure performed.

Laparoscopic bariatric surgery (reduced wound infections and risk of incisional hernias compared with open bariatric surgery, no significant difference in weight loss)

Five RCTs found no significant difference in weight loss between open and laparoscopic bariatric procedures. The RCTs found consistent evidence that laparoscopic surgery reduced the incidence of wound and incisional hernia complications compared with open surgery. They found more limited evidence that ▶

laparoscopic procedures decreased length of hospital stay compared with open procedures; but data are insufficient to draw conclusions about other complication rates.

TRADE OFF BETWEEN BENEFITS AND HARMS

Bariatric surgery (more effective for clinically important weight loss in morbidly obese adults than non-surgical treatment but operative complication rates common)

One RCT and one cohort study in morbidly obese adults identified by three systematic reviews found that bariatric surgery (horizontal gastroplasty, vertical banded gastroplasty, gastric bypass, or gastric banding) was more effective than non-surgical treatment in increasing weight loss in people with morbid obesity. The cohort study found that, on average, bariatric surgery for obesity resulted in weight losses of 25–44 kg after 1–2 years (compared with matched participants who did not have surgery) and sustained weight loss of 20 kg up to 8 years later. The risk of death from bariatric surgery is estimated to be 0–1.5%. Operative and postoperative complications are common and vary with the type of bariatric procedure performed. The reviews identified no RCTs and we found no observational studies of sufficient quality comparing biliopancreatic diversion versus non-surgical treatment.

UNKNOWN EFFECTIVENESS

Biliopancreatic diversion (no studies comparing biliopancreatic diversion versus other bariatric techniques)

Three systematic reviews identified no RCTs and we found no observational studies of sufficient quality comparing biliopancreatic diversion versus other bariatric procedures.

Gastric banding (less effective in reducing weight than gastric bypass; insufficient evidence to assess benefits and harms compared with gastroplasty)

One small RCT identified by a systematic review found limited evidence that gastric banding was less effective than gastric bypass in reducing weight. Two RCTs found inconclusive results regarding weight loss with gastric banding compared with vertical banded gastroplasty. There were no postoperative deaths in either RCT. Postoperative complications were common and varied by type of procedure performed. There is insufficient evidence to recommend one procedure over the other.

Gastroplasty (less effective in reducing weight than gastric bypass; insufficient evidence to assess benefits and harms compared with gastric banding)

Two RCTs found inconclusive results regarding weight loss with vertical banded gastroplasty compared with gastric banding. Five RCTs identified by a systematic review found that horizontal gastroplasty was less effective than gastric bypass for increasing weight loss. Four RCTs identified by the review found that vertical banded gastroplasty was less effective than gastric bypass in increasing weight loss at 1–3 years but another two RCTs found no significant difference between the procedures. Perioperative mortalities were similar for these procedures. Postoperative complications were common and varied by type of procedure performed. There is insufficient evidence to recommend one procedure over another.

Obesity

DEFINITION   Obesity is a chronic condition characterised by an excess of body fat. It is most often defined by the body mass index (BMI), a mathematical formula that is highly correlated with body fat. BMI is weight in kilograms divided by height in metres squared (kg/m^2). Worldwide, adults with BMIs between 25–30 kg/m^2 are categorised as overweight, and those with BMIs above 30 kg/m^2 are categorised as obese.[1,2] Nearly 5 million US adults used prescription weight loss medication between 1996 and 1998. A quarter of users were not overweight. Inappropriate use of prescription medication is more common among women, white people, and Hispanic people.[3] The National Institutes of Health in the USA has issued guidelines for obesity treatment, which indicate that all obese adults (BMI > 30 kg/m^2) and all adults with a BMI of 27 kg/m^2 or more and concomitant risk factors or diseases are candidates for drug treatment.[1] Morbidly obese adults (BMI > 40 kg/m^2) and all adults with a BMI of 35 kg/m^2 or more and concomitant risk factors are candidates for bariatric surgery.

INCIDENCE/ PREVALENCE   Obesity has increased steadily in many countries since 1900. In the UK in 2001, it was estimated that 21% of men and 24% of women were obese.[4] In the past decade alone, the prevalence of obesity in the USA has increased from 22.9% between 1988 and 1994, to 30.5% between 1999 and 2000.[5]

AETIOLOGY/ RISK FACTORS   Obesity is the result of long term mismatches in energy balance where daily energy intake exceeds daily energy expenditure.[6] Energy balance is modulated by a myriad of factors, including metabolic rate, appetite, diet, and physical activity.[7] Although these factors are influenced by genetic traits, the increase in obesity prevalence in the past few decades cannot be explained by changes in the human gene pool, and is more often attributed to environmental changes that promote excessive food intake and discourage physical activity.[7,8] Less commonly, obesity may also be induced by drugs (e.g. high dose glucocorticoids), or be secondary to a variety of neuroendocrine disorders such as Cushing's syndrome and polycystic ovary syndrome.[9]

PROGNOSIS   Obesity is a risk factor for several chronic diseases, including hypertension, dyslipidaemia, diabetes, cardiovascular disease, sleep apnoea, osteoarthritis, and some cancers.[1] The relationship between increasing body weight and mortality is curvilinear, where mortality is highest among adults with very low body weight (BMI < 18.5 kg/m^2) and among adults with the highest body weight (BMI > 35 kg/m^2).[2] Results from five prospective cohort studies and 1991 national statistics suggest that the number of annual deaths attributable to obesity among US adults is about 280 000.[10] Obese adults also have more annual admissions to hospitals, more outpatient visits, higher prescription drug costs, and worse health related quality of life than normal weight adults.[11,12]

Please refer to the Clinical Evidence website for full text and references.

Prevention of cardiovascular events in diabetes

Search date October 2003

Ronald Sigal, Janine Malcolm, and Hilary Meggison

What are the effects of promoting smoking cessation in people with diabetes?

LIKELY TO BE BENEFICIAL

Smoking cessation*

We found no RCTs on promotion of smoking cessation specifically in people with diabetes. Observational evidence and extrapolation from evidence in people without diabetes suggest that promotion of smoking cessation is likely to reduce cardiovascular events.

*No RCT but observational evidence suggests some benefit.

What are the effects of controlling blood pressure in people with diabetes?

BENEFICIAL

Antihypertensive treatment (compared with no antihypertensive treatment)

One systematic review and RCTs have found that blood pressure lowering with antihypertensive agents in people with diabetes and hypertension reduces cardio-vascular morbidity and mortality compared with no antihypertensive treatment.

Lower target blood pressures

Large RCTs including people with diabetes and hypertension have found that control of blood pressure to a target diastolic blood pressure of no more than 80 mm Hg reduces the risk of major cardiovascular events. One RCT in normo-tensive people with diabetes found that intensive blood pressure lowering reduced cerebral vascular events but found no significant difference in cardiovascular death, myocardial infarction, congestive heart failure, or all cause mortality.

TRADE OFF BETWEEN BENEFITS AND HARMS

Different antihypertensive drugs

Systematic reviews and RCTs have found that angiotensin converting enzyme inhibitors, diuretics, β blockers, and calcium channel blockers all reduce cardio-vascular morbidity and mortality in people with diabetes and hypertension. However, there are differences in the types of adverse effects reported with different antihypertensive drugs. RCTs have found that people taking atenolol gained more weight than those taking captopril, an increase in risk of congestive heart failure with lisinopril or amlodipine compared with chlorthalidone, a higher frequency of headache with diltiazem compared with diuretics or β blockers, and a higher rate of withdrawal from treatment because of adverse effects with atenolol compared with losartan.

▶

Prevention of cardiovascular events in diabetes

What are the effects of treating dyslipidaemia in people with diabetes?

BENEFICIAL

Statins

One systematic review and RCTs have found that statins reduce cardiovascular morbidity and mortality compared with placebo.

LIKELY TO BE BENEFICIAL

Aggressive versus moderate lipid lowering with statins

One RCT found that, compared with usual care, treatment with atorvastatin to achieve a target low density lipoprotein below 2.6 mmol/L (< 100 mg/dL) reduces cardiovascular morbidity and mortality. Another RCT found no significant difference between a lower target low density lipoprotein (1.55–2.20 mmol/L) using lovastatin, along with cholestyramine if necessary, and a moderate target low density lipoprotein (3.36–3.62 mmol/L) in 4 year event rate for myocardial infarction and death.

Fibrates

One RCT found that gemfibrozil reduced cardiovascular events over 5 years compared with placebo whereas another smaller RCT found no significant difference. One RCT found that bezafibrate reduced cardiovascular events compared with placebo.

Low versus standard statin dose in older people

One RCT found no significant difference in cardiovascular events between low dose pravastatin (5 mg/day) and standard dose pravastatin (10–20 mg/day) over 4 years.

What are the effects of antiplatelet drugs in people with diabetes?

LIKELY TO BE BENEFICIAL

Adding glycoprotein IIb/IIIa inhibitors to heparin in acute coronary syndromes

We found no RCTs comparing glycoprotein IIb/IIIa inhibitors versus no antiplatelet treatment. One RCT in people presenting with unstable angina or acute myocardial infarction without ST segment elevation found that addition of tirofiban (a glycoprotein IIb/IIIa inhibitor) to heparin reduced the composite outcome of death, myocardial infarction, or refractory ischaemia at 180 days compared with heparin alone. This RCT found no significant difference between tirofiban plus heparin and heparin alone in risk of bleeding in people already taking aspirin.

Clopidogrel

We found no RCTs comparing only clopidogrel versus placebo. One RCT in people with diabetes and with recent ischaemic stroke, myocardial infarction, or established peripheral arterial disease found no significant difference between clopidogrel and aspirin at 28 days in cardiovascular events. This RCT also found a lower proportion of people hospitalised for a bleeding event with clopidogrel than with aspirin.

TRADE OFF BETWEEN BENEFITS AND HARMS

Prophylactic aspirin

One systematic review found that, compared with controls, antiplatelet treatment mainly with aspirin did not significantly reduce the combined risk of non-fatal myocardial infarction, non-fatal stroke, death from a vascular cause, or death from an unknown cause in people with diabetes and cardiovascular disease diagnosis. The review found that antiplatelet treatment was associated with an increase in the risk of major extracranial haemorrhage and haemorrhagic stroke, but the results for people with diabetes were not reported separately.

UNLIKELY TO BE BENEFICIAL

Adding clopidogrel to aspirin in acute coronary syndromes

One RCT in people presenting with unstable angina or non-Q-wave myocardial infarction and also taking aspirin found no significant reduction in cardiovascular events after 12 months with addition of clopidogrel compared with placebo. This RCT also found a higher proportion of major bleeds with addition of clopidogrel than with placebo.

What are the effects of blood glucose control for prevention of cardiovascular disease in diabetes?

LIKELY TO BE BENEFICIAL

Intensive versus conventional glycaemic control

One systematic review found that, compared with conventional glycaemic control, intensive glycaemic control for more than 2 years reduced the occurrence of first major cardiovascular event in people with type 1 diabetes. Two RCTs found no significant difference in cardiovascular morbidity and mortality with intensive compared with conventional glycaemic control in people with type 2 diabetes. These RCTs also found an increase in weight gain and hypoglycaemic episodes with intensive compared with conventional treatment.

Metformin versus diet alone as initial treatment in overweight or obese people with type 2 diabetes

One RCT in overweight or obese people with type 2 diabetes found that intensive treatment with metformin compared with conventional treatment with diet alone reduced myocardial infarction but not stroke over 5 years. This RCT found no significant increase in major hypoglycaemic episodes in the metformin group compared with the diet only group.

What are the effects of treating multiple risk factors in prevention of cardiovascular disease in people with diabetes?

BENEFICIAL

Intensive multiple risk factor treatment

One RCT found that, compared with conventional treatment according to clinical guidelines, intensive treatment of multiple risk factors with strict treatment goals in people with type 2 diabetes and microalbuminuria reduced cardiovascular disease over 8 years. Multiple risk factor treatment included simultaneously targeting diet, exercise, glycaemic control, blood pressure, treatment of microalbuminuria, and antiplatelet treatment. We found no systematic review or RCTs comparing treatment of multiple risk factors with treatment of a single risk factor for cardiovascular outcomes.

What are the effects of revascularisation procedures in people with diabetes?

BENEFICIAL

Coronary artery bypass graft (CABG) compared with percutaneous transluminal coronary angioplasty (PTCA)

One systematic review found that, in people with diabetes, CABG reduces all cause mortality at 4 years after initial revascularisation compared with PTCA, but it found no significant difference at 6.5 years. One large RCT in people with diabetes and multivessel coronary artery disease found that CABG reduces mortality or myocardial infarction within 8 years compared with PTCA. Another smaller RCT found a non-significant reduction in mortality with CABG compared with PTCA at 4 years.

Stent plus glycoprotein IIb/IIIa inhibitors in people undergoing PTCA

RCTs in people with diabetes undergoing PTCA have found that the combination of stent and a glycoprotein IIb/IIIa inhibitor reduces cardiovascular morbidity and mortality compared with stent plus placebo.

TRADE OFF BETWEEN BENEFITS AND HARMS

CABG compared with PTCA plus stent

One RCT in people with diabetes and multivessel coronary artery disease found no significant difference, at time of discharge, between CABG and PTCA plus stent in cardiovascular morbidity or mortality, but found an increase in risk of stroke. However, the same RCT found that, compared with PTCA plus stent, CABG reduced cardiovascular risk at 1 year.

UNKNOWN EFFECTIVENESS

PTCA compared with thrombolysis

We found no systematic review or RCTs comparing PTCA versus thrombolysis for prevention of cardiovascular events in people with diabetes. One RCT, in people with diabetes presenting with an acute myocardial infarction, found no significant difference between PTCA and thrombolysis with alteplase in simple outcome of death or composite outcome of death, reinfarction, or disabling stroke at 30 days.

DEFINITION   **Diabetes mellitus type 1:** See definition under glycaemic control in diabetes: type 1, p 157. **Cardiovascular disease (CVD):** Atherosclerotic disease of the heart and/or the coronary, cerebral, or peripheral vessels leading to clinical events such as acute myocardial infarction, congestive heart failure, sudden cardiac death, stroke, gangrene, and/or need for revascularisation procedures. **Population:** In previous versions of *Clinical Evidence* we attempted to differentiate between primary and secondary prevention in this topic. However, in middle aged and older people with type 2 diabetes this distinction may not be clinically important. We are not aware of any intervention that has been shown to be effective in secondary prevention but ineffective in primary prevention, or vice versa, in people with diabetes. In most cases a large proportion of people with diabetes entered into CVD prevention trials are middle aged and older with additional CVD risk factors, and a large portion of these actually have undiagnosed CVD.

INCIDENCE/   Diabetes mellitus is a major risk factor for CVD. In the USA, a survey of deaths
PREVALENCE   in 1986 suggested that 60–75% of people with diabetes die from cardiovascular causes.[1] The annual incidence of CVD is increased in people with diabetes (men: RR 2–3; women: RR 3–4, adjusted for age and other cardiovascular risk factors).[2] About 45% of middle aged and older white people with diabetes have evidence of coronary artery disease compared with about 25% of people without diabetes in the same populations. In a Finnish ▶

population based cohort study (1059 people with diabetes and 1373 people without diabetes, aged 45–64 years), the 7 year risk of acute myocardial infarction was as high in adults with diabetes without previous cardiac disease (20.2/100 person years) as it was in people without diabetes with previous cardiac disease (18.8/100 person years).[3]

AETIOLOGY/ RISK FACTORS

Diabetes mellitus increases the risk of CVD. Cardiovascular risk factors in people with diabetes include conventional risk factors (age, prior CVD, cigarette smoking, hypertension, dyslipidaemia, sedentary lifestyle, family history of premature CVD) and more diabetes specific risk factors (elevated urinary protein excretion, poor glycaemic control). Conventional risk factors for CVD contribute to an increase in the relative risk of CVD in people with diabetes to about the same extent as in those without diabetes. One prospective cohort study (164 women and 235 men with diabetes [mean age 65 years] and 437 women and 1099 men without diabetes [mean age 61 years] followed for mortality for a mean of 3.7 years after acute myocardial infarction) found that significantly more people with diabetes died compared with people without diabetes (116/399 [29%] with diabetes v 204/1536 [13%] without diabetes; RR 2.2, 95% CI 1.8 to 2.7).[4] It also found that the mortality risk after myocardial infarction associated with diabetes was higher for women than for men (adjusted HR 2.7, 95% CI 1.8 to 4.2 for women v 1.3, 95% CI 1.0 to 1.8 for men). Physical inactivity is a significant risk factor for cardiovascular events in both men and women. Another cohort study (5125 women with diabetes) found that participation in little (< 1 hour/week) or no physical activity compared with physical activity for at least 7 hours a week was associated with doubling of the risk of a cardiovascular event.[5] A third cohort study (1263 men with diabetes, mean follow up 12 years) found that low baseline cardiorespiratory fitness increased overall mortality compared with moderate or high fitness (RR 2.9, 95% CI 2.1 to 3.6), and overall mortality was higher in those reporting no recreational exercise in the previous 3 months than in those reporting any recreational physical activity in the same period (RR 1.8, 95% CI 1.3 to 2.5).[6] The absolute risk of CVD is almost the same in women as in men with diabetes. Diabetes specific cardiovascular risk factors include the duration of diabetes during adulthood (the years of exposure to diabetes before age 20 years add little to the risk of CVD); raised blood glucose concentrations (reflected in fasting blood glucose or HbA1c); and any degree of microalbuminuria (albuminuria 30–299 mg/24 hours).[7] People with diabetes and microalbuminuria have a higher risk of coronary morbidity and mortality than do people with normal levels of urinary albumin and a similar duration of diabetes (RR 2–3).[8,9] Clinical proteinuria increases the risk of mortality from cardiac events in people with type 2 diabetes (RR 2.61, 95% CI 1.99 to 3.43)[10] and type 1 diabetes (RR 9)[7,11,12] compared with people with the same type of diabetes who have normal albumin excretion. An epidemiological analysis of people with diabetes enrolled in the Heart Outcomes Prevention Evaluation cohort study (3498 people with diabetes and at least 1 other cardiovascular risk factor, age > 55 years, of whom 1140 [32%] had microalbuminuria at baseline; 5 years' follow up) found higher risk for major cardiovascular events in those with microalbuminuria (albumin : creatinine ratio [ACR] ≥ 2.0 mg/mmol) than in those without microalbuminuria (adjusted RR 1.97, 95% CI 1.68 to 2.31), and for all cause mortality (RR 2.15, 95% CI 1.78 to 2.60).[13] It also found an association between ACR and the risk of major cardiovascular events (ACR 0.22–0.57 mg/mmol: RR 0.85, 95% CI 0.63 to 1.14; ACR 0.58–1.62 mg/mmol: RR 1.11, 95% CI 0.86 to 1.43; ACR 1.62–1.99 mg/mmol: RR 1.89, 95% CI 1.52 to 2.36).

PROGNOSIS

Diabetes mellitus increases the risk of mortality or serious morbidity after a coronary event (RR 1.5–3.0).[2,3,14,15] This excess risk is partly accounted for by increased prevalence of other cardiovascular risk factors in people with diabetes. A systematic review (search date 1998, 15 prospective cohort studies) found that, in people with diabetes admitted to hospital for acute myocardial infarction, "stress hyperglycaemia" was associated with significantly higher mortality in hospital compared with lower blood glucose levels (RR 1.7, 95% CI 1.2 to 2.4).[16] One large prospective cohort study (91 285 men aged 40–84 years) found higher all cause and coronary heart disease (CHD) mortality at 5 years' follow up in men with diabetes than in men without coronary artery disease or diabetes (age adjusted RR 3.3, 95% CI 2.6 to 4.1 in men with diabetes and without coronary artery disease v RR 2.3, 95% CI 2.0 to 2.6 in healthy people; RR 5.6, 95% CI 4.9 to 6.3 in men with coronary artery disease but without diabetes v RR 2.2, 95% CI 2.0 to 2.4 in healthy people; RR 12.0, 95% CI 9.9 to 14.6 in men with both risk factors v RR 4.7, 95% CI 4.0 to 5.4 in healthy people).[17] Multivariate analysis did not materially alter these associations. Diabetes mellitus alone is associated with a twofold increase in risk for all cause death, with a threefold increase in risk of death from CHD, and, in people with pre-existing CHD, with a 12-fold increase in risk of death from CHD compared with people with neither risk factor.[17]

Please refer to the Clinical Evidence website for full text and references.

Search date December 2003

Birte Nygaard

What are the effects of treatments for clinical (overt) hypothyroidism?

BENEFICIAL

Levothyroxine (L-thyroxine)

We found no RCTs comparing levothyroxine versus placebo, although there is consensus that treatment is beneficial. Treating clinical (overt) hypothyroidism with thyroid hormone (levothyroxine) can induce hyperthyroidism and reduce bone mass in postmenopausal women and increase the risk of atrial fibrillation.

UNKNOWN EFFECTIVENESS

Levothyroxine (L-thyroxine) plus liothyronine (compared with L-thyroxine alone)

Three small RCTs provided insufficient evidence of outcome improvement between a combination of levothyroxine plus liothyronine and levothyroxine alone. Treating clinical (overt) hypothyroidism with thyroid hormone (levothyroxine) can induce hyperthyroidism and reduce bone mass in postmenopausal women and increase the risk of atrial fibrillation.

What are the effects of treatments for subclinical hypothyroidism?

UNKNOWN EFFECTIVENESS

Levothyroxine (L-thyroxine)

One RCT in women with biochemically defined subclinical hypothyroidism found no significant difference between levothyroxine and placebo in overall symptom improvement at 1 year. The RCT may, however, have lacked power to exclude a clinically important difference between treatments. Another RCT found no significant difference in health related quality of life scores between levothyroxine and placebo. One RCT found inconclusive results about the effect of levothyroxine versus placebo on cognitive function in people with subclinical hypothyroidism. One RCT found that levothyroxine improved left ventricular function at 6 months compared with placebo. Treating subclinical hypothyroidism with thyroid hormone can induce hyperthyroidism and reduce bone mass in postmenopausal women and increase the risk of atrial fibrillation.

DEFINITION　Hypothyroidism is characterised by low levels of blood thyroid hormone. **Clinical (overt) hypothyroidism** is diagnosed on the basis of characteristic clinical features consisting of mental slowing, depression, dementia, weight gain, constipation, dry skin, hair loss, cold intolerance, hoarse voice, irregular menstruation, infertility, muscle stiffness and pain, bradycardia, hypercholesterolaemia, combined with a raised blood level of thyroid stimulating hormone (TSH) (serum TSH levels > 12 mU/L), and a low serum thyroxine T_4 level (serum $T_4 < 60$ nmol/L). **Subclinical hypothyroidism** is diagnosed when serum TSH is raised (serum TSH levels > 4 mU/L) but serum thyroxine is normal and there are no symptoms or signs, or only minor symptoms or signs, of thyroid dysfunction. **Primary hypothyroidism** is seen after destruction of the thyroid gland because of autoimmunity (the most common cause), or ▶

Primary hypothyroidism

medical intervention such as surgery, radioiodine, and radiation. **Secondary hypothyroidism** is seen after pituitary or hypothalamic damage, and results in insufficient production of TSH. Secondary hypothyroidism is not covered in this review. **Euthyroid sick syndrome** is diagnosed when tri-iodothyronine (T_3) levels are low, serum thyroxine is low, and TSH levels are normal or low. Euthyroid sick syndrome is not covered in this review.

INCIDENCE/ PREVALENCE

Hypothyroidism is more common in women than in men (in the UK, the female : male ratio is 6 : 1). One study (2779 people in the UK with a median age of 58 years) found the incidence of clinical (overt) hypothyroidism was 40/10 000 women per year and 6/10 000 men per year. The prevalence was 9.3% in women and 1.3% in men.[1] In areas with high iodine intake, the incidence of hypothyroidism can be higher than in areas with normal or low iodine intake. In Denmark, where there is moderate iodine insufficiency, the overall incidence of hypothyroidism is 1.4/10 000 per year increasing to 8/10 000 per year in people older than 70 years.[2] The incidence of subclinical hypothyroidism increases with age. Up to 10% of women over the age of 60 years have subclinical hypothyroidism (evaluated from data from the Netherlands and USA).[3,4]

AETIOLOGY/ RISK FACTORS

Primary thyroid gland failure can occur as a result of chronic autoimmune thyroiditis, radioactive iodine treatment, or thyroidectomy. Other causes include drug adverse effects (e.g. amiodarone and lithium), transient hypothyroidism due to silent thyroiditis, subacute thyroiditis, or postpartum thyroiditis.

PROGNOSIS

In people with subclinical hypothyroidism, the risk of developing overt hypothyroidism is described in the UK Whickham Survey (25 years' follow up; for women: OR 8, 95% CI 3 to 20; for men: OR 44, 95% CI 19 to 104; if both a raised TSH and positive antithyroid antibodies were present; for women: OR 38, 95% CI 22 to 65; for men: OR 173, 95% CI 81 to 370). For women, the survey found an annual risk of 4.3% per year (if both raised serum TSH and antithyroid antibodies were present), 2.6% per year (if raised serum TSH was present alone); the minimum number of people with raised TSH and antithyroid antibodies who would need treating to prevent this progression to clinical (overt) hypothyroidism in one person over 5 years is 5–8.[1] **Cardiovascular disease:** A large cross-sectional study (25 862 people with serum TSH between 5.1–10 mU/L) found significantly higher mean total cholesterol concentrations in hypothyroid people compared with euthyroid people (5.8 v 5.6 mmol/L).[3] Another study (124 elderly women with subclinical hypothyroidism, 931 euthyroid women) found a significantly increased risk of myocardial infarction in women with subclinical hypothyroidism (OR 2.3, 95% CI 1.3 to 4.0) and of aortic atherosclerosis (OR 1.7, 95% CI 1.1 to 2.6).[4] **Mental health:** Subclinical hypothyroidism is associated with depression.[5] People with subclinical hypothyroidism may have depression that is refractory to both antidepressant drugs and thyroid hormone alone. Memory impairment, hysteria, anxiety, somatic complaints, and depressive features without depression have been described in people with subclinical hypothyroidism.[6]

Please refer to the Clinical Evidence website for full text and references.

Search date February 2004
André Curi, Kimble Matos, and Carlos Pavesio

What are the effects of anti-inflammatory eye drops?

Non-steroidal anti-inflammatory drug eye drops

One RCT found no significant difference between non-steroidal anti-inflammatory drug and placebo eye drops in clinical cure rate after 21 days. Three RCTs found no significant difference between non-steroidal anti-inflammatory drug and steroid eye drops in clinical cure rate after 14 or 21 days.

Steroid eye drops

Steroid eye drops have been standard treatment for anterior uveitis since the early 1950s. However, we found insufficient evidence from RCTs about their effects in people with acute anterior uveitis. One small RCT found no significant difference with steroid (betamethasone phosphate/clobetasone butyrate) eye drops compared with placebo eye drops in symptom severity after 14 or 21 days. Two RCTs found no significant difference between prednisolone and rimexolone in the anterior chamber cell count (a marker of disease severity). One RCT found that prednisolone increased the proportion of people with fewer than five anterior chamber cells per examination field compared with loteprednol after 28 days. The results of a second RCT comparing prednisolone with loteprednol were difficult to interpret. RCTs found that rimexolone and loteprednol were less likely than prednisolone to be associated with increased intraocular pressure, although differences were not statistically significant. Three RCTs found no significant difference between steroid and non-steroidal anti-inflammatory drug eye drops in clinical cure rate after 14 or 21 days.

DEFINITION Anterior uveitis is inflammation of the uveal tract, and includes iritis and iridocyclitis. It can be classified according to its clinical course into acute or chronic anterior uveitis, or according to its clinical appearance into granulomatous or non-granulomatous anterior uveitis. **Acute anterior uveitis** is characterised by an extremely painful red eye, often associated with photophobia and occasionally with decreased visual acuity. **Chronic anterior uveitis** is defined as inflammation lasting over 6 weeks. It is usually asymptomatic, but many people have mild symptoms during exacerbations.

INCIDENCE/ PREVALENCE Acute anterior uveitis is rare, with an annual incidence of 12/100 000 population.[1] It is particularly common in Finland (annual incidence 22.6/ 100 000 population, prevalence 68.7/100 000 population), probably because of genetic factors such as the high frequency of HLA-B27 in the Finnish population.[2] It is equally common in men and women, and more than 90% of cases occur in people older than 20 years of age.[2,3]

AETIOLOGY/ RISK FACTORS No cause is identified in 60–80% of people with acute anterior uveitis. Systemic disorders that may be associated with acute anterior uveitis include ankylosing spondylitis, Reiter's syndrome, juvenile chronic arthritis, Kawasaki syndrome, infectious uveitis, Behçet's syndrome, inflammatory bowel disease, interstitial nephritis, sarcoidosis, multiple sclerosis, Wegener's granulomatosis, Vogt-Koyanagi-Harada syndrome, and masquerade syndromes. Acute anterior uveitis also occurs in association with HLA-B27 not linked to any systemic disease, it may be the manifestation of an isolated eye disorder such as Fuchs' iridocyclitis, Posner-Schlossman syndrome, or Schwartz syndrome. Acute anterior uveitis may occur after surgery or as an adverse drug or hypersensitivity reaction.[2,3]

▶

Acute anterior uveitis

PROGNOSIS Acute anterior uveitis is often self limiting, but we found no evidence about how often it resolves spontaneously, in which people, or over what time period. Complications include posterior synechiae, cataract, glaucoma, and chronic uveitis. In a study of 154 people (232 eyes) with acute anterior uveitis (119 people HLA-B27 positive), visual acuity was better than 20/60 in 209/232 eyes (90%), and 20/60 or worse in 23/232 eyes (10%), including worse than 20/200 (classified as legally blind) in 11/232 eyes (5%).[4]

Please refer to the Clinical Evidence website for full text and references.

Search date July 2004
Jennifer Arnold

What are the effects of interventions to prevent progression of age related macular degeneration?

LIKELY TO BE BENEFICIAL

Antioxidant vitamin and zinc supplementation

One systematic review found modest evidence from one large RCT that, in people with early to late age related macular degeneration, antioxidant vitamins plus zinc supplements reduced the risk of progression and vision loss over 6 years compared with placebo.

UNKNOWN EFFECTIVENESS

Laser to drusen

Two RCTs provided insufficient evidence to assess whether laser to drusen decreased incidence of late age related macular degeneration, choroidal neovascularisation, or geographic atrophy. The first RCT found that threshold laser treatment improved visual acuity after 2 years compared with no treatment, but not compared with subthreshold treatment. The second, larger RCT found no significant difference between laser and no treatment in visual acuity after 1 year. However, subgroup analysis found improved visual acuity where laser treatment had reduced the number of drusen by 50% or more. The RCT also found that, in people with unilateral (but not bilateral) drusen, laser increased the short term incidence of choroidal neovascularisation compared with no treatment.

What are the effects of treatments for exudative age related macular degeneration?

BENEFICIAL

Photodynamic treatment with verteporfin

Two systematic reviews in people with age related macular degeneration found that photodynamic treatment with verteporfin reduced the risk of moderate or severe loss of visual acuity and of legal blindness after 1–2 years in people with vision better than 20/100 or 20/200 compared with placebo. Photodynamic treatment with verteporfin was associated with an initial loss of vision and photosensitive reactions in a small proportion of people.

TRADE OFF BETWEEN BENEFITS AND HARMS

Thermal laser photocoagulation

Four large RCTs found that, in people with well demarcated exudative age related macular degeneration, thermal laser photocoagulation reduced severe visual loss after 2–5 years compared with no treatment, but was associated with an immediate and permanent reduction in visual acuity. Choroidal neovascularisation recurred within 3 years in about half of those treated. One small RCT provided insufficient evidence to compare thermal laser photocoagulation versus submacular surgery.

▶

Age related macular degeneration

External beam radiation

Two large, high quality RCTs and one smaller RCT found no significant difference between low dose external beam radiation and observation alone in moderate visual loss. However, one large RCT and one smaller RCT found that low dose external beam radiation reduced the degree of visual loss compared with placebo. Another smaller RCT found no significant difference in visual loss between high dose external beam radiation and observation. We found insufficient evidence on long term safety, although RCTs found no evidence of toxicity to the optic nerve or retina after 12–24 months.

Submacular surgery

Two small RCTs provided insufficient evidence about the effects of submacular surgery.

LIKELY TO BE INEFFECTIVE OR HARMFUL

Subcutaneous interferon alfa-2a

One large RCT found that, compared with placebo, subcutaneous interferon alfa-2a (an antiangiogenesis drug) increased visual loss after 1 year, although the difference was not significant. The RCT also found evidence of serious ocular and systemic adverse effects.

DEFINITION   Age related macular degeneration (AMD) has two clinical stages: **early AMD** marked by drusen and pigmentary change, and usually associated with normal vision; and **late or sight threatening AMD** associated with a decrease in central vision. Late stage AMD has two forms: **atrophic (or dry) AMD,** characterised by geographic atrophy; and **exudative (or wet) AMD**, characterised by choroidal neovascularisation, which eventually causes a disciform scar.

INCIDENCE/   AMD is a common cause of blindness registration in industrialised countries.
PREVALENCE   Atrophic AMD is more common than the more sight threatening exudative AMD, affecting about 85% of people with AMD.[1] Late (sight threatening) AMD is found in about 2% of all people aged over 50 years, and incidence rises with age (0.7–1.4% of people aged 65–75 years; 11–19% of people aged > 85 years).[2–4]

AETIOLOGY/   Proposed hypotheses for the cause of AMD involve vascular factors and
RISK FACTORS oxidative damage coupled with genetic predisposition.[5] Age is the strongest risk factor. Ocular risk factors for the development of exudative AMD include the presence of soft drusen, macular pigmentary change, choroidal neovascularisation in the other eye, and previous cataract surgery.[6] Systemic risk factors include hypertension, smoking, and a family history of AMD.[5,7,8] Hypertension, diet (especially intake of antioxidant micronutrients), and oestrogen are suspected as causal agents, but the effects of these factors remain unproved.[5]

PROGNOSIS   AMD impairs central vision, which is required for reading, driving, face recognition, and all fine visual tasks. **Atrophic AMD** progresses slowly over many years, and time to legal blindness is highly variable (usually about 5–10 years).[9,10] **Exudative AMD** is more often threatening to vision; 90% of people with severe visual loss owing to AMD have the exudative type. This condition usually manifests with a sudden worsening and distortion of central vision. One study estimated (based on data derived primarily from cohort studies) that the risk of developing exudative AMD in people with bilateral soft drusen was 1–5% at 1 year and 13–18% at 3 years.[11] The observed 5 year rate in a population survey was 7%.[12] Most eyes (estimates vary from 60–90%) with exudative AMD progress to legal blindness and develop a central defect (scotoma) in the visual field.[13–16] Peripheral vision is preserved, allowing the person to be mobile and independent. The ability to read with visual aids depends on the size and density of the central scotoma and the degree to which the person retains sensitivity to contrast. Once exudative AMD has developed in one eye, the other eye is at high risk (cumulative estimated incidence: 10% at 1 year, 28% at 3 years, and 42% at 5 years).[17]

Please refer to the Clinical Evidence website for full text and references.

Bacterial conjunctivitis

Search date February 2004

Justine Smith

What are the effects of antibiotics in adults and children with bacterial conjunctivitis?

BENEFICIAL

Antibiotic treatment in culture positive bacterial conjunctivitis

One systematic review and two subsequent RCTs found that antibiotics (polymyxin–bacitracin, ciprofloxacin, ofloxacin, levofloxacin, or moxifloxacin) increase rates of clinical and microbiological cure compared with placebo. Four RCTs found no significant difference between different antibiotics in clinical or microbiological cure. One RCT found that fusidic acid increased clinical cure rate compared with chloramphenicol. One RCT found that topical netilmicin increased clinical cure rate compared with topical gentamicin. One RCT found that topical levofloxacin increased microbiological cure rate, but not clinical cure rate, compared with topical ofloxacin.

LIKELY TO BE BENEFICIAL

Empirical antibiotic treatment of suspected bacterial conjunctivitis

One systematic review found limited evidence from one RCT that topical norfloxacin increased rates of clinical and microbiological improvement or cure after 5 days compared with placebo. RCTs comparing different topical antibiotics versus each other found no significant difference in rates of clinical or microbiological cure. One RCT found no significant difference between topical polymyxin–bacitracin ointment and oral cefixime for clinical or microbiological improvement or cure.

DEFINITION	Conjunctivitis is any inflammation of the conjunctiva, generally characterised by irritation, itching, foreign body sensation, and watering or discharge. Bacterial conjunctivitis may often be distinguished from other types of conjunctivitis by the presence of a yellow–white mucopurulent discharge. There is also usually a papillary reaction (small bumps with fibrovascular cores on the palpebral conjunctiva, appearing grossly as a fine velvety surface). Bacterial conjunctivitis is usually bilateral. Treatment is often based on clinical suspicion that the conjunctivitis is bacterial, without waiting for results of microbiological investigations. In this topic, we have therefore distinguished effects of empirical treatment from effects of treatment in people with culture positive bacterial conjunctivitis. This review covers only non-gonococcal bacterial conjunctivitis.
INCIDENCE/ PREVALENCE	We found no good evidence on the incidence or prevalence of bacterial conjunctivitis.
AETIOLOGY/ RISK FACTORS	Conjunctivitis may be infectious (caused by bacteria or viruses) or allergic. In adults, bacterial conjunctivitis is less common than viral conjunctivitis, although estimates vary widely (viral conjunctivitis has been reported to account for 8–75% of acute conjunctivitis).[1-3] *Staphylococcus* species are the most common pathogens for bacterial conjunctivitis in adults, followed by *Streptococcus pneumoniae* and *Haemophilus influenzae*.[4,5] In children, bacterial conjunctivitis is more common than viral, and is mainly caused by *Haemophilus influenzae*, *Streptococcus pneumoniae*, and *Moraxella catarrhalis*.[6,7] ▶

PROGNOSIS Most bacterial conjunctivitis is self limiting. One systematic review (search date 2001) found clinical cure or significant improvement with placebo within 2–5 days in 64% of people (99% CI 54% to 73%).[8] Some organisms cause corneal or systemic complications, or both. Otitis media may develop in 25% of children with *H influenzae* conjunctivitis,[9] and systemic meningitis may complicate primary meningococcal conjunctivitis in 18% of people.[10]

Please refer to the Clinical Evidence website for full text and references.

Cataract

Search date November 2003

David Allen

What are the effects of surgery for age related cataract without other ocular co-morbidity?

BENEFICIAL

Manual extracapsular extraction (better than intracapsular extraction)

One RCT found that manual extracapsular extraction plus intraocular lens implant improved visual acuity and quality of life compared with intracapsular extraction plus aphakic glasses. The RCT also found a higher rate of complications with intracapsular extraction plus aphakic glasses than with a manual extracapsular extraction plus intraocular lens implant. The RCT and a systematic review of observational studies found that a higher proportion of people had complications with manual extracapsular extraction than with phaco extracapsular extraction.

Phaco extracapsular extraction (better than manual extracapsular extraction)

We found no systematic review or RCTs comparing phaco extracapsular extraction versus no extraction. One RCT identified by a systematic review found improved vision up to 1 year after phaco extracapsular extraction plus foldable posterior chamber intraocular lens implant compared with manual extracapsular extraction plus rigid posterior chamber intraocular lens implant. The RCT and a systematic review of observational studies found that a higher proportion of people had complications with manual extracapsular extraction than with phaco extracapsular extraction.

DEFINITION	**Cataracts** are cloudy or opaque areas in the lens of the eye (which should usually be completely clear). This results in changes that can impair vision. **Age related (or senile) cataract** is defined as cataract occurring in people over 16 years of age in the absence of known mechanical, chemical, or radiation trauma. This chapter covers treatment for age related cataract. It does not cover cataract in people with diabetes mellitus or recurrent uveitis; these conditions can affect the surgical outcome.
INCIDENCE/ PREVALENCE	Cataract accounts for over 40% of blindness worldwide — causing blindness in about 38 million people.[2] In a rural setting in the USA in the 1970s, the prevalence of visually significant cataract ranged from approximately 5% at the age of 65 years to around 50% in people older than 75 years.[3] The incidence of non-age related cataract within this population is so small that this can be taken as the effective incidence of age related cataract.
AETIOLOGY/ RISK FACTORS	Diet, smoking,[4] and exposure to ultraviolet light[5] are thought to be risk factors in the development of age related cataract. In addition, some people may have a genetic predisposition to development of age related cataract.[6]
PROGNOSIS	Age related cataract progresses with age, but at an unpredictable rate. Cataract surgery is indicated when the chances of significant visual improvement outweigh the risks of a poor surgical outcome. It is not dependent on reaching a specific visual acuity standard. Cataract surgery may also be indicated where the presence of cataract makes it hard to treat or monitor concurrent retinal disease, such as diabetic retinopathy.

Please refer to the Clinical Evidence website for full text and references.

What are the effects of treatments for diabetic retinopathy?

BENEFICIAL

Control of diabetes (see glycaemic control in diabetes: type 1, p 157)

Control of hypertension (see primary prevention, [Web only])

Macular photocoagulation in people with clinically significant macular oedema

One large RCT found that laser photocoagulation to the macula reduced visual loss at 3 years in eyes with macular oedema plus mild to moderate diabetic retinopathy compared with no treatment. There was some evidence of greater benefit in eyes with better vision. Subgroup analysis found that focal laser treatment reduced visual loss in eyes with clinically significant macular oedema particularly in people in whom the centre of the macula was involved or imminently threatened.

Peripheral retinal laser photocoagulation in people with preproliferative (*moderate/severe non-proliferative**) retinopathy and maculopathy

RCTs in eyes with preproliferative retinopathy and maculopathy found that peripheral retinal photocoagulation reduced the risk of severe visual loss at 5 years compared with no treatment.

Peripheral retinal laser photocoagulation in people with proliferative retinopathy

RCTs found that peripheral retinal photocoagulation reduced the risk of severe visual loss at 2–3 years compared with no treatment. One RCT in eyes with high risk proliferative diabetic retinopathy found that low intensity argon laser reduced vitreous haemorrhage and macular oedema compared with standard intensity argon laser. It found no significant difference between treatments for visual acuity, although it may have lacked power to detect clinically important effects.

LIKELY TO BE BENEFICIAL

Grid photocoagulation to zones of retinal thickening in people with diabetic maculopathy

One RCT found that grid photocoagulation improved visual acuity in treated eyes at 12 months and at 24 months compared with no treatment. Photocoagulation reduced the risk of moderate visual loss by 50–70% compared with no treatment.

UNKNOWN EFFECTIVENESS

Macular photocoagulation in people with maculopathy but without clinically significant macular oedema

We found no RCTs of macular photocoagulation in this population.

Peripheral retinal laser photocoagulation in people with background or preproliferative (*non-proliferative**) retinopathy without maculopathy

We found no RCTs in people with background or preproliferative retinopathy without maculopathy.

Diabetic retinopathy

What are the effects of treatments for vitreous haemorrhage?

LIKELY TO BE BENEFICIAL

Vitrectomy in people with severe vitreous haemorrhage and proliferative retinopathy (if performed early)

One RCT found that early vitrectomy reduced visual loss at 1, 2, and 3 years in eyes with severe vitreous haemorrhage and proliferative retinopathy compared with deferred (for 1 year) vitrectomy.

UNKNOWN EFFECTIVENESS

Vitrectomy in people with maculopathy

We found no RCTs.

DEFINITION Diabetic retinopathy is characterised by varying degrees of microaneurysms, haemorrhages, exudates *(hard exudates)*, venous changes, new vessel formation, and retinal thickening. It can involve the peripheral retina, the macula, or both. The range of severity of retinopathy includes background *(mild non-proliferative)*, preproliferative *(moderate/severe non-proliferative)*, proliferative, and advanced retinopathy. Involvement of the macula can be focal, diffuse, ischaemic, or mixed.

INCIDENCE/ Diabetic eye disease is the most common cause of blindness in the UK,
PREVALENCE responsible for 12% of registrable blindness in people aged 16–64 years.[1]

AETIOLOGY/ Risk factors include age, duration and control of diabetes, raised blood
RISK FACTORS pressure, and raised serum lipids.[2]

PROGNOSIS Natural history studies from the 1960s found that at least half of people with proliferative diabetic retinopathy progressed to Snellen visual acuity of less than 6/60 *(20/200)* within 3–5 years.[3–5] After 4 years' follow up, the rate of progression to less than 6/60 *(20/200)* visual acuity in the better eye was 1.5% in people with type 1 diabetes, 2.7% in people with non-insulin requiring type 2 diabetes, and 3.2% in people with insulin requiring type 2 diabetes.[6]

*Terms in italics indicate US definitions.

Please refer to the Clinical Evidence website for full text and references.

What are the effects of treatments for established primary open angle glaucoma?

LIKELY TO BE BENEFICIAL

Laser trabeculoplasty plus medical treatment (compared with no initial treatment or medical treatment alone)

One RCT in people with newly diagnosed primary open angle or pseudoexfoliation glaucoma found that initial treatment with laser trabeculoplasty plus topical medical treatment to lower intraocular pressure reduced progression of glaucoma compared with no initial treatment at 6 years. One RCT found that, compared with medical treatment alone, combined treatment with initial laser trabeculoplasty followed by medical treatment reduced intraocular pressure and deterioration in optic disc appearance, and improved visual fields after a mean of 7 years.

Topical medical treatment (some RCTs included people with primary open angle glaucoma or ocular hypertension alone)

One systematic review and one subsequent RCT in people with primary open angle glaucoma or ocular hypertension alone provided limited evidence that medical treatments reduced intraocular pressure compared with placebo or close observation at between 3 months and 5 years' follow up. However, they found no significant difference between medical treatment and placebo in visual field loss at 1–3 years' follow up. However, one large subsequent RCT found that in people with ocular hypertension, but no evidence of glaucomatous damage, topical medical treatment reduced the risk of developing primary open angle glaucoma after 5 years compared with close observation. One RCT found that, compared with medical treatment alone, initial laser trabeculoplasty followed by medical treatment reduced intraocular pressure and deterioration in optic disc appearance, and improved visual fields after a mean of 7 years. Two RCTs found that surgical trabeculectomy reduced both visual field loss and intraocular pressures compared with medical treatment, but found no significant difference between treatments in visual acuity after about 5 years. One RCT in people with primary open angle glaucoma, pigmentary glaucoma, or pseudoexfoliative glaucoma found no significant difference between initial medical treatment and initial surgical trabeculectomy in visual field loss at 5 years. It found that loss of visual acuity was greater with initial surgical trabeculectomy, but the significance of this finding was not reported.

TRADE OFF BETWEEN BENEFITS AND HARMS

Surgical trabeculectomy

Two RCTs found that surgical trabeculectomy reduced visual field loss and intraocular pressure compared with medical treatment, but found no significant difference between treatments in visual acuity after about 5 years. One RCT in people with primary open angle glaucoma, pigmentary glaucoma, or pseudoexfoliation glaucoma found no significant difference between initial medication and initial surgical trabeculectomy in visual field loss at 5 years. It found that loss of visual acuity was greater with surgical trabeculectomy, but the significance of this difference was not reported. Two RCTs found that surgical trabeculectomy reduced intraocular pressure compared with laser trabeculoplasty, but found mixed effects ▶

Glaucoma

for changes in visual acuity and visual field loss after 5–7 years. Surgical trabeculectomy has been reported to be associated with a reduction in central vision.

UNKNOWN EFFECTIVENESS

Laser trabeculoplasty (compared with surgical trabeculectomy)

Two RCTs found that surgical trabeculectomy reduced intraocular pressure compared with laser trabeculoplasty, but found mixed effects for changes in visual acuity after 5–7 years.

What are the effects of lowering intraocular pressure in people with normal tension glaucoma?

LIKELY TO BE BENEFICIAL

Medical treatment

One RCT found that both surgical and medical treatment, either singly or combined, reduced progression of visual field loss after 8 years compared with no treatment.

TRADE OFF BETWEEN BENEFITS AND HARMS

Surgical treatment

One RCT found that both surgical and medical treatment, either singly or combined, reduced progression of visual field loss after 8 years compared with no treatment, but found that surgery increased cataract formation after 8 years.

What are the effects of treatment for acute angle closure glaucoma?

UNKNOWN EFFECTIVENESS

Medical treatment*

We found no placebo controlled RCTs, but consensus suggests that medical treatments are effective for acute angle closure glaucoma. One small RCT found no significant difference in intraocular pressure after 2 hours with low dose pilocarpine versus an intensive pilocarpine regimen versus pilocarpine ocular inserts. We found no RCTs of other medical treatments.

Surgical treatment*

We found no placebo controlled RCTs, but consensus suggests that surgical treatments are effective for acute angle closure glaucoma. One small RCT found no significant difference between surgical iridectomy and laser iridotomy in visual acuity or intraocular pressure after 3 years.

*No placebo controlled RCTs but strong consensus that treatments are effective.

DEFINITION   Glaucoma is a group of diseases characterised by progressive optic neuropathy. It is usually bilateral but asymmetric and may occur at any intraocular pressure. All forms of glaucoma show optic nerve damage (cupping and/or pallor) associated with peripheral visual field loss. **Primary open angle glaucoma** occurs in people with an open anterior chamber drainage angle and no secondary identifiable cause. Knowledge of the natural history of these conditions is incomplete, but it is thought that the problem starts with an intraocular pressure that is too high for the optic nerve. However, in a significant proportion of people with glaucoma (about 40%) intraocular pressure is within the statistically defined normal range. The term ocular hypertension generally applies to eyes with an intraocular pressure greater ►

than the statistical upper limit of normal (about 21 mm Hg). However, only a relatively small proportion of eyes with raised intraocular pressure have an optic nerve that is vulnerable to its effects (about 10%). However, because intraocular pressure is the main and only modifiable risk factor for the disease, studies on the effectiveness of reducing intraocular pressure often include people who have both ocular hypertension and primary open angle glaucoma. Previously, trialists were anxious about withholding active treatment in overt primary open angle glaucoma, and so many placebo or no treatment trials selected people just with ocular hypertension. Trials comparing treatments often include both people with primary open angle glaucoma and people with ocular hypertension, but in these the outcome is usually intraocular pressure alone. **Normal tension glaucoma** occurs in people with intraocular pressures that are consistently below the statistical upper limit of normal (21 mm Hg; 2 standard deviations above the population mean). **Acute angle closure glaucoma** is glaucoma resulting from a rapid and severe rise in intraocular pressure caused by physical obstruction of the anterior chamber drainage angle.

INCIDENCE/ PREVALENCE
Glaucoma occurs in 1–2% of white people aged over 40 years, rising to 5% at 70 years. Primary open angle glaucoma accounts for two thirds of those affected, and normal tension glaucoma for about a quarter.[1,2] In black people glaucoma is more prevalent, presents at a younger age with higher intraocular pressures, is more difficult to control, and is the main irreversible cause of blindness in black populations of African origin.[1,3] Glaucoma related blindness is responsible for 8% of new blind registrations in the UK.[4]

AETIOLOGY/ RISK FACTORS
The major risk factor for developing primary open angle glaucoma is raised intraocular pressure. Lesser risk factors include family history and ethnic origin. The relationship between systemic blood pressure and intraocular pressure may be an important determinant of blood flow to the optic nerve head and, as a consequence, may represent a risk factor for glaucoma.[5] Systemic hypotension, vasospasm (including Raynaud's disease and migraine), and a history of major blood loss have been reported as risk factors for normal tension glaucoma in hospital based studies.[6] Risk factors for acute angle closure glaucoma include family history, female sex, being long sighted, and cataract. A recent systematic review did not find any evidence supporting the theory that routine pupillary dilatation with short acting mydriatics was a risk factor for acute angle closure glaucoma.[7]

PROGNOSIS
Advanced visual field loss is found in about 20% of people with primary open angle glaucoma at diagnosis,[8] and is an important prognostic factor for glaucoma related blindness.[9] Blindness due to glaucoma results from gross loss of visual field or loss of central vision. Once early field defects have appeared, and where the intraocular pressure is greater than 30 mm Hg, untreated people may lose the remainder of the visual field in 3 years or less.[10] As the disease progresses, people with glaucoma have difficulty moving from a bright room to a darker room, and judging steps and kerbs. Progression of visual field loss is often slower in normal tension glaucoma. Acute angle glaucoma leads to rapid loss of vision, initially from corneal oedema and subsequently from ischaemic optic neuropathy.

Please refer to the Clinical Evidence website for full text and references.

Ocular herpes simplex

Search date August 2003

Nigel H Barker

What are the effects of treatments for epithelial keratitis?

BENEFICIAL

Interferons

One systematic review found that topical interferons (alpha or beta) increase healing after 7 and 14 days compared with placebo. The review found no significant difference between a topical interferon and a topical antiviral agent in healing after 7 days, but found that a topical interferon increased healing after 14 days. The review also found that topical interferon plus a topical antiviral agent increased healing compared with a topical antiviral agent alone after 14 days. "Healing" was not clearly defined.

Topical antiviral agents

One systematic review has found that topical antivirals (idoxuridine or vidarabine) increase healing after 14 days compared with placebo, and that trifluridine or aciclovir increase healing compared with idoxuridine after 7 and 14 days. The review has also found that antiviral treatment plus debridement increases healing after 7 days compared with either treatment alone. It found no significant difference in healing at 14 days between antiviral treatment plus debridement and antiviral treatment alone. It also found no significant difference between topical antiviral agents and topical interferon in healing after 7 days, but found that topical interferon increased healing after 14 days. The review also found that adding topical interferon to a topical antiviral agent increased healing compared with the antiviral agent alone. "Healing" was not clearly defined.

UNKNOWN EFFECTIVENESS

Debridement

One systematic review has found no significant difference between debridement and no treatment. The review has also found that debridement plus antiviral treatment improves healing at 7 days compared with either treatment alone. This difference remained significant at 14 days for combined treatment compared with debridement alone.

What are the effects of treatments for stromal keratitis?

BENEFICIAL

Topical corticosteroids

One RCT in people receiving topical antiviral treatment found that topical corticosteroids reduced progression and shortened the duration of stromal keratitis compared with placebo.

UNLIKELY TO BE BENEFICIAL

Oral aciclovir

One RCT in people receiving topical corticosteroids plus topical antiviral treatment found no significant difference between oral aciclovir and placebo in rates of treatment failure at 16 weeks.

What are the effects of treatments to prevent recurrence of ocular herpes simplex?

BENEFICIAL

Long term (1 year) oral aciclovir

One large RCT in people with at least one previous episode of epithelial or stromal keratitis found that long term oral aciclovir reduced recurrence after 1 year compared with placebo.

UNLIKELY TO BE BENEFICIAL

Short term (3 weeks) oral aciclovir

One RCT in people with epithelial keratitis receiving a topical antiviral agent (trifluridine) found no significant difference between short term prophylaxis with oral aciclovir and placebo in the rate of stromal keratitis or iritis at 1 year.

What are the effects of treatments to prevent recurrence of ocular herpes simplex in people with corneal grafts?

LIKELY TO BE BENEFICIAL

Oral aciclovir

One small RCT found limited evidence that prophylactic use of oral aciclovir reduced recurrence and improved graft survival compared with placebo.

DEFINITION Ocular herpes simplex is usually caused by herpes simplex virus type 1 (HSV-1), but also occasionally by type 2 virus (HSV-2). Ocular manifestations of HSV are varied and include blepharitis (inflammation of the eyelids), canalicular obstruction, conjunctivitis, epithelial keratitis, stromal keratitis, iritis, and retinitis. HSV infections are classified as neonatal, primary (HSV in a person with no previous viral exposure), and recurrent (previous viral exposure with humoral and cellular immunity present).

INCIDENCE/ Infections with HSV are usually acquired in early life. A US study found
PREVALENCE antibodies against HSV-1 in about 50% of people with high socioeconomic status and 80% of people with low socioeconomic status by the age of 30 years.[1] However, only about 20–25% of people with HSV antibodies had any history of clinical manifestations of ocular or cutaneous herpetic disease.[2] Ocular HSV is the most common cause of corneal blindness in high income countries and the most common cause of unilateral corneal blindness in the world.[3] A 33 year study of the population of Rochester, Minnesota, found the annual incidence of new cases of ocular herpes simplex was 8.4/100 000 (95% CI 6.9 to 9.9) and the annual incidence of all episodes (new and recurrent) was 20.7/100 000 (95% CI 18.3 to 23.1).[4] The prevalence of ocular herpes was 149 cases/100 000 population (95% CI 115 to 183). Twelve per cent of people had bilateral disease.

AETIOLOGY/ Epithelial keratitis results from productive, lytic viral infection of the corneal
RISK FACTORS epithelial cells. Stromal keratitis and iritis are thought to result from a combination of viral infection and compromised immune mechanisms. Observational evidence (346 people with ocular HSV in the placebo arm of an RCT) has found that the risk of developing stromal keratitis was 4% in people with no previous history of stromal keratitis (RR 1.0) as compared with 32% (RR 10, 95% CI 4.32 to 23.38) with previous stromal keratitis, but that a history of epithelial keratitis was not a risk factor for recurrent epithelial keratitis.[5] Age, sex, ethnicity, and previous experience of non-ocular HSV disease were not associated with an increased risk of recurrence.[5]

Ocular herpes simplex

PROGNOSIS HSV epithelial keratitis tends to resolve within 1–2 weeks. In a trial of 271 people treated with topical trifluorothymidine and randomly assigned to receive either oral aciclovir or placebo, the epithelial lesion had resolved completely or was at least less than 1 mm after 1 week of treatment with placebo in 89% of people and after 2 weeks in 99% of people.[6] Stromal keratitis or iritis occurs in about 25% of people following epithelial keratitis.[7] The effects of HSV stromal keratitis include scarring, tissue destruction, neovascularisation, glaucoma, and persistent epithelial defects. Rate of recurrence of ocular herpes for people with one episode is 10% at 1 year, 23% at 2 years, and 50% at 10 years.[8] The risk of recurrent ocular HSV infection (epithelial or stromal) has also been found to increase with the number of previous episodes reported (2 or 3 previous episodes: RR 1.41, 95% CI 0.82 to 2.42; 4 or more previous episodes: RR 2.09, 95% CI 1.24 to 3.50).[5] Of corneal grafts performed in Australia over a 10 year period, 5% were in people with visual disability or with actual or impending corneal perforation following stromal ocular herpes simplex. The recurrence of HSV in a corneal graft has a major effect on graft survival. The Australian Corneal Graft Registry has found that, in corneal grafts performed for HSV keratitis, there was at least one HSV recurrence in 58% of corneal grafts that failed over a follow up period of 9 years.[9]

Please refer to the Clinical Evidence website for full text and references.

What are the effects of preventive interventions?

Early diagnosis and treatment of sexually transmitted diseases

One RCT has found that early diagnosis and treatment of sexually transmitted diseases reduces the risk of acquiring HIV infection over 2 years.

Postexposure prophylaxis in healthcare workers*

One case control study found limited evidence suggesting that postexposure prophylaxis with zidovudine may reduce the risk of HIV infection over 6 months. Evidence from other settings suggests that combining several antiretroviral drugs is likely to be more effective than zidovudine alone.

*Based on observational studies and indirectly from RCTs in other settings.

Presumptive mass treatment of sexually transmitted diseases

One RCT found no significant difference in the incidence of HIV over 20 months between presumptive mass treatment for sexually transmitted diseases and no treatment.

What are the effects of treatments?

Three antiretroviral drugs regimens (compared with two antiretroviral drugs regimens)

One systematic review has found that, compared with two antiretroviral drug regimens, three drug regimens reduce disease progression or death. Some of the reviewed trials included a non-nucleoside reverse transcriptase inhibitor as a third drug, and some a protease inhibitor.

Two antiretroviral drugs regimens (compared with single antiretroviral drug regimens)

Large RCTs, with a follow up of 1–3 years, have found that two drug regimens (zidovudine plus another nucleoside analogue or protease inhibitor drug) reduce the risk of new AIDS defining illnesses and death compared with zidovudine alone. Adverse events were common in all treatment groups.

Early versus delayed antiretroviral treatment with multidrug regimens

One systematic review compared early versus delayed antiretroviral treatment, but the RCTs were all started when zidovudine was the only drug available. Overall, the systematic review found no significant difference in the risk of AIDS free survival or overall survival with extended follow up. We found no RCTs exploring this question with two or three drug regimens.

▶

HIV infection

Four antiretroviral drugs regimens (compared with three antiretroviral drugs regimens)

We found no systematic review or RCTs comparing four antiretroviral drugs regimens with three antiretroviral drugs regimens for clinical outcomes.

DEFINITION   HIV infection refers to infection with the human immunodeficiency virus type 1 or type 2. Clinically, this is characterised by a variable period (average around 8–10 years) of asymptomatic infection, followed by repeated episodes of illness of varying and increasing severity as immune function deteriorates. The type of illness varies greatly by country, availability of specific treatment for HIV, and prophylaxis for opportunistic infections.

INCIDENCE/   Worldwide estimates suggest that, by June 2001, about 51 million people
PREVALENCE   had been infected with HIV, about 16 million people had died as a result, and about 16<thin>000 new HIV infections were occurring each day.[1] About 90% of HIV infections occur in the developing world.[1] Occupationally acquired HIV infection in healthcare workers has been documented in 95 definite and 191 possible cases, although this is likely to be an underestimate.[2]

AETIOLOGY/   The major risk factor for transmission of HIV is unprotected heterosexual or
RISK FACTORS   homosexual intercourse. Other risk factors include needlestick injury, sharing drug injecting equipment, and blood transfusion. An HIV infected woman may also transmit the virus to her baby. This has been reported in 15–30% of pregnant women with HIV infection. Not everyone who is exposed to HIV will become infected, although risk increases if exposure is repeated, at high dose, or through blood. There is at least a two to five times greater risk of HIV infection among people with sexually transmitted diseases.[3]

PROGNOSIS   Without treatment, about half of people infected with HIV will become ill and die from AIDS over about 10 years. A meta-analysis of 13 cohort studies from Europe and the USA looked at 12 574 treatment naïve people starting highly active antiretroviral therapy with a combination of at least three drugs.[4] During 24 310 person years of follow up, 1094 people developed AIDS or died. Baseline CD4 cell count and baseline HIV-1 viral load were associated with the probability of progression to AIDS or death. Other independent predictors of poorer outcome were advanced age, infection through injection drug use, and a previous diagnosis of AIDS. The CD4 cell count at initiation was the dominant prognostic factor in people starting highly active antiretroviral therapy. Genetic factors have been shown to affect response to antiretroviral treatment, but were not considered in the meta-analysis.[4]

Please refer to the Clinical Evidence website for full text and references.

Search date January 2004

Jimmy Volmink and Unati Mahlat

What are the effects of measures to reduce mother to child transmission of HIV?

BENEFICIAL

Antiretroviral drugs

One systematic review found that zidovudine reduced the incidence of HIV in infants compared with placebo. One RCT identified by the review found that longer courses of zidovudine given to mother and infant reduced the incidence of HIV in infants compared with shorter courses of zidovudine. One RCT found that nevirapine given to the mother and to her newborn reduced the risk of HIV transmission compared with zidovudine. One RCT found no additional advantage in giving nevirapine to the mother and baby when transmission rates were already reduced by mothers receiving standard antiretroviral treatment. One RCT found that zidovudine plus lamivudine given in the antenatal, intrapartum, and postpartum periods, or during the intrapartum and postpartum periods, reduced the risk of transmission of HIV at 6 weeks compared with placebo. One RCT found no significant difference in newborn HIV infection rates between nevirapine monotherapy and zidovudine plus lamivudine given to the mother during labour and to the mother and baby after delivery. However, one RCT found that nevirapine plus zidovudine given twice daily to babies for 7 days after birth reduced HIV transmission at 6 to 8 weeks compared with a single dose of nevirapine given to babies immediately after birth.

LIKELY TO BE BENEFICIAL

Avoiding breast feeding (provided there is access to clean water and health education)

One RCT in women with HIV who had access to clean water and health education found that, compared with breast feeding, formula feeding reduced the incidence of HIV in infants at 24 months without increasing mortality.

Elective caesarean section

One RCT provided limited evidence that elective caesarean section reduced the incidence of HIV in infants at 18 months compared with vaginal delivery.

UNKNOWN EFFECTIVENESS

Immunotherapy

One RCT found no significant difference in HIV transmission to infants from mothers taking zidovudine and either HIV hyperimmune globulin or immunoglobulin without HIV antibody. However, the study may have been too small to detect a clinically important difference.

Vaginal microbicides

One systematic review, which identified no RCTs, provided insufficient evidence to assess the effects of vaginal microbicides on the transmission of HIV to infants.

LIKELY TO BE INEFFECTIVE OR HARMFUL

Vitamin supplements

Three RCTs found that vitamin A supplements given to HIV positive pregnant women had no significant effect on the risk of HIV infection in their infants ▶

HIV: mother to child transmission

compared with either placebo or no vitamin A. One RCT found that multivitamins given to mothers during pregnancy and lactation had no significant effect on HIV infection in their infants compared with placebo.

DEFINITION   Mother to child transmission of HIV infection is defined as transmission of HIV infection from an infected mother to her child during gestation, labour, or through breast feeding in infancy. HIV-1 infection may be transmitted from mother to child,[1] although HIV-2 is rarely transmitted in this way.[2] Infected children usually have no symptoms or signs of HIV at birth, but develop them over subsequent months or years.[3]

INCIDENCE/   A review of 13 cohort studies found that the risk of mother to child
PREVALENCE   transmission of HIV without antiviral treatment is on average about 15–20% in Europe, 15–30% in the USA, and 25–35% in Africa.[4] The risk of transmission is estimated to be 15–30% during pregnancy, with an additional risk of about 10–20% postpartum through breast feeding.[5] UNAIDS estimates that 2.5 million children under the age of 5 years are living with HIV/AIDS. Of these, over 80% are in sub-Saharan Africa.[6] In 2003 alone, an estimated 700 000 children under 15 years of age (75% in sub-Saharan Africa) were newly infected with HIV.[6]

AETIOLOGY/   Transmission of HIV to children is more likely if the mother has a high viral
RISK FACTORS   load.[1,7,8] Women with detectable viraemia (by p24 antigen or culture) have double the risk of transmitting HIV-1 to their infants than those who do not.[1] Prospective studies have also found that breast feeding is a risk factor for mother to child transmission of HIV.[9,10] Other risk factors include sexually transmitted diseases, chorioamnionitis, prolonged rupture of membranes, vaginal mode of delivery, low CD4 count, advanced maternal HIV disease, obstetric events increasing bleeding (episiotomy, perineal laceration, and intrapartum haemorrhage), young maternal age, and history of stillbirth.[6,11–15]

PROGNOSIS   About 25% of infants infected with HIV progress rapidly to AIDS or death in the first year. Some survive beyond 12 years of age.[3] One European study found a mortality of 15% in the first year of life and a mortality of 28% by the age of 5 years.[16] A recent study reported that, in children under 5 years of age in sub-Saharan Africa, HIV accounted for 2% of deaths in 1990 and almost 8% in 1999.[17] Five countries (Botswana, Namibia, Swaziland, Zambia, and Zimbabwe) had rates of HIV attributable mortality in excess of 30/1000 in children under the age of 5 years.

Please refer to the Clinical Evidence website for full text and references.

HIV: prevention of opportunistic infections 193

Search date December 2003

John Ioannidis and David Wilkinson

The absolute benefits of prophylactic regimens for opportunistic infections are probably smaller in people with HIV who are also taking highly active antiretroviral treatment (HAART). The rate of PCP, toxoplasmosis, and other opportunistic infections has been reduced by HAART.

What are the effects of prophylaxis for P carinii pneumonia (PCP) and toxoplasmosis?

LIKELY TO BE BENEFICIAL

Atovaquone

We found no RCTs comparing atovaquone versus placebo. RCTs in people who are either intolerant of or fail to respond to trimethoprim–sulfamethoxazole found that atovaquone is as effective as dapsone or aerosolised pentamidine in preventing *P carinii* pneumonia (PCP). It would be unethical to perform a trial of atovaquone compared with placebo.

Azithromycin (alone or plus rifabutin, compared with rifabutin alone, for PCP prevention)

One RCT found that azithromycin, either alone or in combination with rifabutin, reduced the risk of *P carinii* pneumonia (PCP) compared with rifabutin alone in people receiving standard PCP prophylaxis.

Trimethoprim–sulfamethoxazole for PCP

Systematic reviews found that trimethoprim–sulfamethoxazole reduces the incidence of PCP compared with placebo or pentamidine. Two systematic reviews found that trimethoprim–sulfamethoxazole reduced incidence of PCP compared with dapsone (with or without pyrimethamine), although only one of these reviews found that the reduction was significant. One systematic review and one subsequent RCT found no significant difference between high and low dose trimethoprim–sulfamethoxazole for PCP prophylaxis, although adverse effects were more common with the higher dose.

UNKNOWN EFFECTIVENESS

Trimethoprim–sulfamethoxazole for toxoplasmosis

One RCT found no significant difference between trimethoprim–sulfamethoxazole and placebo for preventing toxoplasmosis. One systematic review has found no significant difference between trimethoprim–sulfamethoxazole and dapsone (with or without pyrimethamine) for preventing toxoplasmosis.

What are the effects of antituberculosis prophylaxis in people with HIV infection?

BENEFICIAL

Antituberculosis prophylaxis versus placebo (in people with positive tuberculin test)

One systematic review found that in people who are HIV and tuberculin skin test positive, antituberculosis prophylaxis drugs reduced the frequency of tuberculosis compared with placebo over 2–3 years. The review found no evidence of benefit in ▶

HIV: prevention of opportunistic infections

people who are HIV positive but tuberculin skin test negative. One RCT found that the benefit of prophylaxis diminished with time after treatment was stopped.

TRADE OFF BETWEEN BENEFITS AND HARMS

Isoniazid for 6–12 months (v combination treatment for 2–3 months — longer treatment regimen, but similar benefits and fewer harms)
RCTs found no evidence of a difference in effectiveness between regimens using combinations of tuberculosis drugs for 2–3 months and those using isoniazid alone for 6–12 months. One RCT found that multidrug regimens increased the number of people with adverse reactions resulting in cessation of treatment.

What are the effects of prophylaxis for disseminated M avium complex (MAC) disease for people without previous MAC disease?

LIKELY TO BE BENEFICIAL

Azithromycin
One RCT found that azithromycin reduced the incidence of *M avium* complex (MAC) compared with placebo. One RCT found that both azithromycin and azithromycin plus rifabutin reduced the incidence of MAC compared with rifabutin alone.

Clarithromycin
One RCT found that clarithromycin reduced the incidence of *M avium* complex (MAC) compared with placebo. One RCT found that both clarithromycin and clarithromycin plus rifabutin reduced the incidence of MAC compared with rifabutin alone.

TRADE OFF BETWEEN BENEFITS AND HARMS

Rifabutin plus macrolides
One RCT found that rifabutin plus clarithromycin reduced the incidence of *M avium* complex (MAC) compared with rifabutin alone. One RCT found that azithromycin plus rifabutin reduced the incidence of MAC compared with azithromycin alone or rifabutin alone. One systematic review and two subsequent RCTs found that toxicity, including uveitis, was more common with combination therapy than with clarithromycin or rifabutin alone.

What are the effects of prophylaxis for disseminated M avium complex (MAC) disease for people with previous MAC disease?

LIKELY TO BE BENEFICIAL

Clarithromycin, rifabutin, and ethambutol (more effective than clarithromycin plus clofazimine)
One RCT found that clarithromycin, rifabutin and ethambutol reduced MAC relapse compared with clarithromycin plus clofazimine.

Ethambutol added to clarithromycin plus clofazimine
One RCT found that adding ethambutol to clarithromycin and clofazimine reduced MAC relapse compared with clarithromycin plus clofazimine.

UNKNOWN EFFECTIVENESS

Rifabutin added to clarithromycin plus ethambutol
One RCT found no significant difference in survival by adding rifabutin to clarithromycin plus ethambutol in people with previous MAC.

LIKELY TO BE INEFFECTIVE OR HARMFUL

Clofazimine added to clarithromycin and ethambutol (higher mortality than clofazimine plus ethambutol)

One RCT found that adding clarithromycin to clofazimine and ethambutol was associated with higher mortality compared with clofazimine plus ethambutol.

What are the effects of prophylaxis for cytomegalovirus (CMV), herpes simplex virus (HSV), and varicella zoster virus (VZV)?

BENEFICIAL

Aciclovir (for HSV and VZV)

One systematic review found that aciclovir reduced HSV and VZV infection, and reduced overall mortality in people at different clinical stages of HIV infection compared with placebo. It found no reduction in CMV.

TRADE OFF BETWEEN BENEFITS AND HARMS

Oral ganciclovir (in people with severe CD4 delpetion)

One RCT found that oral ganciclovir reduced the incidence of cytomegalovirus (CMV) in people with severe CD4 depletion compared with placebo. It found that 26% of people who took ganciclovir developed severe neutropenia. A second RCT found no significant difference in prevention of CMV between ganciclovir and placebo.

UNKNOWN EFFECTIVENESS

Famciclovir (for recurrent HSV)

One small RCT found that famciclovir reduced the rate of viral shedding compared with placebo, but provided insufficient evidence on the effect of famciclovir on herpes simplex virus (HSV) recurrence.

LIKELY TO BE INEFFECTIVE OR HARMFUL

Valaciclovir (less effective than aciclovir for CMV)

One RCT found that valaciclovir versus aciclovir reduced the incidence of CMV, but may be associated with increased mortality.

What are the effects of prophylaxis for invasive fungal disease in people without previous fungal disease?

TRADE OFF BETWEEN BENEFITS AND HARMS

Fluconazole or itraconazole

RCTs in people with advanced HIV disease found that both fluconazole and itraconazole reduced the incidence of invasive fungal infections compared with placebo. One RCT found that fluconazole reduced the incidence of invasive fungal disease and mucocutaneous candidiasis compared with clotrimazole. One RCT found no difference between high and low dose fluconazole. Azoles have been associated with congenital problems and potentially serious interactions with other drugs.

HIV: prevention of opportunistic infections

What are the effects of prophylaxis for invasive fungal disease in people with previous fungal disease?

LIKELY TO BE BENEFICIAL

Itraconazole (for *Penicillium marneffei*)
> Two RCTs found that itraconazole reduced the incidence of relapse of *P marneffei* infection and candidiasis compared with placebo.

LIKELY TO BE INEFFECTIVE OR HARMFUL

Intraconazole (v fluconazole for maintenance treatment of cryptococcal meningitis)
> One RCT found that itraconazole increased the risk of relapse of cryptococcal meningitis compared with fluconazole.

What are the effects of discontinuing prophylaxis against opportunistic pathogens in people on highly active antiretroviral treatment (HAART)?

LIKELY TO BE BENEFICIAL

Discontinuing prophylaxis for MAC in people with CD4 > 100/mm³
Two RCTs in people with CD4 > 100/mm³ taking HAART found that discontinuation of prophylaxis for MAC disease did not increase the incidence of MAC disease.

Discontinuing prophylaxis for PCP and toxoplasmosis in people with CD4 > 200/mm³
One systematic review of two unblinded RCTs in people with CD4 > 200/mm³ taking HAART found that discontinuation of prophylaxis did not increase the incidence of PCP. Two unblinded RCTs found that discontinuation of prophylaxis did not increase the incidence of toxoplasmosis.

UNKNOWN EFFECTIVENESS

Discontinuing prophylaxis for CMV in people with CD4 > 100/mm³
We found insufficient evidence on the effects of discontinuation of maintenance treatment for CMV retinitis or other end organ disease in people with CD4 > 100/mm³ taking HAART.

DEFINITION   Opportunistic infections are intercurrent infections that occur in people infected with HIV. Prophylaxis aims to avoid either the first occurrence of these infections (primary prophylaxis) or their recurrence (secondary prophylaxis, maintenance treatment). This review includes *Pneumocystis carinii* pneumonia (PCP), *Toxoplasma gondii* encephalitis, *Mycobacterium tuberculosis*, *Mycobacterium avium* complex (MAC) disease, cytomegalovirus (CMV) disease (most often retinitis), infections from other herpesviruses (herpes simplex virus [HSV] and varicella zoster virus [VZV]), and invasive fungal disease (*Cryptococcus neoformans*, *Histoplasma capsulatum*, and *Penicillium marneffei*🅖).

INCIDENCE/   The incidence of opportunistic infections is high in people with immune
PREVALENCE   impairment. Data available before the introduction of highly active antiretroviral treatment (HAART) suggest that, with a CD4 < 250/mm³, the 2 year probability of developing an opportunistic infection is 40% for PCP, 22% for CMV, 18% for MAC, 6% for toxoplasmosis, and 5% for cryptococcal meningitis.[1] The introduction of HAART has reduced the rate of opportunistic infections. One cohort study found that the introduction of HAART decreased ▶

the incidence of PCP by 94%, CMV by 82%, and MAC by 64%, as presenting AIDS events. HAART decreased the incidence of events subsequent to the diagnosis of AIDS by 84% for PCP, 82% for CMV, and 97% for MAC.[2]

AETIOLOGY/ RISK FACTORS Opportunistic infections are caused by a wide array of pathogens and result from immune defects induced by HIV. The risk of developing opportunistic infections increases dramatically with progressive impairment of the immune system. Each opportunistic infection has a different threshold of immune impairment, beyond which the risk increases substantially.[1] Opportunistic pathogens may infect the immunocompromised host *de novo*, but usually they are simply reactivations of latent pathogens in such hosts.

PROGNOSIS Prognosis depends on the type of opportunistic infection. Even with treatment they may cause serious morbidity and mortality. Most deaths owing to HIV infection are caused by opportunistic infections.

Please refer to the Clinical Evidence website for full text and references.

Pneumocystis pneumonia in people with HIV

Search date November 2004

Richard Bellamy

What are the effects of first line antipneumocystis treatments for Pneumocystis pneumonia in people infected with HIV?

BENEFICIAL

Atovaquone

We found no RCTs comparing atovaquone versus placebo or no treatment as the first line treatment for *Pneumocystis* pneumonia in people infected with HIV. One RCT found that atovaquone was less effective than trimethoprim–sulfamethoxazole. One RCT found that atovaquone was equally effective as intravenous pentamidine. Adverse effects requiring termination of treatment occurred less frequently with atovaquone than with trimethoprim–sulfamethoxazole or intravenous pentamidine.

Clindamycin–primaquine

We found no RCTs comparing clindamycin–primaquine versus placebo or no treatment as the first line treatment for *Pneumocystis* pneumonia in people infected with HIV. RCTs found clindamycin–primaquine was as effective as trimethoprim–sulfamethoxazole and trimethoprim–dapsone and no significant difference in rates of serious adverse effects.

Pentamidine (aerosolised)

We found no RCTs comparing aerosolised pentamidine versus placebo or no treatment as first line treatment for *Pneumocystis* pneumonia in people infected with HIV. Two RCTs found no significant difference in mortality between aerosolised pentamidine and trimethoprim–sulfamethoxazole, but they found lower rates of serious adverse effects with aerosolised pentamidine. One RCT found no significant difference in mortality or treatment failure between aerosolised and intravenous pentamidine.

Pentamidine (intravenous)

We found no RCTs comparing intravenous pentamidine versus placebo or no treatment as first line treatment for *Pneumocystis* pneumonia in people infected with HIV. Two RCTs found no significant difference in mortality, treatment failure, or adverse effects between intravenous pentamidine and trimethoprim–sulfamethoxazole. However, a third RCT found that intravenous pentamidine increased mortality compared with trimethoprim–sulfamethoxazole. One RCT found no significant difference between intravenous pentamidine and atovaquone, but atovaquone caused fewer adverse effects requiring termination of treatment. One RCT found no significant difference in mortality or treatment failure between intravenous and aerosolised pentamidine.

Trimethoprim–dapsone

We found no RCTs comparing trimethoprim–dapsone versus placebo or no treatment as first line treatment for *Pneumocystis* pneumonia in people infected with HIV. RCTs have found that trimethoprim–dapsone was as effective as trimethoprim–sulfamethoxazole, with similar rates of adverse effects. One RCT found that trimethoprim–dapsone was as effective as clindamycin–primaquine. ▶

◀ **Trimethoprim–sulfamethoxazole (co-trimoxazole)**

We found no RCTs comparing trimethoprim–sulfamethoxazole versus placebo or no treatment as first line treatment for *Pneumocystis* pneumonia in people infected with HIV. One RCT found that trimethoprim–sulfamethoxazole was more effective than atovaquone. Two RCTs found no significant difference in mortality, treatment failure, or adverse effects between intravenous pentamidine and trimethoprim–sulfamethoxazole. However, a third RCT found that trimethoprim-sulfamethoxazole reduced mortality compared with intravenous pentamidine. RCTs have found that trimethoprim–sulfamethoxazole was as effective as clindamycin–primaquine and trimethoprim–dapsone, and aerosolised pentamidine. RCTs have found that adverse events requiring termination of treatment were more frequent with trimethoprim–sulfamethoxazole than atovaquone or aerosolised pentamidine.

What are the effects of adjuvant corticosteroids in people receiving first line antipneumocystis treatments for *Pneumocystis* pneumonia in people infected with HIV?

BENEFICIAL

Adjuvant corticosteroids for moderate to severe *Pneumocystis* pneumonia

One systematic review found that adjuvant corticosteroids reduced mortality when used early in the treatment of moderate to severe *Pneumocystis* pneumonia (see definition below).

UNKNOWN EFFECTIVENESS

Adjuvant corticosteroids for mild *Pneumocystis* pneumonia

We found insufficient evidence on the effects of adjuvant corticosteroids in the early treatment of mild *Pneumocystis* pneumonia in people infected with HIV (see definition below).

What are the effects of treatments for *Pneumocystis* pneumonia in people infected with HIV who have not responded to first line antipneumocystis treatment?

UNKNOWN EFFECTIVENESS

Treatment after failure of first line treatment

We found no systematic review and no RCTs comparing the effectiveness or adverse effects of different treatments after failure of first line treatment for *Pneumocystis* pneumonia in people infected with HIV. One systematic review of controlled studies, case series, and case reports suggested that clindamycin–primaquine may be more effective than alternative treatments in this situation.

DEFINITION   *Pneumocystis* pneumonia (PCP) is caused by the opportunistic fungus *Pneumocystis jiroveci*. The infection occurs in people with impaired immune function. Most cases occur in people infected with HIV, in whom PCP is an AIDS defining illness. The pneumonia is generally classified as **mild** if P_aO_2 is greater than 70 mm Hg on room air, if the alveolar–arterial oxygen gradient is less than 35 mm Hg, or both. It is generally classified as **moderate/severe** if the P_aO_2 is less than 70 mm Hg, if the alveolar–arterial oxygen gradient is greater than 35 mm Hg, or both. This chapter focuses on the treatment of PCP in adults infected with HIV. Prevention of PCP is covered under HIV: prevention of opportunistic infections, p 193.

▶

Pneumocystis pneumonia in people with HIV

INCIDENCE/ PREVALENCE
PCP is the most common AIDS defining illness in developed nations.[1] It is probably also common throughout the developing world, although the prevalence is harder to assess here because of difficulties in making the diagnosis. Before the widespread use of prophylaxis it was estimated that up to 80% of people with AIDS would eventually develop PCP.[2] Widespread use of prophylaxis against PCP and of highly active antiretroviral treatment has dramatically reduced the incidence of this infection (see HIV: prevention of opportunistic infections, p 193).

AETIOLOGY/ RISK FACTORS
Risk factors for PCP include HIV infection, primary immune deficiencies, prematurity, cancer, use of immune suppressants after organ transplantation, and prolonged use of high dose corticosteroids. HIV infection is now responsible for the vast majority of cases of PCP. Among adults with HIV infection, those with a CD4 count below 200 cells per mm^3 are at highest risk, and the median CD4 count at diagnosis of PCP is about 50 cells per mm^3.[3]

PROGNOSIS
It is generally believed that without treatment PCP would almost certainly be fatal in a person with AIDS. For ethical reasons, no studies have examined short term prognosis without treatment. People with AIDS and PCP frequently have other serious opportunistic infections, which can adversely affect their prognosis.

Please refer to the Clinical Evidence website for full text and references.

What are the effects of drug treatments for amoebic dysentery in endemic areas?

LIKELY TO BE BENEFICIAL

Metronidazole*
We found no RCTs comparing metronidazole versus placebo. We found six RCTs comparing metronidazole versus tinidazole. Four RCTs found that tinidazole improved parasite clearance at 30 days compared with metronidazole. One RCT found no significant difference between metronidazole and tinidazole in parasite clearance at 30 days, while one RCT found similar parasite clearance with both treatments at 6 days. Five of the RCTs reported adverse effects; two of these RCTs found more adverse events with metronidazole than with tinidazole, whereas three RCTs found no significant difference in the rates of adverse effects between the two drugs.

Ornidazole
One RCT found that ornidazole improved parasite clearance compared with placebo. Nausea and vomiting were more common with ornidazole than with placebo, but the difference was not significant. Two RCTs found no significant difference between ornidazole and tinidazole or secnidazole for clearing parasites in children with amoebic dysentery.

Secnidazole*
We found no RCTs comparing secnidazole versus placebo. One RCT found no significant difference between secnidazole and ornidazole in clearing parasites in children with amoebic dysentery.

Tinidazole*
We found no RCTs comparing tinidazole versus placebo. We found six RCTs comparing metronidazole versus tinidazole. Four RCTs found that tinidazole improved parasite clearance at 30 days compared with metronidazole. One RCT found no significant difference between metronidazole and tinidazole in parasite clearance at 30 days, while one RCT found similar parasite clearance with both treatments at 6 days. Five of the RCTs reported adverse effects; two of these RCTs found more adverse effects with metronidazole than with tinidazole, whereas three RCTs found no significant difference in the rates of adverse effects between the two drugs. One RCT found no significant difference between tinidazole and ornidazole for clearing parasites in children with amoebic dysentery.

*No placebo controlled RCTs. Categorisation based on consensus and evidence of similar effectiveness among these drugs.

UNKNOWN EFFECTIVENESS

Emetine, paromomycin
We found no RCTs evaluating these interventions for the treatment of amoebic dysentery in endemic areas.

DEFINITION   Amoebic dysentery is caused by a protozoan parasite *Entamoeba histolytica*. Invasive intestinal parasitic infection can result in symptoms of fulminant dysentery, with fever, chills, and bloody or mucous diarrhoea, abdominal discomfort, or diarrhoea containing blood or mucus alternating with periods of constipation or remission. This chapter focuses on amoebic dysentery only, ▶

Amoebic dysentery

and includes populations with both suspected and documented disease in endemic areas (areas in which levels of infection do not exhibit wide fluctuations through time).[1] Extraintestinal amoebiasis (e.g. amoebic liver abscess) and asymptomatic amoebiasis are not covered. The term "amoebic dysentery" encompasses people described as having symptomatic intestinal amoebiasis, amoebic colitis, amoebic diarrhoea, or invasive intestinal amoebiasis.

INCIDENCE/ PREVALENCE
We found no accurate global prevalence data of *E histolytica* infection and amoebic dysentery. Estimates on the prevalence of *Entamoeba* infection range from 1–40% of the population in Central and South America, Africa, and Asia, and from 0.2–10.8% in endemic areas of developed countries such as the USA.[2–5] However, these estimates are difficult to interpret, mainly because infection can remain asymptomatic or go unreported,[6] and because many older reports do not distinguish *E histolytica* from a non-pathogenic, morphologically identical species *Entamoeba dispar*. Development and availability of more sophisticated methods (such as the ELISA based test) to differentiate the two species might give a more accurate estimate of its global prevalence.[7] Infection with *E histolytica* is a common cause of acute diarrhoea. One survey in Egypt found that 38% of people with acute diarrhoea in an outpatient clinic had amoebic dysentery.[8]

AETIOLOGY/ RISK FACTORS
Ingestion of cysts from food or water contaminated with faeces is the main route of *E histolytica* transmission. Low standards of hygiene and sanitation, particularly those related to crowding, tropical climate, contamination of food and water with faeces, and inadequate disposal of faeces all account for the high rates of infection seen in developing countries.[9,10] It has been suggested that some animals, such as dogs, pigs, and monkeys, may act as reservoir hosts to the protozoa, but this has not been proven. In developed countries, risk factors include communal living, oral and anal sex, compromised immune system, and migration or travel from endemic areas.[9,11,12]

PROGNOSIS
Amoebic dysentery may progress to amoeboma, fulminant colitis, toxic megacolon, colonic ulcers, and may lead to perforation.[13] Amoeboma may be mistaken for colonic carcinoma or pyogenic abscess. Amoebic dysentery may also result in chronic carriage and the chronic passing of amoebic cysts. Fulminant amoebic dysentery is reported to have 55–88% mortality.[14,15] It is estimated that over 500 million people are infected with *E histolytica* worldwide.[10] Between 40 000 to 100 000 will die each year, placing it second to malaria in mortality caused by protozoan parasites.[16]

Please refer to the Clinical Evidence website for full text and references.

What are the effects of interventions to prevent chickenpox in healthy adults and children?

BENEFICIAL

Live attenuated vaccine in healthy children

Two RCTs identified by a systematic review found that live attenuated varicella vaccine reduced clinical chickenpox in healthy children compared with placebo, with no significant increase in adverse effects.

LIKELY TO BE BENEFICIAL

Zoster immune globulin versus human serum globulin in healthy children

One small RCT in children exposed to a sibling with chickenpox found that zoster immune globulin reduced the proportion of exposed children with clinical chickenpox at 20 days compared with human immune serum globulin.

UNKNOWN EFFECTIVENESS

Live attenuated vaccine in healthy adults

We found no RCTs in healthy adults on the effects of live attenuated varicella vaccine.

What are the effects of interventions to prevent chickenpox in immunocompromised adults and children?

BENEFICIAL

High dose aciclovir (> 3200 mg/day) In people with HIV infection

One systematic review in people with HIV infection found that high dose aciclovir (at least 3200 mg/day) reduced the risk of clinical chickenpox and reduced all cause mortality over 22 months' treatment compared with placebo.

UNKNOWN EFFECTIVENESS

Aciclovir in people with immunocompromise other than HIV

We found no RCTs on the effects of aciclovir in people with immunocompromise other than HIV.

Live attenuated vaccine in immunocompromised people

We found no RCTs in immunocompromised adults or children on the effects of live attenuated varicella vaccine.

Zoster immune globulin in immunocompromised adults

We found no RCTs on the effects of zoster immune globulin in immunocompromised adults.

Zoster immune globulin versus varicella zoster immune globulin in immunocompromised children

One RCT in immunocompromised children exposed to a sibling with chickenpox found no significant difference in clinical chickenpox with zoster immune globulin compared with varicella zoster immune globulin at 12 weeks.

What are the effects of treatments for chickenpox in healthy adults and children?

BENEFICIAL

Oral aciclovir in healthy people (given < 24 hours of onset of rash)
Two systematic reviews found that oral aciclovir reduced the symptoms of chickenpox in healthy adults and children compared with placebo.

UNKNOWN EFFECTIVENESS

Oral aciclovir in healthy people (given > 24 hours after onset of rash)
One systematic review and one additional RCT found that oral aciclovir given beyond 24 hours after onset of rash did not reduce the symptoms of chickenpox compared with placebo.

What are the effects of treatments for chickenpox in immunocompromised adults and children?

LIKELY TO BE BENEFICIAL

Intravenous aciclovir for treatment of chickenpox in children with malignancy
Two RCTs compared intravenous aciclovir versus placebo in children with cancer. One large RCT found that aciclovir reduces clinical deterioration. The other smaller RCT found no significant difference in clinical deterioration.

UNKNOWN EFFECTIVENESS

Aciclovir in immunocompromised adults
We found no RCTs on the effects of aciclovir in immunocompromised adults.

DEFINITION Chickenpox is caused by primary infection with varicella zoster virus. In healthy people, it is usually a mild self limiting illness, characterised by low grade fever, malaise, and a generalised, itchy vesicular rash.

INCIDENCE/ PREVALENCE Chickenpox is extremely contagious. Over 90% of unvaccinated people become infected, but infection occurs at different ages in different parts of the world: over 80% of people have been infected by the age of 10 years in the USA, the UK, and Japan, but by 30 years of age in India, South East Asia, and the West Indies.[1,2]

AETIOLOGY/ RISK FACTORS Chickenpox is caused by exposure to varicella zoster virus.

PROGNOSIS **Infants and children:** In healthy children the illness is usually mild and self limiting. In the USA, death rates in infants and children (aged 1–14 years) with chickenpox are about 7/100 000 in infants and 1.4/100 000 in children.[3] In Australia, mortality with chickenpox is about 0.5–0.6/100 000 in children aged between 1 and 11 years, and about 1.2/100 000 in infants.[4] Bacterial skin sepsis is the most common complication in children under 5 years of age, and acute cerebellar ataxia is the most common complication in older children; both cause hospital admission in 2–3/10 000 children.[5] **Adults:** Mortality in adults is higher, at about 31/100 000.[3] Varicella pneumonia is the most common complication, causing 20–30 hospital admissions/10 000 adults.[5] Activation of latent varicella zoster virus infection can cause herpes zoster, also known as shingles (see postherpetic neuralgia, p 241). **Cancer chemotherapy:** One case series (77 children with both cancer and chickenpox) found that more children receiving chemotherapy compared with those in remission developed progressive chickenpox with multiple organ involvement (19/60 [32%] with ▶

children receiving chemotherapy v 0/17 [0%] with children in remission) and more children died (4/60 [7%] with children receiving chemotherapy v 0/17 [0%] with children in remission).[6] **HIV infection:** One retrospective case series (45 children with AIDS) found that one in four children with AIDS who acquired chickenpox in hospital developed pneumonia and 5% died.[7] In a retrospective cohort study (73 children with HIV and chickenpox; 83% with symptomatic HIV), infection beyond 2 months occurred in 10 children (14%) and recurrent varicella zoster virus infections occurred in 38 children (55%). There was a strong association between an increasing number of recurrences and low CD4 cell counts.[8] Half of recurrent infections involved generalised rashes and the other half had zoster. **Newborns:** We found no cohort studies of untreated children with perinatal exposure to chickenpox. One cohort study (281 neonates receiving varicella zoster immune globulin because their mothers had developed a chickenpox rash during the month before or after delivery) found that 134 (48%) developed a chickenpox rash and 19 (14%) developed severe chickenpox.[9] Severe chickenpox occurred in neonates of mothers whose rash had started during the 7 days before delivery.

Please refer to the Clinical Evidence website for full text and references.

Infectious diseases

Congenital toxoplasmosis

Search date March 2004

Piero Olliaro

What are the effects on mother and baby of treating toxoplasmosis in pregnancy?

Antiparasitic drugs

Two systematic reviews of studies in women who seroconverted during pregnancy found insufficient evidence on the effects of current antiparasitic treatment compared with no treatment on mother or baby.

DEFINITION Toxoplasmosis is caused by the parasite *Toxoplasma gondii*. Infection is asymptomatic or unremarkable in immunocompetent individuals, but leads to a lifelong antibody response. During pregnancy, toxoplasmosis can be transmitted across the placenta and may cause intrauterine death, neonatal growth retardation, mental retardation, ocular defects, and blindness in later life. Congenital toxoplasmosis (confirmed infection of the fetus or newborn) presents at birth: either as subclinical disease, which may evolve with neurological or ophthalmological disease later in life; or as a disease of varying severity, ranging from mild ocular damage to severe mental retardation.

INCIDENCE/ PREVALENCE Reported rates of toxoplasma seroprevalence vary among and within countries, as well as over time. The risk of primary infection is highest in young people, including young women during pregnancy. We found no cohort studies describing annual seroconversion rates in women of childbearing age nor incidence of primary infection. One systematic review (search date 1996) identified 15 studies that reported rates of seroconversion in non-immune pregnant women ranging from 2.4–16/1000 in Europe and from 2–6/1000 in the USA.[1] France began screening for congenital toxoplasmosis in 1978, and during the period 1980–1995 the seroconversion rate during pregnancy in non-immune women was 4–5/1000.[2]

AETIOLOGY/ RISK FACTORS Toxoplasma infection is usually acquired by ingesting either sporocysts (from unwashed fruit or vegetables contaminated by cat faeces) or tissue cysts (from raw or undercooked meat). The risk of contracting toxoplasma infection varies with eating habits, contact with cats and other pets, and occupational exposure.

PROGNOSIS One systematic review of studies conducted from 1983–1996 found no population based prospective studies of the natural history of toxoplasma infection during pregnancy.[1] One systematic review (search date 1997; 9 controlled, non-randomised studies) found that untreated toxoplasmosis acquired during pregnancy was associated with infection rates in children of between 10–100%.[3] We found two European studies that correlated gestation at time of maternal seroconversion with risk of transmission and severity of disease at birth.[4,5] Risk of transmission increased with gestational age at maternal seroconversion, reaching 70–90% when maternal seroconversion occurred after 30 weeks' gestation. In contrast, the risk of the infant developing clinical disease was highest when maternal seroconversion occurred early in pregnancy. The highest risk of developing early signs of disease (including chorioretinitis and hydrocephaly) was about 10%, recorded when seroconversion occurred between 24 and 30 weeks' gestation.[5] Infants with congenital toxoplasmosis and generalised neurological abnormalities at birth develop mental retardation, growth retardation, blindness or visual defects, seizures, and spasticity. Children with subclinical infection at birth may have cognitive, ▶

motor, and visual deficits, which may go undiagnosed for many years. One case control study (845 school children in Brazil) found mental retardation and retinochoroiditis to be significantly associated with positive toxoplasma serology (population attributable risk 6–9%).[6]

Please refer to the Clinical Evidence website for full text and references.

Dengue fever

Search date November 2004

Marissa M Alejandria

What are the effects of supportive treatments for dengue haemorrhagic fever or dengue shock syndrome in children?

LIKELY TO BE BENEFICIAL

Intravenous fluids*

We found no RCTs comparing intravenous fluids versus placebo or no treatment. It is widely accepted that immediate fluid replacement should be undertaken in a child who has dengue haemorrhagic fever or dengue shock syndrome; it would be considered unethical to test its role in a placebo controlled trial.

*Although we found no direct evidence to support their use, widespread consensus holds that intravenous fluid replacement with crystalloids should be used universally in children with dengue haemorrhagic fever or dengue shock syndrome because these conditions lead to an acute increase in vascular permeability that leads to plasma leakage, resulting in increased haematocrit and decreased blood pressure. Placebo controlled trials would be considered unethical.

UNKNOWN EFFECTIVENESS

Colloids (compared with crystalloids)

Two RCTs found no significant difference in mortality, recurrence of shock, or requirement for further infusions between crystalloids and colloids for acute resuscitation in Vietnamese children with dengue shock syndrome, but they are likely to have been underpowered to detect a clinically important difference.

Adding carbazochrome sodium sulfonate (AC-17) to standard intravenous fluids

One RCT in Thai children with dengue haemorrhagic fever/dengue shock syndrome found no significant difference in the development of shock, pleural effusion, and duration of hospitalization between adding carbazochrome sodium sulfonate and adding placebo to standard intravenous fluids. Another RCT with weak methods in Indonesian children with grade II dengue haemorrhagic fever found limited evidence that adding carbazochrome sodium sulfonate to standard intravenous fluids decreased the occurrence of pleural effusion compared with standard intravenous fluids alone.

Adding corticosteroids to standard intravenous fluids

Two RCTs in Thai and Indonesian children with dengue shock syndrome found no significant difference in mortality between adding corticosteroids to standard fluid replacement and adding placebo to standard fluid replacement. One open label RCT with weak methods in Burmese children with dengue shock syndrome found limited evidence that adding hydrocortisone to intravenous fluids reduced mortality compared with intravenous fluids alone.

Adding intravenous immunoglobulin to standard intravenous fluids

We found no published RCTs on the effects of intravenous immunoglobulin in people with dengue haemorrhagic fever or dengue shock syndrome. One unpublished RCT in Filipino children with dengue shock syndrome found that adding intravenous immunoglobulin to standard intravenous fluids reduced mortality compared with adding placebo to standard intravenous fluids.

DEFINITION Dengue infection is a mosquito borne arboviral infection. The spectrum of dengue virus infection ranges from asymptomatic or undifferentiated febrile illness to dengue fever and dengue haemorrhagic fever or dengue shock syndrome. An important criterion to consider in the diagnosis of dengue infection is history of travel or residence in a dengue endemic area within 2 weeks of the onset of fever. **Dengue fever** is an acute febrile illness whose clinical presentation varies with age. Infants and young children may have an undifferentiated febrile disease with a maculopapular rash. Children aged 15 years or older and adults may have either a mild febrile illness or the classic incapacitating disease also called "breakbone fever" presenting with high fever of sudden onset and non-specific signs and symptoms of severe headache; pain behind the eyes; muscle, bone, or joint pains; nausea; vomiting; and rash. **Dengue haemorrhagic fever** is characterised by four criteria: acute onset of high fever; haemorrhagic manifestations evidenced by positive tourniquet test, skin haemorrhages, mucosal and gastrointestinal tract bleeding; thrombocytopenia; and evidence of plasma leakage manifested by a rise or drop in haematocrit, fluid in the lungs or abdomen, or hypoproteinaemia. Dengue haemorrhagic fever is classified into four grades of severity (see table 1❶).[1] Presence of thrombocytopenia and haemoconcentration differentiates dengue haemorrhagic fever grades I and II from dengue fever. Grades III and IV dengue haemorrhagic fever are considered **dengue shock syndrome.**[1] Plasma leakage is the major pathophysiological feature observed in dengue haemorrhagic fever.

INCIDENCE/ PREVALENCE Dengue fever and dengue haemorrhagic fever are public health problems worldwide, particularly in low-lying areas where *Aedes aegypti*, a domestic mosquito, is present. Cities near to the equator but high in the Andes are free of dengue because *Aedes* mosquitoes do not survive at high altitudes. Worldwide, an estimated 50–100 million cases of dengue fever and hundreds of thousands of dengue haemorrhagic fever occur yearly.[2] Endemic regions are the Americas, South East Asia, western Pacific, Africa, and the eastern Mediterranean. Major global demographic changes and their consequences (particularly increases in the density and geographic distribution of the vector with declining vector control; unreliable water supply systems; increasing non-biodegradable container and poor solid waste disposal; increased geographic range of virus transmission owing to increased air travel; and increased population density in urban areas) are responsible for the resurgence of dengue in the past century.[3,4] The World Health Organization estimates that global temperature rises of 1.0–3.5 °C can increase transmission by shortening the extrinsic incubation period of viruses within the mosquito, adding 20 000–30 000 more fatal cases annually.[5]

AETIOLOGY/ RISK FACTORS Dengue virus serotypes 1–4 (DEN 1, 2, 3, 4) belonging to the flavivirus genus are the aetiologic agents. These serotypes are closely related but antigenically distinct. *Ae aegypti*, the principal vector, transmits the virus to man. Dengue haemorrhagic fever and dengue shock syndrome typically occur in children under the age of 15 years, although dengue fever primarily occurs in adults and older children. Important risk factors influencing who will develop dengue haemorrhagic fever or severe disease during epidemics include the virus strain and serotype, immune status of the host, and age and genetic predisposition. There is evidence that sequential infection or pre-existing antidengue antibodies increases the risk of dengue haemorrhagic fever through antibody dependent enhancement.[3,4,6–8]

PROGNOSIS Dengue fever is an incapacitating disease but prognosis is favourable in previously healthy adults, although dengue haemorrhagic fever and dengue shock syndrome are major causes of hospital admission and mortality in children. Dengue fever is generally self limiting, with less than 1% case fatality. The acute phase of the illness lasts for 2–7 days but the convalescent phase may be prolonged for weeks associated with fatigue and depression, especially ▶

Dengue fever

in adults. Prognosis in dengue haemorrhagic fever and dengue shock syndrome depends on prevention or early recognition and treatment of shock. Case fatality ranges from 2.5% to 5.0%. Once shock sets in, fatality may be as high as 12–44%.[9] In centres with appropriate intensive supportive treatment, fatality can be less than 1%. There is no specific antiviral treatment. The standard treatment is to give intravenous fluids to expand plasma volume. People usually recover after prompt and adequate fluid and electrolyte supportive treatment. The optimal fluid regimen, however, remains the subject of debate. This is particularly important in dengue, where one of the management difficulties is to correct hypovolaemia rapidly without precipitating fluid overload.

Please refer to the Clinical Evidence website for full text and references.

Search date January 2004

Guy de Bruyn

What are the effects of treatments for acute diarrhoea in adults living in developed countries? *New*

LIKELY TO BE BENEFICIAL

Antimotility agents

RCTs found that loperamide hydrochloride and loperamide oxide reduced the duration of diarrhoea and improved symptoms of acute diarrhoeal illness compared with placebo. One RCT found that diphenoxylate atropine reduced rate of bowel actions compared with placebo but found no significant difference in median time to last stool. One RCT found more constipation-like periods in people taking loperamide hydrochloride and loperamide oxide 2 mg than in people taking placebo. However, it found no significant difference in constipation-like periods between loperamide oxide 1 mg and placebo.

TRADE OFF BETWEEN BENEFITS AND HARMS

Antibiotics (empirical use for mild–moderate diarrhoea)

RCTs found that antibiotics reduced the duration of diarrhoea and improved symptoms of acute diarrhoeal illness compared with placebo, and were more effective in eradicating pathogens from stool. One RCT found various self-limiting adverse effects in of people taking antibiotics, but these only led to discontinuation of treatment in people with rash. Bacterial resistance to *Campylobacter* developed in five people taking antibiotics.

UNKNOWN EFFECTIVENESS

Oral rehydration solutions

We found no systematic review or RCTs evaluating the effects of oral rehydration solutions for acute diarrhoea in adults living in developed countries.

What are the effects of treatments for acute mild–moderate diarrhoea in adults from the developed world travelling to developing countries? *New*

LIKELY TO BE BENEFICIAL

Antimotility agents

Two RCTs found that loperamide hydrocholride reduced the duration of diarrhoea compared with placebo. One of these RCTs also found that loperamide alone and trimethoprim–sulfamethoxazole alone were associated with similar durations of diarrhoea but that combination therapy with loperamide plus trimethoprim–sulfamethoxazole reduced the duration of diarrhoea compared with loperamide alone. Two RCTs found no significant difference in improvement of symptoms of acute diarrhoea between loperamide plus ciprofloxacin and ciprofloxacin.

Diarrhoea in adults (acute)

TRADE OFF BETWEEN BENEFITS AND HARMS

Antibiotics (empirical use for mild–moderate diarrhoea)
One systematic review, one subsequent RCT, and one additional RCT found that antibiotics reduced the duration of diarrhoea compared with placebo. The systematic review performed a meta-analysis of five RCTs and reported more adverse effects in people taking antibiotics compared with placebo, but none were judged to be serious.

UNKNOWN EFFECTIVENESS

Oral rehydration solutions
We found no systematic review or RCTs evaluating the effects of oral rehydration solutions on acute mild–moderate diarrhoea in adults from the developed world travelling to developing countries. One RCT found no significant difference in duration or diarrhoea or symptom control between loperamide plus oral rehydration solution and oral rehydration solution alone.

What are the effects of treatments for acute mild–moderate diarrhoea in adults living in developing countries? New

LIKELY TO BE BENEFICIAL

Antimotility agents
RCTs found that lidamidine and loperamide improved symptoms of acute diarrhoea compared with placebo.

UNKNOWN EFFECTIVENESS

Antibiotics (empirical use)
Two RCTs with flawed methods found no significant difference in symptoms of acute mild–moderate diarrhoea between antibiotics and placebo in adults living in developing countries.

Citrate oral rehydration solution (compared with bicarbonate oral rehydration solution)
One RCT found no significant difference in stool output at 48 hours between citrate oral rehydration solution and bicarbonate oral rehydration solution.

What are the effects of treatments for acute severe diarrhoea in adults living in developing countries? New

BENEFICIAL

Amino acid oral rehydration solution
RCTs found modest clinical benefit with amino acid oral rehydration solution compared with standard oral rehydration solution in both in people with cholera and non-cholera diarrhoea.

Rice based oral rehydration solution
One systematic review found that rice based oral rehydration solution (ORS) reduced stool volume compared with standard ORS both in people with cholera and non-cholera diarrhoea. One additional RCT found that rice ORS reduced stool output compared with standard ORS.

Antibiotics (empirical use)

We found no systematic review or RCTs evaluating the effects of empirical use of antibiotics in treating severe diarrhoea in adults living in developing countries.

Antimotility agents

We found no systematic review or RCTs evaluating the effects of antimotility agents in treating severe diarrhoea in adults living in developing countries.

Bicarbonate oral rehydration solution

RCTs found no significant difference in total stool output or duration of diarrhoea between bicarbonate oral rehydration solution and standard or chloride oral rehydration solution.

Intravenous rehydration (compared with nasogastric tube rehydration or oral rehydration solution)

One small RCT found no significant difference in the duration of diarrhoea or total stool volume between enteral rehydration through a nasogastric tube and intravenous rehydration. We found no systematic review or RCTs comparing oral rehydration solution alone versus intravenous rehydration.

Reduced osmolarity oral rehydration solution

Three RCTs found modest and inconsistent effects of reduced osmolarity oral rehydration solution (ORS) on stool volume and duration of diarrhoea compared with standard ORS. Reduced osmolarity ORS was associated with an increased risk of non-symptomatic hyponatremia.

DEFINITION Diarrhoea is watery or liquid stools, usually with an increase in stool weight above 200 g daily and an increase in daily stool frequency. This chapter covers empirical treatment of suspected infectious diarrhoea in adults.

INCIDENCE/ PREVALENCE An estimated 4000 million cases of diarrhoea occurred worldwide in 1996, resulting in 2.5 million deaths.[1] In the USA, the estimated incidence for infectious intestinal disease is 0.44 episodes per person per year (1 episode per person every 2.3 years), resulting in about one consultation with a doctor per person every 28 years.[2] A recent community study in the UK reported an incidence of 19 cases per 100 person years, of which 3.3 cases per 100 person years resulted in consultation with a general practitioner.[3] Both estimates derive from population based studies including both adults and children. The epidemiology of travellers' diarrhoea is not well understood. Incidence is higher in travellers visiting developing countries, but it varies widely by location and season of travel.[4]

AETIOLOGY/ RISK FACTORS The cause of diarrhoea depends on geographical location, standards of food hygiene, sanitation, water supply, and season. Commonly identified causes of sporadic diarrhoea in adults in developed countries include *Campylobacter*, *Salmonella*, *Shigella*, *Escherichia coli*, *Yersinia*, protozoa, and viruses. No pathogens are identified in more than half of people with diarrhoea. In returning travellers, about 50% of episodes are caused by bacteria such as enterotoxigenic *E coli*, *Salmonella*, *Shigella*, *Campylobacter*, *Vibrio*, enteroadherent *E coli*, *Yersinia*, and *Aeromonas*.[5]

Diarrhoea in adults (acute)

PROGNOSIS In developing countries, diarrhoea is reported to cause more deaths in children under 5 years of age than any other condition.[1] Few studies have examined which factors predict poor outcome in adults. In developed countries, death from infectious diarrhoea is rare, although serious complications, including severe dehydration and renal failure, can occur and may necessitate admission to hospital. Elderly people and those in long term care have an increased risk of death.[6]

Please refer to the Clinical Evidence website for full text and references.

What are the effects of immunisation in countries with high endemicity?

BENEFICIAL

Selective immunisation of high risk individuals (evidence only for children born to HBsAg positive mothers)

One non-systematic review of mainly observational studies with both plasma derived and recombinant vaccine, and three RCTs of plasma derived hepatitis B immunisation all found that immunisation prevented chronic carrier state compared with placebo or no treatment in children born to HBsAg positive mothers. One RCT found minor adverse events with immunisation; the other RCTs did not report on adverse events. We found no good evidence in other high risk groups. One cluster RCT found that selective immunisation in high risk individuals was less effective than universal immunisation of infants in preventing chronic carrier state and acute hepatitis events.

Universal immunisation of infants (limited evidence that it may be better than selective immunisation of high risk individuals)

One non-systematic review and four additional and subsequent RCTs provided evidence that universal (both recombinant and plasma derived) hepatitis B immunisation in infants in countries with high endemicity, compared with placebo, reduces acute hepatitis and development of a chronic carrier state for at least 15 years. Observational studies and one RCT found only minor adverse reactions after recombinant hepatitis B immunisation. One cluster RCT found universal immunisation with first plasma and then recombinant vaccine reduced the development of chronic carrier state and acute hepatitis events compared with immunisation of high risk groups.

What are the effects of immunisation in countries with low endemicity?

LIKELY TO BE BENEFICIAL

Selective immunisation of high risk individuals

One systematic review found that, in countries with low endemicity, plasma derived hepatitis B immunisation prevented acute hepatitis B and development of chronic carrier state in healthcare workers at high risk of exposure to bodily fluids. Three RCTs found that plasma derived hepatitis B immunisation prevented acute hepatitis B in homosexual men. One small RCT found no significant difference in hepatitis B events in heterosexual partners of infected people. Three RCTs of plasma derived immunisation in people on regular haemodialysis found potentially conflicting results. Two RCTs from France and Belgium found good protective efficacy against chronic carrier state. However, one large US based RCT found no good evidence of benefit. The systematic review of plasma derived vaccination found no significant difference between immunisation and placebo in the rate and severity of adverse events. One observational study showed a high prevalence of hepatitis B carrier state and low immunisation uptake in young homosexuals despite a national strategy to immunise high risk groups. Surveillance data from a national programme in Japan found that immunisation of neonates (with recombinant hepatitis B vaccine plus hepatitis B immunoglobulin [HBIG]) born to HBsAg ▶

Hepatitis B (prevention)

positive mothers provided 95% protection against the development of a chronic carrier state. We found insufficient evidence to compare the effectiveness of selective immunisation in high risk individuals with other strategies.

Universal immunisation of infants

One historical cohort study found a reduction in the prevalence of hepatitis B chronic carrier state after universal immunisation. We found insufficient evidence to compare its effectiveness with other strategies. Two cohort studies and surveillance data did not report any links between hepatitis B immunisation and serious adverse events.

UNKNOWN EFFECTIVENESS

Comparative effectiveness of different strategies

We found no systematic reviews, RCTs, or observational studies comparing the effectiveness of different immunisation strategies in countries with low endemicity.

Universal immunisation of adolescents

We found insufficient evidence to assess the effects of universal adolescent immunisation, or to compare its effectiveness with other strategies. One observational study suggests minor adverse effects after hepatitis B immunisation in this group.

DEFINITION   Hepatitis B is a viral infectious disease with an incubation period of 40–160 days. Acute hepatitis B infection is characterised by anorexia, vague abdominal discomfort, nausea and vomiting, jaundice, and occasional fever. Illness is associated with deranged liver function tests (especially raised alanine transaminases) and presence of serological markers of acute hepatitis B infection (e.g. hepatitis B surface antigen [HBsAg], antiHBc IgM).[1]

INCIDENCE/   The incidence of acute hepatitis B and prevalence of its chronic carrier state
PREVALENCE   varies widely across the globe. In areas with high endemicity (HBsAg prevalence ≥ 8%, e.g. South East Asia and Africa), more than half of the population becomes infected at some point in their lives.[2] In countries with low endemicity (HBsAg prevalence < 2%, e.g. North America, western Europe, Australia), most of the population do not become infected.[2] Nearly a third of the world population has been infected by hepatitis B at some point, and at least 350 million people (5–6% of world population) are currently chronic carriers of hepatitis B infection.[3]

AETIOLOGY/   In countries with high endemicity, most infections occur during childhood from
RISK FACTORS   an infected mother to her baby (vertical transmission) or from one family member to another (horizontal transmission).[4] Horizontal transmission is thought to be an important route of hepatitis B infection during early childhood, and probably occurs mainly through unnoticed contact with blood from infected family members.[5] In countries with high endemicity, the proportion of chronic HBsAg carriage attributable to vertical transmission has been estimated at 5–50%.[6–8] The proportion of chronic HBsAg carriage attributable to horizontal transmission is not known, although one survey in China found that 27.2% of families had one or more HBsAg positive members.[8] In developed countries, most hepatitis B infection occurs later, from sexual activity, injection drug use, or occupational exposure. Less frequent causes of infection include household contact, regular haemodialysis, transmission from a healthcare professional, and receipt of organs or blood products.[9] The vaccination policy of a country is a large determinant of the risk of developing hepatitis B. Since the development of plasma derived hepatitis B vaccine in the early 1980s, subsequently replaced by recombinant vaccine, many countries have adopted a policy of universal immunisation of all infants. On the basis of disease burden, the World Health Organization recommended that hepatitis B vaccine be incorporated into routine infant and childhood immunisation programmes in countries with

high endemicity by 1995 and in all countries by 1997.[10] However, in many countries with low endemicity, universal immunisation policy remains controversial and has still not been adopted.[11] Some of these countries have adopted a policy of selective immunisation of high risk individuals. Others have adopted a universal adolescent immunisation policy.

PROGNOSIS Hepatitis B infection resolves after the acute infection in 90–95% of cases. In the remainder (5–10%), it may result in several serious sequelae. Massive hepatic necrosis occurs in 1% of people with acute viral hepatitis, leading to a serious and often fatal condition called acute fulminant hepatitis. Between 2% and 10% of those infected as adults become chronic carriers, indicated by HBsAg persistence for more than 6 months. Chronic carriage is more frequent in those infected as children, and reaches up to 90% in those infected during the perinatal period.[1] Between 20% and 25% of chronic carriers develop a progressive chronic liver disease. In about one quarter to one third of cases, this progresses to cirrhosis and hepatocellular carcinoma.[12] These complications usually arise in older adults and are major causes of mortality in populations with high hepatitis B endemicity.[4] Observational studies suggest that in these countries almost 80% of chronic liver disease and cirrhosis is attributed to hepatitis B, and these complications lead to at least 1 million deaths every year worldwide.

Please refer to the Clinical Evidence website for full text and references.

Influenza

Search date July 2003

Lucy Hansen

Conclusions from studies in people with laboratory confirmed influenza may not be extrapolated to people with clinically suspected influenza, who have not had laboratory confirmation of infection with influenza A or B. RCTs provided insufficient evidence to assess the effects of antiviral agents on reducing serious complications of influenza.

What are the effects of antiviral treatment of influenza in adults?

LIKELY TO BE BENEFICIAL

Oral amantadine for early treatment of influenza A in adults (duration of symptoms reduced)

One systematic review and three additional RCTs have found that oral amantadine reduces the duration of influenza A symptoms by about 1 day compared with placebo. We found insufficient evidence about adverse effects in this setting. We found no good evidence of benefit if amantadine is started more than 2 days after symptom onset.

Orally inhaled zanamivir for early treatment of influenza A and B in adults (duration of symptoms reduced)

One systematic review has found that orally inhaled zanamivir reduces the duration of influenza symptoms by about 1 day compared with placebo. Adverse effects were similar in people taking zanamivir and in people taking placebo. We found no good evidence of benefit if zanamivir is started more than 2 days after symptom onset.

Oral oseltamivir for early treatment of influenza A and B in adults (duration of symptoms reduced)

Two RCTs have found that oral oseltamivir reduces the duration of influenza symptoms by about 1 day compared with placebo. Oral oseltamivir increases the incidence of nausea and vomiting compared with placebo. We found no good evidence of benefit if oseltamivir is started more than 1.5 days after symptom onset.

Oral rimantadine for early treatment of influenza A in adults (duration of symptoms reduced)

One systematic review has found that oral rimantadine reduces the duration of influenza A symptoms by about 1 day compared with placebo. We found insufficient evidence about adverse effects in this setting. We found no good evidence of benefit if rimantadine is started more than 2 days after symptom onset.

UNKNOWN EFFECTIVENESS

All antivirals (reduction of serious influenza complications)

We found insufficient evidence about the effects of antiviral agents on reducing serious complications of influenza.

DEFINITION   Influenza is caused by infection with influenza viruses. Uncomplicated influenza is characterised by the abrupt onset of fever, chills, non-productive cough, myalgias, headache, nasal congestion, sore throat, and fatigue.[1] Influenza is usually diagnosed clinically. Not all people infected with influenza viruses become symptomatic. People infected with other pathogens may have ▶

symptoms identical to those of influenza.[2] The percentage of infections resulting in clinical illness can vary from about 40–85%, depending on age and pre-existing immunity to the virus.[3] Influenza can be confirmed by viral culture, immunofluorescence staining, enzyme immunoassay, or rapid diagnostic testing of nasopharyngeal, nasal or throat swab specimens, or by serological testing of paired sera. Some rapid tests detect influenza A only, some detect and distinguish between influenza A and B, whereas others detect but do not distinguish between influenza A and B.

INCIDENCE/
PREVALENCE
In temperate areas of the northern hemisphere, influenza activity typically peaks between late December and early March, whereas in temperate areas of the southern hemisphere influenza activity typically peaks between May and September. In tropical areas, influenza can occur throughout the year.[2] The annual incidence of influenza varies yearly, and depends partly on the underlying level of population immunity to circulating influenza viruses.[1] One localised study in the USA found that serological conversion with or without symptoms occurred in 10–20% a year, with the highest infection rates in people aged under 20 years.[4] Attack rates are higher in institutions and in areas of overcrowding.[5]

AETIOLOGY/
RISK FACTORS
Influenza viruses are transmitted primarily from person to person through respiratory droplets disseminated during sneezing, coughing, and talking.[1,6]

PROGNOSIS
The incubation period of influenza is 1–4 days and infected adults are usually contagious from the day before symptom onset until 5 days after symptom onset. The signs and symptoms of uncomplicated influenza usually resolve within a week, although cough and fatigue may persist.[1] Complications include otitis media, bacterial sinusitis, secondary bacterial pneumonia, and, less commonly, viral pneumonia and respiratory failure. Complications are also caused by exacerbation of underlying disease.[1,2] In the USA each year, over 110 000 admissions to hospital and about 20 000 deaths are related to influenza.[2] The risk of hospitalisation is highest in people 65 years or older, in very young children, and in those with chronic medical conditions.[1,7,8] Over 90% of influenza related deaths during recent seasonal epidemics in the USA have been in people 65 years or older.[1] During influenza pandemics, morbidity and mortality may be high in younger age groups.[1] Severe illness is more common with influenza A infections than with influenza B infections.[1]

Please refer to the Clinical Evidence website for full text and references.

Leprosy

Search date November 2003

Diana Lockwood

What are the effects of preventive interventions?

BENEFICIAL

Bacillus Calmette Guerin (BCG) vaccine

One RCT evaluated four different vaccines and found that the largest effect was with ICRC vaccine and BCG plus killed *M leprae*, followed by BCG alone. The effectiveness of *Mycobacterium w* was only marginal. However, only for BCG alone were the findings corroborated by large controlled clinical trials conducted in different geographical areas with long term follow up. Only one RCT reported on harms of vaccination; it found these to be minimal.

BCG plus killed *Mycobacterium leprae*

One RCT evaluated four different vaccines and found that the largest effect was with ICRC vaccine and BCG plus killed *M leprae*, followed by BCG alone. The effectiveness of *Mycobacterium w* was only marginal. However, only for BCG alone were the findings corroborated by large controlled clinical trials conducted in different geographical areas with long term follow up. Only one RCT reported on harms of vaccination; it found these to be minimal.

LIKELY TO BE BENEFICIAL

ICRC vaccine

One RCT evaluated four different vaccines and found that the largest effect was with ICRC vaccine and BCG plus killed *M leprae*, followed by BCG alone. The effectiveness of *Mycobacterium w* was only marginal. However, only for BCG alone were the findings corroborated by large controlled clinical trials conducted in different geographical areas with long term follow up. Only one RCT reported on harms of vaccination; it found these to be minimal.

UNKNOWN EFFECTIVENESS

Mycobacterium w vaccine

One RCT evaluated four different vaccines and found that the largest effect was with ICRC vaccine and BCG plus killed *M leprae*, followed by BCG alone. The effectiveness of *Mycobacterium w* was only marginal. However, only for BCG alone were the findings corroborated by large controlled clinical trials conducted in different geographical areas with long term follow up. Only one RCT reported on harms of vaccination; it found these to be minimal.

What are the effects of treatments?

BENEFICIAL

Multidrug treatment for multibacillary leprosy*

We found no reliable comparisons of multidrug treatment with rifampicin plus clofazimine plus dapsone versus dapsone alone, or versus dapsone plus rifampicin, in people with multibacillary leprosy. Observational studies found that multidrug treatment improved skin lesions and was associated with a low relapse rate. The evidence on the incidence of adverse effects is poor. Multidrug treatment was not compared with dapsone alone because rising dapsone resistance rates would make such a study unethical.

◀ **Multidrug treatment for paucibacillary leprosy***

We found no reliable comparisons of multidrug treatment with dapsone plus rifampicin versus dapsone alone in people with paucibacillary leprosy, and RCTs would probably be unethical because of rising rates of dapsone resistance. Observational studies found that multidrug treatment improved skin lesions and was associated with a low relapse rate. We found poor evidence on the incidence of adverse effects.

Multiple dose compared with single dose treatment for single skin lesion leprosy

One RCT found that multiple dose treatment with rifampicin monthly plus dapsone daily for 6 months achieved higher cure rates at 18 months than single dose treatment with rifampicin plus minocycline plus ofloxacin. Some improvement occurred in 99% of people in both groups. Adverse effects were similar with both regimens.

*Observational evidence only; RCTs unlikely to be conducted

DEFINITION   Leprosy is a chronic granulomatous disease caused by *Mycobacterium leprae*, primarily affecting the peripheral nerves and skin. The clinical picture depends on the individual's immune response to *M leprae*. At the tuberculoid end of the Ridley–Jopling scale, individuals have good cell mediated immunity and few skin lesions. At the lepromatous end of the scale, individuals have good cell mediated immunity, causing uncontrolled bacterial spread and skin and mucosal infiltration. Peripheral nerve damage occurs across the spectrum. Nerve damage may occur before, during, or after treatment. Some patients have no nerve damage, others develop anaesthesia of the hands and feet, which puts them at risk of developing neuropathic injury. Weakness and paralysis of the small muscles of the hands, feet, and eyes puts patients at risk of developing deformity and contractures. Loss of the fingers and toes is due to repeated injury in a weak, anaesthetic limb. These visible deformities cause stigmatisation. Classification is based on clinical appearance and bacterial index of lesions. The World Health Organization field classification is based on the number of skin lesions: single lesion leprosy (1 lesion), paucibacillary leprosy (2–5 skin lesions), and multibacillary leprosy (> 5 skin lesions).[1]

INCIDENCE/   Worldwide, about 720 000 new cases of leprosy are reported each year,[2] and
PREVALENCE about 2 million people have leprosy related disabilities. Six major endemic countries (India, Brazil, Myanmar, Madagascar, Nepal, and Mozambique) account for 88% of all new cases. Cohort studies show a peak of disease presentation between 10–20 years of age.[3] After puberty there are twice as many cases in males as in females.

AETIOLOGY/   *M leprae* is discharged from the nasal mucosa of people with untreated
RISK FACTORS lepromatous leprosy, and spreads, via the recipient's nasal mucosa, to infect their skin and nerves. It is a hardy organism and has been shown to survive outside human hosts in India for many months.[4] Risk factors for infection include household contact with a person with leprosy. We found no good evidence of an association with HIV infection, nutrition, or socioeconomic status.[5]

PROGNOSIS   Complications of leprosy include nerve damage, immunological reactions, and bacillary infiltration. Without treatment, tuberculoid infection eventually resolves spontaneously. Most people with borderline tuberculoid and borderline lepromatous leprosy gradually develop lepromatous infection. Many people have peripheral nerve damage at the time of diagnosis, ranging from 15% in Bangladesh[6] to 55% in Ethiopia.[7] Immunological reactions can occur with or without antibiotic treatment. Further nerve damage occurs through immune ▶

mediated reactions and neuritis. Erythema nodosum leprosum (type 2 reaction) is an immune complex mediated reaction causing fever, malaise, and neuritis, which occurs in 20% of people with lepromatous leprosy and 5% with borderline lepromatous leprosy.[8] Secondary impairments (wounds, contractures, and digit resorption) occur in 33–56% of people with established nerve damage.[9] We found no recent information on mortality.

Please refer to the Clinical Evidence website for full text and references.

Search date September 2003

Edward Hayes and Paul Mead

What are the effects of measures to prevent Lyme disease?

BENEFICIAL

Prophylactic antibiotics after *Ixodes scapularis* tick bites in Lyme disease endemic areas in North America

One systematic review in people with recognised *I scapularis* tick bites in the preceding 72 hours found that antibiotics reduced the risk of developing clinical Lyme disease compared with placebo, but the difference was not significant. One subsequent large RCT in people who had removed an attached *I scapularis* tick in the preceding 72 hours found that doxycycline reduced the proportion of people with erythema migrans at the site of the tick bite compared with placebo.

What are the effects of antibiotic treatment for Lyme disease arthritis?

LIKELY TO BE BENEFICIAL

Cefotaxime (more effective than penicillin)*

One RCT found weak evidence from a small subgroup analysis of people with Lyme arthritis that cefotaxime increased the proportion of people with full recovery compared with penicillin.
*Based on subgroup analysis of RCTs

Ceftriaxone (more effective than penicillin)*

One RCT found weak evidence from a small subgroup analysis of people with Lyme arthritis that ceftriaxone improved symptoms compared with penicillin.
*Based on subgroup analysis of RCTs

Doxycycline (as effective as amoxicillin plus probenecid)

One RCT in people with Lyme arthritis found no significant difference between doxycycline and amoxicillin plus probenecid in resolution of Lyme arthritis.

Penicillin (more effective than placebo)

One RCT in people with Lyme arthritis has found that penicillin increases resolution of Lyme arthritis compared with placebo.

What are the effects of antibiotic treatments for late neurological Lyme disease?

LIKELY TO BE BENEFICIAL

Cefotaxime (more effective than penicillin)*

One RCT found weak evidence from a small subgroup analysis of people with late Lyme disease that cefotaxime improved symptoms of neuropathy compared with penicillin.
*Based on subgroup analysis of RCTs

UNKNOWN EFFECTIVENESS

Ceftriaxone (in people with late neurological Lyme disease)

One RCT found insufficient evidence from a small subgroup analysis in people with late neurological Lyme disease about effects of ceftriaxone and cefotaxime.

Infectious diseases

Lyme disease

Ceftriaxone (in people with late neurological Lyme disease who had previously been treated)

One RCT in people with previously treated Lyme disease found no significant difference between ceftriaxone and placebo in cognitive functioning at 6 months. It found that ceftriaxone improved fatigue but blinding in this RCT was incomplete.

LIKELY TO BE INEFFECTIVE OR HARMFUL

Ceftriaxone plus doxycycline (in people with late neurological Lyme disease who had been previously treated)

One RCT comparing ceftriaxone plus doxycycline with placebo in people with previously treated Lyme disease and persistent neurological symptoms found no significant difference in health related quality of life at interim analysis at 180 days.

DEFINITION   Lyme disease is an inflammatory illness resulting from infection with spiro-chetes of the *Borrelia burgdorferi* genospecies transmitted to humans by ticks. Some infected people have no symptoms. The characteristic manifestation of early Lyme disease is erythema migrans: a circular rash at the site of the infectious tick attachment that expands over a period of days to weeks in 80–90% of people with Lyme disease. Early disseminated infection may cause secondary erythema migrans, disease of the nervous system (facial palsy or other cranial neuropathies, meningitis, and radiculoneuritis), muscu-loskeletal disease (arthralgia), and, rarely, cardiac disease (myocarditis or transient atrioventricular block). Untreated or inadequately treated Lyme disease can cause late disseminated manifestations weeks to months after infection. These late manifestations include arthritis, polyneuropathy, and encephalopathy. Diagnosis of Lyme disease is based primarily on clinical findings and a high likelihood of exposure to infected ticks. Serological testing is helpful in people with endemic exposure who have clinical findings consist-ent with later stage disseminated Lyme disease.

INCIDENCE/   Lyme disease occurs in temperate regions of North America, Europe, and
PREVALENCE   Asia. It is the most commonly reported vector borne disease in the USA, with over 23 000 cases reported a year.[1] Most cases occur in the north-eastern and north-central states, with a reported annual incidence in endemic states as high as 133/100 000 people.[1] In highly endemic communities, the incidence of Lyme disease may exceed 1000/100 000 people a year.[1] In some countries of Europe, the incidence of Lyme disease has been estimated to be over 100/100 000 people a year.[2] Foci of Lyme disease have been described in northern forested regions of Russia, in China, and in Japan.[3] Transmission cycles of *B burgdorferi* have not been described in tropical areas or in the southern hemisphere.[3]

AETIOLOGY/   Lyme disease is caused by infection with any of the *B burgdorferi* sensu lato
RISK FACTORS genospecies. Virtually all cases of Lyme disease in North America are the result of infection with *B burgdorferi*. In Europe, Lyme disease may be caused by *B burgdorferi*, *B garinii*, or *B afzelii*. The infectious spirochetes are transmitted to humans through the bite of certain *Ixodes* ticks.[3] Humans who have frequent or prolonged exposure to the habitats of infected *Ixodes* ticks are at highest risk of acquiring Lyme disease. Individual risk depends on the likelihood of being bitten by infected tick vectors, which varies with the density of vector ticks in the environment, the prevalence of infection in ticks, and the extent of a person's contact with infected ticks. The risk of Lyme disease is often concentrated in focal areas. In the USA, risk is highest in certain counties within north-eastern and north-central states during the months of April to July.[2] People become infected when they engage in activities in wooded or bushy areas that are favourable habitats for ticks, and deer and rodent hosts. A vaccine based on recombinant outer surface protein Osp-A was licensed for use in the USA but later removed from the market.

▶

PROGNOSIS   Lyme disease is rarely fatal. Untreated Lyme arthritis resolves at a rate of 10–20% a year; over 90% of facial palsies due to Lyme disease resolve spontaneously, and most cases of Lyme carditis resolve without sequelae.[4] However, untreated Lyme disease can result in arthritis (50% of untreated people), meningitis or neuropathies (15% of untreated people), carditis (5–10% of untreated people with erythema migrans), and, rarely, encephalopathy.

Please refer to the Clinical Evidence website for full text and references.

Malaria: prevention in travellers

Search date March 2004

Ashley M Croft

What are the effects of non-drug preventive interventions in adult travellers?

BENEFICIAL

Insecticide treated nets

We found no RCTs in travellers. One systematic review in adult and child residents of malaria endemic settings found that insecticide treated nets reduced the number of mild episodes of malaria and reduced child mortality.

LIKELY TO BE BENEFICIAL

Insecticide treated clothing in adults

Two RCTs in soldiers and refugee householders found that permethrin treated fabric (clothing or sheets) reduced the incidence of malaria.

UNKNOWN EFFECTIVENESS

Aerosol insecticides in adults

We found no RCTs on the effects of aerosol insecticides in preventing malaria in travellers. One large questionnaire survey in travellers found insufficient evidence on the effects of aerosol insecticides in preventing malaria. Two community RCTs in residents of malaria endemic areas found that indoor spraying of aerosol insecticides reduced clinical malaria.

Air conditioning and electric fans in adults

We found no RCTs on the effects of air conditioning or electric fans in preventing malaria in travellers. One large questionnaire survey found that air conditioning reduced the incidence of malaria. One small observational study found that electric ceiling fans reduced total catches of culicine mosquitoes but did not significantly reduce total catches of anopheline mosquitoes in indoor spaces.

Full length clothing in adults

We found no RCTs on the effects of full length clothing in preventing malaria in travellers. One large questionnaire survey in travellers found that wearing trousers and long sleeved shirts reduced the incidence of malaria.

Mosquito coils and vaporising mats in adults

We found no RCTs on the effects of coils and vaporising mats in preventing malaria in travellers. One case-control study of coils in travellers found no evidence of a protective effect against malaria. One RCT of coils and one observational study of pyrethroid vaporising mats found that these devices reduced numbers of culicine mosquitoes in indoor spaces.

Smoke

We found no RCTs on the effects of smoke in preventing malaria. One controlled clinical trial found that smoke repelled mosquitoes during the evening.

Topical (skin applied) insect repellents in adults

We found no RCTs on the effects of topical (skin applied) insect repellents in preventing malaria in travellers. One small crossover RCT found that diethyltoluamide (DEET) preparations protected against mosquito bites. DEET has been reported to cause systemic and skin adverse reactions, particularly with prolonged use.

Acoustic buzzers in adults; biological control measures

We found no RCTs on the effects of these interventions.

What are the effects of drug prophylaxis in adult travellers?

Atovaquone plus proguanil in adults

One RCT in migrants with limited immunity found that atovaquone plus proguanil reduced the proportion of people with malaria compared with placebo. One RCT found no significant difference between atovaquone plus proguanil and chloroquine plus proguanil in preventing malaria. One RCT of atovaquone plus proguanil versus mefloquine found no cases of clinical malaria throughout the trial, but found a higher rate of neuropsychiatric harm with mefloquine than with atovaquone plus proguanil. RCTs comparing adverse effects of atovaquone plus proguanil versus chloroquine plus proguanil found different results. One RCT found that atovaquone plus proguanil reduced adverse effects compared with mefloquine and chloroquine plus proguanil and had similar adverse effect rates compared with doxycycline. Another RCT found no significant difference in adverse events between atovaquone plus proguanil and chloroquine plus proguanil.

Doxycycline in adults

One RCT in soldiers and one RCT in migrants with limited immunity found that doxycycline reduced the risk of malaria compared with placebo. One of the RCTs found that doxycycline was associated with nausea and vomiting, diarrhoea, cough, headache, and unspecified dermatological symptoms over 13 weeks. We found no evidence on long term safety. One RCT found that doxycycline had fewer adverse effects than mefloquine or chloroquine plus proguanil and had similar adverse effect rates compared with atovaquone plus proguanil.

Chloroquine plus proguanil in adults

One RCT found no significant difference between chloroquine plus proguanil and chloroquine plus sulfadoxine plus pyrimethamine in the incidence of *P falciparum* malaria. One RCT found no significant difference between chloroquine plus proguanil and proguanil alone in the incidence of *P falciparum* malaria. One RCT found no significant difference between chloroquine plus proguanil and atovaquone plus proguanil in preventing malaria. RCTs comparing adverse effects of chloroquine plus proguanil versus atovaquone plus proguanil found different results. One RCT found that chloroquine plus proguanil increased adverse effects compared with three other common antimalarial drug regimens (doxycycline, mefloquine, and atovaquone plus proguanil). Another RCT found no significant difference in adverse events between chloroquine plus proguanil and atovaquone plus proguanil.

Mefloquine in adults

One systematic review of one RCT in soldiers found that mefloquine reduced cases of malaria compared with placebo, and found that mefloquine had a protective efficacy of 100%. One RCT of mefloquine versus atovaquone plus proguanil found no cases of clinical malaria throughout the trial, but found a higher rate of neuropsychiatric harm with mefloquine compared with atovaquone plus proguanil. One RCT found that mefloquine had more adverse effects than doxycycline or atovaquone plus proguanil and had similar adverse event rates compared with chloroquine plus proguanil.

Malaria: prevention in travellers

Chloroquine in adults

We found no RCTs on the effects of chloroquine in travellers. One RCT in Austrian workers residing in Nigeria found no significant difference between chloroquine and sulfadoxine plus pyrimethamine in the incidence of malaria after 6–22 months. *P falciparum* resistance to chloroquine is now established in most malaria endemic regions of the world.

Pyrimethamine plus dapsone in adults

We found no RCTs in travellers. One RCT in Thai soldiers found insufficient evidence to compare pyrimethamine plus dapsone versus proguanil plus dapsone. We found limited observational evidence that pyrimethamine plus dapsone may cause agranulocytosis.

LIKELY TO BE INEFFECTIVE OR HARMFUL

Amodiaquine in adults

We found no RCTs on the effects of amodiaquine in preventing malaria in travellers. We found limited observational evidence that amodiaquine may cause neutropenia, liver damage, and hepatitis.

Sulfadoxine plus pyrimethamine in adults

We found no RCTs of sulfadoxine plus pyrimethamine alone. One RCT found no significant difference between chloroquine plus proguanil and chloroquine plus sulfadoxine plus pyrimethamine in the incidence of *P falciparum* malaria. One retrospective observational study suggested that sulfadoxine plus pyrimethamine was associated with severe cutaneous reactions.

What are the effects of antimalaria vaccines?

UNKNOWN EFFECTIVENESS

Vaccines

We found no RCTs of the effects of antimalaria vaccines in travellers. One systematic review of antimalaria vaccines in residents of malaria endemic areas found that the SPf66 vaccine reduced first attacks of malaria compared with placebo.

What are the effects of preventative interventions in child travellers?

UNKNOWN EFFECTIVENESS

Mefloquine in children

We found no RCTs of the effects of mefloquine in preventing malaria in child travellers.

LIKELY TO BE INEFFECTIVE OR HARMFUL

Topical (skin applied) insect repellents containing DEET in children

We found no RCTs on the effects of DEET in preventing malaria in child travellers. Case reports in young children found serious adverse effects with DEET.

What are the effects of interventions in pregnant travellers?

Insecticide treated nets in pregnant travellers

We found no RCTs on the effects of insecticide treated nets in preventing malaria in pregnant travellers. One RCT of pregnant long term residents of a malaria endemic area found insufficient evidence on the effects of permethrin treated nets in preventing malaria.

Antimalaria drugs in pregnant travellers; insecticide treated clothing in pregnant travellers; topical (skin applied) insect repellents in pregnant travellers

We found no RCTs on the effects of these interventions.

What are the effects of antimalaria interventions in airline pilots?

Antimalaria drugs in airline pilots and aircrew

We found no RCTs on the effects of antimalaria drugs in airline pilots.

DEFINITION Malaria is an acute parasitic disease of the tropics and subtropics, caused by the invasion and destruction of red blood cells by one or more of four species of the genus *Plasmodium: P falciparum, P vivax, P ovale,* and *P malariae*.[1] The clinical presentation of malaria varies according to the infecting species, and to the genetics, immune status, and age of the infected person.[2] The most severe form of human malaria is caused by *P falciparum*, in which variable clinical features include spiking fevers, chills, headache, muscular aching and weakness, vomiting, cough, diarrhoea, and abdominal pain; other symptoms related to organ failure may supervene, such as: acute renal failure, generalised convulsions, and circulatory collapse, followed by coma and death.[3,4] *P falciparum* accounts for over 50% of malaria infections in most East Asian countries, over 90% in sub-Saharan Africa, and almost 100% in Hispaniola.[5] Travellers are defined here as visitors from a malaria-free area to a malaria-endemic area, and who stay in the endemic area for less than 1 year.

INCIDENCE/ PREVALENCE Malaria is the most dangerous parasitic disease of humans, infecting around 5% of the world's population, and causing about one million deaths each year.[6] The disease is strongly resurgent, due to the effects of war, climate change, large-scale population movements, increased breeding opportunities for vector mosquitoes, rapidly spreading drug and insecticide resistance, and neglect of public health infrastructure.[1,7] Malaria is currently endemic in over 100 countries, which are visited by over 125 million international travellers each year.[4] Cases of malaria acquired by international travellers from industrialised countries probably number 25 000 annually; of these, about 10 000 are reported, and 150 are fatal.[8]

AETIOLOGY/ RISK FACTORS Humans acquire malaria from sporozoites transmitted by the bite of infected female anopheline mosquitoes.[9] When foraging, blood-thirsty female mosquitoes fly upwind searching for the scent trail of an attractive host.[10] Female anophelines are attracted to their human hosts over a range of between 7 metres to 20 metres, and through a variety of stimuli including exhaled carbon dioxide, lactic acid, other host odours, warmth, and moisture.[11] Larger people tend to be bitten by mosquitoes more than smaller individuals, and adults more often than infants and children.[11,12] Women get significantly more mosquito bites in trials than men.[13] Of about 3200 mosquito species so far described, some 430 belong to the genus Anopheles, and of these, around 70 ▶

Malaria: prevention in travellers

anopheline species are known to transmit malaria, with about 40 species considered important vectors.[14] Malaria transmission does not usually occur at temperatures below 16 °C or above 35 °C, nor at altitudes greater than 3000 metres above sea level at the equator (lower elevations in cooler climates), because sporozoite development in the mosquito cannot take place.[15] The optimum conditions for transmission are a humidity of over 60% and an ambient temperature between 25–30 °C.[16] Most of the important vectors of malaria breed in small temporary collections of fresh surface water exposed to sunlight and with little predation, and in sites such as residual pools in drying river beds.[17] Although rainfall provides breeding sites for mosquitoes, excessive rainfall may wash away mosquito larvae and pupae.[18] Conversely, prolonged droughts may be associated with increased malaria transmission if they reduce the size and flow rates of large rivers sufficiently to produce suitable Anopheles breeding sites.[19] Anopheline mosquitoes vary in their preferred feeding and resting locations, although the majority bite in the evening and at night.[20] The Anopheles mosquito will feed by day only if unusually hungry.[21] Anopheles adults usually fly not more than 2–3 kilometres from their breeding sites, although a flight range of up to 7 kilometres has been observed.[22] Exceptionally, strong winds may carry Anopheles up to 30 kilometres or more.[11] In travellers, malaria risk is related to destination, activity, and duration of travel. A retrospective cohort study (5898 confirmed cases) in Italian travellers between 1989–1997 found the malaria incidence was 1.5/1000 from travel to Africa, 0.11/1000 from travel to Asia, and 0.04/1000 from Central–South America.[23] A survey of 2131 German travellers to sub-Saharan Africa found that solo travellers were at almost a 9-fold greater risk of infection than those on package tours.[24] A case control study (46 cases, 557 controls) reported that a visit to the tropics of more than 21 days doubles the malaria risk compared with visits lasting 21 days or less.[25]

PROGNOSIS Malaria can develop after just one anopheline mosquito bite.[26] Human malaria has a usual incubation period of between 10–14 days (*P falciparum, P vivax,* and *P ovale*) to around 28 days (*P malariae*).[27] Certain strains of *P vivax* and *P ovale* can have a much longer incubation period, of between 6–18 months.[19] Some 90% of malaria attacks in travellers occur at home.[28] People with any fever pattern should be considered to have malaria until proven otherwise, when they have been to endemic areas.[4,6,21,26,29] Once malaria infection occurs, older travellers are at higher risk of poor clinical outcomes and death. In US travellers between 1966–1987, the case fatality rate was 0.4% for people aged 0–19, 2.2% between ages 20–39, 5.8% between ages 40–69, and 30.3% for those aged 70–79.[30] Complications and death from malaria are mainly because of inappropriate therapy, or to delay in the initiation of treatment.[31] If malaria is diagnosed and treated promptly, around 88% of previously healthy travellers will recover completely.[32]

Please refer to the Clinical Evidence website for full text and references.

Search date February 2004

Aika Omari and Paul Garner

What are the effects of antimalarial treatments for complicated falciparum malaria in non-pregnant people?

LIKELY TO BE BENEFICIAL

Artemether (as effective as quinine)

Two systematic reviews and four subsequent RCTs found no significant difference in death rates between artemether and quinine in people with severe malaria. One of the reviews found no significant difference in the speed of coma recovery, fever clearance time, or neurological sequelae between artemether and quinine. The second review found no significant difference in neurological sequelae at recovery between artemether and quinine.

High initial dose quinine (reduced parasite and fever clearance times, but no difference in mortality)

One systematic review of three small RCTs in adults and children, and one subsequent RCT in children, found no significant difference in mortality between quinine regimens with high initial quinine dose and those with no loading dose. The systematic review found that high initial dose quinine reduced parasite and fever clearance times compared with no loading dose. The subsequent RCT found no significant difference between high initial dose and no loading dose for recovery of consciousness or parasite clearance time. One small RCT included in the review found that high initial dose quinine increased transient partial hearing loss compared with no loading dose. Another small RCT in the review found no significant difference between treatments in neurological sequelae.

Quinine*

We found no RCTs comparing quinine with either placebo or no treatment, but international consensus recommends quinine for the treatment of severe falciparum malaria.

*Based on consensus. RCTs would be considered unethical.

UNKNOWN EFFECTIVENESS

Intramuscular versus intravenous quinine

One RCT in children found no significant difference between intramuscular and intravenous quinine in recovery times or death. However, the study may have lacked power to detect clinically important differences between treatments.

Intravenous artesunate versus quinine

One RCT found no significant difference in mortality between intravenous artesunate and quinine, but may have been underpowered to detect a clinically important difference.

Rectal artemisinin and its derivatives

One systematic review of small RCTs found no significant difference in mortality between rectal artemisinin and quinine in people with severe malaria. One RCT found no significant difference in mortality between rectal dihydroartemisinin and quinine. We found no systematic review and no RCTs comparing rectal artesunate versus quinine.

▶

Malaria: severe, life threatening

What are the effects of adjunctive treatment for complicated falciparum malaria in non-pregnant people?

UNKNOWN EFFECTIVENESS

Desferrioxamine mesylate

One systematic review found limited evidence that the risk of persistent seizures in children with cerebral malaria was reduced with desferrioxamine mesylate compared with placebo.

Exchange blood transfusion

One systematic review found no suitable RCTs. A systematic review of case control studies found no significant difference in mortality between exchange transfusion plus antimalarial drugs and antimalarial drugs alone.

Initial blood transfusion

One systematic review found no significant difference in mortality between initial and expectant blood transfusion among clinically stable children (no respiratory distress or cardiac failure) with malarial anaemia, but found that adverse events were more common with initial blood transfusion. The review found no significant difference between transfusion and no transfusion for the combined outcome of death or severe adverse events. Transmission of hepatitis B or HIV was not reported. We found no RCTs examining the effects of transfusion in adults with malaria.

LIKELY TO BE INEFFECTIVE OR HARMFUL

Dexamethasone

One systematic review found no significant difference in mortality between dexamethasone and placebo, but gastrointestinal bleeding and seizures were more common with dexamethasone.

DEFINITION   Malaria is caused by protozoan infection of red blood cells with *Plasmodium falciparum* and comprises a variety of syndromes. This review deals with clinically complicated malaria (i.e. malaria that presents with life threatening conditions, including coma, severe anaemia, renal failure, respiratory distress syndrome, hypoglycaemia, shock, spontaneous haemorrhage, and convulsions). The diagnosis of cerebral malaria should be considered where there is encephalopathy in the presence of malaria parasites. A strict definition of cerebral malaria requires the presence of unrousable coma, and no other cause of encephalopathy (e.g. hypoglycaemia, sedative drugs), in the presence of *P falciparum* infection.[1] This review does not currently cover the treatment of malaria in pregnancy.

INCIDENCE/ PREVALENCE   Malaria is a major health problem in the tropics, with 300–500 million clinical cases occurring annually, and an estimated 1.1–2.7 million deaths each year as a result of severe malaria.[2] Over 90% of deaths occur in children under 5 years of age, mainly from cerebral malaria and anaemia.[2] In areas where the rate of malaria transmission is stable (endemic), those most at risk of acquiring severe malaria are children under 5 years old, because adults and older children have partial immunity, which offers some protection. In areas where the rate of malaria transmission is unstable (non-endemic), severe malaria affects both adults and children. Non-immune travellers and migrants are also at risk of developing severe malaria.

AETIOLOGY/ RISK FACTORS   Malaria is transmitted by the bite of infected female anopheline mosquitoes. Certain genes are associated with resistance to severe malaria. The human leukocyte antigens HLA-Bw53 and HLA-DRB1*1302 protect against severe malaria. However, associations of HLA antigens with severe malaria are limited ▶

to specific populations.[3,4] Haemoglobin S[3] and haemoglobin C[5] are also protective against severe malaria. Genes such as the tumour necrosis factor gene have also been associated with increased susceptibility to severe malaria (see aetiology under malaria: prevention in travellers, p 226).[6]

PROGNOSIS In children under 5 years of age with cerebral malaria, the estimated case fatality of treated malaria is 19%, although reported hospital case fatality may be as high as 40%.[1,7] Neurological sequelae persisting for more than 6 months occur in more than 2% of survivors, and include ataxia, hemiplegia, speech disorders, behavioural disorders, epilepsy, and blindness. Severe malarial anaemia has a case fatality rate higher than 13%.[7] In adults, the mortality of cerebral malaria is 20%; this rises to 50% in pregnancy, and neurological sequelae occur in about 3% of survivors.[8]

Please refer to the Clinical Evidence website for full text and references.

Malaria: uncomplicated, caused by *Plasmodium falciparum*

Search date September 2004

David Taylor-Robinson, Katharine Jones, and Paul Garner

What are the effects of empirical treatment of clinical malaria compared with treatment targeted to those with parasitaemia? New

UNKNOWN EFFECTIVENESS

Empirical treatment versus treatment of microscopy or rapid diagnostic test confirmed uncomplicated malaria New

We found no RCTs comparing empirical treatment versus treatment of malaria confirmed by microscopy or rapid diagnostic tests.

What are the effects of non-artemisinin treatments, compared with amodiaquine or sulfadoxine-pyrimethamine, in people living in endemic areas (excluding South East Asia)? New

TRADE OFF BETWEEN BENEFITS AND HARMS

Chlorproguanil–dapsone (possibly more effective than sulfadoxine–pyrimethamine but with more serious adverse effects) New

We found no RCTs reporting results for day 28 outcomes with chlorproguanil–dapsone compared with sulfadoxine–pyrimethamine. One RCT identified by a systematic review found lower rates of treatment failure at day 14 with chlorproguanil–dapsone compared with sulfadoxine–pyrimethamine. The review found no significant difference in rates of overall and serious adverse events between treatments. One RCT identified by the review found that a higher proportion of people taking chlorproguanil-dapsone had red blood cell disorders compared with sulfadoxine-pyrimethamine. The other RCT found a higher rate of adverse events leading to discontinuation of treatment with chlorproguanil–dapsone compared with sulfadoxine–pyrimethamine. We found no RCTs comparing a 3 day regimen of chlorproguanil–dapsone (with 2.0 mg chlorproguanil) versus amodiaquine.

UNKNOWN EFFECTIVENESS

Sulfadoxine–pyrimethamine plus amodiaquine (no proven benefit compared with sulfadoxine–pyrimethamine or amodiaquine alone) New

One systematic review found no significant difference in rates of day 28 cure or adverse events between sulfadoxine–pyrimethamine plus amodiaquine and sulfadoxine–pyrimethamine alone although one RCT identified by the review found a shorter mean fever clearance time with the combination treatment compared with sulfadoxine–pyrimethamine alone. One additional RCT found higher rates of day 28 cure and mild to moderate adverse events with the combination treatment compared with sulfadoxine–pyrimethamine alone. One systematic review found no significant difference in cure rate at day 28, mean parasite clearance time, and fever clearance time between sulfadoxine–pyrimethamine plus amodiaquine and amodiaquine alone. Three subsequent RCTs found inconsistent results for cure rates and no significant difference in fever clearance times or rate of adverse ▶

events between combination treatment and amodiaquine alone. One RCT found that combination treatment reduced mean parasite clearance time compared with amodiaquine alone.

Sulfadoxine–pyrimethamine plus chloroquine (no proven benefit compared with sulfadoxine–pyrimethamine alone) *New*

We found no RCTs reporting results for day 28 outcomes with sulfadoxine–pyrimethamine plus chloroquine compared with sulfadoxine–pyrimethamine alone. Two small RCTs provided insufficient evidence to determine whether there was any difference in rates of treatment failure at days 21 (first RCT) and 14 (second RCT) between treatments and gave no information on adverse events.

Are artemisinin combination treatments more effective than non-artemisinin treatments in people living in endemic areas? *New*

BENEFICIAL

Artesunate (3 days) plus amodiaquine (more effective than amodiaquine alone) *New*

One systematic review found lower rates of parasitological failure at day 28 and gametocytaemia at day 7 with a 3 day regimen of artesunate plus amodiaquine compared with amodiaquine alone. It found no significant difference in serious adverse events between treatments. Amodiaquine is not used in South East Asia due to multidrug resistance.

Artesunate (3 days) plus sulfadoxine–pyrimethamine (more effective than sulfadoxine–pyrimethamine alone but limited evidence of effectiveness when compared with amodiaquine plus sulfadoxine–pyrimethamine) *New*

One systematic review found that artesunate plus sulfadoxine–pyrimethamine reduced parasitological failure rate at day 28 and gametocytaemia rate at day 7 compared with sulfadoxine–pyrimethamine alone. It found no significant difference in adverse events between treatments. One additional RCT found no significant difference in treatment failure rate at day 28, mean fever clearance time, and adverse events between treatments. However, it found that combination treatment reduced gametocytaemia in people with an absence of gametocytes at study onset compared with sulfadoxine–pyrimethamine alone. One RCT found that artesunate (3 days) plus sulfadoxine–pyrimethamine significantly increased polymerase chain reaction unadjusted parasitological failure rate at day 28 compared with amodiaquine plus sulfadoxine–pyrimethamine. It found no significant difference in polymerase chain reaction adjusted results between treatments. Sulfadoxine-pyrimethamine and amodiaquine are not used in South East Asia due to multidrug resistance.

TRADE OFF BETWEEN BENEFITS AND HARMS

Artesunate (3 days) plus mefloquine (more effective than mefloquine alone) *New*

Two systematic reviews found that artesunate plus mefloquine reduced treatment failure at day 28 compared with mefloquine alone. Two additional RCTs found that combination treatment reduced the proportion of people with gametocytaemia at day 21 compared with mefloquine alone. The first review reported major adverse effects in both groups, including acute psychosis, anxiety, palpitations, and sleep disturbance. The second review found no significant difference in the rates of serious adverse events between treatments. The additional RCTs found no serious ▶

Malaria: uncomplicated, caused by *Plasmodium falciparum*

adverse events. In South East Asia artesunate plus mefloquinine is used due to multidrug resistance. In regions where other non-artimisinins are still effective, choosing artesunate plus mefloquinine involves a trade off between the higher cure associated with mefloquine and its adverse effects.

UNKNOWN EFFECTIVENESS

Artemether–lumefantrine (6 doses) New

We found no RCTs comparing a 6 dose regimen of artemether–lumefantrine versus chloroquine, amodiaquine, sulfadoxine–pyrimethamine, or mefloquine.

Artesunate (3 days) plus chlorproguanil–dapsone New

We found no RCTs comparing a 3 day regimen of artesunate plus chlorproguanil–dapsone versus chlorproguanil–dapsone alone. Chloraproguanil-dapsone should not be used in South East Asia due to multidrug resistance.

Which artemisinin combination treatment is most effective in people living in endemic areas? New

LIKELY TO BE BENEFICIAL

Artemether–lumefantrine (6 doses) (more effective than a 4 dose regimen, but no significant difference compared with 3 day artesunate plus either mefloquine or amodiaquine) New

One RCT found that six doses of artemether–lumefantrine given over 3 days increased treatment cure at 28 days compared with a 4 dose regimen. It found no serious adverse events and no adverse cardiovascular effects. One systematic review found no significant difference in parasitaemia at day 28 between six doses of artemether–lumefantrine and artesunate plus mefloquine. One RCT identified by the review found no significant difference in median parasite or fever clearance times between treatments. The review found no significant difference in mild to moderate or serious adverse events between treatments. One RCT found no significant difference in adequate clinical and parasitological response at day 14 between six doses of artemether–lumefantrine and artesunate plus amodiaquine. However, it found that six doses of artemether–lumefantrine reduced vomiting at days 1 and 2 compared with artesunate plus amodiaquine.

DEFINITION   Malaria is a parasite transmitted by Anopheles mosquitoes. There are four types of human malaria, *falciparum*, *vivax*, *ovale*, and *malariae*, with *falciparum* being the most important cause of illness and death, and also known to develop resistance to antimalarial drugs.[2] This chapter covers treatments only for *falciparum* malaria and a population of adults and children living in endemic malarial areas, who, by definition, are exposed (seasonally or all year round) to malaria. It does not cover treatment of malaria in non-immune travellers, pregnant women, and people infected with HIV. Repeated falciparum malaria infections result in a temporary and incomplete immunity. Therefore, adults living in areas where malaria is common are often found to be "semi-immune", presenting with asymptomatic or chronic forms of malaria, with clinical episodes that are attenuated by their immunity. "**Severe malaria**" is defined as a form of symptomatic malaria with signs of vital organ disturbance (WHO 2000).[2] Any person with symptomatic malaria who does not develop any such signs is defined as having "**uncomplicated malaria**". This chapter assesses the effectiveness of antimalarial drugs only in people with uncomplicated malaria. Table 3❶ provides an overview of the number of RCTs for each treatment and comparison included in this chapter.

Malaria: uncomplicated, caused by *Plasmodium falciparum*

INCIDENCE/ PREVALENCE
Malaria is a major health problem in the tropics, with 300–500 million new clinical cases annually, most of them cases of uncomplicated malaria. An estimated 1.1–2.7 million deaths occur annually as a result of severe *falciparum* malaria.[2]

AETIOLOGY/ RISK FACTORS
The malaria parasite is transmitted by infected Anopheles mosquitoes. Risk factors for developing the disease include exposure to infected mosquitoes (living in an endemic area; housing that allows mosquitoes to enter, and absence of mosquito nets; and living in an area where Anopheles mosquitoes can thrive). Risk factors in relation to severity of the illness relate to host immunity, determined mainly by exposure to the parasite, and therefore varying with level of transmission in the area and the age of the host. Malaria is uncommon in the first 6 months of life (fetal haemoglobin is protective); it is, however, common in children over 6 months of age. In areas of intense transmission, infection is attenuated by host immunity in older age groups, but with less intense transmission morbidity and mortality can be high in adults as well.

PROGNOSIS
Uncomplicated malaria may progress to severe malaria, become chronic, or resolve with effective treatment or the development of improved immunity. The outcome is, therefore, dependent on host immunity and prompt access to effective treatment. In the absence of effective treatment, people with no or low immunity are at increased risk of developing severe malaria (see Malaria: severe, life threatening, p 231) resulting in high morbidity and mortality.

Please refer to the Clinical Evidence website for full text and references.

Infectious diseases

Meningococcal disease

Search date May 2004

Jailson B Correia and C A Hart

What are the effects of interventions to prevent meningococcal disease in contacts and carriers?

LIKELY TO BE BENEFICIAL

Antibiotics for throat carriage (reduce carriage, but unknown effect on risk of disease)

RCTs found that antibiotics reduced throat carriage of meningococci compared with placebo. We found no RCTs or observational evidence examining whether eradicating throat carriage of meningococcus reduces the risk of meningococcal disease.

Prophylactic antibiotics (sulfadiazine) in contacts*

We found no RCTs on the effects of prophylactic antibiotics on the incidence of meningococcal disease among contacts. One observational study suggested that prophylactic sulfadiazine reduced the risk of meningococcal disease over 8 weeks compared with no prophylaxis. We found no evidence regarding which contacts should be treated.

What are the effects of interventions to treat suspected cases before admission to hospital?

UNKNOWN EFFECTIVENESS

Pre-admission parenteral penicillin in suspected cases*

We found no RCTs on the effects of pre-admission parenteral penicillin in suspected meningococcal disease in people of all ages. We found inconclusive evidence from observational studies on the benefit of pre-admission antibiotics. However, it is unlikely that RCTs on pre-admission antibiotics will be performed because of the unpredictably rapid course of disease in some people and the likely risks involved in delaying treatment, combined with a low risk of causing harm.

What are the effects of treatments for meningococcal meningitis on admission in children?

LIKELY TO BE BENEFICIAL

Adding corticosteroids (reduced severe hearing loss in bacterial meningitis of any cause, but no difference in mortality and unknown effectiveness in meningococcal meningitis)

We found no RCTs on adding corticosteroids specifically in children with meningococcal meningitis. One systematic review found no significant difference between adding corticosteroids and adding placebo in mortality in children with bacterial meningitis of any aetiology or in people of all ages with meningococcal meningitis. The review found that, compared with adding placebo, corticosteroids reduced severe hearing loss in children with bacterial meningitis of any aetiology, but it did not specifically assess the effect in children with meningococcal meningitis. The review found no significant difference between adding corticosteroids and adding placebo for short term or long term neurological sequelae in people of all ages with bacterial meningitis of any aetiology, but it did not separately assess the effect in children with meningococcal meningitis. Interpreting the results of available ▶

evidence on the use of corticosteroids in children with meningococcal meningitis demands caution, as age- and pathogen-specific evidence is scarce. In regions where the conjugate vaccine has been introduced, the incidence of *Haemophilus Influenzae* type b (Hib) has fallen dramatically and the applicability of evidence from trials performed prior to this change in epidemiology is questionable. However, decisions on initial treatment such as adding corticosteroids almost always precede knowledge of the specific aetiology.

What are the effects of treatments for meningococcal meningitis on admission in adults?

LIKELY TO BE BENEFICIAL

Adding corticosteroids (reduced mortality in bacterial meningitis of any cause, but unknown effectiveness in meningococcal meningitis)

We found no RCTs on adding corticosteroids specifically in adults with meningococcal meningitis. One systematic review found that, compared with adding placebo, adding corticosteroids reduced mortality in adults with bacterial meningitis of any aetiology. Subgroup analysis for meningococcal meningitis found no significant difference in mortality with adding corticosteroids compared with adding placebo. The review found that, compared with adding placebo, adding corticosteroids reduced neurological sequelae in people with bacterial meningitis of any aetiology, but the difference did not quite reach significance. Subgroup analysis for meningococcal meningitis found no significant difference in neurological sequelae with adding corticosteroids compared with adding placebo. None of the RCTs included in the systematic review were powered to detect a significant effect of corticosteroid treatment in the subgroup of people with meningococcal meningitis, probably due to the lower rates of mortality and sequelae in this group. However, decisions on initial treatment with adding corticosteroids almost always precede knowledge of the specific aetiology.

What are the effects of treatments for meningococcal septicaemia in children?

UNKNOWN EFFECTIVENESS

Adding corticosteroids

We found no RCTs on adding corticosteroids specifically in children with meningococcal septicaemia. Two RCTs found no significant difference in mortality between adding corticosteroids and adding placebo in children with severe sepsis and septic shock of any bacterial aetiology. It is questionable whether evidence from RCTs on severe sepsis and septic shock of any aetiology can be applied to children with meningococcal septicaemia.

What are the effects of treatments for meningococcal septicaemia in adults?

UNKNOWN EFFECTIVENESS

Adding corticosteroids

We found no RCTs on adding corticosteroids specifically in adults with meningococcal septicaemia. One systematic review found no significant difference in overall mortality at 28 days by adding corticosteroids to antibiotics or by adding high dose, short course corticosteroids compared with placebo, but that adding ▶

Meningococcal disease

low dose, longer duration corticosteroids at doses of 300 mg or less of hydrocortisone or equivalent for 5 or more days reduced all cause mortality at 28 days compared with adding placebo in adults with severe sepsis or septic shock of any aetiology. It is questionable whether evidence from RCTs on severe sepsis and septic shock of any aetiology can be applied to adults with meningococcal septicaemia.

*Based on consensus or observational evidence. RCTs unlikely to be conducted.

DEFINITION Meningococcal disease is any clinical condition caused by *Neisseria meningitidis* (the meningococcus) groups A, B, C, W135, or other serogroups. These conditions include purulent conjunctivitis, septic arthritis, meningitis, and septicaemia with or without meningitis. In this chapter we cover meningococcal meningitis and meningococcal septicaemia with or without meningitis.

INCIDENCE/ PREVALENCE Meningococcal disease is sporadic in temperate countries, and is most commonly caused by group B or C meningococci. Annual incidence in Europe varies from fewer than 1 case/100 000 people in France, up to 4–5 cases/100 000 people in the UK and Spain, and in the USA it is 0.6–1.5/ 100 000 people.[1,2] Occasional outbreaks occur among close family contacts, secondary school pupils, military recruits, and students living in halls of residence. Sub-Saharan Africa has regular epidemics in countries lying in the expanded "meningitis belt", reaching 500 cases/100 000 people during epidemics, which are usually due to serogroup A, although recent outbreaks of serogroup W135 cause concern.[3–5] In sub-Saharan Africa, over 90% of cases present with meningitis alone.[3]

AETIOLOGY/ RISK FACTORS The meningococcus colonises and infects healthy people, and is transmitted by close contact, probably by exchange of upper respiratory tract secretions (see table 1❶).[6–14] The risk of transmission is greatest during the first week of contact.[9] Risk factors include crowding and exposure to cigarette smoke.[15] In the UK, children younger than 2 years have the highest incidence of meningococcal disease, with a second peak between ages 15–24 years. There is currently an increased incidence of meningococcal disease among university students, especially among those in their first term and living in catered accommodation,[16] although we found no accurate numerical estimate of risk from close contact in, for example, halls of residence. Close contacts of an index case have a much higher risk of infection than do people in the general population.[9,12,13] The risk of epidemic spread is higher with groups A and C meningococci than with group B meningococci.[6–8,10] It is not known what makes a meningococcus virulent. Certain clones tend to predominate at different times and in different groups. Carriage of meningococcus in the throat has been reported in 10–15% of people; recent acquisition of a virulent meningococcus is more likely to be associated with invasive disease.

PROGNOSIS Mortality is highest in infants and adolescents, and is related to disease presentation and availability of therapeutic resources. In developed countries, case fatality rates have been around 19–25% for septicaemia, 10–12% for meningitis plus septicaemia, and less than 1% in meningitis alone, but an overall reduction in mortality was observed in recent years in people admitted to paediatric intensive care units.[17–21]

Please refer to the Clinical Evidence website for full text and references.

What are the effects of interventions during an acute attack of herpes zoster aimed at preventing postherpetic neuralgia?

LIKELY TO BE BENEFICIAL

Oral antiviral agents (aciclovir, famciclovir, valaciclovir, netivudine)

One systematic review found limited evidence from RCTs that aciclovir given for 7–10 days reduced pain at 1–3 months compared with placebo. One systematic review of one large RCT found that famciclovir reduced mean pain duration after acute herpes zoster compared with placebo. One RCT found that valaciclovir reduced the prevalence of postherpetic neuralgia at 6 months compared with aciclovir. One RCT found time to cessation of postherpetic neuralgia was reduced with aciclovir compared with netivudine. One RCT found no significant difference between valaciclovir and famciclovir in the resolution of postherpetic neuralgia. One systematic review of one RCT found no significant difference in pain between topical idoxuridine and oral aciclovir 1 month after rash healing. One systematic review found insufficient evidence from two RCTs about the effects of corticosteroids plus antiviral agents.

UNKNOWN EFFECTIVENESS

Tricyclic antidepressants (amitriptyline)

One RCT with weak methods provided insufficient evidence on the effects of amitriptyline in preventing postherpetic neuralgia.

UNLIKELY TO BE BENEFICIAL

Topical antiviral agents (idoxuridine) for pain at 6 months

One systematic review of heterogeneous poor quality RCTs found no significant difference in pain between topical idoxuridine and placebo at 6 months. One systematic review of one RCT found no significant difference in pain between topical idoxuridine and oral aciclovir 1 month after rash healing.

LIKELY TO BE INEFFECTIVE OR HARMFUL

Corticosteroids

Systematic reviews found insufficient evidence from RCTs about the effects of corticosteroids alone on postherpetic neuralgia. One systematic review found insufficient evidence from two RCTs about the effects of corticosteroids plus antiviral agents. There is concern that corticosteroids may cause dissemination of herpes zoster.

What are the effects of interventions to relieve established postherpetic neuralgia after the rash has healed?

BENEFICIAL

Gabapentin

Systematic reviews of two RCTs found that gabapentin reduced pain at 8 weeks compared with placebo.

Postherpetic neuralgia

Tricyclic antidepressants

One systematic review of three crossover RCTs found that tricyclic antidepressants increased pain relief in postherpetic neuralgia after 3–6 weeks compared with placebo.

UNKNOWN EFFECTIVENESS

Oral opioids (oxycodone, morphine, methadone, tramadol)

We found no RCTs examining effects of morphine or methadone in people with postherpetic neuralgia. One small crossover RCT found limited evidence that oral oxycodone reduced pain compared with placebo, but was associated with more adverse effects. One systematic review of one small RCT found limited evidence that tramadol reduced pain compared with clomipramine with or without levomepromazine after 6 weeks. One subsequent RCT found limited evidence that tramadol increased pain relief after 6 weeks compared with placebo.

Topical anaesthesia

We found insufficient evidence from three RCTs about the effects of lidocaine (lignocaine).

Topical counterirritants (capsaicin)

Two systematic reviews including the same two RCTs found limited evidence that the topical counterirritant capsaicin improved pain relief in postherpetic neuralgia compared with placebo. One subsequent RCT found no significant difference in pain between capsaicin and placebo. Capsaicin may cause painful skin reactions (including burning, stinging, and erythema).

LIKELY TO BE INEFFECTIVE OR HARMFUL

Dextromethorphan

One systematic review of one small crossover RCT and one subsequent RCT found no evidence that dextromethorphan was more effective than placebo or lorazepam after 3–6 weeks, but found that dextromethorphan was associated with sedation and ataxia at high doses.

DEFINITION Postherpetic neuralgia is pain that sometimes follows resolution of acute herpes zoster and healing of the zoster rash. It can be severe, accompanied by itching, and follows the distribution of the original infection. Herpes zoster is caused by activation of latent varicella zoster virus (human herpes virus 3) in people who have been rendered partially immune by a previous attack of chickenpox. Herpes zoster infects the sensory ganglia and their areas of innervation. It is characterised by pain along the distribution of the affected nerve, and crops of clustered vesicles over the area.

INCIDENCE/ In a UK general practice survey of 3600–3800 people, the annual incidence
PREVALENCE of herpes zoster was 3.4/1000.[1] Incidence varied with age. Herpes zoster was relatively uncommon in people under the age of 50 years (< 2/1000 a year), but rose to 5–7/1000 a year in people aged 50–79 years, and 11/1000 in people aged 80 years or older. In a population based study of 590 cases in Rochester, Minnesota, USA, the overall incidence was lower (1.5/1000) but there were similar increases in incidence with age.[2] Prevalence of postherpetic neuralgia depends on when it is measured after acute infection. There is no agreed time point for diagnosis.

AETIOLOGY/ The main risk factor for postherpetic neuralgia is increasing age. In a UK general
RISK FACTORS practice study (involving 3600–3800 people, 321 cases of acute herpes zoster) there was little risk in those under the age of 50 years, but postherpetic neuralgia developed in over 20% of people who had had acute herpes zoster aged 60–65 years and in 34% of those aged over 80 years.[1] No other risk factor

has been found to predict consistently which people with herpes zoster will experience continued pain. In a general practice study in Iceland (421 people followed for up to 7 years after an initial episode of herpes zoster), the risk of postherpetic neuralgia was 1.8% (95% CI 0.6% to 4.2%) for people under 60 years of age and the pain was mild in all cases.[2] The risk of severe pain after 3 months in people aged over 60 years was 1.7% (95% CI 0% to 6.2%).

PROGNOSIS About 2% of people with acute herpes zoster in the UK general practice survey had pain for more than 5 years.[1] Prevalence of pain falls as time elapses after the initial episode. Among 183 people aged over 60 years in the placebo arm of a UK trial, the prevalence of pain was 61% at 1 month, 24% at 3 months, and 13% at 6 months after acute infection.[3] In a more recent RCT, the prevalence of postherpetic pain in the placebo arm at 6 months was 35% in 72 people over 60 years of age.[4]

Please refer to the Clinical Evidence website for full text and references.

Tuberculosis

Search date August 2003

Paul Garner, Alison Holmes, and Lilia Ziganshina

What are the effects of interventions to prevent tuberculosis in high risk people without HIV infection?

Isoniazid

One systematic review, in people without HIV infection at high risk of tuberculosis, found that, without isoniazid prophylaxis for 6–12 months reduced the risk of active tuberculosis or extra-pulmonary tuberculosis compared with placebo. It also found that a short 6 month course was as effective as a 12 month course. One large RCT found that treatment with isoniazid significantly increased the risk of hepatotoxicity compared with placebo.

What are the effects of different drug regimens in newly diagnosed pulmonary tuberculosis?

Short course chemotherapy (as good as longer courses)

One RCT found that a 6 month regimen of rifampicin plus isoniazid improved relapse rate compared with isoniazid alone. One RCT found no evidence of a difference in relapse rates between short course regimens containing isoniazid (6 months) and longer term (8–9 months) chemotherapy in people with pulmonary tuberculosis. Three RCTs suggested that treatment with pyrazinamide speeds up sputum clearance after 2 months and improves risk of relapse compared with treatment without pyrazinamide.

Intermittent short course chemotherapy (as good as daily treatment)

Two RCTs in people with newly diagnosed tuberculosis found no significant difference in cure rates between daily and two or three times weekly short course chemotherapy regimens. However, the RCTs may have lacked power to exclude a clinically important difference.

Pyrazinamide

RCTs found that, in people with newly diagnosed tuberculosis, chemotherapy regimens containing pyrazinamide speed up sputum clearance in the first 2 months compared with other regimens, but have found limited evidence about effects on relapse rates.

Regimens containing quinolones

We found insufficient evidence about effects of chemotherapy regimens containing quinolones.

Chemotherapy for less than 6 months

One systematic review found limited evidence that reducing duration of treatment to less than 6 months significantly increased relapse rates compared with 12 months treatment.

◄ *What are the effects of different drug regimens in multidrug resistant tuberculosis?*

Comparative benefits of different regimens in multidrug resistant tuberculosis

We found no RCTs comparing different drug regimens for multidrug resistant tuberculosis in people with newly diagnosed tuberculosis.

What are the effects of low level laser therapy in people with tuberculosis?

Laser therapy

One systematic review found insufficient evidence about effects of low level laser therapy in people with tuberculosis.

What are the effects of interventions to improve adherence and screening attendance?

Cash incentives

One systematic review has found that cash incentives improve attendance among people living in deprived circumstances compared with usual care. One subsequent RCT found that cash incentives improved treatment completion in intravenous drug users. Another subsequent RCT found no significant difference in treatment completion with immediate compared with deferred cash incentives.

Community health advisors

One RCT found that consultation with health advisors recruited from the community significantly increased the rate of treatment attendance compared with no consultation.

Defaulter actions

RCTs have found that intensive action (repeated home visits and reminder letters) significantly improves completion of treatment compared with routine action (single reminder letter and home visit) for defaulters.

Health education by a nurse

One RCT found that health education by a nurse improved treatment completion compared with provision of an educational leaflet.

Direct observation treatment

One systematic review found no significant difference in cure rates between any direct observation treatment compared with self treatment. One large RCT, which allowed participants to choose their therapy supervisor, found that direct observation therapy significantly improved both cure rates and cure plus treatment completion rate combined, compared with self treatment. However co-intervention factors may have contributed to better treatment adherence in this study.

►

Tuberculosis

Prompts and contracts to improve reattendance for Mantoux test reading

One RCT in healthy people found that telephone prompts to return for Mantoux test reading slightly increased the number of people who reattended compared with no prompts, but the difference was not significant. One RCT found that healthy people were more likely to reattend for Mantoux test reading after providing either a verbal or written commitment compared with no such commitment.

Health education by a doctor; prompts to adhere to treatment; sanctions for non-adherence; staff training

We found insufficient evidence on the effects of these interventions.

DEFINITION	Tuberculosis is caused by *Mycobacterium tuberculosis* and can affect many organs. Specific symptoms relate to site of infection and are generally accompanied by fever, sweats, and weight loss.
INCIDENCE/ PREVALENCE	About a third of the world's population is infected with *M tuberculosis*. The organism kills more people than any other infectious agent. The World Health Organization estimates that 95% of cases are in developing countries, and that 25% of avoidable deaths in developing countries are caused by tuberculosis.[1]
AETIOLOGY/ RISK FACTORS	Social factors include poverty, overcrowding, homelessness, and inadequate health services. Medical factors include HIV and immunosuppression.
PROGNOSIS	Prognosis varies widely and depends on treatment.[2]

Please refer to the Clinical Evidence website for full text and references.

What are the effects of different doses and osmotic agents for peritoneal dialysis? New

LIKELY TO BE BENEFICIAL

Icodextrin (reduces volume overload compared with 1.36% or 2.27% dextrose solutions) New

Three RCTs in people receiving continuous ambulatory peritoneal dialysis found that 7.5% icodextrin solution for the long dwell increased ultrafiltration (fluid loss) compared with 1.36% or 2.27% dextrose solutions. Two of the RCTs found that 7.5% icodextrin reduced extracellular water or total body water compared with 1.36% or 2.27% dextrose solutions. One of the RCTs found that 7.5% icodextrin reduced left ventricular mass compared with 1.36% dextrose solution. However, one of the RCTs found no significant difference between 7.5% icodextrin solution and 3.86% dextrose solution in mean ultrafiltration during the long dwell.

UNLIKELY TO BE BENEFICIAL

Increased dose dialysis (no more effective than standard dose dialysis in reducing mortality) New

One RCT found no significant difference in mortality between standard dose and increased dose peritoneal dialysis.

What are the effects of different doses and membrane fluxes for haemodialysis? New

UNLIKELY TO BE BENEFICIAL

High membrane flux haemodialysis (no more effective than low membrane flux haemodialysis in reducing mortality) New

One RCT found no significant difference in hospital admission for cardiac causes, or all cause mortality between high membrane flux and low membrane flux (with standard or increased dose haemodialysis).

Increased dose haemodialysis (no more effective than standard dose dialysis in reducing mortality) New

One RCT found no significant difference in hospital admission for cardiac causes or all cause mortality between standard dose haemodialysis and increased dose haemodialysis (at high or low membrane flux).

What are the effects of interventions aimed at preventing secondary complications? New

BENEFICIAL

Sevelamer (reduces progression of coronary artery and aortic calcification compared with calcium salts) New

One RCT found that sevelamer reduced the progression of coronary artery and aortic calcification compared with calcium salts at 52 weeks. It found similar mortality with sevelamer and calcium salts. One crossover RCT found no difference in reduction of serum phosphorus between sevelamer and calcium acetate. Both ▶

End stage renal disease

RCTs found that sevelamer reduced serum low density lipoprotein cholesterol levels and the incidence of hypercalcaemia compared with calcium salts.

LIKELY TO BE BENEFICIAL

Erythropoietin or darbepoetin New

One RCT found no significant difference between darbepoetin α and recombinant human erythropoietin in maintenance of haemoglobin levels at 25–32 weeks. There is consensus based on observational studies that erythropoietin is effective for the treatment of anaemia in people with end stage renal disease.

DEFINITION End stage renal disease (ESRD) is defined as irreversible decline in a person's own kidney function, which is severe enough to be fatal in the absence of dialysis or transplantation. ESRD is included under stage 5 of the National Kidney Foundation Kidney Disease Outcomes Quality Initiative (K/DOQI) classification of chronic kidney disease (CKD), where it refers to individuals with an estimated glomerular filtration rate below 15 mL per minute or 1.73 m^2 body surface area, or those requiring dialysis irrespective of glomerular filtration rate.[1] The reduction or absence of kidney function leads to a host of maladaptive changes including fluid retention (extracellular volume overload), anaemia, disturbances of bone and mineral metabolism, dyslipidaemia, and protein energy malnutrition. **Fluid retention** in people with ESRD contributes significantly to the hypertension, ventricular dysfunction, and excess cardiovascular events observed in this population. **Anaemia** associated with CKD is normocytic and normochromic, and most commonly attributed to reduced erythropoietin synthesis by the affected kidneys. Additional factors such as iron deficiency from frequent phlebotomy, blood retention in the dialyser and tubing, and gastrointestinal bleeding; severe secondary hyperparathyroidism; acute and chronic inflammatory conditions (e.g. infection); and shortened red blood cell survival also contribute to the anaemia. **Disturbances of bone and mineral metabolism**, such as hyperparathyroidism, hyperphosphataemia, and hypo- or hypercalcaemia are common in people with CKD.[1] If untreated, these disturbances can cause pain, pruritus, anaemia, bone loss, and increased fracture risk, and can contribute to hypertension and cardiovascular disease.[2] **Dyslipidaemia** in people with CKD is characterised by high levels of very low density lipoprotein, low levels of high density lipoprotein, and elevated levels of modified low density lipoprotein, and is associated with increased cardiovascular risk.

INCIDENCE/ PREVALENCE The incidence and prevalence of ESRD continues to grow worldwide. According to data collected from 120 countries with dialysis programmes, at the end of 2001, about 1 479 000 people were receiving renal replacement therapy (RRT).[3] Among these individuals, 1 015 000 (69%) received haemodialysis and 126 000 (9%) received peritoneal dialysis, although an additional 338 000 (23%) were living with a kidney transplant.[3] Exact estimates of ESRD incidence and prevalence remain elusive, because international databases of renal registries exclude individuals with ESRD who do not receive RRT.[4] International comparisons of RRT pose similar challenges owing to differences in health care systems, government funding, acceptance of treatment, demographics, and access to care. Worldwide, the highest incidence and prevalence rates are reported from the US and Japan. According to the United States Renal Data System (USRDS) 2003 annual report, there were 93 327 new cases of ESRD in 2001, equivalent to an annual incidence of 336 cases per million population. The prevalence of ESRD in the US in 2002 was 406 081 (1403 cases/million population).[5] Similarly, according to reports published by the Japanese Society for Dialysis Therapy, 252 people per million population started dialysis in 2000. In 2001, there were 1721 people per million population in Japan receiving dialysis, the highest reported prevalence for industrialised nations.[6] In comparison, based on data pooled from the European Renal Association–European Dialysis and Transplant ►

Association Registry and UK Renal Registry, the incidence of RRT in 2000 ranged from 89 cases per million population in Norway to 160 cases per million population in French and Belgium. The prevalence of RRT in 2000 ranged from about 300 cases per million population in Poland to 850 cases per million population in Belgium. In 2000, the Oceania region reported an annual incidence of ESRD of about 90 people per million population in Australia and 107 people per million population in New Zealand. The prevalence of ESRD in 2000 was similar for Australia and New Zealand, about 600 cases per million population.[4,7,8]

AETIOLOGY/ RISK FACTORS The amount of daily proteinuria remains one of the strongest predictors of progression to ESRD.[9–11] Hypertension is a strong independent risk for progression to ESRD, particularly in people with proteinuria.[11,12] Age is also a predictor for FSRD: people over 65 years old have a four to fivefold increase in risk of ESRD compared with people under 65 years old.[13] Additional risk factors for developing ESRD include a history of chronic renal insufficiency, diabetes mellitus, heroin abuse, tobacco or analgesic use, black race, lower socioeconomic status, and a family history of kidney disease.[14–20]

PROGNOSIS The overall prognosis of untreated ESRD remains poor. Most people with ESRD eventually die from complications of cardiovascular disease, infection, or if dialysis is not provided, progressive uraemia (hyperkalaemia, acidosis, malnutrition).[1,5,7,21] Exact mortality estimates, however, are unavailable as international renal registries omit individuals with ESRD who do not receive RRT.[4] Among people receiving RRT, cardiovascular disease is the leading cause of mortality, and accounts for over 40% of deaths in this population.[1,5,7] Extracellular volume overload and hypertension, common among people with CKD, are known predictors of left ventricular hypertrophy and cardiovascular mortality in this population.[22] Even after adjustment for age, gender, ethnicity, and the presence of diabetes, annual cardiovascular mortality remains roughly an order of magnitude higher in people with ESRD compared with the general population, particularly among younger individuals.[1,8]

Please refer to the Clinical Evidence website for full text and references.

Kidney stones

Search date March 2004

Robyn Webber, David Tolley, James Lingeman

What are the effects of treatments for stone removal in people with asymptomatic kidney stones? New

UNKNOWN EFFECTIVENESS

Extracorporeal shockwave lithotripsy (ESWL) in people with asymptomatic renal or ureteric stones New

One RCT found no significant difference in stone free rate at about 1 year between prophylactic extracorporeal shockwave lithotripsy and conservative treatment for people with asymptomatic renal stones less than 15 mm in diameter. However, it found limited evidence that more people required invasive procedures after conservative management. We found no RCTs on extracorporeal shockwave lithotripsy in people with larger renal stones or with ureteric stones.

Percutaneous nephrolithotomy (PCNL) in people with asymptomatic renal or ureteric stones New

We found no RCTs on percutaneous nephrolithotomy in people with asymptomatic renal or ureteric stones.

Ureteroscopy in people with asymptomatic renal or ureteric stones New

We found no RCTs on ureteroscopy in people with asymptomatic renal or ureteric stones.

What are the effects of treatments for the removal of symptomatic renal stones? New

LIKELY TO BE BENEFICIAL

Extracorporeal shockwave lithotripsy (ESWL) in people with renal stones less than 20 mm New

One RCT found that extracorporeal shockwave lithotripsy decreased the stone free rate at 3 months and increased the rate of treatment failure in people with symptomatic renal stones less than 30 mm in diameter compared with percutaneous nephrolithotomy. It found no significant difference in complication rate between extracorporeal shockwave lithotripsy and percutaneous nephrolithotomy, although complications were more frequent with percutaneous nephrolithotomy. We found no RCTs comparing extracorporeal shockwave lithotripsy with ureteroscopy or open nephrolithotomy in people with renal stones. There is consensus that extracorporeal shockwave lithotripsy is the first line treatment in people with renal stones less than 20mm in diameter as it is a less invasive intervention than percutaneous nephrolithotomy.

Percutaneous nephrolithotomy (PCNL) in people with renal stones New

One RCT found that percutaneous nephrolithotomy increased the stone free rate at 3 months and reduced the rate of treatment failure in people with symptomatic renal stones less than 30 mm in diameter compared with extracorporeal shockwave lithotripsy. It found no significant differences in complication rates between percutaneous nephrolithotomy and extracorporeal shockwave lithotripsy, although complications were more frequent with percutaneous nephrolithotomy. We found no RCTs comparing percutaneous nephrolithotomy with conservative management, ureteroscopy, or open nephrolithotomy in people with renal stones.

◄ **UNKNOWN EFFECTIVENESS**

Open nephrolithotomy in people with renal stones New

We found no RCTs on open nephrolithotomy in people with renal stones.

Ureteroscopy in people with renal stones New

We found no RCTs on ureteroscopy in people with renal stones.

What are the effects of treatments for the removal of symptomatic ureteric stones? New

LIKELY TO BE BENEFICIAL

Extracorporeal shockwave lithotripsy (ESWL) in people with mid- and distal ureteric stones New

Three RCTs found that overall stone free rates were lower and the time needed to become stone free longer in people with mid- and distal ureteric stones with extracorporeal shockwave lithotripsy compared with ureteroscopy. However, one RCT found no significant difference in stone free rates between treatments in people with distal ureteric stones of less than 15 mm. One RCT found a lower rate of treatment failure with extracorporeal shockwave lithotripsy compared with ureteroscopy. Three of the RCTs found a lower rate of severe complications with extracorporeal shockwave lithotripsy compared with ureteroscopy.

TRADE OFF BETWEEN BENEFITS AND HARMS

Ureteroscopy in people with mid- and distal ureteric stones New

Three RCTs found that ureteroscopy increased overall stone free rate and decreased the time needed to become stone free in people with mid- and distal ureteric stones compared with extracorporeal shockwave lithotripsy. However, one RCT found no significant difference in stone free rates between treatments in people with distal ureteric stones of less than 15 mm. One RCT found a higher rate of treatment failure with ureteroscopy compared with extracorporeal shockwave lithotripsy. Three RCTs found a higher complication rate with ureteroscopy compared with extracorporeal shockwave lithotripsy.

UNKNOWN EFFECTIVENESS

Extracorporeal shockwave lithotripsy (ESWL) in people with proximal ureteric stones New

We found no RCTs comparing extracorporeal shockwave lithotripsy versus ureteroscopy in people with proximal ureteric stones or comparing extracorporeal shockwave lithotripsy with conservative treatment or ureterolithotomy (open or laparoscopic) in people with ureteric stones.

Ureterolithotomy (open or laparoscopic) in people with ureteric stones New

We found no RCTs on ureterolithotomy (open or laparoscopic) in people with ureteric stones.

Ureteroscopy in people with proximal ureteric stones New

We found no RCTs comparing ureteroscopy versus extracorporeal shockwave lithotripsy in people with proximal ureteric stones or comparing ureteroscopy with conservative treatment, extracorporeal shockwave lithotripsy, or ureterolithotomy (open or laparoscopic) in people with ureteric stones.

Kidney stones

DEFINITION **Nephrolithiasis** is the presence of stones within the kidney; **urolithiasis** is a more general term for stones anywhere within the urinary tract. A third of all kidney stones become clinically evident; typically causing pain, often severe in nature; renal angle tenderness; haematuria; or digestive symptoms (e.g. nausea, vomiting, or diarrhoea).[1] The onset of pain is usually sudden, typically felt in the loin, and radiating to the groin, and genitalia (scrotum or labia). People are typically restless, finding the pain excruciating and describing it as the worst pain ever experienced. Severe ureteric obstruction may cause hydronephrosis or infection. Infection may also occur after invasive procedures for stone removal. Urolithiasis is usually categorised according to the anatomical location of the stones (i.e. renal calyces, renal pelvis, ureteric, bladder, and urethra). Ureteric urolithiasis is described further by stating in which portion (proximal, middle, or distal) the stone is situated. Kidney stones develop when crystals separate from the urine and aggregate within the kidney papillae, the renal pelvis, or the ureter. The most common type of stone contains varying amounts of calcium and oxalate, whereas "struvite" stones contain a mixture of magnesium, ammonium, and phosphate. Struvite stones are associated almost exclusively with infection with urease producing organisms, whilst calcium oxalate stones have several aetiologies. Rarer stones include those formed from uric acid, cysteine, and xanthine, although this list is not exhaustive. The aetiology and chemical composition of a stone may have some bearing on its diagnosis, management, and particularly on prevention of recurrence. Although the choices for surgical management in general remain the same for all types of stone disease, the recognition of a specific cause, such as recurrent infection with a urease producing organism for struvite stones, or cysteinuria for cysteine stones, will inform further management. Diagnosis is usually based on clinical history, supported by investigations with diagnostic imaging. Bleeding within the urinary tract may present with identical symptoms to kidney stones, particularly if there are blood clots present within the renal pelvis or ureter. Several other conditions may also mimic a renal colic and need to be considered for differential diagnosis. These include urinary tract infection (and indeed the two conditions may coexist), analgesic abuse (either renal damage from excessive ingestion of analgesics, or in people with a history of opiate abuse, who may feign a renal colic in an attempt to obtain opiate analgesia). Rarely, people with sickle cell disease may also present with severe abdominal pain, which needs to be distinguished from a renal colic. This chapter assesses the effects of treatments only for the removal of renal and ureteric stones. It excludes pregnant women, in whom some forms of diagnostic procedures and treatments for stone removal are contraindicated, and people with significant comorbidities (including severe cardiovascular and respiratory conditions) who may be at increased risk when having general anaesthesia.

INCIDENCE/ PREVALENCE The peak incidence for stone disease occurs at the ages of 20–40 years, although stones are seen in all age groups.[2] There is a male to female ratio of 3 : 1. Calcium oxalate stones, the most common variety, have a recurrence rate of 10% at 1 year, 35% at 5 years, and 50% at 5 years after the first episode of kidney stone disease in North America.

AETIOLOGY/ RISK FACTORS In many otherwise healthy people the aetiology is uncertain.[3] However, incidence is higher in people with hyperparathyroidism and people with disorders including small bowel dysfunction, urinary tract infection (in particular caused by urease producing organisms) and structural/anatomical abnormalities of the kidney and ureter (including obstruction of the pelviureteric junction, hydronephrotic renal pelvis or calyces, calyceal diverticulum, horseshoe kidney, ureterocele, vesicoureteral reflux, ureteric stricture, or medullary sponge kidney). Other conditions associated with the development of renal stones include gout (especially leading to uric acid calculi) and chronic metabolic acidosis (typically resulting in stones composed of calcium phosphate). Women with a history of ▶

surgical menopause are also at higher risk because of increased bone resorption, and urinary excretion of calcium. Drugs, including some decongestants, diuretics, and anticonvulsants are also associated with an increased risk of stone formation.

PROGNOSIS Most kidney stones pass within 48 hours with expectant treatment (including adequate fluid intake and analgesia). Others may take longer to pass and the observation period can be extended to 3–4 weeks where appropriate. Ureteric stones less than 5 mm in diameter will pass spontaneously in about 90% of people, compared with 50% of ureteric stones between 5 mm and 10 mm.[4] Expectant management is considered on a case to case basis, and only in people with stones which are asymptomatic or very small (although stone size may not correlate with symptom severity), or both, and in people with significant comorbidities (including severe cardiovascular and respiratory conditions, who may be at increased risk when having general anaesthesia), in whom the risks of treatment may outweigh the likely benefits. Stones may migrate regardless of treatment or after treatment for their removal, and may or may not present clinically once in the ureter. Stones blocking the urine flow may lead to hydronephrosis and renal atrophy. They may also result in life threatening complications including urinary infection, perinephric abscess, or urosepsis. Some of these complications may cause kidney damage and compromised renal function.[5] Eventually, 10–20% of all kidney stones need treatment.

Please refer to the Clinical Evidence website for full text and references.

Renal failure (acute)

Search date April 2004

John A Kellum, Martine Leblanc, and Ramesh Venkataraman

What are the effects of interventions to prevent acute renal failure In people at high risk?

Low osmolality contrast media (reduced nephrotoxocity compared with standard media)

One systematic review found that low osmolality contrast media reduced nephrotoxicity in people with underlying renal failure needing contrast investigation compared with standard osmolality contrast media. One subsequent RCT found that non-ionic iso-osmolar contrast medium (iodixanol) reduced contrast media induced nephropathy compared with low osmolar non-ionic contrast medium (iohexol) in people with diabetes.

Acetylcysteine

One systematic review found that N-acetylcysteine plus hydration reduced contrast nephropathy (defined by an increase in serum creatinine) compared with hydration alone in people with chronic renal insufficiency who were having radiocontrast imaging studies. However, N-acetylcysteine may reduce serum creatinine independently of any effect on renal function, so conclusions about clinical efficacy should be interpreted with caution.

Fluids

One RCT of people having elective cardiac catheterisation found that intravenous sodium chloride hydration reduced acute renal failure compared with unrestricted oral fluids 48 hours after catheterisation. One RCT found that hydration with 0.9% sodium chloride infusion reduced contrast nephropathy compared with 0.45% sodium chloride. This effect was greater in women, people with diabetes, and people who received more than 250 mL of contrast. One RCT found inconclusive evidence on the effects of inpatient hydration regimens compared with outpatient hydration regimens.

Lipid formulations of amphotericin B (may cause less nephrotoxicity than standard formulations)

We found no RCTs. Lipid formulations of amphotericin B seem to cause less nephrotoxicity compared with standard formulations, but direct comparisons of long term safety are lacking.

Single dose aminoglycosides (as effective as multiple doses for treating infection, but with reduced nephrotoxicity)

One systematic review and one additional RCT compared single and multiple doses of aminoglycosides and found different results for nephrotoxicity. The systematic review, in people with fever and neutropenia receiving antibiotic treatment including aminoglycosides, found no significant difference in cure rates or nephrotoxicity between once daily compared with three times daily administration of the aminoglycoside. However, the RCT found that single doses of aminoglycosides reduced nephrotoxicity compared with multiple doses in people with fever and receiving antibiotic treatment including an aminoglycoside.

UNLIKELY TO BE BENEFICIAL

Fenoldopam

Five RCTs examined the role of fenoldopam in preventing acute renal failure. Although four small, poor quality, RCTs suggested that fenoldopam may improve renal perfusion and creatinine clearance compared with conventional care, the fifth and largest RCT, which focused on clinical outcomes in people having invasive cardiovascular procedures, found no evidence that it is more effective than conventional care for preventing acute renal failure. Fenoldopam may induce hypotension.

Mannitol

Small RCTs in people with traumatic rhabdomyolysis, or in people who had had coronary artery bypass, vascular, or biliary tract surgery, found that mannitol plus hydration did not reduce acute renal failure compared with hydration alone. One RCT found that mannitol increased the risk of acute renal failure compared with 0.45% sodium chloride infusion, but the difference was not significant.

Theophylline

One RCT in people with adequate hydration found that theophylline did not prevent contrast nephropathy compared with placebo. Three further RCTs, which did not report on the hydration status of participants, found mixed results. Two found that theophylline protected renal function compared with placebo and one found no significant difference. Another RCT found no significant reduction in renal impairment after elective coronary artery bypass surgery with theophylline compared with hydration alone but may have been underpowered to detect a clinically important difference.

LIKELY TO BE INEFFECTIVE OR HARMFUL

Calcium channel blockers for early allograft dysfunction

One RCT found no significant difference between isradipine and placebo in preventing early allograft dysfunction in people receiving cadaveric or living renal transplant. One systematic review limited to people with cadaveric renal transplant found limited evidence from heterogeneous RCTs that calcium channel blockers given in the peri-operative period reduced post-transplant acute tubular necrosis, although it found no significant effect on graft loss, need for haemodialysis, or mortality. We found no RCTs assessing the effects of calcium channel blockers in preventing other forms of acute renal failure. Calcium channel blockers are associated with hypotension and bradycardia.

Dopamine

Two systematic reviews and one subsequent RCT found no significant difference between dopamine and placebo in the development of acute renal failure, the need for dialysis, or death. One RCT found insufficient evidence on the effects of combined dopamine and diltiazem in people having cardiac surgery. Dopamine is associated with serious adverse effects, such as extravasation necrosis, gangrene, and conduction abnormalities.

Loop diuretics

One systematic review and one subsequent RCT found that adding loop diuretics to fluids was not effective and may be harmful in preventing acute renal failure compared with fluids alone in people at high risk of acute renal failure.

Natriuretic peptides

One large RCT found no significant difference between natriuretic peptides and placebo in the prevention of acute renal failure induced by contrast media. ▶

Subgroup analysis in another large RCT found that atrial natriuretic peptide reduced dialysis free survival in non-oliguric people compared with placebo.

What are the effects of treatments for critically ill people with acute renal failure?

LIKELY TO BE BENEFICIAL

High dose continuous renal replacement therapy (reduced mortality compared with low dose)

One RCT found that high dose continuous renal replacement therapy (haemofiltration) reduced mortality compared with low dose continuous therapy. A small prospective study found that intensive (daily) intermittent haemodialysis reduced mortality in people with acute renal failure compared with conventional alternate day haemodialysis. A subsequent small three arm RCT found no significant difference in survival at 28 days between early, low dose haemofiltration; early, high dose haemofiltration; and late, low dose haemofiltration.

UNKNOWN EFFECTIVENESS

Combined diuretics and albumin

We found no RCTs on the effects of intravenous albumin supplementation plus loop diuretics in people with acute renal failure.

Continuous infusion of loop diuretics (compared with bolus injection)

We found no RCTs comparing continuous infusion versus bolus injection of loop diuretics in critically ill people with acute renal failure.

Continuous renal replacement therapy (compared with intermittent renal replacement therapy)

One systematic review found no significant difference between continuous and intermittent renal replacement therapy in mortality, renal death, or dialysis dependence in critically ill adults with acute renal failure.

Synthetic dialysis membranes (compared with cellulose based membranes)

Two systematic reviews provided inconclusive evidence of the effects of synthetic membranes on mortality in critically ill people with acute renal failure compared with cellulose based membranes.

UNLIKELY TO BE BENEFICIAL

Loop diuretics

Underpowered RCTs in people with oliguric renal failure found no significant difference between loop diuretics and placebo on renal recovery, the number of days spent on dialysis, or mortality. Loop diuretics have been associated with toxicity and low renal perfusion.

LIKELY TO BE INEFFECTIVE OR HARMFUL

Dopamine

One systematic review found no significant difference in mortality or need for dialysis between dopamine and placebo. One additional RCT found that low dose dopamine did not reduce renal dysfunction compared with placebo. Dopamine has been associated with important adverse effects, including extravasation necrosis, gangrene, and conduction abnormalities.

◀ **Natriuretic peptides**

RCTs found no significant difference between atrial natriuretic peptide, ularitide (urodilatin), and placebo in dialysis free survival in oliguric and non-oliguric people with acute renal failure. One of the RCTs found that atrial natriuretic peptide may reduce survival in non-oliguric people.

DEFINITION
Acute renal failure is characterised by abrupt and sustained decline in glomerular filtration rate,[1] which leads to accumulation of urea and other chemicals in the blood. Most studies define it biochemically as a serum creatinine of 2–3 mg/dL (200–250 μmol/L), an elevation of more than 0.5 mg/dL (45 μmol/L) over a baseline creatinine below 2 mg/dL, or a twofold increase of baseline creatinine. A recent international, interdisciplinary, consensus panel has classified acute renal failure according to a change from baseline serum creatinine or urine output. The three level classification begins with "Risk", defined by either a 50% increase in serum creatinine or a urine output of less than 0.5 mL/kg/hour for at least 6 hours, and concludes with "Failure", defined by a threefold increase in serum creatinine or a urine output of less than 0.3 mL/kg/hour for 24 hours.[2] Acute renal failure is usually additionally classified according to the location of the predominant primary pathology (prerenal, intrarenal, and postrenal failure). Critically ill people are unstable and at imminent risk of death, which usually implies that they need to be in, or have been admitted to, the intensive care unit.

INCIDENCE/ PREVALENCE
Two prospective observational studies (2576 people) have found that established acute renal failure affects nearly 5% of people in hospital and as many as 15% of critically ill people, depending on the definitions used.[3,4]

AETIOLOGY/ RISK FACTORS
General risk factors: Risk factors for acute renal failure that are consistent across multiple causes include hypovolaemia; hypotension; sepsis; pre-existing renal, hepatic, or cardiac dysfunction; diabetes mellitus; and exposure to nephrotoxins (e.g. aminoglycosides, amphotericin, immunosuppressive agents, non-steroidal anti-inflammatory drugs, angiotensin converting enzyme inhibitors, iv contrast media) (see table 1❶). **Risk factors/aetiology in critically ill people:** Isolated episodes of acute renal failure are rarely seen in critically ill people, but are usually part of multiple organ dysfunction syndromes. Acute renal failure requiring dialysis is rarely seen in isolation (< 5% of people). The kidneys are often the first organs to fail.[9] In the perioperative setting, acute renal failure risk factors include prolonged aortic clamping, emergency rather than elective surgery, and use of higher volumes (> 100 mL) of intravenous contrast media. One study (3695 people) using multiple logistic regression identified the following independent risk factors: baseline creatinine clearance below 47 mL/minute (OR 1.20, 95% CI 1.12 to 1.30), diabetes (OR 5.5, 95% CI 1.4 to 21.0), and a marginal effect for doses of contrast media above 100 mL (OR 1.01, 95% CI 1.00 to 1.01). Mortality of people with acute renal failure requiring dialysis was 36% while in hospital.[5] Prerenal acute renal failure is caused by reduced blood flow to the kidney from renal artery disease, systematic hypotension, or maldistribution of blood flow. Intrarenal acute renal failure is caused by parenchymal injury (acute tubular necrosis, interstitial nephritis, embolic disease, glomerulonephritis, vasculitis, or small vessel disease). Postrenal acute renal failure is caused by urinary tract obstruction. Observational studies (in several hundred people from Europe, North America, and west Africa with acute renal failure) found a prerenal cause in 40–80%, an intrarenal cause in 10–50%, and a postrenal cause in the remaining 10%.[7,8,10–13] Prerenal acute renal failure is the most common type of acute renal failure in people who are critically ill,[7,14] but acute renal failure in this context is usually part of multisystem failure, and most frequently because of acute tubular necrosis resulting from ischaemic or nephrotoxic injury, or both.[15,16]

Renal failure (acute)

◀ **PROGNOSIS** One retrospective study (1347 people with acute renal failure) found that mortality was less than 15% in people with isolated acute renal failure.[17] One recent prospective study (> 700 people) found that, in people with acute renal failure, overall mortality and the need for dialysis were higher in an intensive care unit (ICU) than in a non-ICU setting, despite no significant difference between the groups in mean maximal serum creatinine (need for dialysis: 71% in ICU v 18% in non-ICU; P < 0.001; mortality: 72% in ICU v 32% in non-ICU; P = 0.001).[18] One large study (> 17 000 people admitted to Austrian ICUs) found that acute renal failure was associated with a greater than fourfold increase in mortality.[19] Even after controlling for underlying severity of illness, mortality was still significantly higher in people with acute renal failure (62.8% v 38.5%), suggesting that acute renal failure is independently responsible for increased mortality, even if dialysis is used. However, the exact mechanism that leads to increased risk of death is uncertain.

Please refer to the Clinical Evidence website for full text and references.

What are the effects of treatments?

BENEFICIAL

α Blockers

Systematic reviews have found that α blockers improve lower urinary tract symptom scores compared with placebo. Systematic reviews found limited evidence that different α blockers have similar effects. RCTs found limited evidence that α blockers improved symptom scores compared with the 5α reductase inhibitor finasteride. One RCT found no significant difference between tamsulosin and saw palmetto plant extracts in symptom scores or maximum flow rate after 1 year. Another RCT found limited evidence suggesting that α blockers were less effective than transurethral microwave thermotherapy in improving symptoms over 18 months. We found no RCTs comparing α blockers versus surgical treatment.

5α Reductase inhibitors

One systematic review and additional RCTs have found that 5α reductase inhibitors improve symptom scores and reduce complications compared with placebo. The review found that 5α reductase inhibitors were associated with more adverse events than placebo, including decreased libido, impotence, and ejaculatory dysfunction. RCTs found limited evidence that the 5α reductase inhibitor finasteride was less effective at improving symptom scores than α blockers. One systematic review found no significant difference in symptom scores between finasteride and saw palmetto plant extracts. We found no RCTs comparing 5α reductase inhibitors versus surgical treatment.

Saw palmetto plant extracts

One systematic review has found that saw palmetto plant extracts improve symptom scores compared with placebo. It found no significant difference in symptom scores between saw palmetto plant extracts and the α blocker tamsulosin or the 5α reductase inhibitor finasteride. One RCT found no significant difference in symptom scores between tamsulosin and tamsulosin plus saw palmetto plant extracts.

Transurethral microwave thermotherapy

RCTs found that transurethral microwave thermotherapy reduced symptom scores compared with sham treatment. We found limited evidence that thermotherapy was less effective in relieving short term symptoms than transurethral resection. One RCT found that transurethral microwave thermotherapy improved symptom scores over 18 months compared with α blockers.

Transurethral resection versus no surgery

RCTs found that transurethral resection reduced symptom scores more than watchful waiting, and did not increase the risk of erectile dysfunction or incontinence.

LIKELY TO BE BENEFICIAL

β-Sitosterol plant extract

One systematic review has found that β-sitosterol plant extract improves lower urinary tract symptom scores compared with placebo in the short term. We found no RCTs comparing β-sitosterol plant extract versus other treatments.

▶

Benign prostatic hyperplasia

◄ **UNKNOWN EFFECTIVENESS**

Pygeum africanum

One systematic review found limited evidence that *Pygeum africanum* increased peak urinary flow and reduced residual urine volume at 4–16 weeks compared with placebo. We found no RCTs comparing Pygeum africanum versus other treatments.

Rye grass pollen extract

One systematic review found limited evidence that rye grass pollen extract increased self rated improvement and reduced nocturia at 12–24 weeks compared with placebo. However, the review identified only two small RCTs, from which we were unable to draw reliable conclusions. We found no RCTs comparing rye grass pollen extract versus other treatments.

Transurethral resection versus less invasive surgical techniques

RCTs found no significant difference in symptom scores between transurethral resection and transurethral incision or between transurethral resection and electrical vaporisation. RCTs found limited evidence that transurethral resection improved symptom scores more than visual laser ablation but that transurethral resection may be associated with a higher risk of blood transfusion.

Transurethral resection versus transurethral needle ablation

One RCT found that transurethral resection reduced symptom scores compared with transurethral needle ablation after 1 year, although transurethral needle ablation caused fewer adverse effects.

DEFINITION
Benign prostatic hyperplasia is defined histologically. Clinically, it is characterised by lower urinary tract symptoms (urinary frequency, urgency, a weak and intermittent stream, needing to strain, a sense of incomplete emptying, and nocturia) and can lead to complications, including acute urinary retention.

INCIDENCE/ PREVALENCE
Estimates of the prevalence of symptomatic benign prostatic hyperplasia range from 10–30% for men in their early 70s, depending on how benign prostatic hyperplasia is defined.[1]

AETIOLOGY/ RISK FACTORS
The mechanisms by which benign prostatic hyperplasia causes symptoms and complications are unclear, although bladder outlet obstruction is an important factor.[2] The best documented risk factors are increasing age and normal testicular function.[3]

PROGNOSIS
Community and practice based studies suggest that men with lower urinary tract symptoms can expect slow progression of the symptoms.[4,5] However, symptoms can wax and wane without treatment. In men with symptoms of benign prostatic hyperplasia, rates of acute urinary retention range from 1–2% a year.[5–7]

Please refer to the Clinical Evidence website for full text and references.

Search date July 2004

Thomas Jang and Anthony Schaeffer

What are the effects of treatments for chronic bacterial prostatitis?

LIKELY TO BE BENEFICIAL

α Blockers

We found no RCTs comparing α blockers versus placebo or no treatment. We found limited evidence from one RCT suggesting that adding α blockers to antimicrobials improved symptoms and reduced recurrence compared with antimicrobials alone.

UNKNOWN EFFECTIVENESS

Local injection of antimicrobials

We found no RCTs comparing local injection of antimicrobials with placebo or no treatment. One small RCT found that anal submucosal injection of amikacin improved symptom scores and bacterial eradication rates at 3 months compared with intramuscular amikacin.

Oral antimicrobial drugs

We found no RCTs comparing oral antimicrobial drugs versus placebo or no treatment. Two RCTs found no significant difference between ciprofloxacin and other quinolones (levofloxacin or lomefloxacin) in rates of clinical success or bacteriological cure at 6 months. Retrospective observational studies report cure rates of 0–88% depending on the drug used and the duration of treatment.

Radical prostatectomy

We found no RCTs on the effects of radical prostatectomy.

Transurethral resection

We found no RCTs on the effects of transurethral resection.

What are the effects of treatments for chronic abacterial prostatitis?

LIKELY TO BE BENEFICIAL

α Blockers

Two small RCTs identified by a systematic review and three small subsequent RCTs found limited evidence that α blockers improved quality of life and symptoms compared with placebo. The RCTs may have been too small to detect other clinically important differences.

UNKNOWN EFFECTIVENESS

5α reductase inhibitors

One RCT identified by a systematic review provided insufficient evidence about the effects of 5α reductase inhibitors compared with placebo in men with chronic abacterial prostatitis.

Allopurinol

One RCT identified by a systematic review provided insufficient evidence about the effects of allopurinol compared with placebo in men with chronic abacterial prostatitis.

▶

Chronic prostatitis

Anti-inflammatory medications

One RCT identified by a systematic review provided insufficient evidence about the effects of anti-inflammatory medications compared with placebo or no treatment in men with chronic abacterial prostatitis.

Biofeedback

We found no RCTs on the effects of biofeedback.

Prostatic massage

We found no RCTs on the effects of prostatic massage.

Sitz baths

We found no RCTs on the effects of Sitz baths.

Transurethral microwave thermotherapy

One systematic review found limited evidence from one small RCT suggesting that transurethral microwave thermotherapy improved quality of life at 3 months and symptoms over 21 months compared with sham treatment. However, we were unable to draw reliable conclusions from this one small study.

DEFINITION **Chronic bacterial prostatitis** is characterised by a positive culture of expressed prostatic secretions. It may cause symptoms such as suprapubic, lower back, or perineal pain, or mild urgency, frequency, and dysuria, and may be associated with recurrent urinary tract infections. However, it may also be asymptomatic. **Chronic abacterial prostatitis**, or chronic pelvic pain syndrome (CPPS), is characterised by pelvic or perineal pain in the absence of pathogenic bacteria in expressed prostatic secretions. It is often associated with irritative and obstructive voiding symptoms including urgency, frequency, hesitancy, and poor interrupted flow. Symptoms can also include pain in the suprapubic region, lower back, penis, testes, or scrotum. Chronic abacterial prostatitis may be inflammatory (white cells present in prostatic secretions) or non-inflammatory (white cells absent in prostatic secretions).[1]

INCIDENCE/ PREVALENCE One community based study in the USA (58 955 visits by men ≥ 18 years to office based physicians) estimated that 9% of men have a diagnosis of chronic prostatitis at any one time.[2] Another study found that, of men with genitourinary symptoms, 8% presenting to urologists and 1% presenting to primary care physicians are diagnosed with chronic prostatitis.[3] Most cases of chronic prostatitis are abacterial. Acute bacterial prostatitis, although easy to diagnose, is rare.

AETIOLOGY/ RISK FACTORS Organisms commonly implicated in bacterial prostatitis include *Escherichia coli*, other Gram negative enterobacteriaceae, occasionally *Pseudomonas* species, and rarely Gram positive enterococci. The cause of abacterial prostatitis is unclear, although it has been suggested that it may be caused by undocumented infections with *Chlamydia trachomatis*,[4] *Ureaplasma urealyticum*,[5] *Mycoplasma hominis*,[6] and *Trichomonas vaginalis*.[7] Other factors might also be involved, including inflammation,[8] autoimmunity,[9] hormonal imbalances,[10] pelvic floor tension myalgia,[11] intra-prostatic urinary reflux,[12] and psychological disturbances.[13]

PROGNOSIS The natural history of untreated chronic bacterial and abacterial prostatitis remains ill-defined. Chronic bacterial prostatitis may cause recurrent urinary tract infections in men.[14] Furthermore, several investigators have reported an association between chronic bacterial prostatitis and infertility.[15] The sequelae of chronic abacterial prostatitis are similar to those of chronic bacterial prostatitis. Fertility may be decreased.[16] One study found that chronic abacterial prostatitis had an impact on quality of life similar to that from angina, Crohn's disease, or a previous myocardial infarction.[17]

Please refer to the Clinical Evidence website for full text and references.

Erectile dysfunction

Search date August 2003

Robyn Webber

What are the effects of treatments?

Intracavernosal alprostadil

One large RCT found that intracavernosal alprostadil increased the chances of a satisfactory erection compared with placebo. One small RCT found limited evidence that vacuum devices were as effective as intracavernosal alprostadil injections for rigidity but not for orgasm.

Intraurethral alprostadil

One large RCT (in men who had previously responded to alprostadil) found limited evidence that intraurethral alprostadil (prostaglandin E1) increased the chances of successful sexual intercourse and at least one orgasm over 3 months compared with placebo. About a third of men suffered penile ache. We found no direct comparisons of intraurethral alprostadil versus either intracavernosal alprostadil or oral drug treatments.

Sildenafil

One systematic review and 15 subsequent RCTs have found that sildenafil improves erections and increases rates of successful intercourse compared with placebo. Adverse effects, including headaches, flushing, and dyspepsia, are reported in up to a quarter of men. Deaths have been reported in men on concomitant treatment with oral nitrates.

Yohimbine

One systematic review has found that yohimbine improves self reported sexual function and penile rigidity at 2–10 weeks compared with placebo. Transient adverse effects are reported in up to a third of men.

Topical alprostadil

Two quasi randomised trials found limited evidence that topical alprostadil increased the number of men with erections sufficient for intercourse compared with placebo but was commonly associated with skin irritation.

L-arginine

One small RCT found no significant difference in sexual function between L-arginine and placebo, but it may have been too small to exclude a clinically important difference.

Penile prostheses

We found no RCTs of penile prostheses in men with erectile dysfunction.

Trazodone

One small RCT found no significant difference in erections or libido with trazodone compared with placebo, but it may have been too small to exclude a clinically important difference.

Vacuum devices

Vacuum devices have not been adequately assessed in RCTs. One small RCT found limited evidence that they were as effective as intracavernosal alprostadil (prostaglandin E1) injections for rigidity but not for orgasm.

DEFINITION Erectile dysfunction has largely replaced the term "impotence". It is defined as the persistent inability to obtain or maintain sufficient rigidity of the penis to allow satisfactory sexual performance.

INCIDENCE/ PREVALENCE We found little good epidemiological information, but one cross sectional study found that age is the variable most strongly associated with erectile dysfunction and that up to 30 million men in the USA may be affected.[1] Even among men in their 40s, nearly 40% report at least occasional difficulty obtaining or maintaining erection, whereas this approaches 70% in 70 year olds.

AETIOLOGY/ RISK FACTORS About 80% of cases of erectile dysfunction now are believed to have an organic cause, the rest being psychogenic in origin. Risk factors include increasing age, smoking, and obesity. Erectile problems fall into three categories: failure to initiate; failure to fill, caused by insufficient arterial inflow into the penis to allow engorgement and tumescence because of vascular insufficiency; and failure to store because of veno-occlusive dysfunction. Erectile dysfunction is a recognised adverse effect of a wide variety of pharmaceutical agents.

PROGNOSIS We found no good evidence on prognosis in untreated organic erectile dysfunction.

Please refer to the Clinical Evidence website for full text and references.

Prostate cancer (non-metastatic)

Search date February 2003

Timothy Wilt

What are the effects of treatments for clinically localised prostate cancer?

TRADE OFF BETWEEN BENEFITS AND HARMS

Radical prostatectomy

Two RCTs found no significant difference in death from any cause between radical prostatectomy and watchful waiting in men with clinically detected disease after median follow up of 6.2 and 23 years. The larger of the RCTs found that radical prostatectomy reduced death due to prostate cancer and metastases at 6 years compared with watchful waiting. Two small RCTs found that radical prostatectomy reduced the risk of treatment failure compared with external beam radiation. Radical prostatectomy carries the risks of major surgery and of sexual and urinary dysfunction.

Watchful waiting

Two RCTs found no significant difference in overall survival between watchful waiting and radical prostatectomy in men with clinically detected disease after median follow up of 6 and 23 years. The larger RCT found that radical prostatectomy reduced death rates due to prostate cancer and metastases at 6 years compared with watchful waiting. One RCT found that radical prostatectomy increased erectile dysfunction compared with watchful waiting but found no significant difference in quality of life after 12 months.

UNKNOWN EFFECTIVENESS

Androgen suppression

We found no RCTs of early androgen suppression on length or quality of life in men with asymptomatic, clinically localised prostate cancer. One RCT identified by a systematic review found limited evidence that oestrogen decreased prostate cancer related deaths compared with watchful waiting. It found no significant difference in overall survival. One preliminary report of three large ongoing RCTs in men with localised or locally advanced prostate cancer found that bicalutamide plus standard care reduced rates of radiological progression and bone metastases at 2–3 years compared with standard care alone. There was no significant difference between treatments in overall survival.

External beam radiation

We found no RCTs comparing external beam radiation versus watchful waiting. Two RCTs found that external beam radiation increased the risk of treatment failure compared with radical prostatectomy. Two small RCTs found no significant difference between conformal radiotherapy and conventional radiotherapy in overall survival or tumour control at 3–5 years. One systematic review found limited evidence that conformal radiotherapy with dose escalation reduced acute and late treatment related morbidity compared with conventional radiotherapy for men with T1 or T2 low or intermediate risk prostate cancer.

Androgen suppression in asymptomatic men with raised prostate specific antigen concentrations after early treatment; brachytherapy; cryosurgery

We found no RCTs on the effects of these interventions.

What are the effects of treatments for locally advanced prostate cancer?

BENEFICIAL

Immediate androgen suppression after radical prostatectomy and pelvic lymphadenectomy in men with node positive prostate cancer (compared with radical prostatectomy and deferred androgen suppression)

One small RCT in men with node positive prostate cancer found that immediate androgen suppression compared with deferred androgen suppression after radical prostatectomy and pelvic lymphadenectomy reduced mortality over a median of 7 years' follow up.

LIKELY TO BE BENEFICIAL

Androgen suppression initiated at diagnosis

RCTs found no significant difference in overall survival between androgen suppression with bicalutamide and no androgen suppression in men with localised or locally advanced prostate cancer at 2–10 years. The RCTs found that bicalutamide reduced objective progression compared with no bicalutamide. One systematic review found that early androgen suppression increased survival at 10 years compared with deferred treatment in men with locally advanced prostate cancer but found no significant difference in survival at 5 years. One RCT found limited evidence that immediate androgen suppression reduced complications compared with deferred androgen suppression.

Early androgen suppression in addition to external beam radiation (improves survival compared with radiation and deferred androgen suppression)

RCTs found limited evidence that androgen suppression initiated at diagnosis plus external beam radiation improved long term survival compared with radiation alone or radiation plus deferred androgen suppression. One RCT found limited evidence that immediate androgen suppression reduced complications compared with deferred androgen suppression.

DEFINITION   Prostatic cancer is staged according to two systems: the tumour, node, metastasis (TNM) classification system and the American urologic staging system❶. Non-metastatic prostate cancer can be divided into clinically localised disease and locally advanced disease. Clinically localised disease is prostate cancer thought, after clinical examination, to be confined to the prostate gland. Locally advanced disease is prostate cancer that has spread outside the capsule of the prostate gland but has not yet spread to other organs. Metastatic disease is prostate cancer that has spread outside the prostate gland to either local, regional, or systemic lymph nodes, seminal vesicles, or to other body organs (e.g. bone, liver, brain) and is not connected to the prostate gland. We consider clinically localised and locally advanced disease here. Metastatic disease is covered in a separate chapter (see prostate cancer [metastatic], [Web only]).

INCIDENCE/
PREVALENCE   Prostate cancer is the sixth most common cancer in the world and the third most common cancer in men. In 2000, an estimated 513 000 new cases of prostate caner were diagnosed and about 250 000 deaths were attributed to prostate cancers worldwide. Prostate cancer is uncommon under the age of 50 years. About 85% of men with prostate cancer are diagnosed after the age of 65 years. Autopsy studies suggest that the prevalence of subclinical prostate cancer is high at all ages: 30% for men aged 30–39 years, 50% for men aged 50–59 years, and more than 75% for men older than 85 years. ▶

Prostate cancer (non-metastatic)

Incidence varies widely by ethnic group and around the world. The highest rates occur in men of black ethnic group living in the USA and the lowest among men living in China.[1]

AETIOLOGY/ RISK FACTORS
Risk factors for prostate cancer include increasing age, family history of prostate cancer, black race, and possibly higher dietary consumption of fat and meat, low intake of lycopene (from tomato products), low intake of fruit, and high dietary calcium. In the USA, black men have about a 60% higher incidence than white men.[2] The prostate cancer incidence for black men living in the USA is about 90/100 000 in men aged less than 65 years and about 1300/100 000 in men aged 65–74 years. For white men, incidence is about 44/100 000 in men aged less than 65 years and 900/100 000 in men aged 65–74 years.[2]

PROGNOSIS
The chance that men with well to moderately differentiated, palpable, clinically localised prostate cancer will remain free of symptomatic progression is 70% at 5 years and 40% at 10 years.[3] The risk of symptomatic disease progression is higher in men with poorly differentiated prostate cancer.[4] One retrospective analysis of a large surgical series in men with clinically localised prostate cancer found that the median time from the increase in prostate specific antigen (PSA) concentration to the development of metastatic disease was 8 years.[5] Time to PSA progression, PSA doubling time, and Gleason score were predictive of the probability and time to development of metastatic disease. Once men developed metastatic disease, the median actuarial time to death was less than 5 years.[5] Morbidity from local or regional disease progression includes haematuria, bladder obstruction, and lower extremity oedema. The age adjusted prostate cancer specific mortality in the USA for all men aged 65 years and older has decreased by about 15% (244 deaths/100 000 to 207 deaths/100 000) from 1991–1997. The reasons for this are unclear, although inaccurate death certification, PSA screening, and earlier, more intensive treatment, including radical prostatectomy, radiotherapy, and androgen suppression, have been suggested. However, regions of the USA and Canada where PSA testing and early treatment are more common have similar prostate cancer mortality to regions with lower testing and early treatment rates.[6] Similarly, countries with low rates of PSA testing and treatment, such as the UK, have similar age adjusted prostate cancer mortality to countries with high rates of testing and treatment, such as the USA.[7]

Please refer to the Clinical Evidence website for full text and references.

Search date September 2004

Chandra Shekhar Biyani and Günter Janetschek

What are the effects of treatments in men with varicocele?

UNKNOWN EFFECTIVENESS

Embolisation

We found no RCTs comparing embolisation with no treatment or sclerotherapy. Three RCTs provided insufficient evidence on the effects of embolisation for improving fertility in men with varicocele compared with ligation techniques. We found no evidence examining the effects of embolisation on pain or discomfort caused by varicocele.

Expectant management

One systematic review of poor quality, heterogeneous RCTs in couples with male factor subfertility found no consistent evidence of difference in pregnancy rate between expectant management and surgical ligation or sclerotherapy. The review found no RCTs comparing expectant management with embolisation. We found no evidence examining the effects of expectant management on pain or discomfort caused by varicocele.

Sclerotherapy

One RCT found no significant difference in pregnancy rate between sclerotherapy and no treatment. We found no evidence examining the effects of sclerotherapy on pain or discomfort caused by varicocele.

Surgical ligation

One systematic review and additional RCTs provided insufficient evidence on the effects of different surgical ligation techniques in pregnancy rate compared with no treatment, embolisation or each other. We found no RCTs comparing surgical ligation with sclerotherapy. We found no evidence examining the effects of ligation on pain or discomfort caused by varicocele.

DEFINITION　Varicocele is a dilation of the pampiniform plexus of the spermatic cord. Severity is commonly graded as follows: **grade 0**, only demonstrable by technical investigation; **grade 1**, palpable or visible only on Valsalva manoeuvre (straining); **grade 2**, palpable but not visible when standing upright at room temperature; and **grade 3**, visible when standing upright at room temperature. Varicocele is unilateral and left sided in at least 85% of cases. In most of the remaining cases, the condition is bilateral. Unilateral right sided varicocele is rare. Many men who have a varicocele have no symptoms. Symptoms may include testicular ache or discomfort and distress about cosmetic appearance. The condition is widely believed to be associated with male factor infertility, which is the most common reason for referral for treatment. However, evidence for a causal relationship is sparse.[1]

INCIDENCE/　We found few data on the prevalence of varicocele. Anecdotally, it has been
PREVALENCE　estimated that about 10–15% of men and adolescent boys in the general population have varicocele.[1] One multicentre study found that, in couples with subfertility, the prevalence of varicocele in male partners was about 12%.[2] In men with abnormal semen analysis, the prevalence of varicocele was about 25%.

AETIOLOGY/　We found no reliable data on epidemiological risk factors for varicocele, such as
RISK FACTORS　a family history or environmental exposures. Anatomically, varicoceles are caused by dysfunction of the valves in the spermatic vein, which allows pooling ▶

of blood in the pampiniform plexus. This is more likely to occur in the left spermatic vein than in the right because of normal anatomical asymmetry.

PROGNOSIS Varicocele is believed to be associated with subfertility, although reliable evidence is sparse. The natural history of varicocele is unclear.

Please refer to the Clinical Evidence website for full text and references.

Search date December 2003
Janet Treasure and Ulrike Schmidt

What are the effects of treatments in anorexia nervosa?

UNKNOWN EFFECTIVENESS

Inpatient versus outpatient treatment setting in anorexia nervosa

One small RCT found no significant difference between outpatient treatment and inpatient treatment for increasing weight and improving Morgan Russell scale global scores at 1, 2, and 5 years in people who did not need emergency intervention.

Psychotherapy

Small RCTs provided insufficient evidence to compare psychotherapy versus treatment as usual, dietary counselling, or each other.

Selective serotonin reuptake inhibitors

Three small RCTs provided insufficient evidence about the effects of selective serotonin reuptake inhibitors compared with placebo or no treatment in people with anorexia nervosa.

Zinc

One small RCT found limited evidence that zinc may improve daily body mass index gain compared with placebo in people managed in an inpatient setting. However, we were unable to draw reliable conclusions from this small study.

LIKELY TO BE INEFFECTIVE OR HARMFUL

Cisapride

One small RCT found no significant difference between cisapride and placebo in weight gain at 8 weeks. Use of cisapride has been restricted in many countries because of concern about cardiac irregularities, including ventricular tachycardia, torsades de pointes, and sudden death.

Cyproheptadine

Two RCTs in inpatient settings found no significant difference between cyproheptadine and placebo in weight gain.

Neuroleptic drugs

We found no RCTs. The QT interval may be prolonged in people with anorexia nervosa, and many neuroleptic drugs (haloperidol, pimozide, sertindole, thioridazine, chlorpromazine, and others) also increase the QT interval. Prolongation of the QT interval may be associated with increased risk of ventricular tachycardia, torsades de pointes, and sudden death.

Tricyclic antidepressants

Two small RCTs found no evidence of benefit with amitriptyline compared with placebo. One RCT found that amitriptyline was associated with more adverse effects, such as drowsiness, dry mouth, and blurred vision. The QT interval may be prolonged in people with anorexia nervosa, and tricyclic antidepressants (amitriptyline, protriptyline, nortriptyline, doxepin, and maprotiline) also increase the QT interval. Prolongation of the QT interval may be associated with increased risk of ventricular tachycardia, torsades de pointes, and sudden death.

Anorexia nervosa

What are the effects of interventions to prevent or treat complications of anorexia nervosa?

UNKNOWN EFFECTIVENESS

Oestrogen treatment

We found no RCTs on the effects of oestrogen treatment on fracture rates in people with anorexia nervosa. Two small RCTs found no significant difference between oestrogen and placebo or no treatment in bone mineral density in people with anorexia nervosa.

DEFINITION
Anorexia nervosa is characterised by a refusal to maintain weight at or above a minimally normal weight (< 85% of expected weight for age and height, or body mass index < 17.5 kg/m^2), or a failure to show the expected weight gain during growth. In association with this, there is often an intense fear of gaining weight, preoccupation with weight, denial of the current low weight and its adverse impact on health, and amenorrhoea. Two subtypes of anorexia nervosa, binge–purge and restricting, have been defined.[1]

INCIDENCE/ PREVALENCE
A mean incidence in the general population of 19/100 000 a year in females and 2/100 000 a year in males has been estimated from 12 cumulative studies.[2] The highest rate was in female teenagers (age 13–19 years), where there were 50.8 cases/100 000 a year. A large cohort study screened 4291 Swedish school children, aged 16 years, by weighing and subsequent interview, and found the prevalence of anorexia nervosa (defined using DSM-III and DSM-III-R criteria) to be 7/1000 for girls and 1/1000 for boys.[3] Little is known of the incidence or prevalence in Asia, South America, or Africa.

AETIOLOGY/ RISK FACTORS
Anorexia nervosa has been related to family, biological, social, and cultural factors. Studies have found that anorexia nervosa is associated with a family history of anorexia nervosa (adjusted HR 11.4, 95% CI 1.1 to 89.0), bulimia nervosa (adjusted HR 3.5, 95% CI 1.1 to 14.0),[4] depression, generalised anxiety disorder, obsessive compulsive disorder, or obsessive compulsive personality disorder (adjusted RR 3.6, 95% CI 1.6 to 8.0).[5] A twin study suggested that anorexia nervosa may be related to genetic factors but it was unable to estimate reliably the contribution of non-shared environmental factors.[6] Specific aspects of childhood temperament thought to be related include perfectionism, negative self evaluation, and extreme compliance.[7] Perinatal factors include prematurity, particularly if the baby was small for gestational age (prematurity: OR 3.2, 95% CI 1.6 to 6.2; prematurity and small for gestational age: OR 5.7, 95% CI 1.1 to 28.7).[8]

PROGNOSIS
One prospective study followed up 51 people with teenage-onset anorexia nervosa, about half of whom received no or minimal treatment (< 8 sessions). After 10 years, 14/51 people (27%) had a persistent eating disorder, three (6%) had ongoing anorexia nervosa, and six (12%) had experienced a period of bulimia nervosa. People with anorexia nervosa were significantly more likely to have an affective disorder than controls matched for sex, age, and school (lifetime risk of affective disorder 96% in people with anorexia v 23% in controls; ARI 73%, 95% CI 60% to 85%). Obsessive compulsive disorder was, similarly, significantly more likely in people with anorexia nervosa compared with controls (30% v 10%; ARI 20%, 95% CI 10% to 41%). However, in 35% of people with obsessive compulsive disorder and anorexia nervosa, obsessive compulsive disorder preceded the anorexia. About half of all participants continued to have poor psychosocial functioning at 10 years (assessed using the Morgan Russell scale and Global Assessment of Functioning Scale).[9] A summary of treatment studies (68 studies published between 1953 and 1989, 3104 people, length of follow up 1–33 years) found that 43% of people recover completely (range ▶

7–86%), 36% improve (range 1–69%), 20% develop a chronic eating disorder (range 0–43%), and 5% die from anorexia nervosa (range 0–21%).[10] Favourable prognostic factors include an early age at onset and a short interval between onset of symptoms and the beginning of treatment. Unfavourable prognostic factors include vomiting, bulimia, profound weight loss, chronicity, and a history of premorbid developmental or clinical abnormalities. The all cause standardised mortality ratio of eating disorders (anorexia nervosa and bulimia nervosa) has been estimated at 538, about three times higher than that of other psychiatric illnesses.[11] The average annual mortality was 0.59% a year in females in ten eating disorder populations (1322 people) with a minimum follow up of 6 years.[12] The mortality was higher for people with lower weight and with older age at presentation. Young women with anorexia nervosa are at an increased risk of fractures later in life.[13]

Please refer to the Clinical Evidence website for full text and references.

Bipolar disorder

Search date August 2003

John Geddes

What are the effects of treatments in mania?

BENEFICIAL

Lithium

One RCT in people with bipolar type I disorder experiencing a manic episode identified by a systematic review found that lithium increased the proportion of people who responded after 3–4 weeks compared with placebo. One systematic review found that lithium increased the proportion of people who had remission of manic symptoms at 3 weeks compared with chlorpromazine. It found no significant difference in symptoms at 3–6 weeks between lithium and haloperidol, valproate, carbamazepine or clonazepam. One RCT identified by the systematic review found that lithium was less effective than risperidone in reducing manic symptoms at 4 weeks. RCTs found no significant difference in symptoms at 4 weeks between lithium and olanzapine or lamotrigine. Another RCT identified by a systematic review found that lithium plus olanzapine increased the proportion of people who responded at 3–6 weeks compared with placebo. Lithium can cause a range of adverse effects, including gastrointestinal disturbances, fine tremor, renal impairment, polydipsia, leucocytosis, weight gain, oedema, and hypothyroidism. The RCTs provided insufficient evidence about how the adverse effects of lithium compared with those of other antipsychotic drugs.

Olanzapine

One systematic review and one subsequent RCT in people with bipolar type I disorder found that olanzapine increased the proportion of people who responded at 3–6 weeks compared with placebo, both as monotherapy and in combination with lithium or valproate. One RCT found no significant difference in symptoms at 28 days between olanzapine and lithium. RCTs identified by a systematic review found that olanzapine was more effective in reducing symptoms than valproate, but was also more likely to cause adverse effects such as sedation and weight gain. The acceptability of olanzapine may be limited by weight gain.

Valproate

One systematic review in people with bipolar type I disorder experiencing a manic episode found that valproate increased the proportion of people who responded over 3 weeks compared with placebo but caused more dizziness. It found no significant difference in response rates at 1–6 weeks between valproate and lithium, haloperidol, or carbamazepine. It found that valproate was less effective in reducing manic symptoms than olanzapine, but was also less likely to cause adverse effects such as sedation and weight gain. One RCT identified by a systematic review found that valproate plus olanzapine increased the proportion of people who responded at 3–6 weeks compared with placebo.

LIKELY TO BE BENEFICIAL

Carbamazepine

RCTs in people with bipolar type I disorder experiencing a manic episode identified by a systematic review found no significant difference in manic symptoms at 4–6 weeks between carbamazepine and lithium or valproate. The review provided insufficient evidence to assess adverse effects of carbamazepine.

▶

Clonazepam

We found no RCTs comparing clonazepam versus placebo in people with mania. RCTs in people with bipolar type I disorder experiencing a manic episode identified by a systematic review suggest that clonazepam may be as effective as lithium in improving manic symptoms at 1–4 weeks. The review provided insufficient evidence to assess adverse effects of clonazepam.

Haloperidol

We found no RCTs comparing haloperidol versus placebo in people with mania. RCTs in people with bipolar type I disorder experiencing a manic episode identified by a systematic review found no significant difference in manic symptoms at 1–3 weeks between haloperidol and lithium or valproate, although haloperidol was associated with more extrapyramidal adverse effects and sedation than valproate.

Risperidone

We found no RCTs comparing risperidone alone versus placebo. One RCT in people with mania taking lithium, valproate, or carbamazepine found no significant difference in symptoms between adding risperidone and placebo and found that adding risperidone increased extrapyramidal adverse effects. Another RCT in people with bipolar type I disorder experiencing a manic episode found that risperidone reduced manic symptoms at 4 weeks compared with lithium.

Ziprasidone

One RCT found that ziprasidone increased the proportion of people who responded at 3 weeks compared with placebo, but caused sedation, headaches, dizziness, and akathisia.

UNKNOWN EFFECTIVENESS

Chlorpromazine

One very small RCT in people with mania found limited evidence that chlorpromazine may improve manic symptoms over 7 weeks more than placebo or imipramine. One systematic review found that fewer people had remission of symptoms at 3 weeks with chlorpromazine than with lithium. The review and RCT provided insufficient evidence to assess adverse effects of chlorpromazine.

Gabapentin

One RCT in people with bipolar type I disorder experiencing a manic or mixed episode already taking lithium or valproate found that adding gabapentin was less effective in reducing manic symptoms over 10 months than placebo. Gabapentin was associated with somnolence, dizziness, diarrhoea, and memory loss.

Lamotrigine

We found no RCTs comparing lamotrigine versus placebo in people with mania. One RCT in people with bipolar type I disorder experiencing a manic episode identified by a systematic review found no significant difference in manic symptoms at 4 weeks between lamotrigine and lithium. The review provided insufficient evidence to assess adverse effects of lamotrigine.

Quetiapine

One RCT in adolescents found that quetiapine increased the proportion of people who responded at 6 weeks compared with placebo, but caused sedation.

Topiramate

One systematic review identified no RCTs of topiramate in people with mania.

What are the effects of treatments in bipolar depression?

Antidepressants

Systematic reviews found that antidepressants improved depressive symptoms at the end of the trial (unspecified) compared with placebo. They found no significant difference between selective serotonin reuptake inhibitors and tricyclic antidepressants in the proportion of people who responded, although people taking selective serotonin reuptake inhibitors were more likely to respond. The reviews and one subsequent RCT found no significant difference in symptoms between monoamine oxidase inhibitors and tricyclic antidepressants or between selective serotonin reuptake inhibitors and serotonin noradrenaline reuptake inhibitors. Antidepressants are associated with manic switching and the reviews and subsequent RCT suggested that tricyclic antidepressants are more likely to induce mania than selective serotonin reuptake inhibitors.

Lamotrigine

One RCT in people with bipolar type I disorder experiencing a depressive episode identified by a systematic review found that lamotrigine increased the proportion of people who responded over 7 weeks compared with placebo. Lamotrigine increased the proportion of people with headache compared with placebo.

Carbamazepine

One systematic review identified no RCTs of sufficient quality to assess carbamazepine in people with bipolar depression.

Lithium

One systematic review identified no RCTs of sufficient quality to assess lithium in people with bipolar depression.

Psychological treatments

We found no systematic review or RCTs of psychological treatments in people with bipolar depression.

Topiramate

One systematic review identified no RCTs of topiramate in people with bipolar depression. One subsequent RCT in people taking lithium or valproate found no significant difference in symptoms at 8 weeks between adding topiramate and adding bupropion. The RCT found that a third of people taking topiramate and a fifth of people taking bupropion withdrew because of adverse effects, including anxiety, increase or decrease in appetite, blurred vision, backache, headache, and nausea.

Valproate

We found no systematic review or RCTs of valproate in people with bipolar depression.

What are the effects of interventions to prevent relapse of mania or bipolar depression?

Lithium

Systematic reviews and subsequent RCTs found that lithium reduced relapse over 2 years compared with placebo. They found no significant difference in relapse ▶

between lithium and valproate, carbamazepine, or lamotrigine. RCTs found that more people had overall adverse effects (not specified) with lithium than with placebo, and that lithium may increase hypothyroidism. They found that lithium caused more polyuria, thirst, and diarrhoea than valproate but less sedation and infection. More people taking lithium than carbamazepine had adverse effects, including blurred vision, difficulty concentrating, thirst, hand tremor and muscle weakness, but more people taking carbamazepine had increased appetite. RCTs also found that fewer people taking lithium than lamotrigine had headaches.

LIKELY TO BE BENEFICIAL

Carbamazepine

We found no RCTs comparing carbamazepine versus placebo for preventing relapse. One systematic review and one subsequent RCT found no significant difference between carbamazepine and lithium in the proportion of people who relapsed over 1–3 years. The review and subsequent RCT found that carbamazepine was associated with fewer adverse effects than lithium.

Cognitive therapy

Two RCTs found that cognitive therapy reduced relapse over 6–12 months compared with usual care. Another RCT found no significant difference between cognitive therapy and usual care in the proportion of people who relapsed over 6 months, although fewer people receiving cognitive therapy relapsed. The RCT is likely to have been underpowered to detect a clinically important difference between treatments. The RCTs provided insufficient evidence to assess adverse effects of cognitive therapy.

Education to recognise symptoms of relapse

One RCT found limited evidence that an educational programme to recognise symptoms of relapse reduced manic relapse over 18 months, but that it may increase depressive episodes.

Lamotrigine (reduced relapse of bipolar depressive episodes)

Three RCTs found that lamotrigine reduced relapse compared with placebo. However, secondary analyses in two of the RCTs suggested that lamotrigine protected against depressive relapse, but not manic relapse. RCTs found no significant difference between lamotrigine and lithium in the proportion of people who relapsed and found that more people taking lamotrigine than lithium had headaches.

Valproate

One RCT identified by a systematic review found that valproate reduced relapse over 12 months compared with placebo. One systematic review found no significant difference between lithium and valproate in relapse over 12 months. The review found that valproate cause more sedation and infection than lithium but less polyuria, thirst, and diarrhoea.

UNKNOWN EFFECTIVENESS

Antidepressant drugs

One systematic review and one subsequent RCT provided insufficient evidence to assess antidepressants in preventing relapse of bipolar disorder.

Bipolar disorder

Family focused psychoeducation

One RCT found that 21 sessions of family focused psychoeducation reduced relapse over 12 months compared with two family sessions plus crisis management. Another RCT found that family focused psychoeducation may reduce relapse compared with individual focused therapy. The RCTs gave no information on adverse effects.

DEFINITION
Bipolar disorder (bipolar affective disorder, manic depressive disorder) is characterised by marked mood swings between mania (mood elevation) and bipolar depression that cause significant personal distress or social dysfunction, and are not caused by drugs or known physical disorders. **Bipolar type I disorder** is diagnosed when episodes of depression are interspersed with mania or mixed episodes. **Bipolar type II disorder** is diagnosed when depression is interspersed with less severe episodes of elevated mood that do not lead to dysfunction or disability (hypomania). Bipolar disorder has been subdivided in several further ways).[1]

INCIDENCE/ PREVALENCE
One 1996 cross-national community based study (38 000 people) found lifetime prevalence rates of bipolar disorder ranging from 0.3% in Taiwan to 1.5% in New Zealand.[2] It found that men and women were at similar risk, and that the age at first onset ranged from 19–29 years (average of 6 years earlier than first onset of major depression).

AETIOLOGY/ RISK FACTORS
The cause of bipolar disorder is uncertain, although family and twin studies suggest a genetic basis.[3] The lifetime risk of bipolar disorder is increased in first degree relatives of a person with bipolar disorder (40–70% for a monozygotic twin; 5–10% for other first degree relatives). If the first episode of mania occurs in an older adult, it may be secondary mania due to underlying medical or substance induced factors.[4]

PROGNOSIS
Bipolar disorder is a recurring illness and one of the leading causes of worldwide disability, especially in the 15–44 year age group.[3] One 4 year inception cohort study (173 people treated for a first episode of mania or mixed affective disorder) found that 93% of people no longer met criteria for mania at 2 years (median time to recover from a syndrome 4.6 weeks), but that only 36% had recovered to premorbid function.[4] It found that 40% of people had a recurrent manic (20%) or depressive (20%) episode within 2 years of recovering from the first episode. A meta-analysis, comparing observed suicide expected rates of suicide in an age and sex matched sample of the general population, found that the lifetime prevalence of suicide was about 2%, or 15 times greater than expected, in people with bipolar disorder.[5]

Please refer to the Clinical Evidence website for full text and references.

What are the effects of treatments?

LIKELY TO BE BENEFICIAL

Cognitive behavioural therapy for bulimia nervosa (CBT-BN)

One RCT found that CBT-BN improved remission rate, and reduced bulimic symptoms and depression compared with remaining on a waiting list. One RCT found no significant difference in remission of binge vomiting between guided self help CBT and CBT-BN after about 1 year. One RCT found no significant difference in remission rate or symptoms between cognitive behavioural therapy plus exposure response prevention and CBT-BN. One systematic review identified two RCTs, which found that interpersonal psychotherapy (IPT) was as effective as cognitive behavioural therapy for bulimia nervosa. One RCT found no significant difference between hypnobehavioural therapy (HBT) and CBT-BN for bulimia behavioural symptoms. One RCT found no clinically important difference in binge frequency between motivational enhancement therapy (MET) and CBT-BN. Two RCTs found no significant difference in remission or symptoms between CBT-BN and fluoxetine. Two RCTs comparing tricyclic antidepressants versus CBT-BN found mixed results. One found that imipramine improved remission compared with CBT-BN, and the other found no significant difference in remission rate between CBT-BN and desipramine. Two RCTs found no significant difference in remission rates or symptoms between CBT-BN and CBT-BN plus tricyclic antidepressants. Two RCTs found no significant difference in remission rates or symptoms between CBT-BN and CBT-BN plus fluoxetine.

Combination treatment (antidepressants plus cognitive behavioural therapy as effective as either treatment alone)

Two RCTs found no significant difference in remission rates or symptoms between CBT-BN plus tricyclic antidepressants and CBT-BN or tricyclic antidepressants alone. Two RCTs found no significant difference in remission rates or symptoms between CBT-BN plus fluoxetine and CBT-BN or fluoxetine alone. One RCT found no significant difference in remission rates between unguided self help CBT plus fluoxetine and unguided self help CBT or fluoxetine alone.

Monoamine oxidase inhibitors

One systematic review identified three RCTs, which found that monoamine oxidase inhibitors improved remission rates compared with placebo.

Selective serotonin reuptake inhibitors (evidence limited to fluoxetine)

Three RCTs have found that fluoxetine 60 mg daily improves remission compared with placebo. Two RCTs found no significant difference in remission or symptoms between CBT-BN and fluoxetine. We found no RCTs of other serotonin reuptake inhibitors (fluvoxamine, paroxetine, sertraline, or citalopram).

Tricyclic antidepressants

One systematic review found that tricyclic antidepressants (desipramine and imipramine) improved bulimic symptoms and reduced binge eating compared with placebo. Two RCTs comparing tricyclic antidepressants versus CBT-BN found mixed results. One found that imipramine improved remission compared with CBT-BN, and the other found no significant difference in remission rate between CBT-BN and desipramine.

▶

Cognitive orientation therapy

We found no RCTs of cognitive orientation therapy in people with bulimia nervosa.

Cognitive behavioural therapy plus exposure response prevention (CBT-ERP)

One RCT found no significant difference in vomiting frequency between CBT-ERP and waiting list, although it found that CBT-ERP improved depression scores compared with being on a waiting list. The RCT found no significant difference in remission rate or symptoms between CBT-ERP and CBT-BN.

Dialectical behavioural therapy

We found limited evidence from one small RCT that dialectical behavioural therapy improves bulimic symptoms compared with being on a waiting list.

Guided self help cognitive behavioural therapy

One RCT found no significant difference in behavioural symptoms between face to face or telephone guided self help cognitive behavioural therapy and waiting list. One RCT found no significant difference in remission of binge vomiting between guided self help CBT and CBT-BN after about 1 year. One RCT found no significant difference in remission between unguided and guided self help CBT.

Interpersonal psychotherapy (as effective as cognitive behavioural therapy for bulimia nervosa)

We found no RCTs comparing interpersonal psychotherapy versus no treatment, placebo, or waiting list control. One systematic review identified two RCTs, which found no significant difference in abstinence from binge eating between interpersonal psychotherapy and cognitive behavioural therapy for bulimia nervosa.

Hypnobehavioural therapy

One RCT found limited evidence that hypnobehavioural therapy (HBT) improved abstinence from bingeing and purging compared with waiting list. The same RCT found no significant difference between HBT and CBT for bulimia behavioural symptoms.

Motivational enhancement therapy

We found no RCTs comparing motivational enhancement therapy (MET) versus no treatment, placebo, or waiting list. One RCT found no clinically important difference in binge frequency between MET and CBT-BN.

Pure or unguided self help cognitive behavioural therapy

Two RCTs found no significant difference in remission or reduction in binge-purge frequency between pure or unguided self help CBT and waiting list. One RCT found no significant difference in remission between unguided and guided self help CBT. One RCT found no significant difference in remission between unguided self help CBT and fluoxetine alone or unguided self help CBT plus fluoxetine.

Mirtazapine; nefazodone; reboxetine; venlafaxine

We found no RCTs.

What are the effects of discontinuing treatment with antidepressants in people with remission?

UNLIKELY TO BE BENEFICIAL

Discontinuing fluoxetine

One RCT has found that continuing fluoxetine 60 mg daily is more effective than discontinuing fluoxetine and substituting placebo for maintaining a reduction in vomiting frequency in people who have responded well to an initial 8 week course of fluoxetine.

DEFINITION   Bulimia nervosa is an intense preoccupation with body weight and shape, with regular episodes of uncontrolled overeating of large amounts of food (binge eating) associated with use of extreme methods to counteract the feared effects of overeating. If a person also meets the diagnostic criteria for anorexia nervosa, then the diagnosis of anorexia nervosa takes precedence.[1] Bulimia nervosa can be difficult to identify because of extreme secrecy about binge eating and purgative behaviour. Weight may be normal but there is often a history of anorexia nervosa or restrictive dieting. Some people alternate between anorexia nervosa and bulimia nervosa. Some RCTs included people with subthreshold bulimia nervosa or a related eating disorder, binge eating disorder. Where possible, only results relevant to bulimia nervosa are reported in this review.

INCIDENCE/   In community based studies, the prevalence of bulimia nervosa is between
PREVALENCE   0.5% and 1.0% in young women, with an even social class distribution.[2–4] About 90% of people diagnosed with bulimia nervosa are women. The numbers presenting with bulimia nervosa in industrialised countries increased during the decade that followed its recognition in the late 1970s and "a cohort effect" is reported in community surveys,[2,5,6] implying an increase in incidence. The prevalence of eating disorders such as bulimia nervosa is lower in non-industrialised populations,[7] and varies across ethnic groups. African-American women have a lower rate of restrictive dieting than white American women, but have a similar rate of recurrent binge eating.[8]

AETIOLOGY/   Young women from the developed world who restrict their dietary intake are at
RISK FACTORS   greatest risk of developing bulimia nervosa and other eating disorders. One community based case control study compared 102 people with bulimia nervosa with 204 healthy controls and found higher rates of the following in people with the eating disorder: obesity, mood disorder, sexual and physical abuse, parental obesity, substance misuse, low self esteem, perfectionism, disturbed family dynamics, parental weight/shape concern, and early menarche.[9] Compared with a control group of 102 women who had other psychiatric disorders, women with bulimia nervosa had higher rates of parental problems and obesity.[9]

PROGNOSIS   A 10 year follow up study (50 people with bulimia nervosa from a placebo-controlled trial of mianserin treatment) found that 52% receiving placebo had fully recovered, and only 9% continued to experience full symptoms of bulimia nervosa.[10] A larger study (222 people from a trial of antidepressants and structured, intensive group psychotherapy) found that, after a mean follow up of 11.5 years, 11% still met criteria for bulimia nervosa, whereas 70% were in full or partial remission.[11] Short term studies found similar results: about 50% of people made a full recovery, 30% made a partial recovery, and 20% continued to be symptomatic.[12] There are few consistent predictors of longer term outcome. Good prognosis has been associated with shorter illness duration, a younger age of onset, higher social class, and a family history of alcohol abuse.[10] Poor prognosis has been associated with a history of substance misuse,[13] premorbid and paternal obesity,[14] and, in some studies, personality ▶

Bulimia nervosa

disorder.[15–18] One study (102 women) of the natural course of bulimia nervosa found that 31% still had the disorder at 15 months and 15% at 5 years.[19] Only 28% received treatment during the follow up period. In an evaluation of response to cognitive behavioural therapy, early progress (by session 6) best predicted outcome.[20] A subsequent systematic review of the outcome literature found no consistent evidence to support early intervention and a better prognosis.[21]

Please refer to the Clinical Evidence website for full text and references.

Deliberate self harm (and attempted suicide)

Search date October 2004

G Mustafa Soomro

We found little RCT evidence for any intervention in people who have deliberately self harmed. Most RCTs and meta-analyses of small RCTs are likely to have been underpowered to detect clinically important differences between interventions.

What are the effects of treatments for deliberate self harm and attempted suicide in adolescents and adults?

UNKNOWN EFFECTIVENESS

Continuity of care

One systematic review identified one RCT, which found limited evidence that follow up after hospital treatment with the same therapist may increase repetition of deliberate self harm compared with follow up with a different therapist over 3 months. However, the difference between groups may be explained by a higher level of risk factors for repetition in the group receiving follow up with the same therapist.

Dialectical behavioural therapy

One systematic review including one RCT found limited and equivocal evidence that dialectical behavioural therapy may reduce the proportion of people who repeat deliberate self harm over 12 months compared with usual care.

Emergency card

One systematic review found no significant difference in the proportion of people who repeated deliberate self harm over 12 months between emergency card (allowing emergency admission or contact with a doctor) and usual care.

Flupentixol depot injection

One systematic review including one small RCT found that flupentixol depot injection reduced the proportion of people who repeated deliberate self harm over 6 months compared with placebo. However, we were unable to draw reliable conclusions from this small study. Typical antipsychotics such as flupentixol are associated with a wide range of adverse effects.

Hospital admission

One systematic review found no significant difference between hospital admission and immediate discharge in the proportion of people who repeated deliberate self harm over 16 weeks.

Intensive outpatient follow up plus outreach

One systematic review found no significant difference in the proportion of people who repeated deliberate self harm over 4–12 months between intensive outpatient follow up plus outreach and usual care.

Manual assisted cognitive behavioural therapy

One RCT found no significant difference in repeat self harm rates at 1 year between manual assisted cognitive therapy and usual treatment (problem solving approaches, dynamic psychotherapy, short term counselling, or referral to a general practitioner or a voluntary group).

Mianserin

One systematic review provided insufficient evidence to assess mianserin.

Deliberate self harm (and attempted suicide)

Nurse led case management

One RCT found no significant difference between nurse led case management and usual care in the proportion of people who were admitted to emergency departments for episodes of deliberate self harm over 12 months.

Paroxetine

One systematic review, including one RCT in people who had previously deliberately self harmed, receiving concurrent psychotherapy, found no significant difference between paroxetine and placebo in the proportion of people who repeated self harm over 12 months. It found that paroxetine increased diarrhoea and tremor compared with placebo. Paroxetine, like other selective serotonin re-uptake inhibitors, has been linked to suicidal ideation. In clinical trials in children and adolescents with depression it showed higher rates of suicide related events. Abrupt withdrawal of SSRIs should be avoided. Withdrawal side-effects include headache, nausea, paraesthesia, dizziness and anxiety. Extrapyramidal reactions (including orofacial dystonias) and withdrawal syndrome have been reported more commonly with paroxetine than with other SSRIs.

Problem solving therapy

One systematic review of small RCTs found no significant difference between problem solving therapy and usual care in the proportion of people who repeated deliberate self harm over 6–12 months. A second systematic review found that problem solving therapy reduced symptoms of depression, anxiety, and hopelessness, and improved problems compared with usual care.

Psychodynamic interpersonal therapy

One RCT found that brief psychodynamic interpersonal therapy for 4 weeks reduced repetition of deliberate self harm, depression, and suicidal ideation over 6 months compared with usual care. However, we were unable to draw reliable conclusions from this single RCT.

Telephone contact

One RCT found no significant difference between telephone contact at 4 and 8 months and usual care in repetition of deliberate self harm, global functioning, and suicidal ideation over 12 months.

UNLIKELY TO BE BENEFICIAL

General practice based guidelines

One large cluster randomised trial comparing the use of general practitioner guidelines for management of deliberate self harm versus usual care found no significant difference in the proportion of people who repeated deliberate self harm over 12 months or in the time to repetition of self harm.

DEFINITION Deliberate self harm is an acute non-fatal act of self harm carried out deliberately in the form of an acute episode of behaviour by an individual with variable motivation.[1] The intention to end life may be absent or present to a variable degree. Other terms used to describe this phenomenon are "attempted suicide" and "parasuicide". For the purpose of this chapter the term deliberate self harm will be used throughout. Common methods of deliberate self harm include self cutting and self poisoning, such as overdosing on medicines. Some acts of deliberate self harm are characterised by high suicidal intent, meticulous planning (including precautions against being found out), and severe lethality of the method used. Other acts of deliberate self harm are characterised by no or low intention of suicide, lack of planning and concealing of the act, and low lethality of the method used. The related term of "suicide" is defined as an act with a fatal outcome that is deliberately initiated and performed by the person with the knowledge or expectation of its fatal outcome.[1]

This review focuses on recent deliberate self harm, in all age groups, as the main presenting problem and excludes RCTs in which deliberate self harm is assessed as an outcome associated with other disorders, such as depression or borderline personality disorder. Deliberate self harm is not defined in the *Diagnostic and statistical manual of mental disorders* (DSM IV)[2] or the *International classification of mental and behavioural disorders* (ICD-10).[3]

INCIDENCE/ PREVALENCE
Based on data from 16 European countries between 1989–1992, the lifetime prevalence of deliberate self harm in people treated in hospital and other medical facilities, including general practice settings, is estimated at about 3% for women and 2% for men.[4] Over the last 50 years there has been a rise in the incidence of deliberate self harm in the UK.[4] A reasonable current estimate is about 400/100 000 population a year.[5] In two community studies in the USA, 3–5% of responders said that they had made an attempt at deliberate self harm at some time.[6] Self poisoning using organophosphates is particularly common in developing countries.[7] A large hospital (catering for 900 000 people) in Sri Lanka reported 2559 adult hospital admissions and 41% occupancy of medical intensive care beds for deliberate self harm with organophosphates over 2 years.[8] An international survey using representative community samples of adults (aged 18–64 years) reported lifetime prevalence of self reported suicide attempts of 3.82% in Canada, 5.93% in Puerto Rico, 4.95% in France, 3.44% in West Germany, 0.72% in Lebanon, 0.75% in Taiwan, 3.2% in Korea, and 4.43% in New Zealand.[6]

AETIOLOGY/ RISK FACTORS
Familial, biological, and psychosocial factors may contribute to deliberate self harm. Evidence for genetic factors includes a higher risk of familial suicide and greater concordance in monozygotic than dizygotic twins for deliberate self harm.[9] Evidence for biological factors includes reduced cerebrospinal fluid 5-hydroxyindole acetic acid levels and a blunted prolactin response to the fenfluramine challenge test, indicating a reduction in the function of serotonin in the central nervous system.[10] People who deliberately self harm and attempt suicide also show traits of impulsiveness and aggression, inflexible and impulsive cognitive style, and impaired decision making and problem solving.[11] Deliberate self harm is more likely to occur in women, young adults, and people who are single or divorced, of low education level, unemployed, disabled, or suffering from a psychiatric disorder,[12] particularly depression,[13] substance misuse,[14] borderline and antisocial personality disorders,[15] severe anxiety disorders,[16] and physical illness.[17]

PROGNOSIS
Suicide is highest during the first year after deliberate self harm.[18] One systematic review found median rates of repetition of 16% (interquartile range [IQR] 12% to 25%) within the first year, 21% (IQR 12% to 30%) within 1–4 years, and 23% (IQR 11% to 32%) within 4 years or longer. It found median mortality from suicide after deliberate self harm of 1.8% (IQR 0.8% to 2.6%) within the first year, 3.0% (IQR 2.0% to 4.4%) within 1–4 years, 3.4% (IQR 2.5% to 6.0%) within 5–10 years, and 6.7% (IQR 5.0% to 11.0%) within 9 years or longer.[18] Repetition of deliberate self harm is more likely in people aged 25–49 years who are unemployed, divorced, from lower social class, or who suffer from substance misuse, depression, hopelessness, powerlessness, personality disorders, have unstable living conditions or live alone, have a criminal record, previous psychiatric treatment, a history of stressful traumatic life events, or a history of coming from a broken home or of family violence.[12] Factors associated with risk of suicide after deliberate self harm are aged over 45 years, male sex, being unemployed, retired, separated, divorced, or widowed, living alone, poor physical health, psychiatric disorder (particularly depression, alcoholism, schizophrenia, and sociopathic personality disorder), high suicidal intent in current episode including leaving a written note, violent method used in current episode, and history of previous deliberate self harm.[19]

Please refer to the Clinical Evidence website for full text and references.

Dementia

Search date Februry 2004

James Warner, Rob Butler, and Pradeep Arya

People in RCTs of treatments for dementia are often not representative of people with dementia. Few RCTs are conducted in primary care and few are conducted in people with types of dementia other than Alzheimer's disease.

What are the effects of treatments on cognitive symptoms of dementia?

Donepezil

One systematic review in people with mild to moderate Alzheimer's disease and one subsequent RCT in people with moderate to severe Alzheimer's disease found that donepezil improved cognitive function and global clinical state at up to 52 weeks compared with placebo in people with mild to severe Alzheimer's disease. The review found no significant difference in patient rated quality of life at 12 or 24 weeks between donepezil and placebo. One large RCT identified by the review found that donepezil delayed the median time to "clinically evident functional decline" by 5 months compared with placebo. One open label RCT in people with mild to moderate Alzheimer's disease found no significant difference in cognitive function at 12 weeks between donepezil and rivastigmine, although fewer people taking donepezil withdrew from the trial for any cause. One RCT in people with Alzheimer's disease found no significant difference between galantamine and donepezil in cognitive function or adverse effects at 1 year. One systematic review in people with vascular dementia found that donepezil improved cognitive function compared with placebo at 24 weeks.

Galantamine

RCTs found that galantamine improved cognitive function and global clinical state over 6 months compared with placebo in people with Alzheimer's disease or vascular dementia. One RCT in people with Alzheimer's disease found no significant difference between donepezil and galantamine in cognitive function or adverse effects at 1 year.

Ginkgo biloba

RCTs found limited evidence that ginkgo biloba improved cognitive function over 24–26 weeks compared with placebo in people with Alzheimer's disease or vascular dementia. Preparations of gingo biloba available without prescription differ in terms of purity and concentrations of active ingredients compared with the high purity extract (EGb 761) used in most RCTs.

Memantine

Two RCTs identified by a systematic review found that memantine improved cognitive function at 12–28 weeks compared with placebo in people with mild to moderate vascular dementia. Subsequent RCTs found that memantine improved global clinical outcome and reduced care dependence at 12–28 weeks in people with more severe Alzheimer's disease or vascular dementia.

Reality orientation

One systematic review of small RCTs found that reality orientation improved cognitive function compared with no treatment in people with various types of dementia.

TRADE OFF BETWEEN BENEFITS AND HARMS

Physostigmine

One RCT in people with Alzheimer's disease found limited evidence that slow release physostigmine improved cognitive function over 12 weeks compared with placebo, but adverse effects, including nausea, vomiting, diarrhoea, dizziness, and stomach pain, were common.

Rivastigmine

One systematic review and one additional RCT found that rivastigmine improved cognitive function compared with placebo in people with Alzheimer's disease or Lewy body dementia, but adverse effects such as nausea, vomiting, and anorexia were common. Subgroup analysis from one RCT in people with Alzheimer's disease found limited evidence that people with vascular risk factors may respond better to rivastigmine than those without. One open label RCT in people with mild to moderate Alzheimer's disease found no significant difference in cognitive function at 12 weeks between rivastigmine and donepezil, although more people taking rivastigmine withdrew from the trial for any cause.

Tacrine

Two systematic reviews found limited evidence that tacrine improved cognitive function and global state at 3–36 weeks compared with placebo in people with Alzheimer's disease, but adverse effects, including nausea, vomiting, diarrhoea, anorexia, and abdominal pain, were common.

UNKNOWN EFFECTIVENESS

Lecithin

Small, poor RCTs identified by a systematic review provided insufficient evidence to assess lecithin in people with Alzheimer's disease.

Music therapy

Poor studies identified by a systematic review provided insufficient evidence to assess music therapy in people with dementia.

Nicotine

One systematic review found no RCTs of sufficient quality on the effects of nicotine in people with dementia.

Non-steroidal anti-inflammatory drugs

One RCT in people with Alzheimer's disease found no significant difference in cognitive function after 25 weeks' treatment with diclofenac plus misoprostol compared with placebo. Another RCT in people with Alzheimer's disease found insufficient evidence to compare indometacin versus placebo in people with Alzheimer's disease. A third RCT found no significant difference between naproxen or rofecoxib and placebo in cognitive function at 1 year.

Reminiscence therapy

One systematic review found insufficient evidence to assess reminiscence therapy in people with dementia.

Selegiline

One systematic review found that, in people with mild to moderate Alzheimer's disease, selegiline for 2–4 months improved cognitive function compared with placebo. It found no significant difference in global clinical state or activities of daily living. RCTs assessing outcomes beyond 4 months found no significant difference between selegiline and placebo.

Dementia

Vitamin E

One RCT in people with moderate to severe Alzheimer's disease found limited evidence of no significant difference in cognitive function after 2 years' treatment with vitamin E compared with placebo. However, it found limited evidence that vitamin E reduced mortality, institutionalisation, loss of ability to perform activities of daily living, and the proportion of people who developed severe dementia.

UNLIKELY TO BE BENEFICIAL

Oestrogen

One systematic review found insufficient evidence that oestrogen with or without progestogen improved cognitive symptoms in postmenopausal women with dementia. However, there is concern that oestrogen treatment may increase the risk of developing breast cancer and cardiovascular events.

What are the effects of treatments on behavioural and psychological symptoms of dementia?

LIKELY TO BE BENEFICIAL

Carbamazepine

One RCT found that carbamazepine reduced agitation and aggression over 6 weeks compared with placebo in people with various types of dementia and behavioural and psychological symptoms.

Reality orientation

One systematic review of small RCTs found that reality orientation improved behaviour compared with no treatment in people with various types of dementia.

TRADE OFF BETWEEN BENEFITS AND HARMS

Haloperidol

One systematic review in people with various types of dementia plus behavioural and psychological symptoms found no significant difference in agitation at 6–16 weeks between haloperidol and placebo. However, it found that haloperidol may reduce aggression. It found that haloperidol increased the frequency and severity of extrapyramidal symptoms compared with placebo. Another systematic review in people with various types of dementia plus behavioural and psychological symptoms found limited evidence that haloperidol and risperidone were similarly effective in reducing agitation over 12 weeks but that haloperidol caused more frequent and more severe extrapyramidal symptoms. Two RCTs in people with agitated behaviour associated with dementia found no significant difference in agitation between trazodone and haloperidol, but may have been too small to exclude a clinically important difference.

Olanzapine

One RCT identified by a systematic review in nursing home residents with Alzheimer's disease or Lewy body dementia plus behavioural and psychological symptoms found that low and medium doses of olanzapine reduced agitation, hallucinations, and delusions over 6 weeks compared with placebo. Olanzapine has been associated with cerebrovascular adverse effects.

Risperidone

One systematic review and one subsequent RCT in people with various types of dementia, primarily Alzheimer's disease, all with behavioural and psychological symptoms, found that risperidone improved symptoms over 12 weeks compared with placebo. Another systematic review in people with various types of dementia plus aggressive behaviours found limited evidence that risperidone and haloperidol were similarly effective in reducing agitation over 12 weeks but that risperidone caused fewer and less severe extrapyramidal symptoms. Risperidone has been associated with cerebrovascular adverse events.

UNKNOWN EFFECTIVENESS

Sodium valproate

One RCT found limited evidence that sodium valproate reduced agitation over 6 weeks compared with placebo in people with dementia plus behavioural and psychological problems. Another RCT found no significant difference in aggressive behaviour over 8 weeks between sodium valproate and placebo.

Trazodone

We found no RCTs comparing trazodone versus placebo. One small RCT in people with agitated behaviour associated with dementia found no significant difference in agitation over 9 weeks between trazodone and haloperidol. Another small RCT in people with Alzheimer's disease and agitated behaviour found no significant difference in outcomes over 16 weeks among trazodone, haloperidol, behaviour management techniques, and placebo. The RCTs may have been underpowered to detect a clinically important difference.

Donepezil; galantamine

RCTs provided inconclusive evidence about the effects of donepezil or galantamine compared with placebo on behavioural and psychiatric symptoms in people with mild to moderate Alzheimer's disease.

DEFINITION **Dementia** is characterised by chronic, global, non-reversible impairment in cerebral function. It usually results in loss of memory (initially of recent events), loss of executive function (such as the ability to make decisions or sequence complex tasks), and changes in personality. **Alzheimer's disease** is a type of dementia characterised by an insidious onset and slow deterioration, and involves speech, motor, personality, and executive function impairment. It should be diagnosed after other systemic, psychiatric, and neurological causes of dementia have been excluded clinically and by laboratory investigation. **Vascular dementia** is multi-infarct dementia involving a stepwise deterioration in executive function with or without language and motor dysfunction occurring as a result of cerebral arterial occlusion. It usually occurs in the presence of vascular risk factors (diabetes, hypertension, and smoking). Characteristically, it has a more sudden onset and stepwise progression than Alzheimer's disease. **Lewy body dementia** is a type of dementia involving insidious impairment of executive function with Parkinsonism, visual hallucinations, fluctuating cognitive abilities, and increased risk of falls or autonomic failure.[1,2] Careful clinical examination of people with mild to moderate dementia and the use of established diagnostic criteria accurately identifies 70–90% of cases confirmed at postmortem.[3,4]

INCIDENCE/ PREVALENCE About 6% of people aged over 65 years and 30% of people aged over 90 years have some form of dementia.[5] Dementia is rare before the age of 60 years. Alzheimer's disease and vascular dementia (including mixed dementia) are each estimated to account for 35–50% of dementia, and Lewy body dementia is estimated to account for up to 20% of dementia in the elderly, varying with geographical, cultural, and racial factors.[1,5–9]

AETIOLOGY/ RISK FACTORS **Alzheimer's disease:** The cause of Alzheimer's disease is unclear. A key pathological process is deposition of abnormal amyloid in the central nervous system.[10] Most people with the relatively rare condition of early onset Alzheimer's disease (before age 60 years) show an autosomal dominant inheritance owing to mutations in presenilin or amyloid precursor protein genes. Several ▶

genes (*APP*, *PS-1*, and *PS-2*) have been identified. Later onset dementia is sometimes clustered in families, but specific gene mutations have not been identified. Head injury, Down's syndrome, and lower premorbid intellect may be risk factors for Alzheimer's disease. **Vascular dementia:** Vascular dementia is related to cardiovascular risk factors, such as smoking, hypertension, and diabetes. **Lewy body dementia:** The cause of Lewy body dementia is unknown. Brain acetylcholine activity is reduced in many forms of dementia, and the level of reduction correlates with cognitive impairment. Many treatments for Alzheimer's disease enhance cholinergic activity.[1,6]

PROGNOSIS **Alzheimer's disease:** Alzheimer's disease usually has an insidious onset with progressive reduction in cerebral function. Diagnosis is difficult in the early stages. Median life expectancy after diagnosis is 5–6 years.[11] **Vascular dementia:** We found no reliable data on prognosis. **Lewy body dementia:** People with Lewy body dementia have an average life expectancy of about 6 years after diagnosis.[5] Behavioural problems, depression, and psychotic symptoms are common in all types of dementia.[12,13] Eventually, most people with dementia find it difficult to perform simple tasks without help.

Please refer to the Clinical Evidence website for full text and references.

Rob Butler, Stuart Carney, Andrea Cipriani, John Geddes, Simon Hatcher, Jonathan Price, and Michael Von Korff

Mild to moderate depression: We found no reliable direct evidence that one type of treatment (drug or non-drug) is superior to another in improving symptoms of depression. However, we found strong evidence that some treatments are effective, whereas the effectiveness of others remains uncertain.

Severe depression: Of the interventions examined, prescription antidepressant drugs and electroconvulsive therapy are the only treatments for which there is good evidence of effectiveness in severe depressive disorders. We found no RCTs comparing drug and non-drug treatments in severe depressive disorders.

What are the effects of treatments in mild to moderate or severe depression?

BENEFICIAL

Prescription antidepressant drugs (tricyclic antidepressants [including low dose tricyclic antidepressants], selective serotonin reuptake inhibitors, monoamine oxidase inhibitors, reboxetine, or venlafaxine) versus placebo in mild to moderate and severe depression

Systematic reviews and subsequent RCTs in people aged 16 years or over in primary and secondary care found that prescription antidepressant drugs (tricyclic antidepressants [including low dose tricyclic antidepressants], selective serotonin reuptake inhibitors, monoamine oxidase inhibitors, or venlafaxine) were effective for treatment of all grades of depressive disorders compared with placebo. Two RCTs in people admitted to hospital with severe depression found that reboxetine increased the proportion of people who responded at 4–6 weeks compared with placebo. One RCT in people with major depressive disorder provided insufficient evidence to assess the effects of reboxetine compared with placebo on depressive symptoms, although it found that reboxetine improved social functioning over 8 weeks. One systematic review in people aged 55 years or over with all grades of depressive disorder found that tricyclic antidepressants, selective serotonin reuptake inhibitors, or monoamine oxidase inhibitors reduced the proportion of people who failed to recover over 26–49 days compared with placebo. The reviews gave little information on severe adverse effects of antidepressant drugs compared with placebo. Evidence of publication bias has been found in the RCTs of selective serotonin reuptake inhibitors and the efficacy and safety of these drugs is currently under review by the regulatory authorities in several countries.

Tricyclic antidepressants versus other prescription antidepressant drugs

Three systematic reviews found no significant difference in outcomes with different kinds of antidepressant drug (tricyclic antidepressants, selective serotonin reuptake inhibitors, or monoamine oxidase inhibitors). One systematic review found no significant difference between tricyclic antidepressants and venlafaxine in the proportion of people who responded over 1–12 months. Another systematic review suggested that tricyclic antidepressants were more effective than monoamine oxidase inhibitors in people with severe depressive disorders, but may be less effective in atypical depressive disorders with biological features such as increased sleep, and increased appetite. A third systematic review found that tricyclic antidepressants were associated with higher rates of adverse effects than selective serotonin reuptake inhibitors, but the difference was small. Two RCTs, primarily in people with severe depression, found no significant difference in symptoms at 4 ▶

weeks between desipramine or imipramine and reboxetine, but results were sensitive to outcome scales used. One systematic review found no significant difference between low dosage tricyclics and standard dosage tricyclics in the proportion of responders at 6–8 weeks.

Selective serotonin reuptake inhibitors and related drugs versus other prescription antidepressant drugs

Three systematic reviews found no significant difference in outcomes with tricyclic antidepressants, selective serotonin reuptake inhibitors, or monoamine oxidase inhibitors, although one systematic review found that selective serotonin reuptake inhibitors were less effective than venlafaxine in increasing the proportion of people who responded. RCTs in people with major depression found similar response rates at 6 weeks between fluoxetine and reboxetine, but found that reboxetine may be slightly more effective in improving social functioning. One systematic review found that selective serotonin reuptake inhibitors were associated with fewer adverse effects than tricyclic antidepressants, but the difference was small. Another systematic review and one retrospective cohort study found no strong evidence that fluoxetine was associated with increased risk of suicide compared with tricyclic antidepressants or placebo. One RCT and observational data suggested that abrupt withdrawal of selective serotonin reuptake inhibitors was associated with symptoms including dizziness and rhinitis, and that these symptoms are more likely with drugs with a short half life, such as paroxetine. Evidence of publication bias has been found in the RCTs of selective serotonin reuptake inhibitors and the efficacy and safety of these drugs is currently under review by the regulatory authorities in several countries.

Monoamine oxidase inhibitors versus other prescription antidepressant drugs

Systematic reviews found no significant difference in outcomes with different kinds of antidepressant drug (tricyclic antidepressants, selective serotonin reuptake inhibitors, or monoamine oxidase inhibitors). One systematic review found that monoamine oxidase inhibitors were less effective than tricyclic antidepressants in people with severe depressive disorders. However, they may be more effective in atypical depressive disorders with biological features such as increased sleep and increased appetite.

Venlafaxine versus other prescription antidepressant drugs

One systematic review found no significant difference between venlafaxine and tricyclic antidepressants in the proportion of people who responded over 1 month to 1 year and found that venlafaxine increased the proportion of people who responded compared with selective serotonin reuptake inhibitors.

Cognitive therapy (in mild to moderate depression)

One systematic review in younger and older adults found that cognitive therapy improved symptoms compared with no treatment. Three systematic reviews in younger and older adults with mild to moderate depression found that psychological therapies (mainly interpersonal psychotherapy and cognitive therapy) increased the proportion of people who were in remission over 10–34 weeks compared with control (usual care, usual care plus pill placebo or supportive therapy). These reviews did not report results for cognitive therapy alone compared with control. One systematic review found limited evidence that cognitive therapy was more effective than interpersonal therapy in improving recovery rates but this difference disappeared when low quality studies were excluded or if studies which relied on advertising or similar techniques to recruit people were excluded. One systematic review of poor quality RCTs in people aged 55 years or over with mild to moderate depression found no significant difference in symptoms between psychological treatments (such as cognitive therapy or cognitive behavioural therapy) and no treatment. It also found no significant difference in symptoms between psychological treatments and similar but non-specific attention.

Electroconvulsive therapy (in moderate to severe depression)

One systematic review in people with moderate to severe depressive disorder, many of whom were inpatients, found that electroconvulsive therapy improved symptoms over 1–6 weeks' treatment compared with simulated electroconvulsive therapy or antidepressant drugs. The review found that bilateral electroconvulsive therapy improved symptoms compared with unilateral electroconvulsive therapy and that high dose electroconvulsive therapy was more effective than low dose. The degree of reported short term cognitive impairment seemed to be inversely related to treatment efficacy. Another systematic review provided insufficient evidence to assess electroconvulsive therapy in older adults. Because electroconvulsive therapy may be unacceptable to some people and, because it is a short term treatment, there is consensus that it should normally be reserved for people who cannot tolerate or have not responded to antidepressant drug treatment, although it may be useful when a rapid response is required.

Interpersonal psychotherapy (In mild to moderate depression)

Two systematic reviews in younger and older adults with mild to moderate depression found that both psychological therapies (mainly interpersonal psychotherapy and cognitive therapy) increased the proportion of people who were in remission over 10–34 weeks compared with control (usual care, usual care plus pill placebo or supportive therapy). These reviews did not report results for interpersonal therapy alone compared with control. One RCT identified by a third review found that interpersonal therapy increased response rates compared with usual care. One systematic review found limited evidence that interpersonal therapy was less effective than cognitive therapy in improving recovery rates but this difference disappeared when low quality studies were excluded or if studies which relied on advertising or similar techniques to recruit people were excluded.

LIKELY TO BE BENEFICIAL

Combining prescription antidepressant drugs and psychological treatments (in mild to moderate and severe depression)

One non-systematic review of RCTs in people aged 18–80 years found that, in people with severe depression, adding antidepressant drug treatment to interpersonal psychotherapy or to cognitive therapy improved symptoms compared with either psychological treatment alone. The review found no significant difference in symptoms in people with mild to moderate depression. However, subsequent RCTs in younger and older adults with mild to moderate depression found that combining antidepressant drugs plus psychological treatments improved symptoms more than either antidepressant drugs or psychological treatments alone. One RCT in older adults with mild to moderate depression found that cognitive behavioural therapy plus desipramine improved symptoms more than desipramine alone.

Non-directive counselling (in mild to moderate depression)

One systematic review in people aged 18 years or over with recent onset psychological problems, including depression, found that brief, non-directive counselling in primary care reduced symptom scores in the short term (< 6 months) in people with mild to moderate depression compared with usual care. However, it found no significant difference in scores in the long term (> 6 months). ▶

Depressive disorders

Reboxetine versus other antidepressant drugs (in mild to moderate or severe depression)

Two RCTs, primarily in people with severe depression, found no significant difference in symptoms at 4 weeks between reboxetine and desipramine or imipramine, but results were sensitive to outcome scales used. RCTs in people with major depression found similar response rates at 6 weeks between reboxetine and fluoxetine, and found that reboxetine may slightly improve social functioning.

Problem solving therapy (in mild to moderate depression)

One systematic review in younger and older adults with mild to moderate depression in primary care found that psychological therapies (including problem solving therapy) improved outcomes compared with usual care. The review did not report results of problem solving therapy alone in people with moderate depression. It found no significant difference between problem solving therapy and usual care in symptoms at 6–11 weeks in people with mild depression or dysthymia. One large subsequent RCT found that problem solving therapy increased the proportion of people who were not depressed at 6 months compared with usual care. However, it found no significant difference at 1 year. Another smaller RCT found no significant difference in symptoms at 8 or 26 weeks between problem solving therapy and usual care.

St John's Wort (in mild to moderate depression)

Two systematic reviews and one subsequent RCT in people with mild to moderate depressive disorders found that St John's Wort (*Hypericum perforatum*) improved depressive symptoms over 4–12 weeks compared with placebo. However, two subsequent RCTs found no significant difference in symptoms at 8 weeks between St John's Wort and placebo. RCTs found no significant difference in symptoms between St John's Wort and prescription antidepressant drugs. The results of the RCTs should be interpreted with caution because many of the RCTs did not use standardised preparations of St John's Wort, and doses of antidepressant drugs varied. One subsequent RCT in people aged 18 years or over with major depressive disorder found no significant difference in depressive symptoms at 8 weeks between a standardised preparation of St John's Wort and sertraline, but it is likely to have been underpowered to detect a clinically important difference.

UNKNOWN EFFECTIVENESS

Befriending (in mild to moderate depression)

One small RCT provided insufficient evidence to assess befriending in people with mild to moderate despression.

Bibliotherapy (in mild to moderate depression)

One systematic review of RCTs in younger and older adults recruited by advertisement found limited evidence that bibliotherapy may reduce mild depressive symptoms compared with waiting list control or usual care. It is unclear whether people in the RCTs identified by the review are clinically representative of people with depressive disorders. Another RCT in people with depression found that bibliotherapy may improve symptoms over 2–6 months compared with antidepressant drugs.

Exercise (in mild to moderate depression)

One systematic review in younger and older adults found limited evidence from poor RCTs that exercise may improve symptoms compared with no treatment, and may be as effective as cognitive therapy. One poor RCT in older adults identified by the review found limited evidence that exercise may be as effective as antidepressant drugs in improving symptoms and may reduce relapse over 10 months. ▶

◄ **Psychological treatments (cognitive therapy, interpersonal psychotherapy, non-directive counselling, and problem solving therapy) in severe depression**

> RCTs provided insufficient evidence to assess psychological treatments in severe depression.

What are the effects of interventions in treatment resistant depression?

UNKNOWN EFFECTIVENESS

Lithium augmentation

> RCTs provided insufficient evidence to assess augmentation of prescription anti-depressant drug treatment with lithium in younger and older adults with treatment resistant depression.

Pindolol augmentation

> RCTs provided insufficient evidence to assess augmentation of prescription anti-depressant drug treatment with pindolol in younger and older adults with treatment resistant depression.

Which interventions reduce relapse rates?

BENEFICIAL

Continuing prescription antidepressant drugs (reduced risk of relapse after recovery in people with mild to moderate depression)

> One systematic review found that continuing prescription antidepressant drug treatment after recovery reduced the proportion of people who relapsed over 1–3 years compared with placebo. The effect of continuing antidepressants was independent of the underlying risk of relapse, the duration of treatment before randomisation, or the duration of previous antidepressant treatment. RCTs in people aged over 60 years found that continued treatment with dosulepin (dothiepin) or citalopram after recovery reduced the risk of relapse over 1–2 years compared with placebo, but may increase the risk of ischaemic heart disease.

UNKNOWN EFFECTIVENESS

Cognitive therapy (weak evidence that may reduce relapse over 1–2 years after stopping treatment in people with mild to moderate depression compared with antidepressant drugs)

> One systematic review in younger and older adults with mild to moderate depression found limited evidence by combining relapse rates across different RCTs that cognitive therapy may reduce the risk of relapse over 1–2 years after stopping treatment compared with antidepressant drugs. One small RCT found that, in people with residual depressive symptoms after antidepressant drug treatment, cognitive therapy for 2 years after the initial depressive episode reduced relapse rates compared with continuing antidepressant drugs. We found no systematic review or RCTs specifically in older adults. ►

Depressive disorders

◄ **Relapse prevention programme (improved symptoms over 1 year after recovery in people with mild to moderate depression but no significant difference in relapse rates)**

One large RCT in people who had recovered after 8 weeks of antidepressant treatment found that a relapse prevention programme improved depressive symptoms over 1 year compared with usual care. However, it found no significant difference in relapse rates.

What are the effects of interventions to improve delivery of treatments?

BENEFICIAL

Care pathways (in mild to moderate depression)

One systematic review and four subsequent RCTs in people aged over 18 years with mild to moderate or major depression found that the effectiveness of treatment for depression (antidepressant drugs or cognitive behavioural therapy) may be improved by several care pathways, including collaborative working between primary care clinicians and psychiatrists, intensive patient education, case management, and telephone support. They also found that that clinical practice guidelines and educational strategies without other organisational processes improved neither detection nor outcome of depression compared with usual care. One RCT in people aged over 60 years with major depression, dysthymic depression, or both, treated in a variety of primary care clinics found that collaborative care was more effective than usual care in reducing depressive symptoms.

DEFINITION
Depressive disorders are characterised by persistent low mood, loss of interest and enjoyment, and reduced energy. They often impair day to day functioning. Most of the RCTs assessed in this review classify depression using the Diagnostic and Statistical Manual of Mental Disorders (DSM-IV)[1] or the International Classification of Mental and Behavioural Disorders (ICD-10).[2] DSM-IV divides depression into major depressive disorder or dysthymic disorder. Major depressive disorder is characterised by one or more major depressive episodes (i.e. at least 2 weeks of depressed mood or loss of interest accompanied by at least 4 additional symptoms of depression). Dysthymic disorder is characterised by at least 2 years of depressed mood for more days than not, accompanied by additional symptoms that do not reach the criteria for major depressive disorder.[1] ICD-10 divides depression into mild to moderate or severe depressive episodes.[2] Mild to moderate depression is characterised by depressive symptoms and some functional impairment. Treatment resistant depression is defined as an absence of clinical response to treatment with a tricyclic antidepressant at a minimum dose of 150 mg daily of imipramine (or equivalent drug) for 4–6 weeks.[3] Severe depression is characterised by additional agitation or psychomotor retardation with marked somatic symptoms.[2] In this review, we use both DSM-IV and ICD-10 classifications, but treatments are considered to have been assessed in severe depression if the RCT included inpatients. **Older adults:** Older adults are generally defined as people aged 65 years or older. However, some of the RCTs of older people in this review included people aged 55 years or over. The presentation of depression in older adults may be atypical: low mood may be masked and anxiety or memory impairment may be the principal presenting symptoms. Dementia should be considered in the differential diagnosis of depression in older adults.[4] This review does not cover intervention in women with postnatal depression (see postnatal depression, p 410) or seasonal affective disorder. ▶

INCIDENCE/ PREVALENCE
Depressive disorders are common, with a prevalence of major depression between 5% and 10% of people seen in primary care settings.[5] Two to three times as many people may have depressive symptoms but do not meet DSM-IV criteria for major depression. Women are affected twice as often as men. Depressive disorders are the fourth most important cause of disability worldwide and they are expected to become the second most important cause by 2020.[6,7] **Older adults:** Between 10% and 15% of older people have depressive symptoms, although major depression is relatively rare in older adults.[8]

AETIOLOGY/ RISK FACTORS
The causes are uncertain but include both childhood events and current psychosocial adversity.

PROGNOSIS
About half of people suffering a first episode of major depressive disorder experience further symptoms in the next 10 years.[9] **Older adults:** One systematic review (search date 1996, 12 prospective cohort studies, 1268 people, mean age 60 years) found that the prognosis may be especially poor in elderly people with a chronic or relapsing course of depression.[10] Another systematic review (search date 1999, 23 prospective cohort studies in people aged >65 years, including 5 identified by the first review) found that depression in older people was associated with increased mortality (15 studies; pooled OR 1.73, 95% CI 1.53 to 1.95).[11]

Please refer to the Clinical Evidence website for full text and references.

Generalised anxiety disorder

Search date February 2004

Christopher Gale and Mark Oakley-Browne

What are the effects of treatments?

LIKELY TO BE BENEFICIAL

Antidepressants (imipramine, opipramol, paroxetine, and venlafaxine)

One systematic review found that antidepressants (imipramine, paroxetine, and venlafaxine) improved symptoms over 4–28 weeks compared with placebo. One subsequent RCT found that paroxetine increased response rates compared with placebo. One RCT found no significant difference in response rates between venlafaxine and placebo at 24 weeks. One RCT found that opipramol increased response rate after 28 days compared with placebo. RCTs found no significant difference among these antidepressants or between antidepressants and benzodiazepines or buspirone. RCTs and observational studies have found that antidepressants are associated with sedation, dizziness, nausea, falls, and sexual dysfunction.

Buspirone

RCTs found that buspirone improved symptoms over 4–9 weeks compared with placebo. RCTs found no significant difference in symptoms over 6–8 weeks between buspirone and antidepressants, diazepam, or hydroxyzine, but the studies may have lacked power to detect clinically important differences among treatments.

Cognitive behavioural therapy

Two systematic reviews and three subsequent RCTs found that cognitive behavioural therapy (using a combination of interventions, such as exposure, relaxation, and cognitive restructuring) improved anxiety and depression over 4–12 weeks compared with waiting list control, anxiety management alone, relaxation alone, or non-directive psychotherapy. Three subsequent RCTs found no significant difference in symptoms at 13 weeks, 6 months, or 24 months between cognitive therapy and applied relaxation.

Hydroxyzine

Three RCTs comparing hydroxyzine versus placebo found different results. Two RCTs found that, compared with placebo, hydroxyzine improved symptoms of anxiety at 4 or 12 weeks, but a third RCT found no significant difference in the proportion of people with improved symptoms of anxiety at 5 weeks. One of the RCTs found that hydroxyzine increased somnolence and headaches compared with placebo. One RCT found no significant difference between hydroxyzine and bromazepam in the proportion of people who responded after 6 weeks. Another RCT found no significant difference between hydroxyzine and buspirone in the proportion of people who responded after 4 weeks.

TRADE OFF BETWEEN BENEFITS AND HARMS

Benzodiazepines

One systematic review and one subsequent RCT found that benzodiazepines reduced symptoms over 2–9 weeks compared with placebo. RCTs found no significant difference in symptoms over 3–8 weeks between alprazolam and bromazepam or mexazolam, or between benzodiazepines and buspirone, hydroxyzine, abecarnil, or antidepressants. RCTs and observational studies found that benzodiazepines increased the risk of dependence, sedation, industrial accidents, and road traffic accidents. If used in late pregnancy or while breast feeding, ▶

benzodiazepines may cause adverse effects in neonates. One systematic review of poor quality RCTs provided insufficient evidence to assess long term treatment with benzodiazepines.

Kava

One systematic review in people with a variety of anxiety disorders, including generalised anxiety disorder, found that kava reduced symptoms of anxiety over 1–24 weeks compared with placebo. It is unclear whether results of the review can be extrapolated to people with generalised anxiety disorder. Observational evidence suggests that kava may be associated with hepatotoxicity.

Trifluoperazine

One large RCT found that trifluoperazine reduced anxiety after 4 weeks compared with placebo, but caused more drowsiness, extrapyramidal reactions, and other movement disorders.

UNKNOWN EFFECTIVENESS

Abecarnil

One RCT found limited evidence that low dose abecarnil improved symptoms compared with placebo. Another RCT found no significant difference in symptoms at 6 weeks between abecarnil and placebo or diazepam. Both RCTs found that abecarnil increased drowsiness compared with placebo.

Applied relaxation

We found no RCTs comparing applied relaxation versus placebo or no treatment. Three RCTs found no significant difference in symptoms at 13 weeks, 6 months, or 24 months between applied relaxation and cognitive behavioural therapy.

β Blockers

We found no RCTs on the effects of β blockers in people with generalised anxiety disorder.

DEFINITION Generalised anxiety disorder (GAD) is defined as excessive worry and tension about every day events and problems, on most days, for at least 6 months, to the point where the person experiences distress or has marked difficulty in performing day to day tasks.[1] It may be characterised by the following symptoms and signs: increased motor tension (fatigability, trembling, restlessness, and muscle tension); autonomic hyperactivity (shortness of breath, rapid heart rate, dry mouth, cold hands, and dizziness); and increased vigilance and scanning (feeling keyed up, increased startling, and impaired concentration), but not panic attacks.[1] One non-systematic review of epidemiological and clinical studies found marked reduction of quality of life and psychosocial functioning in people with anxiety disorders (including GAD).[2] It also found that people with GAD have low overall life satisfaction and some impairment in ability to fulfil roles, social tasks, or both.[2]

INCIDENCE/ PREVALENCE One overview of observational studies found that the prevalence of GAD among adults in the community was 1.5–3.0%.[3] It found that 3–5% of adults have had GAD in the past year and 4–7% had had GAD during their lives. The US National Comorbidity Survey found that over 90% of people diagnosed with GAD had a comorbid diagnosis, including dysthymia (22%), depression (39–69%), somatisation, other anxiety disorders, bipolar disorder, or substance abuse.[4] The Harvard–Brown Anxiety Research Program also found that only 30/180 (17%) people had GAD alone.[5] Subgroup analysis suggested that 46/122 people (38%) with GAD had comorbid personality disorder.[6] A systematic review of the comorbidity of eating disorders and anxiety disorders (search date 2001, 2 observational studies, 55 people) found a lifetime prevalence of GAD among people with anorexia nervosa of 24% in one study and 31% in the other.[7] The lifetime prevalence of GAD in the control group of

Generalised anxiety disorder

one of the studies (44 people) was 2%. The reliability of the measures used to diagnose GAD in epidemiological studies is unsatisfactory.[8,9] One US study, with explicit diagnostic criteria (DSM-III-R), estimated that 5% of people will develop GAD at some time during their lives.[9] A recent cohort study of people with depressive and anxiety disorders found that 49% of people initially diagnosed with GAD retained this diagnosis over 2 years.[10] The incidence of GAD in men is half the incidence in women[11] and is lower in older people.[12] A non-systematic review (20 observational studies in younger and older adults) suggested that autonomic arousal to stressful tasks was decreased in older people, and that older people became accustomed to stressful tasks more quickly than younger people.[13]

AETIOLOGY/ RISK FACTORS GAD is believed to be associated with an increase in the number of minor stressors, independent of demographic factors,[14,15] but this finding is also common in people with other diagnoses.[10] One non-systematic review (5 case control studies) of psychological sequelae to civilian trauma found that rates of GAD reported in four of the five studies were significantly increased compared with a control population (rate ratio 3.3, 95% CI 2.0 to 5.5).[16] One systematic review (search date 1997) of cross-sectional studies found that bullying (or peer victimisation) was associated with a significant increase in the incidence of GAD (effect size 0.21, CI not reported).[17] Genetic factors are also implicated. One systematic review (search date not reported, 2 family studies, 45 index cases, 225 first degree relatives) found a significant association between GAD in the index cases and in their first degree relatives (OR 6.1, 95% CI 2.5 to 14.9).[18] The review also identified three twin studies (13 305 people), which estimated that 32% (95% CI 24% to 39%) of the variance in liability to GAD was explained by genetic factors.

PROGNOSIS One systematic review found that 25% of adults with GAD will be in full remission after 2 years, and 38% will have a remission after 5 years.[3] The Harvard–Brown anxiety research program reported 5 year follow up of 167 people with GAD.[19] In this period, the weighed probability for full remission was 38% and for at least partial remission was 47%; the probability of relapse from full remission was 27% and relapse from partial remission was 39%.

Please refer to the Clinical Evidence website for full text and references.

Mental health

What are the effects of initial treatments in adults?

BENEFICIAL

Behavioural therapy

We found no RCTs comparing behavioural therapy versus no treatment. One systematic review and subsequent RCTs have found that behavioural therapy improves symptoms compared with relaxation. The review and one subsequent RCT found no significant difference in symptoms over 4–16 weeks between behavioural therapy and cognitive therapy. One subsequent RCT found limited evidence that group behavioural therapy improved symptoms after 12 weeks compared with group cognitive behavioural therapy.

Cognitive or cognitive behavioural therapy

We found no RCTs comparing cognitive therapy versus no treatment. One RCT found that cognitive behavioural group therapy improved symptoms and quality of life compared with no treatment after 12 weeks. One systematic review and one subsequent RCT found no significant difference in symptoms over 4–16 weeks between behavioural therapy and cognitive therapy. Another subsequent RCT found limited evidence that group behavioural therapy improved symptoms over 12 weeks compared with group cognitive behavioural therapy.

Serotonin reuptake inhibitors (citalopram, clomipramine, fluoxetine, fluvoxamine, paroxetine, sertraline)

RCTs have found that selective and non-selective serotonin reuptake inhibitors (citalopram, clomipramine, fluoxetine, fluvoxamine, paroxetine) improve symptoms compared with placebo. Two systematic reviews found inconsistent results about the effects of sertraline compared with placebo. RCTs have found that selective and non-selective serotonin reuptake inhibitors (citalopram, clomipramine, fluoxetine, fluvoxamine, paroxetine, sertraline) improve symptoms compared with tricyclic antidepressants or monoamine oxidase inhibitors. RCTs have found no consistent evidence of a difference in efficacy among serotonin reuptake inhibitors, but have found that the non-selective serotonin reuptake inhibitor clomipramine is associated with more adverse effects than selective serotonin reuptake inhibitors.

UNKNOWN EFFECTIVENESS

Behavioural or cognitive therapy plus serotonin reuptake inhibitors (compared with behavioural or cognitive therapy alone)

RCTs provided insufficient evidence to assess the effects of adding serotonin reuptake inhibitors to behavioural or cognitive therapy.

Electroconvulsive therapy

We found no RCTs of electroconvulsive therapy in people with obsessive compulsive disorder.

Venlafaxine

One RCT provided insufficient evidence to compare vanlafaxine versus clomipramine.

▶

Obsessive compulsive disorder

What are the best forms of maintenance treatment in adults?

Optimum duration of treatment with serotonin reuptake inhibitors

RCTs provided insufficient evidence to define the optimum duration of treatment with serotonin reuptake inhibitors.

What are the effects of treatments in adults who have not responded to initial treatment with serotonin reuptake inhibitors?

Addition of antipsychotics to serotonin reuptake inhibitors

Three small RCTs in people unresponsive to serotonin reuptake inhibitors found that the addition of antipsychotics improved symptoms compared with placebo.

DEFINITION Obsessive compulsive disorder involves obsessions, compulsions, or both, that are not caused by drugs or a physical disorder, and which cause significant personal distress or social dysfunction.[1,2] The disorder may have a chronic or an episodic course. **Obsessions** are recurrent and persistent ideas, images, or impulses that cause pronounced anxiety and that the person perceives to be self produced. **Compulsions** are repetitive behaviours or mental acts performed in response to obsessions or according to certain rules, which are aimed at reducing distress or preventing certain imagined dreaded events. People with obsessive compulsive disorder may have insight into their condition, in that obsessions and compulsions are usually recognised and resisted. There are minor differences in the criteria for obsessive compulsive disorder between the third, revised third, and fourth editions of the *Diagnostic and Statistical Manual* (DSM-III, DSM-III-R, and DSM-IV)[1] and *The ICD-10 Classification of Mental and Behavioural Disorders.*[2]

INCIDENCE/ PREVALENCE One national, community based survey of obsessive compulsive disorder in the UK (1993, 10 000 people) found that 1% of men and 1.5% of women reported symptoms in the past month.[3] An epidemiological catchment area (ECA) survey carried out in the USA in 1984 (about 10 000 people) found age and sex standardised annual prevalence of obsessive compulsive disorder in people aged 26–64 years of 1.3%, and lifetime prevalence of 2.3%.[4] Subsequent cross national surveys using methodology comparable to ECA found age and sex standardised annual and lifetime prevalence in people aged 26–64 years as follows: Canada (survey size about 2200 people), annual prevalence 1.4% (SE 0.25), and lifetime prevalence 2.3% (SE 0.32); Puerto Rico (survey size about 1200 people), annual prevalence 1.8% (SE 0.39), and lifetime prevalence 2.5% (SE 0.46); Germany (survey size 4811 people), annual prevalence 1.6% (SE 0.57), and lifetime prevalence 2.1% (SE 0.66); Taiwan (survey size about 7400 people), annual prevalence 0.4% (SE 0.07), and lifetime prevalence 0.7% (SE 0.10); Korea (survey size about 4000 people), annual prevalence 1.1% (SE 0.10), and lifetime prevalence 1.9% (SE 0.20); and New Zealand (survey size about 1200 people), annual prevalence 1.1% (SE 0.31), and lifetime prevalence 2.2% (SE 0.42).[4]

AETIOLOGY/ RISK FACTORS The cause of obsessive compulsive disorder is uncertain. Behavioural, cognitive, genetic, and neurobiological factors have been implicated.[5-11] Risk factors include a family history of obsessive compulsive disorder, being single (which ▶

could be a consequence of the disorder), and belonging to a higher socioeconomic class.[12] Other risk factors include cocaine abuse, female sex, not being in paid employment, past history of alcohol dependence, affective disorder, and phobic disorder.[4]

PROGNOSIS One study (144 people followed for a mean of 47 years) found that an episodic course of obsessive compulsive disorder was more common during the initial years (about 1–9 years), but a chronic course was more common afterwards.[13] Over time, the study found that 39–48% of people had symptomatic improvement. A 1 year prospective cohort study found 46% of people had an episodic course and 54% had a chronic course.[14]

Please refer to the Clinical Evidence website for full text and references.

Panic disorder

Search date September 2003

Shailesh Kumar and Mark Oakley-Browne

What are the effects of drug treatments?

BENEFICIAL

Selective serotonin reuptake inhibitors

Systematic reviews and one additional RCT have found that selective serotonin reuptake inhibitors improve symptoms in panic disorder compared with placebo. One subsequent RCT found that discontinuation of sertraline in people with a good response increased exacerbation of symptoms. A second subsequent RCT found that paroxetine plus cognitive behavioural therapy improved symptoms compared with placebo plus cognitive behavioural therapy.

Tricyclic antidepressants (imipramine)

One systematic review, one subsequent RCT, and one additional RCT have found that imipramine improves symptoms compared with placebo. One subsequent RCT found that imipramine reduced relapse rates over 12 months.

TRADE OFF BETWEEN BENEFITS AND HARMS

Benzodiazepines

One systematic review and one additional RCT have found that alprazolam reduces the number of panic attacks and improves symptoms compared with placebo. However, benzodiazepines are associated with a wide range of adverse effects, both during and after treatment.

UNKNOWN EFFECTIVENESS

Buspirone

We found insufficient evidence to assess the effects of buspirone.

Monoamine oxidase inhibitors

We found no RCTs on the effects of monoamine oxidase inhibitors.

DEFINITION A panic attack is a period in which there is sudden onset of intense apprehension, fearfulness, or terror often associated with feelings of impending doom. Panic disorder occurs when there are recurrent, unpredictable attacks followed by at least 1 month of persistent concern about having another panic attack, worry about the possible implications or consequences of the panic attacks, or a significant behavioural change related to the attacks.[1] The term panic disorder excludes panic attacks attributable to the direct physiological effects of a general medical condition, a substance, or another mental disorder. Panic disorder is sometimes categorised as being with or without agoraphobia.[1] Alternative categorisations focus on phobic anxiety disorders and specify agoraphobia with or without panic disorder.[2]

INCIDENCE/ PREVALENCE Panic disorder often starts at around 20 years of age (between late adolescence and the mid 30s).[3] Lifetime prevalence is 1–3%, and panic disorder is more common in women than in men.[4] An Australian community study found 1 month prevalence rates for panic disorder (with or without agoraphobia) of 0.4% using International Classification of Diseases (ICD)-10 diagnostic criteria, and of 0.5% using Diagnostic and Statistical Manual (DSM)-IV diagnostic criteria.[5]

AETIOLOGY/ RISK FACTORS Stressful life events tend to precede the onset of panic disorder,[6,7] although a negative interpretation of these events in addition to their occurrence has been suggested as an important casual factor.[8] Panic disorder is associated with ▶

major depression,[9] social phobia, generalised anxiety disorder, obsessive compulsive disorder,[10] and a substantial risk of drug and alcohol abuse.[11] It is also associated with avoidant, histrionic, and dependent personality disorders.[10]

PROGNOSIS   The severity of symptoms in people with panic disorder fluctuates considerably, and patients commonly experience periods of no attacks, or only mild attacks with few symptoms. There is often a long delay between the initial onset of symptoms and presentation for treatment. Recurrent attacks may continue for several years, especially if associated with agoraphobia. Reduced social or occupational functioning varies among people with panic disorder and is worse in people with associated agoraphobia. Panic disorder is also associated with an increased rate of attempted, but unsuccessful, suicide.[12] One study analysing data from RCTs and systematic reviews found that co-existence of anxiety and depressive features adversely affected treatment response at 12 years compared with treatment of panic disorder alone.[13]

Please refer to the Clinical Evidence website for full text and references.

Post-traumatic stress disorder

Search date January 2004

Jonathan Bisson

What are the effects of preventive interventions?

Multiple session cognitive behavioural therapy in people with acute stress disorder

Two small RCTs in people with acute stress disorder after a traumatic event (accident or non-sexual assault) found that five sessions of cognitive behavioural therapy reduced the proportion of people with post-traumatic stress disorder after 6 months compared with supportive counselling.

Hydrocortisone

One small RCT in people in intensive care with septic shock provided insufficient evidence to assess hydrocortisone in preventing post-traumatic stress disorder.

Multiple session cognitive behavioural therapy in all people exposed to a traumatic event

One RCT found that four sessions of cognitive behavioural therapy in people with psychological distress following physical injury reduced post-traumatic stress symptoms at 13 months compared with no psychological intervention. However, it found no significant difference in the proportion of people meeting the DSM-IV diagnostic criteria for post-traumatic stress disorder. One RCT in bus drivers who had been attacked in the past 5 months found that cognitive behavioural therapy improved measures of anxiety and intrusive symptoms at 6 months compared with standard care. However, it found no significant difference in measures of depression or avoidance symptoms. One RCT provided insufficient evidence to assess cognitive behavioural therapy plus educational techniques in preventing post-traumatic stress disorder in road traffic accident survivors. Another small RCT provided insufficient evidence to compare memory structuring versus supportive listening in road traffic accident survivors.

Multiple session collaborative trauma support

Two RCTs provided insufficient evidence to assess multiple session collaborative trauma support interventions involving emotional, social, and practical support in people exposed to a traumatic event in the past 24 hours to 1 week.

Multiple session education

We found no systematic review or RCTs assessing effects of multiple session education alone. One RCT provided insufficient evidence to assess educational techniques plus cognitive behavioural therapy in preventing post-traumatic stress disorder in road traffic accident survivors.

Propranolol

One small RCT provided insufficient evidence to assess propranolol in preventing post-traumatic stress disorder in people with early symptoms of post-traumatic stress disorder after a traumatic event.

Single session group debriefing

We found no RCTs comparing single session group debriefing with no debriefing. One RCT found that early group debriefing (within 10 hours of the traumatic event) reduced post-traumatic stress disorder compared with delayed group debriefing (after 48 hours).

▶

Temazepam

One small RCT provided insufficient evidence to assess temazepam in preventing post-traumatic stress disorder in people with acute stress disorder or early symptoms of post-traumatic stress disorder after road traffic accident, industrial accident, or non-sexual assault.

UNLIKELY TO BE BENEFICIAL

Single session individual debriefing

One systematic review of RCTs in people who had been exposed to a traumatic event in the previous month found no significant difference between a single session of individual psychological debriefing and no debriefing in the incidence of post-traumatic stress disorder at 3 months or 1 year.

Supportive counselling

Two RCTs in people with acute stress disorder after a traumatic event (road traffic accident or non-sexual assault) found that supportive counselling was less effective than five sessions of cognitive behavioural therapy in reducing the proportion of people with post-traumatic stress disorder after 6 months.

What are the effects of treatments?

BENEFICIAL

Cognitive behavioural therapy

RCTs found that cognitive behavioural therapy improved post-traumatic stress disorder symptoms, anxiety, and depression immediately after treatment and at up to 1 year compared with no treatment or supportive counselling. RCTs provided no consistent evidence of a difference in symptoms between cognitive behavioural therapy and eye movement desensitisation and reprocessing.

Eye movement desensitisation and reprocessing

RCTs found that eye movement desensitisation and reprocessing improved symptoms compared with no treatment, but provided no consistent evidence of a difference in symptoms between eye movement desensitisation and reprocessing and cognitive behavioural therapy.

LIKELY TO BE BENEFICIAL

Fluoxetine

One RCT found that fluoxetine improved symptoms compared with placebo at 3 months. One small RCT found no significant difference between fluoxetine and placebo in response rate at 3 months, but is likely to have been underpowered to detect a clinically important difference.

Paroxetine

Two RCTs found that paroxetine improved response rate compared with placebo at 3 months. One smaller RCT found no significant difference between paroxetine and placebo in response rate at 3 months, but may have been underpowered to detect a clinically important difference.

Sertraline

Three RCTs found that sertraline reduced symptoms at 3–7 months compared with placebo. Two small RCTs found no significant difference between sertraline and placebo in symptoms at up to 3 months, but were likely to be underpowered to detect a clinically important difference between groups. One RCT provided insufficient evidence to compare sertraline with nefazodone.

Post-traumatic stress disorder

Affect management
We found insufficient evidence about the effects of this intervention in improving symptoms.

Benzodiazepines
One systematic review identified no RCTs of sufficient quality in people with post-traumatic stress disorder.

Brofaromine
We found insufficient evidence about the effects of this intervention in improving symptoms.

Carbamazepine
We found no RCTs of carbamazepine in people with post-traumatic stress disorder.

Drama therapy
We found insufficient evidence about the effects of this intervention in improving symptoms.

Eclectic psychotherapy
We found insufficient evidence about the effects of this intervention in improving symptoms.

Group therapy
We found insufficient evidence about the effects of this intervention in improving symptoms.

Hypnotherapy
We found insufficient evidence about the effects of this intervention in improving symptoms.

Inpatient treatment programmes
We found insufficient evidence about the effects of this intervention in improving symptoms.

Internet based psychotherapy
We found insufficient evidence about the effects of this intervention in improving symptoms.

Lamotrigine
One RCT provided insufficient evidence to assess lamotrigine in people with post-traumatic stress disorder.

Mirtazapine
We found insufficient evidence about the effects of this intervention in improving symptoms.

Nefazodone
We found insufficient evidence about the effects of this intervention in improving symptoms.

Olanzapine
We found no good quality RCTs that assessed olanzapine in people with post-traumatic stress disorder.

Phenelzine
We found insufficient evidence about the effects of this intervention in improving symptoms.

◀ Propranolol

We found no RCTs of propranolol in people with post-traumatic stress disorder.

Psychodynamic psychotherapy

We found insufficient evidence about the effects of this intervention in improving symptoms.

Risperidone

We found no RCTs of risperidone in people with post-traumatic stress disorder.

Supportive psychotherapy

We found insufficient evidence about the effects of this intervention in improving symptoms.

Tricyclic antidepressants

RCTs provided insufficient evidence to assess imipramine or amitriptyline in people with post-traumatic stress disorder.

DEFINITION   **Post-traumatic stress disorder (PTSD)** can occur after any major traumatic event. Symptoms include upsetting thoughts and nightmares about the traumatic event, avoidance behaviour, numbing of general responsiveness, increased irritability, and hypervigilance.[1] To fulfil the *Diagnostic and statistical manual of mental disorders* (DSM-IV) criteria for PTSD, an individual must have been exposed to a traumatic event; have at least one re-experiencing, three avoidance, and two hyperarousal phenomena; have had the symptoms for at least 1 month; and the symptoms must cause clinically important distress or reduced day to day functioning.[1] People with sub-syndromal PTSD have all the criteria for PTSD except one of the re-experiencing, avoidance, or hyperarousal phenomena. **Acute stress disorder** occurs within the first month after a major traumatic event and requires the presence of symptoms for at least 2 days. It is similar to PTSD but dissociative symptoms are required to make the diagnosis. Treatments for PTSD may have similar effects, regardless of the traumatic event that precipitated PTSD. However, great caution should be applied when generalising from one type of trauma to another.

INCIDENCE/   One large cross-sectional study in the USA found that 1/10 (10%) women and
PREVALENCE   1/20 (5%) men experience PTSD at some stage in their lives.[2]

AETIOLOGY/   Risk factors include major trauma, such as rape, a history of psychiatric
RISK FACTORS disorders, acute distress and depression after the trauma, lack of social support, and personality factors.[3]

PROGNOSIS   One large cross-sectional study in the USA found that over a third of people with previous PTSD continued to satisfy the criteria for PTSD 6 years after initial diagnosis.[2] However, cross-sectional studies provide weak evidence about prognosis.

Please refer to the Clinical Evidence website for full text and references.

Schizophrenia

Search date April 2004

Zia Nadeem, Andrew McIntosh, and Stephen Lawrie

Most evidence is from systematic reviews of RCTs that report disparate outcomes. There is a need for larger RCTs, over longer periods, with well designed end points, including standardised, validated symptom scales. No intervention has been found to reduce negative symptoms consistently.

What are the effects of drug treatments for positive and negative symptoms?

TRADE OFF BETWEEN BENEFITS AND HARMS

Amisulpride*

Two systematic reviews found that amisulpride improved symptoms more than standard antipsychotic drugs. One review found that extrapyramidal adverse effects were less likely with amisulpride than with standard antipsychotic drugs. One RCT found no significant difference in symptoms between amisulpride and olanzapine. One systematic review found no significant difference in symptoms between amisulpride and risperidone.

Chlorpromazine*

One systematic review found that, compared with placebo, chlorpromazine reduced the proportion of people with no improvement or with worse severity of illness at 6 months on a psychiatrist rated scale. The review found that, compared with placebo, chlorpromazine caused more adverse effects, such as sedation, acute dystonia, and parkinsonism.

Clozapine*

One systematic review found that clozapine improved symptoms over 4–10 weeks compared with standard antipsychotic drugs (predominantly haloperidol and chlorpromazine) and was less likely to lead to antipsychotic induced movement disorders. RCTs provided insufficient evidence to compare clozapine versus other, newer antipsychotic drugs. RCTs found that clozapine may be associated with blood dyscrasias.

Depot bromperidol decanoate*

One systematic review of three small RCTs found no significant difference between depot bromperidol decanoate and haloperidol or fluphenazine decanoate in the proportion of people who needed additional medication, left the trial early, or had movement disorders over 6–12 months. The review may have lacked power to detect a clinically important difference.

Depot haloperidol decanoate*

One small RCT identified by a systematic review found no significant difference between depot haloperidol decanoate and oral haloperidol in global clinical state at 4 months, but it may have been too small to exclude a clinically important difference. Haloperidol is associated with acute dystonia, akathisia, and parkinsonism.

Haloperidol*

One systematic review found that haloperidol increased physician rated global improvement at 6 and 24 weeks compared with placebo, but was associated with acute dystonia, akathisia, and parkinsonism.

Olanzapine*

One systematic review found no significant difference in psychotic symptoms between olanzapine and standard antipsychotic drugs. The review and one subsequent RCT found that olanzapine was associated with fewer extrapyramidal adverse effects than standard antipsychotic drugs. RCTs found no clear difference in symptoms or adverse effects between olanzapine, amisulpride, risperidone, and clozapine.

Pimozide*

One systematic review found no significant difference between pimozide and standard antipsychotic drugs in global clinical impression, and found that pimozide decreased sedation but increased tremor. It found no overall difference in cardio-vascular adverse effects such as rise or fall in blood pressure or dizziness between pimozide and standard antipsychotic drugs. Pimozide has been associated with sudden cardiac death at doses above 20 mg daily.

Risperidone*

One large systematic review found that risperidone improved symptoms more than standard antipsychotic drugs (mainly haloperidol). One small additional RCT found no significant difference between risperidone and haloperidol in responders over 8 weeks. One systematic review found that risperidone decreased extrapyramidal side effects and the need for antiparkinsonian medication, but increased weight gain, compared with standard antipsychotic drugs. Systematic reviews found no significant difference in symptoms between risperidone and other new antipsychotic drugs (olanzapine, sulpiride, and clozapine).

Thioridazine*

One systematic review found that thioridazine improved global mental state compared with placebo over 3–12 months.

Zotepine*

One systematic review found weak evidence that zotepine increased the proportion of people with a clinically important improvement in symptoms compared with standard antipsychotic drugs, and reduced akasthesia, dystonia, and rigidity. This finding was not robust because removal of a single RCT from the analysis meant that the difference between zotepine and standard antipsychotic drugs was no longer significant.

Loxapine*; molindone*; quetiapine*; sulpiride*; ziprasidone*

Systematic reviews found no significant difference between these newer antipsychotic drugs and standard antipsychotic drugs in symptom improvement, and that they have different profiles of adverse effects.

*These drugs are beneficial in schizophrenia but all have important harms, which may include parkinsonism, dystonia, cholinergic effects, and weight gain.

UNKNOWN EFFECTIVENESS

Perazine

One weak RCT found no significant difference in global clinical impression over 28 days between perazine and haloperidol. Two small RCTs provided insufficient evidence to compare perazine versus zotepine, and one small RCT found no significant difference in mental state at 28 days between perazine and amisulpride. Three RCTs found no significant difference in extrapyramidal effects over 28 days between perazine and zotepine or amisulpride.

Schizophrenia

What are the effects of interventions to reduce relapse rates?

BENEFICIAL

Continuation of antipsychotic drugs for at least 6 months after an acute episode

Systematic reviews found that continuing antipsychotic drugs for at least 6 months after an acute episode reduced relapse rates compared with no treatment or placebo. Eight systematic reviews found no significant difference in relapse rates among antipsychotic drugs. One systematic review found that clozapine reduced relapse rates over 12 weeks compared with standard antipsychotic drugs. Another review found that fewer people taking depot zuclopenthixol decanoate relapsed over 12 weeks to 1 year compared with people taking other depot preparations. A third review found that bromperidol increased the proportion of people who relapsed compared with haloperidol or fluphenazine. One additional RCT found that risperidone reduced relapse over 2.2 years compared with haloperidol.

Multiple session family interventions

One systematic review found that multiple session family interventions reduced relapse rates at 12 months compared with usual care, single session family interventions, or psychoeducational interventions.

Psychoeducational interventions

One systematic review found that psychoeducation reduced relapse rates at 9–18 months compared with usual care.

UNKNOWN EFFECTIVENESS

Cognitive behavioural therapy

Limited evidence from a systematic review of two RCTs found no significant difference in relapse rates between cognitive behavioural therapy plus standard care and standard care alone.

Social skills training

One systematic review of small RCTs provided insufficient evidence to assess the effect of social skills training on relapse rates.

What are the effects of treatments in people resistant to standard treatment?

BENEFICIAL

Clozapine (compared with standard antipsychotic drugs)

One systematic review in people resistant to standard antipsychotic drugs found that clozapine improved symptoms after 12 weeks and after 2 years compared with standard antipsychotic drugs. One systematic review found no significant difference in symptoms between clozapine and other new antipsychotic drugs in people resistant to standard antipsychotic drugs.

UNKNOWN EFFECTIVENESS

Olanzapine

Small RCTs identified by a systematic review found no significant difference in psychotic symptoms over 8 weeks between olanzapine and chlorpromazine or between olanzapine and clozapine.

What are the effects of interventions to improve adherence?

LIKELY TO BE BENEFICIAL

Behavioural therapy

One small RCT found limited evidence that behavioural interventions improved adherence to antipsychotic medication compared with usual treatment. Two RCTs found limited evidence that behavioural interventions improved adherence more than psychoeducational therapy.

Compliance therapy

Two RCTs found limited evidence that compliance therapy increased adherence to antipsychotic drugs at 6 and 18 months compared with supportive or non-specific counselling.

Psychoeducational interventions

One systematic review found limited evidence that psychoeducational interventions improved adherence to antipsychotic medication compared with usual care. Two RCTs found limited evidence that psychoeducational interventions improved adherence less than behavioural therapy.

UNKNOWN EFFECTIVENESS

Multiple session family interventions

One systematic review found that "compliance with medication" over 9–24 months was higher in people who received multiple family interventions compared with usual care, single family interventions, or psychoeducational interventions, but the difference was not statistically significant.

DEFINITION	Schizophrenia is characterised by the positive symptoms of auditory hallucinations, delusions, and thought disorder, and by the negative symptoms of demotivation, self neglect, and reduced emotion.[1] People are defined as being resistant to standard antipsychotic drugs if, over the preceding 5 years, they have not had a clinically important improvement in symptoms after 2–3 regimens of treatment with standard antipsychotic drugs for at least 6 weeks (from at least 2 classes at doses equivalent to or greater than 1000 mg/day chlorpromazine) and they have had no period of good functioning.[2,3] About 30% (10–45%) of people with schizophrenia meet these criteria.[3]
INCIDENCE/ PREVALENCE	Onset of symptoms typically occurs in early adult life (average age 25 years) and is earlier in men than in women.[4,5] Prevalence worldwide is 2–4/1000. One in 100 people will develop schizophrenia in their lifetime.
AETIOLOGY/ RISK FACTORS	Risk factors include a family history (although no major genes have been identified), obstetric complications, developmental difficulties, central nervous system infections in childhood, cannabis use, and acute life events.[4] The precise contributions of these factors and ways in which they may interact are unclear.
PROGNOSIS	About three quarters of people suffer recurrent relapse and continued disability, although the proportion of people who improved significantly increased after the mid-1950s (mean 48.5% from 1956–1985 v 35.4% from 1895–1956).[6] Outcome may be worse in people with insidious onset and delayed initial treatment, social isolation, or a strong family history; in people living in industrialised countries; in men; and in people who misuse drugs.[5] Drug treatment is generally successful in treating positive symptoms, but up to a third ▶

of people derive little benefit, and negative symptoms are notoriously difficult to treat. About half of people with schizophrenia do not adhere to treatment in the short term. The figure is even higher in the longer term.[7]

Please refer to the Clinical Evidence website for full text and references.

What are the effects of treatment strategies for acute ankle ligament ruptures?

BENEFICIAL

Functional treatment (early mobilisation with use of an external support)

One systematic review and one subsequent RCT found limited evidence that functional treatment reduced the risk of the ankle giving way compared with minimal treatment. One systematic review and one subsequent RCT found that, compared with immobilisation, functional treatment improved symptoms and functional outcomes at short (< 6 weeks), intermediate (6 weeks to 1 year), or long term (> 1 year) follow up. However, effects were found to be less marked at long term follow up, or if only results from high quality trials were analysed. One systematic review and one subsequent RCT provided insufficient evidence to compare functional treatment versus surgery. One systematic review and three additional RCTs provided insufficient evidence to compare different functional treatments.

LIKELY TO BE BENEFICIAL

Immobilisation

There is consensus that immobilisation is more effective than no treatment; however one systematic review and one subsequent RCT found that, compared with functional treatment, immobilisation was associated with less improvement in symptoms and functional outcomes at either short (< 6 weeks), intermediate (6 weeks to 1 year), or long term (> 1 year) follow up. Effects were less marked at long term follow up, or if only results from high quality trials were analysed. One systematic review found no significant difference between immobilisation and surgery in pain, swelling, recurrence, or subjective instability. However, the review found that compared with immobilisation, surgery improved stability and increased the proportion of people able to return to sports. One systematic review found insufficient evidence to compare immobilisation versus physiotherapy.

Surgery

One systematic review found no significant difference between surgery and immobilisation in pain, swelling, recurrence, or subjective instability. However, the review found that surgery increased the proportion of people able to return to sports and increased ankle stability compared with immobilisation. Other systematic reviews and one subsequent RCT provided insufficient evidence to compare surgery versus functional treatment or conservative treatment (including both immobilisation and functional treatment).

UNKNOWN EFFECTIVENESS

Diathermy

One systematic review found insufficient evidence on the effects of diathermy compared with placebo on walking ability and reduction in swelling.

Homeopathic ointment

One small RCT found limited evidence that homeopathic ointment improved outcome based on a "composite criteria of treatment success" compared with placebo.

Ankle sprain

Cold treatment

One RCT found no significant difference in symptoms between cold pack placement and placebo (simulated treatment). One RCT found no significant difference between ice treatment plus physiotherapy and physiotherapy alone. One RCT found less oedema with cold pack placement compared with heat or a contrast bath at 3–5 days after injury.

Ultrasound

One systematic review found no significant difference between ultrasound and sham ultrasound in the general improvement of symptoms or the ability to walk or bear weight at 7 days. Three RCTs found no significant difference between ultrasound and other treatments.

DEFINITION Ankle sprain is an injury of the lateral ligament complex of the ankle joint. The injury is graded on the basis of severity.[1–5] Grade I is a mild stretching of the ligament complex without joint instability; grade II is a partial rupture of the ligament complex with mild instability of the joint (such as isolated rupture of the anterior talofibular ligament); and grade III involves complete rupture of the ligament complex with instability of the joint. Practically, this gradation may be considered as purely theoretical, because it has no therapeutic or prognostic consequences.[6] Unless otherwise stated, studies included in this topic did not specify the grades of injury included, or included a wide range of grades.

INCIDENCE/ PREVALENCE Ankle sprain is a common problem in acute medical care, occurring at a rate of about one injury per 10 000 people a day.[7] Injuries of the lateral ligament complex of the ankle form a quarter of all sports injuries.[7]

AETIOLOGY/ RISK FACTORS The usual mechanism of injury is inversion and adduction (usually referred to as supination) of the plantar flexed foot. Predisposing factors are a history of ankle sprains and specific malalignment, like crus varum and pes cavo-varus.

PROGNOSIS Some sports (e.g. basketball, football/soccer, and volleyball) are associated with a particularly high incidence of ankle injuries. Pain is the most frequent residual problem, often localised on the medial side of the ankle.[4] Other residual complaints include mechanical instability, intermittent swelling, and stiffness. People with more extensive cartilage damage have a higher incidence of residual complaints.[4] Long term cartilage damage can lead to degenerative changes, especially if there is persistent or recurrent instability. Every further sprain has the potential to add new damage.

Please refer to the Clinical Evidence website for full text and references.

What are the effects of conservative treatments?

UNKNOWN EFFECTIVENESS

Night splints

One systematic review found no reliable RCTs comparing night splints with any other or no treatment.

Orthoses to treat hallux valgus in adults

One RCT in adults found that, orthoses reduced pain compared with no treatment at 6 months but not at 1 year and that orthoses were less effective at improving outcomes than chevron osteotomy.

LIKELY TO BE INEFFECTIVE OR HARMFUL

Antipronatory orthoses in children

One RCT in children found that antipronatory orthoses increased deterioration in metatarsophalangeal joint angles after 3 years compared with no treatment, although the difference was not statistically significant.

What are the effects of surgery?

LIKELY TO BE BENEFICIAL

Chevron osteotomy (more effective than no treatment or orthoses but insufficient evidence to compare with other metatarsal osteotomies)

One systematic review found conflicting evidence on the effects of chevron osteotomy compared with other metatarsal osteotomies. One RCT found that chevron osteotomy improved outcomes compared with orthoses or no treatment after 1 year.

UNKNOWN EFFECTIVENESS

Chevron osteotomy plus Akin osteotomy

One systematic review identified one small RCT comparing chevron osteotomy plus Akin osteotomy and Akin osteotomy plus distal soft tissue reconstruction, which found no significant difference in outcomes between treatments at 1 year. However, this trial may have lacked power to detect a clinically significant difference.

Chevron osteotomy plus adductor tenotomy

One systematic review found no evidence that adductor tenotomy plus chevron osteotomy improved outcomes compared with chevron osteotomy alone.

Different methods of bone fixation (standard fixation, absorbable pin fixation, screw fixation plus early weight bearing, suture fixation plus delayed weight bearing)

One small RCT identified by a systematic review found no significant difference between standard fixation and absorbable pin fixation in clinical or radiological outcomes; however, it may have lacked power to detect a clinically significant difference. A second small RCT identified by the review found that screw fixation plus early weight bearing reduced time to return to work and social activity compared with suture fixation and later weight bearing, but found no significant difference in radiological outcomes.

Bunions

Keller's arthroplasty

We found no RCTs comparing Keller's arthroplasty versus no treatment. One systematic review found insufficient evidence from limited RCTs on the effects of Keller's arthroplasty compared with other types of operation.

What are the effects of postoperative care?

UNKNOWN EFFECTIVENESS

Continuous passive motion

One systematic review provided insufficient evidence on the effects of continuous passive motion.

Early weight bearing

One systematic review provided insufficient evidence on the effects of early weight bearing.

Slipper casts

One systematic review provided insufficient evidence on the effects of plaster slipper casts.

DEFINITION **Hallux valgus** is a deformity of the great toe, whereby the hallux (great toe) moves towards the second toe, overlying it in severe cases. This abduction (movement away from the midline of the body) is usually accompanied by some rotation of the toe so that the nail is facing the midline of the body (valgus rotation). With the deformity, the metatarsal head becomes more prominent and the metatarsal is said to be in an adducted position as it moves towards the midline of the body.[1] Radiological criteria for hallux valgus vary, but a commonly accepted criterion is to measure the angle formed between the metatarsal and the abducted hallux. This is called the metatarsophalangeal joint angle or hallux abductus angle and it is considered abnormal when it is greater than 14.5°.[2] **Bunion** is the lay term used to describe a prominent and often inflamed metatarsal head and overlying bursa. Symptoms include pain, limitation in walking, and problems with wearing normal shoes.

INCIDENCE/ PREVALENCE The prevalence of hallux valgus varies in different populations. In a recent study of 6000 UK school children aged 9–10 years, 2.5% had clinical evidence of hallux valgus, and 2% met both clinical and radiological criteria for hallux valgus. An earlier study found hallux valgus in 48% of adults.[2] Differences in prevalence may result from different methods of measurement, varying age groups, or different diagnostic criteria (e.g. metatarsal joint angle > 10° or > 15°).[3]

AETIOLOGY/ RISK FACTORS Nearly all population studies have found that hallux valgus is more common in women. Footwear may contribute to the deformity, but studies comparing people who wear shoes with those who do not have found contradictory results. Hypermobility of the first ray and excessive foot pronation are associated with hallux valgus.[4]

PROGNOSIS We found no studies that looked at the progression of hallux valgus. While progression of deformity and symptoms is rapid in some people, others remain asymptomatic. One study found that hallux valgus is often unilateral initially, but usually progresses to bilateral deformity.[2]

Please refer to the Clinical Evidence website for full text and references.

Search date January 2004

Nigel Ashworth

What are the effects of drug treatments?

BENEFICIAL

Local corticosteroid injection (short term)

Two small RCTs found that local corticosteroid injection (methylprednisone, hydro-cortisone) improved symptoms after 4–6 weeks compared with placebo or no treatment. One small RCT found that local betamethasone injection improved symptoms after 1 month compared with betamethasone injection into the deltoid. One small RCT found no significant difference between local methylprednisone injection and oral prednisone in symptoms after 2 weeks, but found that local methylprednisone injection improved symptoms after 8 and 12 weeks.

Oral corticosteroids (short term)

Three small RCTs found that oral prednisone improved symptoms after 2 weeks, and two of the three RCTs found the improvement was maintained at 4–8 weeks. We found no RCTs that measured the effects of oral corticosteroids on symptoms in the longer term. One small RCT found no significant difference in symptoms at 2 weeks between local methylprednisone injection and oral prednisone, but found that local methylprednisone injection improved symptoms after 8 and 12 weeks.

One RCT found that oral prednisone reduced symptoms compared with a non-steroidal anti-inflammatory drug (tenoxicam) and with a diuretic (trichlorme-thiazide) after 4 weeks.

UNKNOWN EFFECTIVENESS

Non-steroidal anti-inflammatory drugs

One small RCT found no significant difference between tenoxicam and placebo in symptoms after 2 or 4 weeks. However, the RCT may have lacked power to detect a clinically important difference. One RCT found that oral prednisone reduced symptoms compared with a non-steroidal anti-inflammatory drug (tenoxicam) after 4 weeks. One RCT found no significant difference in symptoms between a diuretic (trichlormethiazide) and a non-steroidal anti-inflammatory drug (tenoxi-cam) at 4 weeks.

Pyridoxine

One small RCT found a similar improvement in symptoms with pyridoxine com-pared with placebo or no treatment after 10 weeks. The RCT may have been too small to detect a clinically important difference between treatments. One small RCT found no significant difference between pyridoxine and placebo in nocturnal pain, numbness, or tingling after 12 weeks.

Local corticosteroid injection (long term); oral corticosteroids (long term)

We found no RCTs on the effects of these interventions.

UNLIKELY TO BE BENEFICIAL

Diuretics

One small RCT found no significant difference between trichlormethiazide and placebo in symptoms after 2 or 4 weeks. One RCT found no significant difference between bendrofluazide and placebo in the proportion of people with no improve-ment in symptoms after 4 weeks. One RCT found no significant difference in ▶

Carpal tunnel syndrome

symptoms between a diuretic (trichlormethiazide) and a non-steroidal anti-inflammatory drug (tenoxicam) at 4 weeks. One RCT found that oral prednisone reduced symptoms compared with a diuretic (trichlormethiazide) after 4 weeks.

What are the effects of non-drug treatments?

UNKNOWN EFFECTIVENESS

Nerve and tendon gliding exercises

One small RCT found no significant difference between nerve and tendon gliding exercises plus neutral angle wrist splint and neutral angle wrist splint alone in symptom severity or function 8 weeks after the end of 4 weeks of treatment.

Therapeutic ultrasound

One RCT found that ultrasound increased the proportion of wrists with satisfactory improvement or complete remission of symptoms after 6 months compared with placebo. One RCT found no significant difference in symptom severity between high or low intensity ultrasound compared with placebo after 2 weeks.

Wrist splints

One RCT found that a nocturnal hand brace improved symptoms after 2 and 4 weeks compared with no treatment. One small RCT found no significant difference in symptoms after 2 weeks between neutral angle compared with 20° extension wrist splinting. One small RCT found no significant difference in symptoms at 6 weeks between full time compared with night time only neutral angle wrist splinting.

What are the effects of surgical treatments?

TRADE OFF BETWEEN BENEFITS AND HARMS

Endoscopic carpal tunnel release versus open carpal tunnel release

One systematic review and subsequent RCTs found no consistent difference in symptoms up to 12 months after surgery or time taken to return to work between endoscopic and open carpal tunnel release. Harms resulting from endoscopic and open carpal tunnel release vary between RCTs. One systematic review and two RCTs comparing the interventions suggests that endoscopic carpal tunnel release may cause more transient nerve problems, whereas open carpal tunnel release may cause more wound problems.

Surgery versus placebo or non-surgical intervention

We found no RCTs comparing surgery with placebo. One small RCT identified by a systematic review and one subsequent RCT found that surgery increased symptom resolution compared with splinting at 12–15 months. One systematic review and five subsequent RCTs provided no clear evidence of a difference in symptoms or time taken to return to work between endoscopic and open carpal tunnel release up to 12 months after the operation. Harms resulting from endoscopic and open carpal tunnel release vary among RCTs. One systematic review and two RCTs comparing the interventions suggests that endoscopic carpal tunnel release may cause more transient nerve problems, whereas open carpal tunnel release may cause more wound problems.

UNLIKELY TO BE BENEFICIAL

Internal neurolysis in conjunction with open carpal tunnel release

RCTs identified by a systematic review found no significant difference in symptoms between open carpal tunnel release alone and open carpal tunnel release plus internal neurolysis in symptoms.

What are the effects of postoperative treatments?

LIKELY TO BE INEFFECTIVE OR HARMFUL

Wrist splinting after carpal tunnel release surgery

Two RCTs in people after carpal tunnel release surgery found no significant difference between wrist splinting and no splinting in grip strength or in the proportion of people who considered themselves "cured" at 2–4 weeks. A third RCT found that splinting increased pain at 1 month and the time to return to work compared with no splinting.

DEFINITION
Carpal tunnel syndrome is a neuropathy caused by compression of the median nerve within the carpal tunnel.[1] Classical symptoms of carpal tunnel syndrome include numbness, tingling, burning, or pain in at least two of the three digits supplied by the median nerve (i.e. the thumb, index, and middle fingers).[2] The American Academy of Neurology has described diagnostic criteria that rely on a combination of symptoms and physical examination findings.[3] Other diagnostic criteria include results from electrophysiological studies.[2]

INCIDENCE/ PREVALENCE
A general population survey in Rochester, Minnesota, found the age adjusted incidence of carpal tunnel syndrome to be 105 (95% CI 99 to 112) cases per 100 000 person years.[4,5] Age adjusted incidence rates were 52 (95% CI 45 to 59) cases for men and 149 (95% CI 138 to 159) cases for women per 100 000 person years. The study found incidence rates increased from 88 (95% CI 75 to 101) cases per 100 000 person years in 1961–1965 to 125 (95% CI 112 to 138) cases per 100 000 person years in 1976–1980. Incidence rates of carpal tunnel syndrome increased with age for men, whereas for women they peaked between the ages of 45–54 years. A general population survey in the Netherlands found prevalence to be 1% for men and 7% for women.[6] A more comprehensive study in southern Sweden found the general population prevalence for carpal tunnel syndrome was 3% (95% CI 2% to 3%).[7] As in other studies, the overall prevalence in women was higher than in men (male to female ratio 1 : 1.4); however, among older people, the prevalence in women was almost four times that in men (age group 65–74 years: men 1%, 95% CI 0% to 4%; women 5%, 95% CI 3% to 8%).

AETIOLOGY/ RISK FACTORS
Most cases of carpal tunnel syndrome have no easily identifiable cause (idiopathic).[4] Secondary causes of carpal tunnel syndrome include the following: space occupying lesions (tumours, hypertrophic synovial tissue, fracture callus, and osteophytes); metabolic and physiological (pregnancy, hypothyroidism, rheumatoid arthritis); infections; neuropathies (associated with diabetes mellitus or alcoholism); and familial disorders.[4] One case control study found that risk factors in the general population included repetitive activities requiring wrist extension or flexion, obesity, very rapid dieting, shorter height, hysterectomy without oopherectomy, and recent menopause.[8]

PROGNOSIS
One observational study (carpal tunnel syndrome defined by symptoms and electrophysiological study results) found that 34% of people with idiopathic carpal tunnel syndrome without treatment had complete resolution of symptoms (remission) within 6 months of diagnosis.[9] Remission rates were higher for younger age groups, for women versus men, and for pregnant versus ▶

Carpal tunnel syndrome

non-pregnant women. A more recent observational study of untreated idiopathic carpal tunnel syndrome also demonstrated that symptoms may spontaneously resolve in some people. The main positive prognostic indicators were short duration of symptoms and young age, whereas bilateral symptoms and a positive Phalen's test were indicators of a poorer prognosis.[10]

Please refer to the Clinical Evidence website for full text and references.

Search date November 2003

Steven Reid, Trudie Chalder, Anthony Cleare, Matthew Hotopf, and Simon Wessely

What are the effects of treatments?

BENEFICIAL

Cognitive behavioural therapy

One systematic review found that cognitive behavioural therapy administered by highly skilled therapists in specialist centres improved quality of life and physical functioning compared with standard medical care or relaxation therapy. One additional multicentre RCT found that cognitive behavioural therapy administered by less experienced therapists may also be effective compared with guided support groups or no interventions.

Graded aerobic exercise

RCTs found that a graded aerobic exercise programme improved measures of fatigue and physical functioning compared with flexibility and relaxation training or general advice. One RCT found that an educational package to encourage graded exercise improved measures of physical functioning, fatigue, mood, and sleep at 1 year compared with written information alone.

UNKNOWN EFFECTIVENESS

Dietary supplements

One small RCT found no significant difference between a nutritional supplement (containing multivitamins, minerals, and coenzymes) and placebo in fatigue severity or functional impairment at 10 weeks.

Evening primrose oil

One small RCT found no significant difference between evening primrose oil and placebo in depression scores at 3 months.

Magnesium (intramuscular)

One small RCT found that intramuscular magnesium injections improved symptoms at 6 weeks compared with placebo. However, we were unable to draw reliable conclusions from this small study.

Antidepressants; corticosteroids; oral nicotinamide adenine dinucleotide

RCTs provided insufficient evidence about the effects of these interventions in people with chronic fatigue syndrome.

UNLIKELY TO BE BENEFICIAL

Immunotherapy

Small RCTs provided limited evidence that immunoglobulin G modestly improved physical functioning and fatigue at 3–6 months compared with placebo, but it was associated with considerable adverse effects. Small RCTs provided insufficient evidence on the effects of interferon alfa or aciclovir compared with placebo. One RCT found that staphylococcus toxoid improved symptoms at six months compared with placebo, although it is associated with local reaction and could cause anaphylaxis.

Prolonged rest

We found no RCTs on the effects of prolonged rest. Indirect observational evidence in healthy volunteers and in people recovering from a viral illness suggests that prolonged rest may perpetuate or worsen fatigue and symptoms.

Chronic fatigue syndrome

DEFINITION Chronic fatigue syndrome (CFS) is characterised by severe, disabling fatigue and other symptoms, including musculoskeletal pain, sleep disturbance, impaired concentration, and headaches. Two widely used definitions of CFS, from the US Centers for Disease Control and Prevention (CDC, current criteria issued in 1994, which superseded CDC criteria issued in 1988)[1] and from Oxford, UK,[2] were developed as operational criteria for research❶. There are important differences between these definitions. The UK criteria insist upon the presence of mental fatigue, whereas the US criteria include a requirement for several physical symptoms, reflecting the belief that CFS has an underlying immunological or infective pathology.

INCIDENCE/ PREVALENCE Community and primary care based studies have reported the prevalence of CFS to be up to 3%, depending on the criteria used.[3,4] Systematic population surveys have found similar prevalences of CFS in people of different socio-economic status and in all ethnic groups.[4,5]

AETIOLOGY/ RISK FACTORS The cause of CFS is poorly understood. Women are at higher risk than men (RR 1.3–1.7 depending on diagnostic criteria used).[6]

PROGNOSIS Studies have focused on people attending specialist clinics. A systematic review of studies of prognosis (search date 1996) found that children with CFS had better outcomes than adults: 54–94% of children showed definite improvement (after up to 6 years' follow up), whereas 20–50% of adults showed some improvement in the medium term and only 6% returned to premorbid levels of functioning.[7] Despite the considerable burden of morbidity associated with CFS, we found no evidence of increased mortality. The systematic review found that outcome was influenced by the presence of psychiatric disorders (depression and anxiety) and beliefs about causation and treatment.[7]

Please refer to the Clinical Evidence website for full text and references.

Fracture prevention in postmenopausal women

Search date January 2004

Olivier Bruyère, John Edwards, and Jean-Yves Reginster

What are the effects of treatments to prevent fractures in postmenopausal women?

BENEFICIAL

Alendronate

Two systematic reviews in postmenopausal women found that alendronate reduced vertebral and non-vertebral fractures compared with placebo at 1–4 years.

Parathyroid hormone

One RCT in women with prior vertebral fractures found that parathyroid hormone reduced the proportion of women with vertebral and non-vertebral fractures compared with placebo. Another RCT in women with osteoporosis found that parathyroid hormone plus oestrogen reduced vertebral fractures compared with oestrogen alone after 3 years.

Raloxifene

One large RCT in postmenopausal women with osteoporosis found that raloxifene reduced vertebral fractures compared with placebo, but no significant difference was found in non-vertebral fractures. We found no RCTs examining the effects of other selective oestrogen receptor modulators.

Risedronate

One systematic review in postmenopausal women found that compared with control (placebo, calcium, or calcium plus vitamin D) risedronate reduced vertebral and non-vertebral fractures at 4 years.

LIKELY TO BE BENEFICIAL

Calcitonin

One systematic review in postmenopausal women found that calcitonin reduced vertebral fractures compared with placebo at 1–5 years after treatment, but found no significant difference between calcitonin and placebo in non-vertebral fractures.

Calcium plus vitamin D

One large RCT in women aged 69–106 years living in nursing homes found that calcium plus vitamin D3 reduced hip fractures and all non-vertebral fractures over 18 months to 3 years compared with placebo. One smaller RCT in women and men aged 65 years or older found that calcium plus vitamin D3 reduced non-vertebral fractures at 3 years compared with placebo, but found no significant difference in hip fractures. Another smaller RCT in postmenopausal women found no significant difference between calcium plus vitamin D3 and placebo in hip fractures after 2 years. The two smaller RCTs may have lacked power to detect clinically important differences.

Etidronate

One systematic review in postmenopausal women found that etidronate reduced vertebral fractures compared with control (placebo, calcium, or calcium plus vitamin D) over 2 years, but found no significant difference in non-vertebral fractures.

Fracture prevention in postmenopausal women

Vitamin D analogue (calcitriol)

One systematic review found limited evidence from two small RCTs in postmenopausal women that calcitriol reduced vertebral fractures over 3 years compared with placebo.

UNKNOWN EFFECTIVENESS

Environmental manipulation

We found no systematic review and no RCTs assessing environmental manipulation alone.

Exercise

Three RCTs found no significant difference in falls resulting in fracture at 8 months to 1 year between exercise (advice to walk briskly three times weekly, balance and strength exercises plus walking, or low-intensity exercise plus incontinence care) and control. One small RCT in postmenopausal women found no significant difference between a 2 year back strengthening exercise programme and usual care in vertebral fractures over 10 years.

Hip protectors

One systematic review in elderly community dwelling or nursing home residents found no significant difference in hip fractures at 6 months to 2 years between hip protectors and no protectors in RCTs where individuals were randomised. However, the review found that hip protectors reduced fractures at 11–19 months in RCTs that used cluster analysis. The systematic review found no significant difference in pelvic fractures at 6 months to 2 years between hip protectors and no hip protectors in RCTs where individuals were randomised, but in RCTs with cluster analysis, the review found that hip protectors were associated with a reduction in pelvic fractures at 11–19 months. The review found no significant difference between hip protectors and no hip protectors in the rate of other fractures.

UNLIKELY TO BE BENEFICIAL

Calcium alone

One systematic review in postmenopausal women found no significant difference between calcium supplementation and placebo in vertebral or non-vertebral fractures at 1.5–4 years.

Vitamin D alone

One large RCT in postmenopausal women and two large RCTs in postmenopausal women and elderly men provided no evidence of a difference between vitamin D3 and placebo in hip, vertebral, and non-vertebral fractures after 2–5 years.

LIKELY TO BE INEFFECTIVE OR HARMFUL

Hormone replacement therapy

We found insufficient evidence of benefit, but reliable evidence of harm. One systematic review in postmenopausal women found that hormone replacement therapy reduced vertebral fractures compared with control. However, another systematic review and two subsequent RCTs in postmenopausal women found no significant difference in vertebral fractures. Two systematic reviews and two subsequent RCTs provided insufficient evidence about the effects of hormone replacement therapy on non-vertebral fractures. One large RCT of oestrogen plus progestin versus placebo for primary prevention of coronary heart disease in healthy postmenopausal women was stopped because hormonal treatment increased risks of invasive breast cancer, coronary events, stroke, and pulmonary embolism.

DEFINITION   This topic covers interventions to prevent fractures in postmenopausal women. Fractures may be symptomatic or asymptomatic. A fracture is a break or disruption of bone or cartilage. Symptoms and signs may include immobility, pain, tenderness, numbness, bruising, joint deformity, joint swelling, limb deformity, and limb shortening.[1] Diagnosis is usually based on a typical clinical picture combined with results from an appropriate imaging technique. Usually, in trials dealing with osteoporosis, menopause is considered to be present 12 months after the last menstruation.

INCIDENCE/   The lifetime risk of fracture in white women is 20% for the spine, 15% for the
PREVALENCE   wrist, and 18% for the hip.[2] The incidence of postmenopausal fracture increases with age.[3] One observational study found that age specific incidence rates for postmenopausal fracture of the hip increased exponentially beyond the age of 50 years.[4]

AETIOLOGY/   Fractures usually arise from trauma. General risk factors include those associ-
RISK FACTORS ated with increased risks of falling (such as ataxia, drug and alcohol intake, loose carpets), age, osteoporosis, bony metastases, and other bone disorders. Postmenopausal women are at increased risk of fracture because of hormone related bone loss. Risk factors for fractures in postmenopausal women include increasing age; low body mass index; time since menopause; alcohol consumption; smoking; some endocrine diseases, such as hyperparathyroidism or thyroid disease; and steroid use, among others.

PROGNOSIS   Fractures may result in pain, short or long term disability, haemorrhage, thromboembolic disease (see thromboembolism, p 33), shock, and death. Vertebral fractures are associated with pain, physical impairment, muscular atrophy, changes in body shape, loss of physical function, and lower quality of life.[5] About 20% of women die in the first year after a hip fracture, representing an increase in mortality of 12–20% compared with women of similar age and no hip fracture. Half of elderly women who had been independent become partly dependent after hip fracture. A third become totally dependent.

Please refer to the Clinical Evidence website for full text and references.

Gout

Search date June 2004

Martin Underwood

What are the effects of treatments for acute gout?

UNKNOWN EFFECTIVENESS

Colchicine (oral)

One small RCT provided limited evidence that colchicine improved pain in people with gout. However, we were unable to draw reliable conclusions from this small RCT. The high incidence of adverse effects in people taking colchicine precludes its use as routine treatment.

Corticosteroids

We found no RCTs on the effects of intra-articular, parenteral, or oral corticosteroids in people with gout.

Non-steroidal anti-inflammatory drugs

One small RCT provided limited evidence that tenoxicam reduced short term pain and tenderness in people with gout compared with placebo. However, this study was too small to provide reliable conclusions. We found no RCTs comparing other non-steroidal anti-inflammatory drugs with placebo in people with gout. Five RCTs found no significant difference in effectiveness between different non-steroidal anti-inflammatory drugs. However, these RCTs may have lacked power to detect clinically relevant differences. Two equivalence studies found no difference in pain between etoricoxib and indometacin, but found that indometacin was associated with more adverse effects. The adverse effects of non-steroidal anti-inflammatory drugs include gastrointestinal ulceration and haemorrhage, and for at least some COX-2 inhibitors, increased cardiovascular risk.

What are the effects of treatments to prevent gout in people with prior acute episodes?

UNKNOWN EFFECTIVENESS

Advice to lose weight

We found no RCTs on the effects of advice to lose weight to prevent attacks of gout in people with prior episodes.

Advice to reduce alcohol intake

We found no RCTs on the effects of advice to reduce alcohol intake to prevent attacks of gout in people with prior episodes.

Advice to reduce dietary intake of purines

We found no RCTs on the effects of advice to reduce dietary intake of purines to prevent attacks of gout in people with prior episodes.

Allopurinol

We found no RCTs on the effects of allopurinol to prevent attacks of gout in people with prior episodes.

Benzbromarone

We found no RCTs on the effects of benzbromarone to prevent attacks of gout in people with prior episodes.

Colchicine
We found no RCTs on the effects of colchicine in preventing attacks of gout in people with prior episodes.

Probenecid
We found no RCTs on the effects of probenecid to prevent attacks of gout in people with prior episodes.

Sulphinpyrazone
We found no RCTs on the effects of sulphinpyrazone to prevent attacks of gout in people with prior episodes.

DEFINITION Gout is a syndrome caused by deposition of urate crystals.[1] It typically presents as an acute monoarthritis of rapid onset. The first metatarsophalangeal joint is the most commonly affected joint (podagra). Gout also affects other joints: joints in the foot, ankle, knee, wrist, finger, and elbow are the most frequently affected. Crystal deposits (tophi) may develop around hands, feet, elbows, and ears. Diagnosis is usually made clinically. The American College of Rheumatology (ACR) criteria for diagnosing gout are as follows: (1) characteristic urate crystals in joint fluid; (2) a tophus proved to contain urate crystals; or (3) the presence of six or more defined clinical laboratory and x ray phenomena).[2] We have included studies of people meeting the ACR criteria, studies in which the diagnosis was made clinically, and studies that used other criteria.

INCIDENCE/ PREVALENCE Gout is more common in older people and men.[3] In people aged 65–74 years in the UK, the prevalence is about 50/1000 in men and about 9/1000 in women.[4] The annual incidence of gout in people aged over 50 years in the USA is 1.6/1000 for men and 0.3/1000 for women.[5] One 12 year longitudinal study of 47 150 male health professionals with no previous history of gout estimated that annual incidence of gout ranged from 1/1000 for those aged 40–44 years to 1.8/1000 for those aged 55–64 years.[6] Gout may be more common in some non-white ethnic groups.[3] A pooled analysis of two cohort studies of former medical students found the annual incidence of gout to be 3.1/1000 in black men and 1.8/1000 in white men.[7] After correcting for the higher prevalence of hypertension among black men, which is a risk factor for gout, the relative risk of gout in black men compared with white men was 1.30 (95% CI 0.77 to 2.19).

AETIOLOGY/ RISK FACTORS Urate crystals form when serum urate concentration exceeds 0.42 mmol/L.[8] Serum urate concentration is the principal risk factor for a first attack of gout,[9] although 40% of people have normal serum urate concentration during an attack of gout.[8,10–12] A cohort study of 2046 men followed for about 15 years found that the annual incidence is about 0.4% in men with a urate concentration of 0.42–0.47 mmol/L, rising to 4.3% when serum urate concentration is 0.45–0.59 mmol/L.[13] A 5 year longitudinal study of 223 asymptomatic men with hyperuricaemia estimated 5 year cumulative incidence of gout to be 10.8% for those with baseline serum urate of 0.42–0.47 mmol/L, 27.7% for baseline urate 0.48–0.53 mmol/L, and 61.1% for baseline urate levels of 0.54 mmol/L or more.[9] The study found that a 0.6 mmol/L difference in baseline serum urate increased the odds of an attack of gout by a factor of 1.8 (OR adjusted for other risk factors for gout: 1.84, 95% CI 1.24 to 2.72). One 12 year longitudinal study (47 150 male health professionals with no history of gout)[6,14] estimated that the relative risk of gout from one additional daily serving of different foods (weekly for seafood) was: meat 1.21 (95% CI 1.04 to1.41), seafood (fish, lobster, and shellfish) 1.07 (95% CI 1.01 to 1.12), purine rich vegetables 0.97 (95% CI 0.79 to 1.19), low fat dairy products 0.79 (95% CI 0.71 to 0.87), and high fat dairy products 0.99 (95% CI 0.89 to 1.10).[6] Alcohol consumption of greater than 14.9 g daily significantly increased the risk of gout compared with no alcohol consumption (compared ▶

Gout

with no alcohol consumption: RR for 15.0 g/day to 29.9 g/day: 1.49, 95% CI 1.14 to 1.94; RR for 30.0 g/day to 49.9 g/day: 1.96, 95% CI 1.48 to 2.60; RR for ≥ 50 g/day: 2.53, 95% CI 1.73 to 3.70).[14] The longitudinal study also estimated the relative risk of an additional serving of beer (355 mL, 12.8 g alcohol), wine (118 mL, 11.0 g alcohol), and spirits (44 mL, 14.0 g alcohol). It found that an extra daily serving of beer or spirits was significantly associated with gout, but an extra daily serving of wine was not (RR for 355 mL/day beer: 1.49, 95% CI 1.32 to 1.70; RR for 44 mL/day spirits: 1.15, 95% CI 1.04 to 1.28; RR for 118 mL/day wine: 1.04, 95% CI 0.88 to 1.22). Other suggested risk factors for gout include obesity, insulin resistance, dyslipidaemia, hypertension, and cardiovascular disorders.[15,16]

PROGNOSIS We found few reliable data about prognosis or complications of gout. One study found that 3/11 (27%) people with untreated gout of the first metatarsophalangeal joint experienced spontaneous resolution after 7 days.[17] A case series of 614 people with gout who had not had treatment to reduce urate levels, and could recall the interval between first and second attacks, reported recurrence rates of 62% after 1 year, 78% after 2 years, and 84% after 3 years.[18] An analysis of two prospective cohort studies of 371 black and 1181 white male former medical students followed up for about 30 years found no significant difference in risk of coronary heart disease in men who had developed gout compared with men who had not (RR 0.85, 95% CI 0.40 to 1.81).[19]

Please refer to the Clinical Evidence website for full text and references.

Musculoskeletal disorders

What are the effects of drug treatments?

UNKNOWN EFFECTIVENESS

Analgesics
We found no systematic review or RCTs on the use of analgesics for treatment of people with symptomatic herniated lumbar discs.

Antidepressants
We found no systematic review or RCTs on the use of antidepressants for treatment of people with symptomatic herniated lumbar discs.

Muscle relaxants
We found no systematic review or RCTs on the use of muscle relaxants for treatment of people with symptomatic herniated lumbar discs.

UNLIKELY TO BE BENEFICIAL

Epidural corticosteroid injections
One systematic review found limited evidence that epidural corticosteroid injections increased global improvement compared with placebo. However, one subsequent RCT found no significant difference between epidural corticosteroid injections plus conservative treatment and conservative treatment alone in pain, mobility, or people returning to work at 6 months. Another subsequent RCT found no significant difference between epidural corticosteroid injection and control injection in pain, disability, or self rated improvement after 35 days.

Non-steroidal anti-inflammatory drugs
One systematic review found no significant difference in overall improvement between non-steroidal anti-inflammatory drugs and placebo in people with sciatica caused by disc herniation.

What are the effects of non-drug treatments?

LIKELY TO BE BENEFICIAL

Spinal manipulation
One RCT identified by a systematic review in people with sciatica caused by disc herniation found that spinal manipulation increased self perceived improvement after 2 weeks compared with a placebo of infrequent infrared heat. Another RCT identified by the review, comparing spinal manipulation, manual traction, exercise, and corsets, found no significant difference among groups in self perceived improvement after 1 month. One subsequent RCT found that spinal manipulation increased the proportion of people with improved symptoms compared with traction. Concerns exist regarding possible further herniation from spinal manipulation in people who are surgical candidates.

UNKNOWN EFFECTIVENESS

Acupuncture
One systematic review found insufficient evidence on the effects of acupuncture in people with herniated lumbar discs.

▶

Musculoskeletal disorders

Herniated lumbar disc

Advice to stay active

One systematic review of conservative treatments for sciatica caused by lumbar disc herniation found no RCTs on advice to stay active.

Exercise therapy

One systematic review of one RCT found no significant difference in global improvement between isometric exercise and manual traction in people with sciatica caused by disc herniation.

Heat or ice

One systematic review identified no RCTs of heat or ice for sciatica caused by lumbar disc herniation.

Massage

One systematic review identified no RCTs of massage in people with symptomatic lumbar disc herniation.

UNLIKELY TO BE BENEFICIAL

Bed rest

One systematic review of conservative treatment found no RCTs on bed rest in people with symptomatic herniated discs. One subsequent RCT in people with sciatica found no significant difference between bed rest and watchful waiting for 2 weeks in people's perceived improvement, mean pain scores, mean disability scores, or mean satisfaction scores after 12 weeks.

What are the effects of surgery?

LIKELY TO BE BENEFICIAL

Microdiscectomy (as effective as standard discectomy)

We found no RCTs comparing microdiscectomy versus conservative treatment. Three RCTs found no significant difference in clinical outcomes between microdiscectomy and standard discectomy. One RCT found no significant difference in satisfaction or pain between video-assisted arthroscopic microdiscectomy and standard discectomy at about 30 months, although postoperative recovery was slower with standard discectomy. We found insufficient evidence on the effects of automated percutaneous discectomy compared with microdiscectomy.

Standard discectomy (short term benefit)

One RCT found that standard discectomy increased self reported improvement at 1 year, but not at 4 and 10 years, compared with conservative treatment (physiotherapy). Three RCTs found no significant difference in clinical outcomes between standard discectomy and microdiscectomy. Adverse effects were similar with both procedures. One RCT found no significant difference in satisfaction or pain between standard discectomy and video-assisted arthroscopic microdiscectomy at about 30 months, although post-operative recovery was slower with standard discectomy.

UNKNOWN EFFECTIVENESS

Automated percutaneous discectomy

We found no RCTs comparing automated percutaneous discectomy versus either conservative treatment or standard discectomy. We found insufficient evidence on the clinical effects of automated percutaneous discectomy compared with microdiscectomy.

Laser discectomy

We found no systematic review or RCTs on the use of laser discectomy for treatment of people with symptomatic herniated lumbar discs.

DEFINITION Herniated lumbar disc is a displacement of disc material (nucleus pulposus or annulus fibrosis) beyond the intervertebral disc space.[1] The diagnosis can be confirmed by radiological examination; however, magnetic resonance imaging findings of herniated disc are not always accompanied by clinical symptoms.[2,3] This review covers treatment of people who have clinical symptoms relating to confirmed or suspected disc herniation. It does not include treatment of people with spinal cord compression or people with cauda equina syndrome, which requires emergency intervention. The management of non-specific acute low back pain, p 336 and chronic low back pain, p 339 are covered elsewhere in *Clinical Evidence*.

INCIDENCE/ PREVALENCE The prevalence of symptomatic herniated lumbar disc is about 1–3% in Finland and Italy, depending on age and sex.[4] The highest prevalence is among people aged 30–50 years,[5] with a male to female ratio of 2 : 1.[6] In people aged between 25 and 55 years, about 95% of herniated discs occur at the lower lumbar spine (L4–L5 level); disc herniation above this level is more common in people over 55 years of age.[7,8]

AETIOLOGY/ RISK FACTORS Radiographical evidence of disc herniation does not reliably predict low back pain in the future or correlate with symptoms; 19–27% of people without symptoms have disc herniation on imaging.[2,9] Risk factors for disc herniation include smoking (OR 1.7, 95% CI 1.0 to 2.5), weight bearing sports (e.g. weight lifting, hammer throw etc), and certain work activities such as repeated lifting. Driving motor vehicles is also associated with increased risk (OR 1.7, 95% CI 0.2 to 2.7).[6,10,11] This may be because the resonant frequency of the spine is similar to that of certain vehicles.

PROGNOSIS The natural history of disc herniation is difficult to determine because most people take some form of treatment for their back pain, and a formal diagnosis is not always made.[6] Clinical improvement is usual in most people, and only about 10% of people still have sufficient pain after 6 weeks to consider surgery. Sequential magnetic resonance images have shown that the herniated portion of the disc tends to regress over time, with partial to complete resolution after 6 months in two thirds of people.[12]

Please refer to the Clinical Evidence website for full text and references.

Leg cramps

Search date February 2004

Gavin Young

What are the effects of treatments for idiopathic leg cramps?

BENEFICIAL

Quinine

One systematic review has found that quinine reduces the frequency of nocturnal leg cramp attacks compared with placebo over 4 weeks. We found no evidence about the optimal dose of quinine or length of treatment.

LIKELY TO BE BENEFICIAL

Quinine plus theophylline

One small RCT found limited evidence that quinine plus theophylline reduced the number of nights affected by leg cramps compared with quinine alone over 2 weeks.

UNKNOWN EFFECTIVENESS

Analgesics; antiepileptic drugs; compression hosiery

We found no RCTs on the effects of these interventions on idiopathic leg cramps.

UNLIKELY TO BE BENEFICIAL

Vitamin E

One small RCT found no significant difference between vitamin E and placebo in the number of nights disturbed by leg cramps.

What are the effects of treatments for leg cramps in pregnancy?

LIKELY TO BE BENEFICIAL

Magnesium salts

One systematic review identified one small RCT in pregnant women, which found that magnesium tablets (primarily magnesium lactate, magnesium citrate) reduced leg cramps compared with placebo after 3 weeks.

UNKNOWN EFFECTIVENESS

Calcium salts

One systematic review identified two RCTs that compared calcium versus vitamin C or no treatment. The RCTs found different results.

Multivitamins and mineral supplements

One systematic review identified one small RCT in pregnant women, which found no significant difference between a multivitamin plus mineral tablet and placebo in leg cramps in the ninth month of pregnancy.

Sodium chloride

One systematic review found insufficient evidence about the effects of sodium chloride on leg cramps in pregnancy.

◀ **DEFINITION**   Leg cramps are involuntary, localised, and usually painful skeletal muscle contractions, which commonly affect calf muscles. Leg cramps typically occur at night and usually last only seconds to minutes. Leg cramps may be idiopathic (of unknown cause) or related to a definable process or condition such as pregnancy, renal dialysis, or venous insufficiency.

INCIDENCE/   Leg cramps are common and their incidence increases with age. About half of
PREVALENCE   people attending a general medicine clinic have had leg cramps within 1 month of their visit, and over two thirds of people over 50 years of age have experienced leg cramps.[1]

AETIOLOGY/   Very little is known about the causes of leg cramps. Risk factors include
RISK FACTORS   pregnancy, exercise, salt depletion, renal dialysis, electrolyte imbalances, peripheral vascular disease (both venous and arterial), peripheral nerve injury, polyneuropathies, motor neuron disease, muscle diseases, and certain drugs. Other causes of acute calf pain include trauma, deep venous thrombosis (see thromboembolism, p 33), and ruptured Baker's cyst.

PROGNOSIS   Leg cramps may cause severe pain and sleep disturbance.

Please refer to the Clinical Evidence website for full text and references.

Low back pain (acute)

Search date October 2003

Maurits van Tulder and Bart Koes

What are the effects of treatments?

BENEFICIAL

Advice to stay active

Two systematic reviews and one subsequent RCT found that advice to stay active increased the rate of recovery, reduced pain, reduced disability, and reduced time spent off work compared with advice to rest in bed or bed rest.

Non-steroidal anti-inflammatory drugs

One systematic review and one additional RCT have found that non-steroidal anti-inflammatory drugs increased overall improvement after 1 week and reduced the need for additional analgesics compared with placebo. One systematic review and additional RCTs have found no significant difference among non-steroidal anti-inflammatory drugs or between non-steroidal anti-inflammatory drugs and other treatments (paracetamol, opioids, muscle relaxants, and non-drug treatments) in pain relief.

LIKELY TO BE BENEFICIAL

Behavioural therapy

One RCT found that cognitive behavioural therapy reduced acute low back pain and disability compared with traditional care or electromyographic biofeedback.

Multidisciplinary treatment programmes (for subacute low back pain)

We found no RCTs in people with acute low back pain. One systematic review in people with subacute low back pain found limited evidence that multidisciplinary treatment, including a workplace visit, reduced sick leave compared with usual care.

TRADE OFF BETWEEN BENEFITS AND HARMS

Muscle relaxants

Systematic reviews have found that muscle relaxants improve symptoms (including pain and muscle tension) and increase mobility compared with placebo, but found no significant difference in outcomes among muscle relaxants. Adverse effects in people using muscle relaxants were common and included dependency, drowsiness, and dizziness.

UNKNOWN EFFECTIVENESS

Acupuncture

We found no RCTs of acupuncture specifically in people with acute low back pain.

Analgesics (paracatemol, opioids)

We found no placebo controlled RCTs. Systematic reviews have found no consistent difference between analgesics and non-steroidal anti-inflammatory drugs in reducing pain.

Back schools

One systematic review found limited evidence that back schools increased rates of recovery and reduced sick leave compared with placebo in the short term. The review found no significant difference in outcomes between back school and physiotherapy, and found that back school increased pain and sick leave compared with McKenzie exercises.

◀ **Epidural steroid injections**

One RCT found that epidural steroids increased the proportion of people who were pain free compared with subcutaneous lidocaine (lignocaine) injections after 3 months. A second RCT found no significant difference in the proportion of people cured or improved between epidural steroids and epidural saline, epidural bupivacaine, or dry needling.

Lumbar supports

We found no RCTs on the effects of lumbar supports.

Massage

One systematic review found insufficient evidence from one RCT about the effects of massage compared with spinal manipulation or electrical stimulation.

Spinal manipulation

Systematic reviews found conflicting evidence on the effects of spinal manipulation.

Traction

RCTs found conflicting evidence on the effects of traction.

Colchicine; electromyographic biofeedback; temperature treatments (short wave diathermy, ultrasound, ice, heat); transcutaneous electrical nerve stimulation

We found insufficient evidence on the effects of these interventions.

UNLIKELY TO BE BENEFICIAL

Back exercises

Systematic reviews and additional RCTs have found either no significant difference between back exercises and conservative or inactive treatments in pain or disability, or have found that back exercises increase pain or disability.

LIKELY TO BE INEFFECTIVE OR HARMFUL

Bed rest

Systematic reviews have found that bed rest could be worse than no treatment, advice to stay active, back exercises, physiotherapy, spinal manipulation, or non-steroidal anti-inflammatory drugs. One systematic review has found that adverse effects of bed rest include joint stiffness, muscle wasting, loss of bone mineral density, pressure sores, and venous thromboembolism.

DEFINITION   Low back pain is pain, muscle tension, or stiffness localised below the costal margin and above the inferior gluteal folds, with or without leg pain (sciatica),[1] and is designated as acute when it persists for less than 12 weeks.[2] Non-specific low back pain is low back pain not attributed to a recognisable pathology (such as infection, tumour, osteoporosis, rheumatoid arthritis, fracture, or inflammation).[1] This review excludes low back pain or sciatica with symptoms or signs at presentation that suggest a specific underlying condition.

INCIDENCE/   Over 70% of people in developed countries will experience low back pain at
PREVALENCE   some time in their lives.[3] Each year, 15–45% of adults suffer low back pain, and 1/20 (5%) people present to hospital with a new episode. Low back pain is most common between the ages of 35–55 years.[3]

AETIOLOGY/   Symptoms, pathology, and radiological appearances are poorly correlated. Pain
RISK FACTORS is non-specific in about 85% of people. About 4% of people with low back pain in primary care have compression fractures and about 1% have a tumour. The ▶

Low back pain (acute)

prevalence of prolapsed intervertebral disc is about 1–3%.[3] Ankylosing spond-ylitis and spinal infections are less common.[4] Risk factors for the development of back pain include heavy physical work, frequent bending, twisting, lifting, and prolonged static postures. Psychosocial risk factors include anxiety, depression, and mental stress at work.[3,5]

PROGNOSIS Acute low back pain is usually self limiting (90% of people recover within 6 weeks), although 2–7% develop chronic pain. One study found recurrent pain accounted for 75–85% of absenteeism from work.[6]

Please refer to the Clinical Evidence website for full text and references.

What are the effects of oral drug treatments?

LIKELY TO BE BENEFICIAL

Analgesics

One RCT found that tramadol (an opioid) decreased pain and increased function at 7 weeks compared with placebo. One RCT found that a combination of tramadol and paracetamol (acetaminophen) decreased pain and increased function at 3 months compared with placebo. One RCT found no significant difference between paracetamol and diflusinal in the proportion of people who rated the treatment as good or excellent. One RCT found no significant difference in pain relief between a parenteral non-steroidal anti-inflammatory drug and a parenteral opioid analgesic.

Antidepressants

One systematic review found that antidepressants decreased pain compared with placebo, but found no consistent difference in function. One RCT found that maproteline increased pain relief compared with paroxetine. Four additional RCTs found no significant difference in depression between antidepressants and placebo, and two additional RCTs found that antidepressants improved depression in people with chronic low back pain.

Non-steroidal anti-inflammatory drugs

One small RCT found that naproxen reduced pain compared with placebo. One systematic review and one subsequent RCT found no significant differences in symptoms between different non-steroidal anti-inflammatory drugs. One RCT identified by the review found no significant difference between diflunisal and paracetamol in the proportion of people who rated the treatment as good or excellent. One RCT found no significant difference in pain relief between a parenteral non-steroidal anti-inflammatory drug and a parenteral opioid analgesic. Two RCTs found that COX 2 inhibitors decreased pain and improved function at 4–12 weeks compared with placebo, but effects were small.

TRADE OFF BETWEEN BENEFITS AND HARMS

Muscle relaxants

Two RCTs identified by a systematic review found that tetrazepam reduced pain and increased overall improvement after 10–14 days compared with placebo. Two RCTs identified by a systematic review found that non-benzodiazepines (flupirtine and tolperisone) increased overall improvement at 7–21 days, but found no significant difference for pain. Adverse effects of muscle relaxants include dizziness and drowsiness.

What are the effects of injection therapy?

UNKNOWN EFFECTIVENESS

Epidural steroid injections

We found no systematic reviews or RCTs in people with chronic back pain who did not have sciatica.

Local injections

One systematic review found no significant difference between local injections (local anaesthetic and corticosteroids) and placebo in short term pain relief.

Low back pain (chronic)

◄ **LIKELY TO BE INEFFECTIVE OR HARMFUL**

Facet joint injections

One RCT identified by a systematic review found no significant difference in pain relief and disability between corticosteroid and saline injections after 1 and after 3 months. Adverse effects include infection, haemorrhage, chemical meningitis. and neurological damage.

What are the effects of non-drug treatments?

BENEFICIAL

Multidisciplinary treatment programmes

One systematic review has found that intensive multidisciplinary biopsychosocial rehabilitation with functional restoration reduced pain and improved function compared with inpatient or outpatient non-multidisciplinary treatments or usual care. The review found no significant difference between less intensive multidisciplinary treatments and non-multidisciplinary treatment or usual care in pain or function.

LIKELY TO BE BENEFICIAL

Back schools

One systematic review and one subsequent RCT found limited evidence that back schools reduced pain and disability compared with inactive treatments (waiting list control, placebo gel, or written advice) or no treatment within 6 months, although results suggested that benefits may not persist in the longer term. Three RCTs identified by the review compared back schools with other treatments and found mixed results.

Behavioural therapy

One systematic review found that behavioural therapy reduced pain and improved functional status and behavioural outcomes compared with no treatment, placebo, or waiting list control. The review and one subsequent RCT provided no evidence of a difference in functional status, pain, or behavioural outcomes between different types of behavioural therapy. The review found insufficient evidence to compare behavioural therapy with other treatments.

Exercise

RCTs found insufficient evidence on the effects of different types of exercise, or exercise compared with other treatments.

Physical conditioning programmes (cognitive behavioural approach plus physical training)

Two RCTs identified by a systematic review found that physical conditioning programmes (consisting of a cognitive behavioural approach plus physical training) reduced sick days overall but not the risk of being off work at 12 months compared with general practitioner care.

Spinal manipulative therapy

One systematic review found that spinal manipulative therapy reduced pain in the short and long term and improved short term function compared with sham manipulation, but found no significant difference in long term function (> 6 weeks). The systematic review found no significant difference in pain or function between spinal manipulative therapy and general practitioner care, physical therapy, exercises, or back school. Two subsequent RCTs compared spinal manipulation with exercise and found that spinal manipulation reduced pain at ►

6–12 months, but found different results for function. One of the RCTs found that spinal manipulation increased return to work at 12 months compared with exercise therapy.

UNKNOWN EFFECTIVENESS

Acupuncture

Two systematic reviews and two subsequent RCTs found insufficient evidence about the effects of acupuncture compared with placebo or no treatment. One systematic review and one subsequent RCT found limited evidence that acupuncture reduced pain intensity and increased overall improvement compared with transcutaneous electrical nerve stimulation.

Electromyographic biofeedback

One systematic review found no significant difference in pain relief or functional status between electromyographic biofeedback and placebo or waiting list control, but found insufficient evidence on the effects of electromyographic biofeedback compared with other treatments.

Lumbar supports

We found insufficient evidence on the effects of lumbar supports.

Massage

One systematic review found insufficient evidence about effects of massage compared with inactive treatments or other treatments.

Transcutaneous electrical nerve stimulation

One systematic review found no significant difference in pain relief between transcutaneous electrical nerve stimulation and sham stimulation.

LIKELY TO BE INEFFECTIVE OR HARMFUL

Traction

One systematic review and two additional RCTs found no significant difference between traction and placebo or between traction plus massage and interferential treatment treatments in pain relief or functional status.

DEFINITION Low back pain is pain, muscle tension, or stiffness localised below the costal margin and above the inferior gluteal folds, with or without leg pain (sciatica),[1] and is defined as chronic when it persists for 12 weeks or more (see definition of low back pain [acute], p 336).[2] Non-specific low back pain is low back pain not attributed to a recognisable pathology (such as infection, tumour, osteoporosis, rheumatoid arthritis, fracture, or inflammation).[1] This review excludes low back pain or leg pain with symptoms or signs at presentation that suggest a specific underlying condition. People with sciatica (lumbosacral radicular syndrome) or pain due to herniated discs are also excluded.

INCIDENCE/ PREVALENCE Over 70% of people in developed countries will experience low back pain at some time in their lives.[3] Each year, 15–45% of adults suffer low back pain, and 1/20 people present to hospital with a new episode. About 2–7% of patients with acute low back pain will go on to become chronic. Low back pain is most common between the ages of 35–55 years.[3]

AETIOLOGY/ RISK FACTORS Symptoms, pathology, and radiological appearances are poorly correlated. Pain is non-specific in about 85% of people. About 4% of people with low back pain in primary care have compression fractures and about 1% have a tumour. The prevalence of prolapsed intervertebral disc is about 1–3%.[3] Ankylosing spondylitis and spinal infections are less common.[4] This chapter only covers non-specific chronic low back pain. Risk factors for the development of back pain include heavy physical work, frequent bending, twisting, lifting, and prolonged ▶

Low back pain (chronic)

static postures. Psychosocial risk factors include anxiety, depression, and mental stress at work.[3,5] Having a previous history of low back pain and a longer duration of the present episode are significant risk factors for chronicity. A recently published systematic review of prospective cohort studies found that some psychological factors (distress, depressive mood, and somatisation) are associated with an increased risk of chronic low back pain.[6] Individual and workplace factors have also been reported to be associated with the transition to chronic low back pain.[7]

PROGNOSIS   Generally, the clinical course of an episode of low back pain seems to be favourable, and most pain will resolve within 2 weeks. Back pain among primary care patients typically has a recurrent course characterised by variation and change, rather than an acute, self limiting course.[8] Most back pain patients will have experienced a previous episode, and acute attacks often occur as exacerbations of chronic low back pain. In general, recurrences will occur more frequently and be more severe if patients had frequent or long lasting low back pain complaints in the past. The course of sick leave due to low back pain is similarly favourable. One study reported that 67% of patients with sick leave due to low back pain will have returned to work within a week, and 90% within 2 months. However, the longer the period of sick leave the less likely the return to work becomes. Less than half of the low back pain patients who have been off work for 6 months will return to work. After 2 years of work absenteeism, the chance to return to work is virtually zero.[9]

Please refer to the Clinical Evidence website for full text and references.

Search date May 2004

Allan Binder

What are the effects of treatments for people with uncomplicated neck pain without severe neurological deficit?

The evidence about the effects of individual interventions for neck pain is often contradictory because of the poor quality of the RCTs, the tendency for interventions to be given in combination, and for RCTs to be conducted in diverse groups. This lack of consistency in study design makes it difficult to isolate which intervention may be of use in which type of neck pain.

LIKELY TO BE BENEFICIAL

Exercise

Systematic reviews and subsequent RCTs, primarily in people with chronic uncomplicated neck pain, found that strengthening exercise or active physical treatment including exercise reduced pain compared with usual care including drug treatment, stress management, or no specific exercise programme. RCTs identified by several systematic reviews provided insufficient evidence about the effects of exercise compared with traction. The reviews identified one RCT in people with chronic neck pain that compared low technology strengthening exercises plus manipulation, high technology strengthening exercises, and manipulation alone. It found that low technology strengthening exercises plus manipulation improved participant satisfaction, objective strength, and range of movement at 11 weeks compared with manipulation alone. At 1 and 2 years it found that both low technology strengthening exercises plus manipulation and high technology strengthening exercises improved pain and patient satisfaction compared with manipulation alone. The 2 year follow up was in a subset of participants only. Another RCT identified by a systematic review found no significant difference in pain after treatment or at 12 months among exercise, manipulation, or mobilisation. A third RCT found that exercise was less effective in improving pain than mobilisation in people with neck pain for over 2 weeks.

Manipulation

One systematic review found no significant difference in symptoms between manipulation and usual care in people with subacute or chronic neck or back pain. The meta-analysis performed by the review may have been underpowered to detect a clinically important difference. One RCT found limited evidence that manipulation may be more effective in reducing pain at 1 year than less active physical treatment (massage, pulsed electrical field treatment, and slight traction). We found one RCT in people with chronic neck pain that compared manipulation plus low technology strengthening exercises, high technology strengthening exercises, and manipulation alone. It found that manipulation plus low technology strengthening exercises improved pain and objective range of movement at 11 weeks compared with manipulation alone. At 1 and 2 years it found that both manipulation plus low technology strengthening exercises and high technology strengthening exercises improved pain and patient satisfaction compared with manipulation alone. The 2 year follow up was in a subset of participants only. Two RCTs provided insufficient evidence to compare manipulation versus mobilisation in people with uncomplicated neck pain.

Manipulation plus exercise

One RCT in people with chronic neck pain found that manipulation plus strengthening exercise improved pain and objective range of movement at 11 weeks ▶

compared with either treatment alone. At 1 and 2 years the difference in outcomes remained significant with manipulation plus strengthening exercise compared with manipulation alone but not compared with exercise alone. The 2 year follow up was in a subset of participants only.

Mobilisation

One RCT found that mobilisation improved symptoms compared with usual care (drug treatment) or exercise in people with neck pain for over 2 weeks. Another RCT identified by several systematic reviews found no significant difference in pain after treatment or at 12 months among mobilisation, manipulation, or exercise. A third RCT identified by several systematic reviews found limited evidence that manual treatment (mobilisation or manipulation) may be more effective in reducing pain at 1 year than less active physical treatment. Two RCTs provided insufficient evidence to compare mobilisation versus manipulation in people with uncomplicated neck pain. Weak RCTs, some identified by systematic reviews, provided insufficient evidence to compare mobilisation versus acupuncture or transcutaneous electrical nerve stimulation in people with uncomplicated neck pain.

UNKNOWN EFFECTIVENESS

Acupuncture

Systematic reviews of weak RCTs provided insufficient evidence about the effects of acupuncture compared with a range of other treatments, including sham acupuncture, sham transcutaneous electrical nerve simulation, diazepam, traction, short wave diathermy, and mobilisation in people with acute or chronic uncomplicated neck pain.

Biofeedback

Three systematic reviews identified no RCTs of biofeedback in people with uncomplicated neck pain.

Drug treatments (analgesics, non-steroidal anti-inflammatory drugs, antidepressants, or muscle relaxants)

We found insufficient evidence on the effects of analgesics, non-steroidal anti-inflammatory drugs, antidepressants, or muscle relaxants for neck pain, although they are widely used. Several drugs used to treat neck pain are associated with well documented adverse effects.

Heat or cold

Two systematic reviews identified no RCTs of sufficient quality of heat or cold in people with uncomplicated neck pain. One large RCT of people with chronic neck and back pain found that heat combined with other physical treatment was less effective in improving outcomes than manipulation or mobilisation.

Multimodal treatment

One RCT identified by a systematic review provided insufficient evidence to assess multimodal treatment in people with uncomplicated neck pain.

Pulsed electromagnetic field treatment

One RCT identified by several systematic reviews provided insufficient evidence to compare pulsed electromagnetic field treatment versus sham treatment in people with uncomplicated neck pain. RCTs in people with chronic neck and back pain identified by another systematic review found that pulsed electromagnetic field treatment combined with other physical treatments was less effective in improving outcomes than manipulation or mobilisation.

Soft collars and special pillows
We found no RCTs of sufficient quality on the effects of soft collars or special pillows in people with uncomplicated neck pain.

Spray and stretch
One RCT identified by several systematic reviews provided insufficient evidence about the effects of spray and stretch in people with uncomplicated neck pain.

Traction
Systematic reviews in people with acute or chronic neck pain provided insufficient evidence about the effects of traction compared with a range of other physical treatments, including sham traction, placebo tablets, exercise, acupuncture, heat, collar, and analgesics. Systematic reviews identified no RCTs of sufficient quality comparing traction versus manipulation or mobilisation.

Transcutaneous electrical nerve stimulation
Five systematic reviews identified no RCTs of sufficient quality of transcutaneous electrical nerve stimulation in people with uncomplicated neck pain.

UNLIKELY TO BE BENEFICIAL

Patient education
Two RCTs in people with chronic neck, back, or shoulder pain found no significant difference among patient education (individual advice, pamphlets, or group instruction) with or without analgesics and no treatment, stress management, and cognitive behavioural therapy.

What are the effects of treatments for acute whiplash injury?
The evidence about the effects of individual interventions for neck pain is often contradictory because of the poor quality of the RCTs, the tendency for interventions to be given in combination, and for RCTs to be conducted in diverse groups. This lack of consistency in study design makes it difficult to isolate which intervention may be of use in which type of neck pain.

LIKELY TO BE BENEFICIAL

Early mobilisation
Four RCTs identified by several systematic reviews provided limited evidence that early mobilisation reduced pain compared with immobilisation or rest plus a collar.

Early return to normal activity
One RCT in people with acute whiplash identified by one systematic review provided limited evidence that advice to "act as usual" plus anti-inflammatory drugs improved some symptoms (including pain during daily activities, neck stiffness, memory, concentration, and headache) at 6 months compared with immobilisation plus 14 days' sick leave. It found no significant difference in neck range or sick leave and found that a similar proportion of people had severe neck pain.

Multimodal treatment
One RCT identified by a systematic review found that multimodal treatment reduced pain at 1 and 6 months compared with physical treatments.

UNKNOWN EFFECTIVENESS

Drug treatments (analgesics, non-steroidal anti-inflammatory drugs, antidepressant drugs, or muscle relaxants
Two systematic reviews identified no RCTs of drug treatments in people with acute whiplash injury.

Neck pain

Exercise

One RCT found no significant difference between two home exercise programmes in pain or disability.

Pulsed electromagnetic field treatment

One small RCT identified by two systematic reviews found limited evidence that electromagnetic field treatment reduced pain after 4 weeks but not after 3 months compared with sham treatment.

What are the effects of treatments for chronic whiplash injury?

The evidence about the effects of individual interventions for neck pain is often contradictory because of the poor quality of the RCTs, the tendency for interventions to be given in combination, and for RCTs to be conducted in diverse groups. This lack of consistency in study design makes it difficult to isolate which intervention may be of use in which type of neck pain.

LIKELY TO BE BENEFICIAL

Percutaneous radiofrequency neurotomy

One RCT identified by a systematic review found limited evidence that percutaneous radiofrequency neurotomy reduced pain after 27 weeks compared with sham treatment in people with chronic whiplash injury.

UNKNOWN EFFECTIVENESS

Multimodal treatment

One small RCT found no difference between multimodal treatment and physical treatments in disability, pain, or range of movement at the end of treatment or at 3 months but it may have been too small to detect a clinically important difference.

Physical treatments

One small RCT found no significant difference between physical treatments alone and multimodal treatment in disability, pain, or range of movement at the end of treatment or at 3 months but it may have been too small to detect a clinically important difference.

What are the effects of treatments for neck pain with radiculopathy?

The evidence about the effects of individual interventions for neck pain is often contradictory because of the poor quality of the RCTs, the tendency for interventions to be given in combination, and for RCTs to be conducted in diverse groups. This lack of consistency in study design makes it difficult to isolate which intervention may be of use in which type of neck pain.

UNKNOWN EFFECTIVENESS

Drug treatments (epidural steroid injections, analgesics, non-steroidal anti-inflammatory drugs, or muscle relaxants)

We found no RCTs examining the effects of analgesics, non-steroidal anti-inflammatory drugs, or muscle relaxants in people with neck pain with radiculopathy. Two RCTs found limited evidence that cervical steroid epidural injections may improve pain from baseline in people with chronic neck pain with or without radiculopathy.

◀ **Surgery versus conservative treatment**

One RCT found no significant difference in pain at 1 year between surgery and conservative treatment in people with neck pain with radiculopathy.

DEFINITION   In this chapter we have differentiated uncomplicated neck pain from whiplash, although many studies, particularly in people with chronic pain (duration > 3 months), do not specify which types of people are included. Most studies of acute pain (duration < 3 months) are confined to whiplash. Uncomplicated neck pain is defined as pain with a postural or mechanical basis, often called cervical spondylosis. It does not include pain associated with fibromyalgia. Uncomplicated neck pain may include some people with a traumatic basis for their symptoms, but not people for whom pain is specifically stated to have followed sudden acceleration — deceleration injuries to the neck, that is, whiplash. Whiplash is commonly seen in road traffic accidents or sports injuries. It is not accompanied by radiographic abnormalities or clinical signs of nerve root damage. Neck pain often occurs in combination with limited movement and poorly defined neurological symptoms affecting the upper limbs. The pain can be severe and intractable, and can occur with radiculopathy or myelopathy. We have included under radiculopathy those studies involving people with predominantly radicular symptoms arising in the cervical spine.

INCIDENCE/   About two thirds of people will experience neck pain at some time in their
PREVALENCE   lives.[1,2] Prevalence is highest in middle age. In the UK about 15% of hospital based physiotherapy and in Canada 30% of chiropractic referrals are for neck pain.[3,4] In the Netherlands neck pain contributes up to 2% of general practitioner consultations.[5]

AETIOLOGY/   The aetiology of uncomplicated neck pain is unclear. Most uncomplicated neck
RISK FACTORS pain is associated with poor posture, anxiety and depression, nerve strain, occupational injuries, or sporting injuries. With chronic pain, mechanical and degenerative factors (often referred to as cervical spondylosis) are more likely. Some neck pain results from soft tissue trauma, most typically seen in whiplash injuries. Rarely, disc prolapse and inflammatory, infective, or malignant conditions affect the cervical spine and present with neck pain with or without neurological features.

PROGNOSIS   Neck pain usually resolves within days or weeks but can recur or become chronic. In some industries, neck related disorders account for as much time off work as low back pain (see low back pain [acute], p 336).[6] The proportion of people in whom neck pain becomes chronic depends on the cause but is thought to be about 10%,[1] similar to low back pain. Neck pain causes severe disability in 5% of affected people.[2] Whiplash injuries are more likely to cause disability than neck pain because of other causes; up to 40% of sufferers reported symptoms even after 15 years' follow up.[7] Factors associated with a poorer outcome after whiplash are not well defined.[8] The incidence of chronic disability after whiplash varies among countries, although reasons for this variation are unclear.[9]

Please refer to the Clinical Evidence website for full text and references.

Musculoskeletal disorders

Non-steroidal anti-inflammatory drugs

Search date January 2004

Peter C Gøtzsche

Are there any important differences between available non-steroidal anti-inflammatory drugs (NSAIDs)?

UNKNOWN EFFECTIVENESS

Choice between different NSAIDs

Systematic reviews found no important differences in efficacy between different NSAIDs. Cyclo-oxygenase-2 (COX 2) inhibitors reduce gastroscopically diagnosed ulcers compared with other NSAIDs, but the reduction in clinical effects was less marked and COX 2 inhibitors may increase the risk of myocardial infarction.

UNLIKELY TO BE BENEFICIAL

NSAIDs in increased doses

Systematic reviews found that benefits of NSAIDs increased towards a maximum value at high doses. Recommended doses are close to creating the maximum benefit. In contrast, three systematic reviews found no ceiling for adverse effects, which increased in an approximately linear fashion with dose.

What are the effects of co-treatments to reduce the risk of gastrointestinal adverse effects of NSAIDs?

LIKELY TO BE BENEFICIAL

H_2 blockers in people who cannot avoid NSAIDs

One systematic review in people who had taken NSAIDs for 3 months found that H_2 blockers reduced endoscopically diagnosed gastric and duodenal ulcers compared with placebo. One weak RCT found limited evidence that misoprostol reduced the number of people with NSAID induced gastric ulcers compared with 300 mg ranitidine daily.

Omeprazole in people who cannot avoid NSAIDs

One systematic review in people who had taken NSAIDs for at least 3 months found that omeprazole reduced endoscopically diagnosed gastric and duodenal ulcers compared with placebo.

TRADE OFF BETWEEN BENEFITS AND HARMS

Misoprostol in people who cannot avoid NSAIDs

One systematic review in people who had taken NSAIDs for at least 3 months found that misoprostol reduced gastric or duodenal ulcers compared with placebo. However, RCTs found that misoprostol increased clinical gastrointestinal adverse events, such as diarrhoea and abdominal pain compared with placebo. One RCT found no significant difference in the number of people taking NSAIDS and with proven gastric ulceration or erosion in successful response to treatment with misoprostol compared with omeprazole.

▶

What are the effects of topical NSAIDS?

BENEFICIAL

Topical NSAIDs in acute and chronic pain conditions
One systematic review in people with acute and chronic pain conditions found that topical NSAIDs reduced pain compared with placebo.

UNKNOWN EFFECTIVENESS

Topical versus systemic NSAIDs or alternative analgesics
One systematic review found no high quality RCTs of topical NSAIDs compared with oral forms of the same NSAID, or with paracetamol.

DEFINITION
Non-steroidal anti-inflammatory drugs (NSAIDs) have anti-inflammatory, analgesic, and antipyretic effects, and inhibit platelet aggregation. The drugs have no documented effect on the course of musculoskeletal diseases, such as osteoarthritis (Web only).

INCIDENCE/ PREVALENCE
NSAIDs are widely used. Almost 10% of people in the Netherlands used a non-aspirin NSAID in 1987, and the overall use was 11 defined daily doses per 1000 population per day.[1] In Australia in 1994, overall use was 35 defined daily doses per 1000 population per day, with 36% of the people receiving NSAIDs for osteoarthritis, 42% for sprain and strain or low back pain, and 4% for rheumatoid arthritis; 35% were aged over 60 years.[2]

Please refer to the Clinical Evidence website for full text and references.

Plantar heel pain and fasciitis

Search date August 2004

Fay Crawford

What are the effects of treatments for plantar heel pain?

UNKNOWN EFFECTIVENESS

Casted orthoses (custom made insoles)

One systematic review found no RCTs comparing the effects of casted orthoses versus placebo or no treatment. One RCT found no significant difference in pain between heel pad plus orthoses and corticosteroid injection plus local anaesthesia plus non-steroidal anti-inflammatory drugs. One RCT found that orthoses plus heel pads reduced pain compared with heel pads plus paracetamol at 8 weeks. One RCT found that heel pads plus stretching reduced pain compared with custom made orthoses plus stretching at 8 weeks. One RCT found that stretching plus heel pad (silicone insert, rubber insert, or felt insert) improved symptoms compared with stretching alone at 8 weeks. One RCT found no significant difference in pain between orthoses plus stretching (Achilles tendon stretching and plantar fascia stretching) and stretching alone after 8 weeks. One RCT provided insufficient evidence to compare orthoses versus night splints.

Corticosteroid injection (in the short term)

One systematic review identified no RCTs comparing short term effects of corticosteroid injections versus placebo, orthoses, heel pads, analgesic medication, or corticosteroid injection plus local anaesthesia. Observational studies found a high rate of plantar fascia rupture and other complications associated with corticosteroid injections, which may lead to chronic disability in some people.

Corticosteroid injection plus local anaesthetic injection in the short term (with or without non-steroidal anti-inflammatory drugs or heel pads)

One systematic review identified no RCTs comparing short term effects of corticosteroid injections plus local anaesthesia versus placebo or no treatment. RCTs provided insufficient evidence about clinically important short term effects of corticosteroids plus local anaesthesia (alone or combined with non-steroidal anti-inflammatory drugs or heel pads) compared with other treatments. Observational studies found a high rate of plantar fascia rupture and other complications associated with corticosteroid injections, which may lead to chronic disability in some people.

Extracorporeal shock wave therapy

One systematic review and four subsequent RCTs of extracorporeal shock wave therapy in people with heel pain found insufficient evidence to assess the effect on pain of extracorporeal shock wave therapy compared with placebo. Two RCTs found limited evidence that high dose extracorporeal shock wave therapy reduced pressure pain and walking pain scores compared with low dose therapy. However, the clinical importance of these effects is unclear.

Heel pads and heel cups

One systematic review found no RCTs on the effects of heel pads and heel cups compared with placebo, no treatment, or corticosteroid injection. One RCT found no significant difference in pain relief between heel pads and heel pads plus corticosteroid injection. One RCT provided insufficient evidence about clinically important effects of heel pads compared with corticosteroids plus local anaesthesia (alone or combined with non-steroidal anti-inflammatory drugs or heel pads). One RCT found that stretching plus heel pad (silicone insert, rubber insert, or felt insert) improved symptoms compared with stretching alone at 8 weeks. One RCT ▶

found that heel pads plus stretching reduced pain compared with custom made orthoses plus stretching at 8 weeks. One RCT found that heel pads plus orthoses reduced pain compared with heel pads plus paracetamol at 8 weeks.

Lasers

One small RCT identified by a systematic review found no significant difference between laser treatment and placebo.

Local anaesthetic injection

One systematic review identified no RCTs comparing local anaesthesia versus placebo or no treatment. One RCT found that combining local anaesthetic with a corticosteroid injection compared with local anaesthetic injection alone slightly improved pain score at 1 month. However, it found no significant difference in pain thereafter. The clinical importance of this result is unclear.

Night splints plus non-steroidal anti-inflammatory drugs

One RCT found no significant difference in pain between a night splint plus non-steroidal anti-inflammatory drugs and non-steroidal anti-inflammatory drugs alone after 3 months. There was insufficient evidence from one RCT comparing night splints versus orthoses.

Stretching exercises

One systematic review identified no RCTs comparing stretching exercises versus no treatment in people with heel pain. One RCT found no significant difference in pain between stretching alone (Achilles tendon stretching and plantar fascia stretching) and stretching plus orthoses after 8 weeks. One RCT found that stretching plus heel pad (silicone insert, rubber insert, or felt insert) improved symptoms compared with stretching alone at 8 weeks. One RCT found no significant difference in pain between sustained and intermittent Achilles tendon stretching exercises. One RCT found that plantar fascia stretching plus heel pad was more effective at reducing morning heel pain than Achilles tendon stretching plus heel pad.

Surgery

One systematic review found no RCTs of surgery for heel pain.

Ultrasound

One small RCT identified by a systematic review found no significant difference in pain between ultrasound and sham ultrasound.

LIKELY TO BE INEFFECTIVE OR HARMFUL

Corticosteroid injection in the medium to long term (with or without heel pad)

One systematic review identified no RCTs comparing medium to long term effects of corticosteroid injections versus placebo, orthoses, heel pads, analgesic medication, or corticosteroid injection plus local anaesthesia. One small RCT provided insufficient evidence about the long term effects of corticosteroid injection plus heel pad compared with placebo plus heel pad. Observational studies found a high rate of plantar fascia rupture and other complications associated with corticosteroid injections, which may lead to chronic disability in some people.

Corticosteroid injection plus local anaesthetic injection in the medium to long term (with or without non-steroidal anti-inflammatory drugs or heel pads)

One systematic review identified no RCTs comparing medium to long term effects of corticosteroid injections plus local anaesthesia versus placebo or no treatment. RCTs identified by the review provided insufficient evidence about clinically important long term effects of corticosteroids plus local anaesthesia (alone or combined with non-steroidal anti-inflammatory drugs or heel pads) compared with other

Plantar heel pain and fasciitis

treatments. Observational studies have found a high rate of plantar fascia rupture and other complications associated with corticosteroid injections, which may lead to chronic disability in some people.

DEFINITION   Plantar heel pain is soreness or tenderness of the heel that is restricted to the sole of the foot. It often radiates from the central part of the heel pad or the medial tubercle of the calcancum, but may extend along the plantar fascia into the medial longitudinal arch of the foot. Severity may range from an irritation at the origin of the plantar fascia, which is noticeable on rising after rest, to an incapacitating pain. This review excludes clinically evident underlying disorders, for example, infection, calcaneal fracture, and calcaneal nerve entrapment, which may be distinguished clinically — a calcaneal fracture may present after trauma, and calcaneal nerve entrapment gives rise to shooting pains and feelings of "pins and needles" on the medial aspect of the heel.

INCIDENCE/ PREVALENCE   The incidence and prevalence of plantar heel pain is uncertain. Plantar heel pain primarily affects those in mid to late life.[1]

AETIOLOGY/ RISK FACTORS   Unknown.

PROGNOSIS   One systematic review found that almost all of the included trials reported an improvement in discomfort regardless of the intervention received (including placebo), suggesting that the condition is at least partially self limiting.[1] A telephone survey of 100 people treated conservatively (average follow up 47 months) found that 82 people had resolution of symptoms, 15 had continued symptoms but no limitations of activity or work, and three had persistent bilateral symptoms that limited activity or changed work status.[2] Thirty one people said that they would have seriously considered surgical treatment at the time that medical attention was sought.

Please refer to the Clinical Evidence website for full text and references.

What are the effects of treatments for primary Raynaud's phenomenon?

TRADE OFF BETWEEN BENEFITS AND HARMS

Nifedipine

Six RCTs found that nifedipine reduced the frequency and severity of attacks over 4–12 weeks compared with placebo, and was rated by participants as more effective than placebo in improving overall symptoms. The RCTs found that nifedipine was associated with higher rates of adverse effects compared with placebo, including flushing, headache, oedema, and tachycardia.

UNKNOWN EFFECTIVENESS

Amlodipine

We found no satisfactory RCTs of the effects of amlodipine.

Diltiazem

We found no satisfactory RCTs of the effects of diltiazem.

Exercise

We found no satisfactory RCTs of the effects of exercise.

Inositol nicotinate

Two RCTs provided insufficient evidence to assess inositol nicotinate.

Keeping warm

We found no satisfactory RCTs of the effects of keeping warm.

Moxisylyte (thymoxamine)

We found no satisfactory RCTs of the effects of moxisylyte (thymoxamine).

Naftidrofuryl oxalate

One RCT found that, compared with placebo, naftidrofuryl oxalate reduced the duration and intensity of Raynaud's attacks over 2 months and reduced the impact of attacks on daily activities. However, we were unable to draw reliable conclusions from this single study.

Nicardipine

One RCT found that nicardipine decreased the frequency of Raynaud's attacks over 8 weeks after crossover compared with placebo, but found no significant difference in the severity of attacks. Another RCT found no significant difference in frequency, severity, or duration of attacks with nicardipine compared with placebo, but it is likely to have been too small to detect a clinically important difference in outcomes.

Prazosin

One small crossover RCT found limited evidence that prazosin reduced the number and duration of attacks over 6 weeks after crossover compared with placebo, but found no significant difference in the severity of attacks. However, we were unable to draw reliable conclusion from this single study.

Raynaud's phenomenon (primary)

DEFINITION Raynaud's phenomenon is episodic vasospasm of the peripheral arteries, causing pallor followed by cyanosis and redness with pain and sometimes paraesthesia, and, rarely, ulceration of the fingers and toes (and in some cases of the ears or nose). Primary or idiopathic Raynaud's phenomenon (Raynaud's disease) occurs without an underlying disease. Secondary Raynaud's phenomenon (Raynaud's syndrome) occurs in association with an underlying disease — usually connective tissue disorders such as scleroderma, systemic lupus erythematosus, rheumatoid arthritis, or polymyositis. This review excludes secondary Raynaud's phenomenon.

INCIDENCE/ PREVALENCE The prevalence of primary Raynaud's phenomenon varies by gender, country, and exposure to workplace vibration. One large US cohort study (4182 people) found symptoms in 9.6% of women and 8.1% of men, of whom 81% had primary Raynaud's phenomenon.[1] Smaller cohort studies in Spain have estimated the prevalence of Raynaud's phenomenon to be 3.7–4.0%, of which 90% is primary Raynaud's phenomenon.[2,3] One cohort study in Japan (332 men, 731 women) found symptoms of primary Raynaud's phenomenon in 3.4% of women and 3.0% of men.[4]

AETIOLOGY/ RISK FACTORS The cause of primary Raynaud's phenomenon is unknown.[5] There is evidence for genetic predisposition,[6,7] most likely in those people with early onset Raynaud's phenomenon (aged < 40 years).[8] One prospective observational study (424 people with Raynaud's phenomenon) found that 73% of sufferers first developed symptoms before age 40 years.[8] Women are more at risk than men (OR 3.0, 95% CI 1.2 to 7.8, in 1 US case control study [235 people]).[9] The other known risk factor is occupational exposure to vibration from tools (symptoms developed in about 8% with exposure v 2.7% with no exposure in 2 cohorts from Japan).[10,11] People who are obese may be less at risk.[9] Symptoms are often worsened by cold or emotion.

PROGNOSIS Attacks may last from several minutes to a few hours. One systematic review (search date 1996, 10 prospective observational studies, 639 people with primary Raynaud's phenomenon) found that 13% of long term sufferers later manifested an underlying disorder such as scleroderma.[12]

Please refer to the Clinical Evidence website for full text and references.

What are the effects of treatments?

Shoulder pain is not a specific diagnosis. Well designed, double blind RCTs of specific interventions in specific shoulder disorders are needed. Systematic reviews have found RCTs mostly with poor methods, and pronounced heterogeneity of study populations and outcome measures. We found insufficient evidence on the effects of most interventions in people with non-specific shoulder pain.

LIKELY TO BE BENEFICIAL

Laser treatment

One systematic review found three small RCTs. Two of the RCTs found that laser improved pain after 2–3 weeks compared with placebo, and one RCT found no significant difference at 8 weeks between treatments, although it may have lacked power to detect a difference. One additional RCT found that laser significantly increased recovery rates at 1 month compared with placebo.

Physiotherapy (manual treatments and exercises)

One RCT in people with mixed shoulder disorders found that physiotherapy improved function at 4 weeks compared with no treatment. One RCT in people with rotator cuff disease found that a supervised exercise regimen plus advice on pain management improved pain and function compared with no exercise regimen at 6 months and 2.5 years. One RCT in people with adhesive capsulitis found that intra-articular steroids improved pain and function at 6 weeks compared with physiotherapy, although the magnitude of effect declined by 12 months.

Surgical arthroscopic decompression/forced manipulation

One RCT found that arthroscopic decompression by experienced surgeons followed by physiotherapy improved pain and function compared with sham laser but not compared with supervised exercises at 6 months and 2.5 years. One small RCT found that forced manipulation plus intra-articular hydrocortisone injection increased recovery rate at 3 months compared with intra-articular hydrocortisone injection alone.

UNKNOWN EFFECTIVENESS

Arthroscopic laser subacromial decompression

One systematic review found no RCTs on arthroscopic laser subacromial decompression.

Electrical stimulation

Three small RCTs provided insufficient evidence about the effects of electrical stimulation in people with shoulder pain.

Extracorporeal shock wave therapy

Small and limited RCTs provided insufficient evidence about the effects of extracorporeal shock wave therapy compared with sham treatment or no treatment in people with non-calcifying rotator cuff tendinosis and chronic supraspinatus tendinosis. There was limited evidence of benefit in people with calcific tendinitis.

Ice

One small RCT provided insufficient evidence about the effects of ice.

Shoulder pain

Intra-articular corticosteroid injection

We found inconclusive evidence about the effects of intra-articular steroids, with or without local anaesthetic or physiotherapy, compared with placebo or physiotherapy alone in people with shoulder pain.

Intra-articular guanethidine

We found no systematic review or RCTs of intra-articular guanethidine in people with non-arthritic shoulder pain.

Multidisciplinary biopsychosocial rehabilitation

One systematic review found no good quality RCTs of multidisciplinary biopsychosocial rehabilitation in people with shoulder pain.

Oral corticosteroids

Two small RCTs found no evidence of reduced pain or improved abduction with oral corticosteroids compared with placebo or no treatment at 4–8 months. Adverse effects of corticosteroids are well documented (see rheumatoid arthritis [Web only], and asthma, p 432).

Oral non-steroidal anti-inflammatory drugs

One systematic review and one additional RCT provided insufficient evidence to draw reliable conclusions about the effects of oral non-steroidal anti-inflammatory drugs compared with placebo in people with non-specific shoulder pain.

Phonophoresis

We found no RCTs solely in people with shoulder pain.

Subacromial corticosteroid injection

We found no RCTs comparing subacromial injection of steroids versus placebo. Three small RCTs in people with rotator cuff tendinitis and one small RCT in people with subacromial impingement provided insufficient evidence to compare the clinical effects of corticosteroid plus lidocaine versus lidocaine alone. One RCT found no significant difference between subacromial steroid plus lidocaine and physiotherapyin terms of disability or successful outcome at 6 months in people attending their general practitioner because of a new episode of unilateral shoulder pain, but found that steroid injection increased the need for repeat consultation or other intervention.

Transdermal glyceryl trinitrate

We found no reliable RCTs.

Paracetamol or opiates; topical or intra-articular non-steroidal anti-inflammatory drugs

We found no RCTs about these interventions.

UNLIKELY TO BE BENEFICIAL

Ultrasound

One RCT identified by a systematic review found that ultrasound significantly improved pain and quality of life at the end of treatment (6 weeks) in people with calcific tendinitis, but found no significant difference at 9 months. Four other RCTs identified by the review found no significant difference between ultrasound and sham ultrasound, but may have been too small to detect a clinically important difference.

DEFINITION Shoulder pain arises in or around the shoulder from the glenohumeral, acromioclavicular, sternoclavicular, "subacromial", and scapulothoracic articulations, and surrounding soft tissues. Regardless of the disorder, pain is the most common reason for consulting a practitioner. In adhesive capsulitis (frozen shoulder), pain is associated with pronounced restriction of movement. For most shoulder disorders, diagnosis is based on clinical features, with imaging studies playing a role in some people. Post-stroke shoulder pain is not addressed in this chapter.

INCIDENCE/ Each year in primary care in the UK, about 1% of adults aged over 45 years
PREVALENCE present with a new episode of shoulder pain.[1] Prevalence is uncertain, with estimates from 4–20%.[2-6] One community survey (392 people) found a 1 month prevalence of shoulder pain of 34%.[7] A second community survey (644 people aged ≥ 70 years) reported a point prevalence of 21%, with a higher frequency in women than men (25% v 17%).[8] Seventy per cent of cases involved the rotator cuff. One survey of 134 people in a community based rheumatology clinic found that 65% of cases were rotator cuff lesions; 11% were caused by localised tenderness in the pericapsular musculature; 10% acromioclavicular joint pain; 3% glenohumeral joint arthritis; and 5% were referred pain from the neck.[9] One survey found that, in adults, the annual incidence of frozen shoulder was about 2%, with those aged 40–70 years most commonly affected.[10] The age distribution of specific shoulder disorders in the community is unknown.

AETIOLOGY/ Rotator cuff disorders are associated with excessive overloading, instability of
RISK FACTORS the glenohumeral and acromioclavicular joints, muscle imbalance, adverse anatomical features (narrow coracoacromial arch and a hooked acromion), cuff degeneration with ageing, ischaemia, and musculoskeletal diseases that result in wasting of the cuff muscles.[11 14] Risk factors for frozen shoulder include female sex, older age, shoulder trauma, surgery, diabetes, cardiorespiratory disorders, cerebrovascular events, thyroid disease, and hemiplegia.[10,15,16] Arthritis of the glenohumeral joint can occur in numerous forms, including primary and secondary osteoarthritis, rheumatoid arthritis, and crystal arthritides.[11]

PROGNOSIS One survey in an elderly community found that most people with shoulder pain were still affected 3 years after the initial survey.[17] One prospective cohort study of 122 people in primary care found that 25% of people with shoulder pain reported previous episodes and 49% reported full recovery at 18 months' follow up.[18]

Please refer to the Clinical Evidence website for full text and references.

Tennis elbow

Search date April 2003

Willem Assendelft, Sally Green, Rachelle Buchbinder, Peter Struijs, and Nynke Smidt

---

What are the effects of treatments?

BENEFICIAL

Topical non-steroidal anti-inflammatory drugs for short term pain relief

One systematic review has found that topical non-steroidal anti-inflammatory drugs improve pain in the short term compared with placebo. Minor adverse effects have been reported. We found no RCTs comparing oral versus topical non-steroidal anti-inflammatory drugs.

LIKELY TO BE BENEFICIAL

Oral non-steroidal anti-inflammatory drugs for short term pain relief

One systematic review found limited evidence that an oral non-steroidal anti-inflammatory drug reduced pain and improved function compared with placebo in the short term, although we found limited evidence that it was less effective than corticosteroid injection in the short term.

TRADE OFF BETWEEN BENEFITS AND HARMS

Corticosteroid injections

One systematic review and subsequent RCTs of corticosteroid injections found limited evidence of a short term improvement in symptoms with steroid injections compared with placebo, a local anaesthetic, orthoses (elbow strapping), physiotherapy, or oral non-steroidal anti-inflammatory drugs. We found no good evidence on long term effects of corticosteroids compared with placebo, local anaesthetic, physiotherapy (mobilisation plus massage) or elbow strapping, and found limited evidence that corticosteroid injection was less effective than physiotherapy or oral non-steroidal anti-inflammatory drugs in the long term.

UNKNOWN EFFECTIVENESS

Acupuncture

We found insufficient evidence from small, methodologically weak RCTs about effects of needle acupuncture, laser acupuncture, or electro-acupuncture) in people with tennis elbow.

Exercise and mobilisation

One small RCT identified by a systematic review found limited evidence that exercise reduced symptoms at 8 weeks compared with ultrasound plus friction massage. However, we were unable to draw reliable conclusions from this small study.

Non-steroidal anti-inflammatory drugs for longer term pain relief

We found insufficient evidence to assess the longer term effects of oral or topical non-steroidal anti-inflammatory drugs, although one RCT found that non-steroidal anti-inflammatory drugs were more effective than corticosteroid injections in the long term.

Orthoses

One systematic review found insufficient evidence about the effects of orthoses (braces) compared with placebo or physiotherapy. It found limited evidence of s short term improvement in symptoms compared with corticosteroid injections.

▶

◀ **Surgery**

One systematic review found no RCTs of surgical treatment.

UNLIKELY TO BE BENEFICIAL

Extracorporeal shock wave therapy

One systematic review and one subsequent RCT found no significant difference in symptoms between extracorporeal shock wave therapy and sham treatment at 3 months.

DEFINITION Tennis elbow has many analogous terms, including lateral elbow pain, lateral epicondylitis, rowing elbow, tendonitis of the common extensor origin, and peritendinitis of the elbow. Tennis elbow is characterised by pain and tenderness over the lateral epicondyle of the humerus and pain on resisted dorsiflexion of the wrist, middle finger, or both. For the purposes of this review, tennis elbow is restricted to lateral elbow pain or lateral epicondylitis.

INCIDENCE/ Lateral elbow pain is common (population prevalence 1–3%).[1] Peak inci-
PREVALENCE dence is at 40–50 years of age and for women of 42–46 years of age the incidence increases to 10%.[2,3] The incidence of lateral elbow pain in general practice is 4–7/1000 people a year.[3–5]

AETIOLOGY/ Tennis elbow is considered to be an overload injury, typically after minor and
RISK FACTORS often unrecognised trauma of the extensor muscles of the forearm. Despite the title tennis elbow, tennis is a direct cause in only 5% of those with lateral epicondylitis.[6]

PROGNOSIS Although lateral elbow pain is generally self limiting, in a minority of people symptoms persist for 18 months to 2 years and in some cases for much longer.[7] The cost is therefore high, both in terms of lost productivity, and healthcare use. In a general practice trial of an expectant waiting policy, 80% of the people with elbow pain of already greater than 4 weeks' duration had recovered after 1 year.[8]

Please refer to the Clinical Evidence website for full text and references.

Altitude sickness

Search date status January 2004

David Murdoch

What are the effects of interventions to prevent acute mountain sickness?

Acetazolamide

One systematic review and one subsequent RCT found that acetazolamide reduced the incidence of acute mountain sickness compared with placebo. The review found that acetazolamide caused polyuria and/or paraesthesia in over a third of people. We found no RCTs of sufficient quality comparing acetazolamide versus dexamethasone.

Dexamethasone

One systematic review and further RCTs found that dexamethasone was more effective than placebo for preventing acute mountain sickness. However, the review found that adverse effects (including depression) occurred in a quarter of people on withdrawal of dexamethasone. We found no RCTs of sufficient quality comparing dexamethasone versus acetazolamide.

Slow ascent (or acclimatisation)*

We found no RCTs evaluating different rates of ascent or acclimatisation. One non-randomised trial, observational studies, and consensus opinion suggest that slower ascent reduces the risk of acute mountain sickness compared with more rapid ascent.

What are the effects of treatments for acute mountain sickness?

Descent compared with resting at the same altitude*

We found no RCTs on the effects of descent compared with resting at the same altitude in people with acute mountain sickness. Consensus opinion suggests that people with acute mountain sickness should descend if possible. However, we found no RCTs examining the effects of different distances of descent, or about the balance of risks and benefits in people who might find it difficult to descend.

Dexamethasone

One small RCT in climbers with symptoms and signs of acute mountain sickness found that dexamethasone reduced mean acute mountain sickness scores compared with placebo.

Acetazolamide

We found no RCTs of sufficient quality on the effects of acetazolamide compared with placebo for treating people with acute mountain sickness.

*Although we found no RCTs on the effects of these interventions, there is a general consensus that they are effective.

DEFINITION
Altitude sickness (or high altitude illness) includes acute mountain sickness, high altitude pulmonary oedema, and high altitude cerebral oedema. Acute mountain sickness typically occurs at altitudes greater than 2500 metres (about 8000 feet) and is characterised by the development of some or all of the symptoms of headache, weakness, fatigue, listlessness, nausea, insomnia, and suppressed appetite. Symptoms may take days to develop or may occur within hours, depending on the rate of ascent and the altitude attained. More severe forms of altitude sickness have been identified. High altitude pulmonary oedema is characterised by symptoms and signs typical of pulmonary oedema, such as shortness of breath, coughing, and production of frothy or blood stained sputum. High altitude cerebral oedema is characterised by confusion, ataxia, and decreasing conscious level. This review covers only acute mountain sickness.

INCIDENCE/ PREVALENCE
The incidence of acute mountain sickness increases with absolute height attained and with the rate of ascent. One survey in Taiwan (93 people ascending above 3000 metres) found that 27% of people experienced acute mountain sickness.[1] One survey in the Himalayas (278 unacclimatised hikers at 4243 metres) found that 53% of people developed acute mountain sickness.[2] One survey in the Swiss Alps (466 climbers at 4 altitudes between 2850 metres and 4559 metres) found the prevalence of two or more symptoms of acute mountain sickness to be 9% of people at 2850 metres; 13% of people at 3050 metres; 34% of people at 3650 metres; and 53% of people at 4559 metres.[3]

AETIOLOGY/ RISK FACTORS
The Himalayan study identified the rate of ascent and absolute height attained as the only risk factors.[2] It found no evidence of a difference in risk between men and women, or that previous episodes of altitude experience, load carried, or recent respiratory infections affected risk. However, the study was too small to exclude these as risk factors or to quantify risks reliably. One systematic review of RCTs (search date 1999) comparing prophylactic agents versus placebo found that, among people receiving placebo, the incidence of acute mountain sickness was higher with a faster rate of ascent (54% of people at a mean ascent rate of 91 metres/hour; 73% at a mean ascent rate of 1268 metres/hour; 89% at a simulated ascent rate in a hypobaric chamber of 1647 metres/hour).[4] One survey in Switzerland (827 mountaineers ascending to 4559 metres) examined the effects of susceptibility, pre-exposure, and ascent rate on acute mountain sickness.[5] In this study, pre-exposure was defined as having spent more than 4 days above 3000 metres in the preceding 2 months, and slow ascent was defined as ascending in more than 3 days. It found that in susceptible people (who had previously had acute mountain sickness at high altitude) the prevalence of acute mountain sickness was 58% with rapid ascent and no pre-exposure, 29% with pre-exposure only, 33% with slow ascent only, and 7% with both pre-exposure and slow ascent.[5] In non-susceptible people, the corresponding values were 31%, 16%, 11%, and 4%. The overall odds ratio for developing acute mountain sickness in susceptible compared with non-susceptible people was 2.9, 95% CI 2.1 to 4.1.[5]

PROGNOSIS
We found no reliable data on prognosis. It is widely held that if no further ascent is attempted, the symptoms of acute mountain sickness tend to resolve over a few days. We found no reliable data about long term sequelae in people whose symptoms have completely resolved.

Please refer to the Clinical Evidence website for full text and references.

Epilepsy

Search date November 2003

Anthony Marson and Sridharan Ramaratnam

Should single seizures be treated?

TRADE OFF BETWEEN BENEFITS AND HARMS

Antiepileptic drugs after a single seizure

RCTs found that treatment of a single seizure with antiepileptic drugs reduced seizure recurrence at 2 years compared with no treatment. However, we found no evidence that treatment alters long term prognosis. Long term antiepileptic drug treatment is potentially harmful.

What are the effects of monotherapy in newly diagnosed partial epilepsy?

BENEFICIAL

Antiepileptic monotherapy in partial epilepsy*

We found no placebo controlled RCTs of the main antiepileptic drugs (carbamazepine, phenobarbital, phenytoin, sodium valproate) used as monotherapy in people with partial epilepsy, but widespread consensus holds that these drugs are effective. Systematic reviews found no reliable evidence on which to base a choice among drugs in terms of seizure control. Systematic reviews found that phenobarbital was more likely to be withdrawn than phenytoin or carbamazepine.

What are the effects of monotherapy in newly diagnosed generalised epilepsy?

BENEFICIAL

Antiepileptic monotherapy in generalised epilepsy*

We found no placebo controlled trials of the main antiepileptic drugs (carbamazepine, phenobarbital, phenytoin, sodium valproate), but widespread consensus holds that these drugs are effective. Systematic reviews found insufficient evidence on which to base a choice among these drugs in terms of seizure control.

Does the addition of second line drugs benefit people with drug resistant partial epilepsy?

BENEFICIAL

Addition of second line drugs (gabapentin, levetiracetam, lamotrigine, oxcarbazepine, tiagabine, topiramate, vigabatrin, or zonisamide) for drug resistant partial epilepsy

Systematic reviews in people with drug resistant partial epilepsy found that adding gabapentin, levetiracetam, lamotrigine, oxcarbazepine, tiagabine, topiramate, vigabatrin, or zonisamide to usual treatment reduced seizure frequency compared with adding placebo. The reviews found that adding any of the drugs increased the frequency of adverse effects compared with adding placebo. We found no good evidence from RCTs on which to base a choice among drugs.

▶

Which people in remission from seizures are at risk of relapse on withdrawal of drug treatment?

Antiepileptic drug withdrawal for people in remission

One RCT in people who had been seizure free for at least 2 years found that further seizures were more likely if people stopped treatment than if they continued antiepileptic medication. Clinical predictors of relapse after drug withdrawal included age, seizure type, number of antiepileptic drugs being taken, whether seizures had occurred since antiepileptic drugs were started, and the period of remission before drug withdrawal.

What are the effects of behavioural and psychological treatments for people with epilepsy?

Educational programmes

One RCT found that a 2 day educational programme reduced seizure frequency at 6 months compared with waiting list control. However, it found no significant difference in health related quality of life. RCTs found that educational packages improved knowledge and understanding of epilepsy, adjustment to epilepsy, and psychosocial functioning compared with control.

Biofeedback

One systematic review provided insufficient evidence about the effects of electro-encephalographic biofeedback.

Cognitive behavioural therapy

Two small RCTs provided insufficient evidence about the effects of cognitive behavioural therapy in people with epilepsy.

Family counselling

One small RCT with methodological weaknesses provided insufficient evidence about the effects of family counselling.

Relaxation plus behavioural modification therapy

One systematic review provided insufficient evidence about the effects of combined relaxation and behavioural modification treatment on seizures.

Relaxation therapy

Systematic reviews provided insufficient evidence on the effects of relaxation therapy in people with epilepsy.

Yoga

One systematic review provided insufficient evidence about effects of yoga in people with epilepsy.

Epilepsy

What are the effects of surgery in people with drug resistant temporal lobe epilepsy? New

BENEFICIAL

Temporal lobectomy* New

One RCT identified by a systematic review found that temporal lobectomy improved seizure control and quality of life after 1 year compared with continued medical treatment in people with poorly controlled temporal lobe epilepsy. There is consensus that temporal lobectomy is beneficial for people with drug resistant temporal lobe epilepsy.

LIKELY TO BE BENEFICIAL

Amygdalohippocampectomy* New

We found no systematic review and no RCTs that examined the effect of amygdalohippocampectomy for people with drug resistant temporal lobe epilepsy. However, there is consensus that amygdalohippocampectomy is likely to be beneficial for people with drug resistant temporal lobe epilepsy.

UNKNOWN EFFECTIVENESS

Lesionectomy New

We found no systematic review and no RCTs that examined the effects of lesionectomy in people with drug resistant temporal lobe epilepsy thought to be caused by a known cerebral lesion.

*Categorisation based on consensus.

DEFINITION	Epilepsy is a group of disorders rather than a single disease. Seizures can be classified by type as partial (categorised as simple partial, complex partial, and secondary generalised tonic clonic seizures), or generalised (categorised as generalised tonic clonic, absence, myoclonic, tonic, and atonic seizures).[1]
INCIDENCE/ PREVALENCE	Epilepsy is common, with an estimated prevalence in the developed world of 5–10/1000, and an annual incidence of 50/100 000 people.[2] About 3% of people will be given a diagnosis of epilepsy at some time in their lives.[3]
AETIOLOGY/ RISK FACTORS	Epilepsy can also be classified by cause.[1] Idiopathic generalised epilepsies (such as juvenile myoclonic epilepsy or childhood absence epilepsy) are largely genetic. Symptomatic epilepsies result from a known cerebral abnormality; for example, temporal lobe epilepsy may result from a congenital defect, mesial temporal sclerosis, or a tumour. Cryptogenic epilepsies are those that cannot be classified as idiopathic or symptomatic and in which no causative factor has been identified, but is suspected.
PROGNOSIS	For most people with epilepsy the prognosis is good. About 70% go into remission, defined as being seizure free for 5 years on or off treatment. This leaves 20–30% who develop chronic epilepsy, which is often treated with multiple antiepileptic drugs.[4] About 60% of untreated people have no further seizures in the 2 years after their first seizure.[5]

Please refer to the Clinical Evidence website for full text and references.

Search date March 2004

Joaquim Ferreira and Cristina Sampaio

We found few RCTs that assessed long term effects of drug treatments for essential tremor.

What are the effects of drug treatments in people with essential tremor of the hand?

LIKELY TO BE BENEFICIAL

Propranolol

Small RCTs found that propranolol for up to 1 month improved clinical scores, tremor amplitude, and self evaluation of severity at up to 6 weeks compared with placebo. One RCT comparing propranolol versus clonidine found that the initial improvement in tremor from baseline was similar with both drugs and was maintained throughout follow up for 1 year. RCTs provided insufficient evidence to compare propranolol versus other β blockers.

Topiramate (improved tremor scores after 2 weeks' treatment but associated with appetite suppression, weight loss, and paraesthesia)

One RCT found limited evidence that topiramate improved observer rated tremor score after 2 weeks' treatment compared with placebo but was associated with adverse effects, including appetite suppression, weight loss, and paraesthesia. The clinical importance of the difference in tremor score is uncertain. We found no RCTs addressing long term outcomes.

TRADE OFF BETWEEN BENEFITS AND HARMS

Phenobarbital (improved tremor at 5 weeks but associated with depression and cognitive adverse effects)

One small RCT found that phenobarbital improved tremor at 5 weeks compared with placebo. However, another two RCTs found no significant difference in tremor scores at 4–5 weeks between phenobarbital and placebo. Phenobarbital is associated with depression and cognitive and behavioural adverse effects.

Primidone (improved tremor and function at 5 weeks compared with placebo and at 1 year compared with baseline but associated with depression and cognitive adverse effects)

Three small, short term RCTs found limited evidence that primidone improved tremor and functional ability over 4–10 weeks compared with placebo. One RCT comparing different doses of primidone found that it improved tremor from baseline at 1 year with no significant difference in outcome between groups. Primidone is associated with depression and cognitive and behavioural adverse effects.

Botulinum A toxin–haemagglutinin complex (improves clinical rating scales at 4–12 weeks but associated with hand weakness)

Two RCTs in people with essential hand tremor found that botulinum A toxin–haemagglutinin complex improved clinical rating scales at 4–12 weeks. They found no consistent improvement in motor tasks or functional disability. Hand weakness, which is dose dependent and transient, is a frequent adverse effect. We found no RCTs addressing long term outcomes.

Benzodiazepines

Two small short term RCTs found weak evidence that alprazolam may improve tremor and function at 2–4 weeks compared with placebo. However, we were unable to draw reliable conclusions about effects. One very small RCT provided insufficient evidence to compare clonazepam versus placebo. Adverse effects with benzodiazepines, including dependency, sedation and cognitive and behavioural effects, have been well described for other conditions (see panic disorder, p 304).

Calcium channel blockers (dihydropyridine)

Poor quality RCTs provided insufficient evidence to compare the dihydropyridine calcium channel blockers nicardipine and nimodipine versus placebo.

Carbonic anhydrase inhibitors

Small RCTs provided insufficient evidence to assess methazolamide or acetazolamide in people with essential tremor. We found no RCTs addressing long term outcomes.

Clonidine

One RCT found no significant difference between clonidine and placebo in essential hand tremor. However, the study lacked power to rule out a clinically important difference. Another RCT comparing clonidine versus propranolol found that the initial improvement in tremor from baseline was similar with both drugs and was maintained throughout follow up for 1 year.

Flunarizine

One small RCT found weak evidence that flunarizine reduced the symptoms of essential hand tremor after 1 months' treatment compared with placebo.

Gabapentin

Small RCTs provided insufficient evidence to compare gabapentin versus placebo. We found no RCTs addressing long term outcomes.

Isoniazid *New*

One RCT found no significant difference between isoniazid and placebo in essential hand tremor, but it may have lacked power to detect a clinically important difference. We found no RCTs addressing long term outcomes.

β Blockers other than propranolol (atenolol, metoprolol, nadolol, pindolol, and sotalol)

Three small RCTs found weak evidence that atenolol or sotalol improved symptoms and self evaluated measures of tremor at 5 days to 4 weeks compared with placebo. One small RCT found no significant difference in symptoms between metoprolol and placebo and another small RCT found that pindolol worsened tremor amplitude compared with placebo. A third very small RCT provided insufficient evidence to compare nadolol versus placebo. RCTs provided insufficient evidence to compare other β blockers versus propranolol.

Mirtazapine *New*

One RCT in people taking antitremor drugs such as propranolol, found no significant difference in tremor between adding mirtazapine and placebo and found that adverse effects were frequent.

DEFINITION   Tremor is a rhythmic, mechanical oscillation of at least one body region. The term essential tremor is used when there is either a persistent bilateral tremor of hands and forearms, or an isolated tremor of the head without abnormal posturing, and when there is no evidence that the tremor arises from another identifiable cause. The diagnosis is not made if there are abnormal neurological signs; known causes of enhanced physiological tremor; a history or signs of psychogenic tremor; sudden change in severity; primary orthostatic tremor; isolated voice tremor; isolated position specific or task specific tremors; and isolated tongue, chin, or leg tremor.[1]

INCIDENCE/   Essential tremor is one of the most common movement disorders throughout
PREVALENCE   the world, with a prevalence of 0.4–3.9% in the general population.[2]

AETIOLOGY/   Essential tremor is sometimes inherited with an autosomal dominant pattern.
RISK FACTORS   About 40% of people with essential tremor have no family history. Alcohol ingestion provides symptomatic benefit in 50–70% of people.[3]

PROGNOSIS   Essential tremor is a persistent and progressive condition. It usually begins during early adulthood and the severity of the tremor increases slowly. Only a small proportion of people with essential tremor seek medical advice, but the proportion in different surveys varies from 0.5–11%.[2] Most people with essential tremor are only mildly affected. However, most of the people who seek medical care are disabled to some extent, and most are socially handicapped by the tremor.[3] A quarter of people receiving medical care for the tremor change jobs or retire because of essential tremor induced disability.[4,5]

Please refer to the Clinical Evidence website for full text and references.

Migraine headache

Search date August 2003

Luis E Morillo

What are the effects of drug treatment?

BENEFICIAL

Eletriptan

One systematic review and subsequent RCTs have found that eletriptan increases headache relief at 2 hours compared with placebo. One systematic review and subsequent RCTs have found that eletriptan 40 and 80 mg increases headache relief at 2 hours compared with sumatriptan 50 and 100 mg. One RCT has found that eletriptan 40 and 80 mg increases headache relief at 2 hours compared with ergotamine plus caffeine.

Ibuprofen

Five RCTs have found that ibuprofen improves migraine symptoms compared with placebo.

Naratriptan

One systematic review and subsequent RCTs have found that naratriptan increases headache relief at 2 hours compared with placebo. One systematic review has found that sumatriptan 100 mg increases headache relief at 2 hours compared with naratriptan 2.5 mg. However, one subsequent RCT found no significant difference in headache recurrence. One RCT found no significant difference between naratriptan 2.5 mg and zolmitriptan 2.5 mg in headache relief at 4 hours. One RCT identified by a systematic review found that naratriptal reduced headache relief at 2 hours compared with nizatriptan.

Rizatriptan

One systematic review and subsequent RCTs have found that rizatriptan improves headache relief compared with placebo. Two RCTs found no significant difference between rizatriptan and zolmitriptan in headache relief at 2 hours. One RCT identified by a systematic review has found that rizatriptan increases headache relief at 2 hours compared with naratriptan. One RCT has found that rizatriptan increases headache relief and reduces nausea and vomiting at 2 hours compared with ergotamine plus caffeine.

Salicylates

RCTs have found that oral or intravenous salicylates (alone or in combination with metoclopramide, paracetamol, or caffeine) increase headache relief compared with placebo. One RCT found no significant difference between aspirin and paracetamol plus codeine in headache relief. One RCT found no significant difference between aspirin plus metoclopramide and sumatriptan in headache relief. One RCT has found that oral lysine acetylsalicylate plus metoclopramide increases headache relief and reduces nausea and vomiting at 2 hours compared with ergotamine plus caffeine. One RCT found no significant difference in headache relief between aspirin plus metoclopramide and zolmitriptan.

Sumatriptan

Systematic reviews and subsequent RCTs have found that subcutaneous, oral, or intranasal sumatriptan increases headache relief compared with placebo. RCTs found no significant difference in headache relief between sumatriptan and aspirin plus metoclopramide, tolfenamic acid, or zolmitriptan. RCTs have found that oral or nasal sumatriptan increase headache relief compared with oral or nasal ergotamine. One systematic review has found that sumatriptan 100 mg increases headache relief at 2 hours compared with naratriptan 2.5 mg. However, one subsequent RCT found no significant difference in headache recurrence. One systematic review and subsequent RCTs have found that eletriptan 40 and 80 mg increases headache relief at 2 hours compared with sumatriptan 50 and 100 mg.

Zolmitriptan

One systematic review and two subsequent RCTs have found that oral zolmitriptan increases headache relief compared with placebo. One systematic review and two subsequent RCTs found no significant difference between zolmitriptan and sumatriptan in headache relief. One RCT found no significant difference in headache relief between aspirin plus metoclopramide and zolmitriptan. One RCT found no significant difference between naratriptan 2.5 mg and zolmitriptan 2.5 mg in headache relief at 4 hours.

LIKELY TO BE BENEFICIAL

Diclofenac

RCTs have found that oral or intramuscular diclofenac improves headache symptoms compared with placebo. One RCT has found that intramuscular diclofenac improves migraine symptoms compared with intramuscular paracetamol.

Ergotamine

One systematic review found limited evidence from four RCTs that ergotamine (with or without caffeine) improved headache relief compared with placebo. One overview of harms suggested that ergotamine increased nausea and vomiting compared with placebo. RCTs have found that ergotamine (or its derivatives, with or without caffeine and cyclizine) is less effective for migraine symptoms than sumatriptan. They found limited evidence that it was less effective than naproxen. RCTs found that ergotamine plus caffeine reduced headache relief and increased nausea and vomiting at 2 hours compared with oral lysine acetylsalicylate plus metoclopramide and rizatriptan.

Naproxen

Three small RCTs have found that naproxen reduces migraine symptoms compared with placebo. Two RCTs have found that naproxen reduces symptoms compared with ergotamine (with or without caffeine plus cyclizine). However, one further RCT found no significant difference between naproxen and ergotamine in pain relief after 1 hour.

Tolfenamic acid

RCTs found limited evidence that tolfenamic acid improved duration and severity of headache compared with placebo. RCTs found no significant difference in symptom relief between tolfenamic acid and sumatriptan or paracetamol.

DEFINITION   Migraine is a primary headache disorder manifesting as recurring attacks usually lasting for 4–72 hours and involving pain of moderate to severe intensity, often with nausea, sometimes vomiting, and/or sensitivity to light, sound, and other sensory stimuli. The 1988 International Headache Society criteria include separate criteria for migraine with and migraine without associated aura.[1] Unless stated otherwise, RCTs used International Headache Society criteria for migraine with or without aura.

INCIDENCE/   Migraine is common worldwide. Prevalence has been reported to be 5–25%
PREVALENCE   in women and 2–10% in men. Overall, the highest incidence for migraine without aura has been reported between the ages of 10 and 11 years (10/1000 person years). The peak incidence of migraine without aura in males is between ages 10 and 11 years (10/1000 person years) and in females between ages 14 and 17 years (19/1000 person years).[2] The incidence of migraine with aura peaks in males at about age 5 years (7/1000 ▶

person years) and in females at about age 12–13 years (14/1000 person years).[2] Female prevalence of migraine with or without aura has a declining trend after age 45–50 years.

AETIOLOGY/ RISK FACTORS Data from independent representative samples from Canada,[3,4] the USA,[5,6] several countries in Latin America,[7] several countries in Europe,[8-11] Hong Kong,[12] and Japan[13] show a female to male predominance and a peak in middle aged women. Migraine has been reported to be 50% more likely in people with a family history of migraine.[14]

PROGNOSIS Acute migraine is self limiting and only rarely results in permanent neurological complications. Chronic recurrent migraine may cause disability through pain, and may affect daily functioning and quality of life.

Please refer to the Clinical Evidence website for full text and references.

We found no evidence from RCTs that any treatment alters long term outcome in multiple sclerosis.

What are the effects of interventions aimed at reducing relapse rates and disability?

LIKELY TO BE BENEFICIAL

Glatiramer acetate

One RCT in people with relapsing and remitting multiple sclerosis found that glatiramer acetate reduced relapse rates over 2 years compared with placebo but found no effect on disability. We found no good quality RCTs in people with secondary progressive multiple sclerosis.

Interferon beta

Two RCTs in people experiencing a first demyelinating event found that interferon beta-1a decreased the risk of conversion to clinically definite multiple sclerosis over 2–3 years compared with placebo. One systematic review in people with active relapsing remitting multiple sclerosis found limited evidence that interferon beta-1a/b reduced exacerbations and disease progression over 2 years compared with placebo. One subsequent RCT in people with relapsing remitting multiple sclerosis found that interferon beta-1b reduced the proportion of people with relapse over 2 years compared with interferon beta-1a. Three RCTs provided insufficient evidence to assess the effects of interferon beta on disease progression in people with secondary progressive multiple sclerosis.

UNKNOWN EFFECTIVENESS

Azathioprine

One systematic review in people with relapsing and remitting or progressive multiple sclerosis comparing azathioprine versus placebo or no treatment found a modest reduction in relapse rates over 2 years but no evidence of a difference in disability. However, we were unable to draw reliable conclusions because of clinical heterogeneity among the included RCTs.

Intravenous immunoglobulin

One RCT in people with relapsing and remitting multiple sclerosis found that intravenous immunoglobulin reduced disability over 2 years compared with placebo. However, the clinical importance of this reduction is unclear. We found no good quality RCTs in people with secondary progressive multiple sclerosis.

Methotrexate

One small RCT provided insufficient evidence to assess the effects of methotrexate in reducing relapse rates and disability in people with multiple sclerosis.

TRADE OFF BETWEEN BENEFITS AND HARMS

Mitoxantrone

One RCT in people with worsening, relapsing, remitting, or progressive multiple sclerosis found that mitoxantrone reduced progression of disability over 2 years compared with placebo. One small RCT in people with active multiple sclerosis found limited evidence that mitoxantrone plus methylprednisolone reduced relapse over 6 months compared with methylprednisolone alone. However, mitoxantrone is associated with leukopenia, menstrual disorders, and arrhythmia. ▶

Multiple sclerosis

What are the effects of treatments for acute relapse?

LIKELY TO BE BENEFICIAL

Corticosteroids (methylprednisolone or corticotrophin)
One systematic review in people with multiple sclerosis requiring treatment for acute exacerbations found that corticosteroids (methylprednisolone or corticotrophin) improved symptoms compared with placebo within the first 5 weeks of treatment. The optimal dose, route, and duration of treatment are unclear.

UNKNOWN EFFECTIVENESS

Plasma exchange
One small RCT provided insufficient evidence to assess plasma exchange in people with acute relapses of multiple sclerosis.

What are the effects of treatments for fatigue?

UNKNOWN EFFECTIVENESS

Amantadine
Four poor quality RCTs identified by two systematic reviews provided insufficient evidence to assess amantadine in people with multiple sclerosis related fatigue.

Behaviour modification
We found no RCTs on the effects of behavioural modification treatment in people with multiple sclerosis related fatigue.

Exercise
Two weak RCTs provided insufficient evidence to assess exercise in people with multiple sclerosis related fatigue.

Pemoline
Two poor quality RCTs identified by a systematic review provided insufficient evidence to assess the effects of pemoline compared with placebo on multiple sclerosis related fatigue.

What are the effects of treatments for spasticity?

UNKNOWN EFFECTIVENESS

Botulinum toxin
One small RCT provided insufficient evidence about the effects of botulinum toxin on functional outcomes in people with spasticity due to multiple sclerosis.

Intrathecal baclofen
One small crossover RCT provided insufficient evidence to assess functional effects of intrathecal baclofen in people with spasticity due to multiple sclerosis.

Oral drug treatments
One systematic review provided insufficient evidence about the effects of oral baclofen, dantrolene, or tizanidine on functional outcomes in people with spasticity due to multiple sclerosis.

Physiotherapy
Two small RCTs provided insufficient evidence to assess physiotherapy in people with spasticity due to multiple sclerosis. One of the RCTs found limited evidence that twice weekly hospital or home based physiotherapy for 8 weeks briefly ▶

improved mobility compared with no physiotherapy. The other, in people with progressive multiple sclerosis, found no significant difference between early versus delayed physiotherapy in mobility or activities of daily living.

What are the effects of multidisciplinary care?

UNKNOWN EFFECTIVENESS

Inpatient rehabilitation

Two small RCTs provided insufficient evidence to assess inpatient rehabilitation in people with multiple sclerosis. Both RCTs found short term functional benefit but no reduction in neurological impairment. Longer term effects are uncertain.

Outpatient rehabilitation

Two small RCTs provided insufficient evidence to assess outpatient rehabilitation in people with multiple sclerosis.

DEFINITION Multiple sclerosis is a chronic inflammatory disease of the central nervous system. Diagnosis requires evidence of lesions that are separated in both time and space, and the exclusion of other inflammatory, structural, or hereditary conditions that might give a similar clinical picture. The disease takes three main forms: relapsing and remitting multiple sclerosis, characterised by episodes of neurological dysfunction interspersed with periods of stability; primary progressive multiple sclerosis, in which progressive neurological disability occurs from the outset; and secondary progressive multiple sclerosis, in which progressive neurological disability occurs later in the course of the disease.

INCIDENCE/ PREVALENCE Prevalence varies with geography and racial group; it is highest in white populations in temperate regions.[1] In Europe and North America, prevalence is 1/800 people, with an annual incidence of 2–10/100 000, making multiple sclerosis the most common cause of neurological disability in young adults. Age of onset is broad, peaking between 20 and 40 years.[2]

AETIOLOGY/ RISK FACTORS The cause remains unclear, although current evidence suggests that multiple sclerosis is an autoimmune disorder of the central nervous system resulting from an environmental stimulus in genetically susceptible individuals. Multiple sclerosis is currently regarded as a single disorder with clinical variants, but there is some evidence that it may consist of several related disorders with distinct immunological, pathological, and genetic features.[1,3]

PROGNOSIS In 90% of people, early disease is relapsing and remitting. Although some people follow a relatively benign course over many years, most develop secondary progressive disease, usually 6–10 years after onset. In 10% of people, initial disease is primary progressive. Apart from a minority of people with "aggressive" multiple sclerosis, life expectancy is not greatly affected and the disease course is often of more than 30 years' duration.

Please refer to the Clinical Evidence website for full text and references.

Neurological disorders

Parkinson's disease

Search date May 2004

Carl Clarke and A Peter Moore

What are the effects of drug treatments in people with early stage Parkinson's disease?

LIKELY TO BE BENEFICIAL

Selegiline

RCTs found that selegiline improved the symptoms of Parkinson's disease and delayed the need for levodopa compared with placebo. One of the RCTs found limited evidence of increased mortality in people treated with selegiline.

TRADE OFF BETWEEN BENEFITS AND HARMS

Dopamine agonists (reduced dyskinesia and motor fluctuations compared with levodopa*, but were associated with increased treatment withdrawal and poorer motor scores)

One systematic review and one subsequent RCT (published only as an abstract) found that dopamine agonist monotherapy reduced the incidence of dyskinesias and motor complications compared with levodopa monotherapy. However, the subsequent RCT found that dopamine agonist monotherapy was associated with poorer motor scores than levodopa monotherapy, and an increased risk of treatment withdrawal. There is consensus that levodopa improves motor function, but that dyskinesias and fluctuations in motor response are related to long term levodopa treatment and are irreversible.

Levodopa* (more effective at improving motor scores but increased dyskinesia and motor fluctuations compared with dopamine agonists)

We found no placebo controlled RCTs, although experience suggests that levodopa improves motor function, but that dyskinesias and fluctuations in motor response are related to long term levodopa treatment and are irreversible.

Dopamine agonists plus levodopa* (reduced dyskinesia compared with levodopa alone, but increased disability)

One systematic review and subsequent RCTs found that dopamine agonists plus levodopa reduced dyskinesia compared with levodopa alone. However, some of the RCTs found that levodopa alone improved motor impairments and disability compared with dopamine agonists plus levodopa. One subsequent RCT found no significant difference between lisuride (lysuride) plus levodopa and levodopa alone in motor complications at 5 years. One RCT found that pramipexole plus rescue levodopa increased somnolence and hallucinations compared with levodopa alone. There is consensus that levodopa improves motor function, but that dyskinesias and fluctuations in motor response are related to long term levodopa treatment and are irreversible.

UNLIKELY TO BE BENEFICIAL

Modified release levodopa* (no more effective than immediate release levodopa)

Two RCTs in people with early Parkinson's disease found no significant difference between modified and immediate release levodopa in dyskinesia, motor fluctuations, and motor impairment after 5 years. The first RCT found no significant difference between UPDRS activities of daily living score at five years. The second RCT found that modified release co-careldopa improved the activities of daily living score and was better tolerated than immediate release co-careldopa.

What are the effects of adding a dopamine agonist in people with motor complications from levodopa?

TRADE OFF BETWEEN BENEFITS AND HARMS

Adding a dopamine agonist to levodopa*

Systematic reviews found that in people with response fluctuations to levodopa, certain dopamine agonists reduced "off" time, improved motor impairment and activities of daily living, and reduced levodopa dose, but increased dopaminergic adverse effects and dyskinesia.

What are the effects of surgery in people with later Parkinson's disease?

TRADE OFF BETWEEN BENEFITS AND HARMS

Pallidal surgery

One systematic review found that unilateral pallidotomy improved motor examination and activities of daily living compared with medical treatment. There is a high incidence of adverse effects with pallidotomy. One RCT found insufficient evidence to assess the effects of pallidotomy compared with those of deep brain stimulation. We found no RCTs comparing pallidal deep brain stimulation versus medical treatment. Three RCTs found insufficient evidence to assess the effects of pallidal deep brain stimulation compared with those of subthalamic deep brain stimulation. Adverse effects are probably less frequent with pallidal deep brain stimulation than with pallidotomy.

UNKNOWN EFFECTIVENESS

Subthalamic surgery

One systematic review found no RCTs comparing subthalamic deep brain stimulation versus medical treatment. One small RCT comparing subthalamic deep brain stimulation versus pallidal deep brain stimulation found no significant difference in motor scores.

Thalamic surgery

Systematic reviews identified no RCTs comparing thalamic surgery versus medical treatment. One RCT found that thalamic deep brain stimulation improved functional status and caused fewer adverse effects compared with thalamotomy. Case series found that, in 14–23% of people, thalamotomy was associated with permanent complications, including speech disturbance, apraxia, or death.

What are the effects of rehabilitation treatments in people with Parkinson's disease?

UNKNOWN EFFECTIVENESS

Occupational therapy

One systematic review provided insufficient evidence to assess the effects of occupational therapy in later Parkinson's disease.

Physiotherapy

Two systematic reviews and a subsequent small crossover RCT found insufficient evidence of the effects of physiotherapy in Parkinson's disease.

◄ **Speech and language therapy for speech disturbance**

One systematic review provided insufficient evidence to assess the effects of speech and language therapy for speech disturbance in later Parkinson's disease.

Swallowing therapy for dysphagia

We found no RCTs of swallowing therapy for dysphagia.

*We have used the term "levodopa" to refer to a combination of levodopa and a peripheral decarboxylase inhibitor.

DEFINITION	Idiopathic Parkinson's disease is an age related neurodegenerative disorder, which is associated with a combination of asymmetrical bradykinesia, hypokinesia, and rigidity, sometimes combined with rest tremor and postural changes. Clinical diagnostic criteria have a sensitivity of 80% and a specificity of 30% (likelihood ratio +ve test 1.14, –ve test 0.67) compared with the gold standard of diagnosis at autopsy.[1] The primary pathology is progressive loss of cells that produce the neurotransmitter dopamine from the substantia nigra in the brainstem. Treatment aims to replace or compensate for the lost dopamine. A good response to treatment supports, but does not confirm, the diagnosis. Several other catecholaminergic neurotransmitter systems are also affected in Parkinson's disease. There is no consistent definition of early and late stage Parkinson's disease. In this chapter we consider people with early stage disease to be those who have not yet developed motor complications associated with long term levodopa treatment (such as dyskinesias and motor fluctuations, also known as "on/off" fluctuations). Late stage Parkinson's disease is taken to mean that motor complications of long term levodopa treatment are present.
INCIDENCE/ PREVALENCE	Parkinson's disease occurs worldwide with equal incidence in both sexes. In 5–10% of people who develop Parkinson's disease, the condition appears before the age of 40 years (young onset), and the mean age of onset is about 65 years. Overall age adjusted prevalence is 1% worldwide and 1.6% in Europe, rising from 0.6% at age 60–64 years to 3.5% at age 85–89 years.[2,3]
AETIOLOGY/ RISK FACTORS	The cause is unknown. Parkinson's disease may represent different conditions with a final common pathway. People may be affected differently by a combination of genetic and environmental factors (viruses, toxins, 1-methyl-4-phenyl-1,2,3,6-tetrahydropyridine, well water, vitamin E, and smoking).[4–7] First degree relatives of affected people may have twice the risk of developing Parkinson's disease (17% chance of developing the condition in their lifetime) compared with people in the general population.[8–10] However, purely genetic varieties probably affect a small minority of people with Parkinson's disease.[11,12] The parkin gene on chromosome 6 may be associated with Parkinson's disease in families with at least one member with young onset Parkinson's disease, and multiple genetic factors, including the tau gene on chromosome 17q21, may be involved in idiopathic late onset disease.[13,14]
PROGNOSIS	Parkinson's disease is currently incurable. Disability is progressive and associated with increased mortality (RR of death compared with matched control populations ranges from 1.6–3.0).[15] Treatment can reduce symptoms and slow progression but it rarely achieves complete control. The question of whether treatment reduces mortality remains controversial.[16] Levodopa seemed to reduce mortality in the UK for 5 years after its introduction, before a "catch up" effect was noted and overall mortality rose toward previous levels. This suggested a limited prolongation of life.[17] An Australian cohort study followed 130 people treated for 10 years.[18] The standardised mortality ratio was 1.58 (P < 0.001). At 10 years, 25% had been admitted to a nursing home and only four were still employed. The mean duration of disease until death was 9.1 years. In a similar Italian cohort study conducted over 8 years, the relative risk of death for affected people compared with healthy controls was 2.3 (95% ►

CI 1.60 to 3.39).[19] Age at initial census date was the main predictor of outcome (for people aged < 75 years: RR of death 1.80, 95% CI 1.04 to 3.11; for people aged > 75 years: RR of death 5.61, 95% CI 2.13 to 14.80).

Please refer to the Clinical Evidence website for full text and references.

Trigeminal neuralgia

Search date November 2003

Joanna M Zakrzewska and Benjamin C Lopez

What are the effects of treatments?

LIKELY TO BE BENEFICIAL

Carbamazepine

One systematic review of three crossover RCTs found that carbamazepine increased pain relief compared with placebo, but also increased adverse effects (drowsiness, dizziness, constipation, and ataxia). One small RCT provided insufficient evidence to compare tizanidine versus carbamazepine. One RCT found that carbamazepine was less effective than pimozide in reducing pain over 8 weeks, but was associated with fewer adverse effects (including hand tremors, memory impairment, and involuntary movements). One systematic review identified one RCT of tocainide versus carbamazepine that was of insufficient quality.

TRADE OFF BETWEEN BENEFITS AND HARMS

Pimozide

One RCT found that pimozide reduced pain over 8 weeks compared with carbamazepine, but increased adverse effects (including hand tremors, memory impairment, and involuntary movements). Cardiac toxicity and sudden death have been reported with pimozide.

UNKNOWN EFFECTIVENESS

Combined streptomycin and lidocaine nerve block

Small RCTs provided insufficient evidence about the effects of nerve block using streptomycin plus lidocaine compared with nerve block using lidocaine alone.

Baclofen; lamotrigine; other drugs (phenytoin, clonazepam, sodium valproate, gabapentin, mexiletine, oxcarbazepine, topiramate); peripheral laser treatment; stereotactic radiosurgery; tizanidine

We found insufficient evidence about the effects of these interventions.

Cryotherapy of peripheral nerves; nerve block; peripheral acupuncture; peripheral injection of alcohol; peripheral injection of phenol; peripheral neurectomy; peripheral radiofrequency thermocoagulation

We found no RCTs about the effects of these interventions.

UNLIKELY TO BE BENEFICIAL

Proparacaine eye drops

One RCT found no significant difference in pain at 30 days between placebo and a single application of proparacaine hydrochloride eye drops to the eye on the same side as the pain.

LIKELY TO BE INEFFECTIVE OR HARMFUL

Tocainide

One systematic review found one RCT of tocainide versus carbamazepine, which was of insufficient quality. The use of tocainide is limited by considerable harms (including serious haematological effects).

▶

DEFINITION   Trigeminal neuralgia is a characteristic pain in the distribution of one or more branches of the fifth cranial nerve. The diagnosis is made on the history alone, based on characteristic features of the pain.[1-3] It occurs in paroxysms with each pain, lasting a few seconds to 2 minutes. The frequency of paroxysms is highly variable, ranging from hundreds of attacks a day to long periods of remission that can last years. Between paroxysms, the person is asymptomatic. The pain is severe and described as intense, sharp, superficial, stabbing, shooting, like an electric shock. In any individual, the pain has the same character in different attacks. It is triggered by light touch in a specific area or by eating, talking, washing the face, or cleaning the teeth. Other causes of facial pain may need to be excluded.[1-3] In trigeminal neuralgia the neurological examination is usually normal.[1-3]

INCIDENCE/   Most evidence about the incidence and prevalence of trigeminal neuralgia is
PREVALENCE   from the USA.[4] The annual incidence (when age adjusted to 1980 age distribution of the USA) is 5.9/100 000 women and 3.4/100 000 men. The incidence tends to be slightly higher in women at all ages. The incidence increases with age. In men aged over 80 years the incidence is 45.2/100 000.[5] Other published surveys are small. One questionnaire survey of neurological disease in a single French village found one person with trigeminal neuralgia among 993 people.[6]

AETIOLOGY/   The cause of trigeminal neuralgia remains unclear.[7,8] It is more common in
RISK FACTORS people with multiple sclerosis (RR 20.0, 95% CI 4.1 to 59.0).[5] Hypertension is a risk factor in women (RR 2.1, 95% CI 1.2 to 3.4) but the evidence is less clear for men (RR 1.53, 95% CI 0.30 to 4.50).[5] A study in the USA found that people with trigeminal neuralgia smoked less, consumed less alcohol, had fewer tonsillectomies, and were less likely than matched controls to be Jewish or an immigrant.[9]

PROGNOSIS   One study found no reduction of 10 year survival with trigeminal neuralgia.[10] We found no evidence about the natural history of trigeminal neuralgia. The illness is characterised by recurrences and remissions. Many people have periods of remission with no pain for months or years.[8] Anecdotal reports suggest that in many people it becomes more severe and less responsive to treatment with time.[11] Most people with trigeminal neuralgia are initially managed medically, and a proportion eventually have a surgical procedure.[8] We found no good evidence about the proportion of people who require surgical treatment for pain control. Anecdotal evidence indicates that pain relief is better after surgery than with medical treatment.[8,11]

Please refer to the Clinical Evidence website for full text and references.

Aphthous ulcers (recurrent)

Search date April 2004

Stephen Porter and Crispian Scully CBE

What are the effects of treatments for recurrent aphthous ulcers?

LIKELY TO BE BENEFICIAL

Chlorhexidine

RCTs found that chlorhexidine gluconate mouth rinses reduced the severity of each episode of ulceration, but did not affect the incidence of ulceration. Limited evidence from one RCT suggested that 0.2% chlorhexidine gel may reduce the incidence and duration of ulceration compared with a control preparation. RCTs found that chlorhexidine reduced the mean severity of pain compared with an inert preparation.

UNKNOWN EFFECTIVENESS

Topical corticosteroids

Small RCTs found that topical corticosteroids reduced the number of ulcer days compared with control preparations. RCTs found no consistent effect of topical corticosteroids on the incidence of new ulcers compared with control preparations. They found weak evidence that topical corticosteroids may reduce the duration and pain of ulcers and hasten pain relief without causing notable local or systemic adverse effects.

UNLIKELY TO BE BENEFICIAL

Hexitidine

Limited evidence from RCTs found no significant difference in any of the reported outcomes between hexitidine mouthwash or a proprietary antibacterial mouthwash and control mouthwashes.

DEFINITION Recurrent aphthous ulcers are superficial and rounded, painful mouth ulcers usually occurring in recurrent bouts at intervals of a few days to a few months.[1]

INCIDENCE/ PREVALENCE The point prevalence of recurrent aphthous ulcers in Swedish adults has been reported as 2%.[1] Prevalence may be 5–10% in some groups of children. Up to 66% of young adults give a history consistent with recurrent aphthous ulceration.

AETIOLOGY/ RISK FACTORS The causes of aphthous ulcers remain unknown. Associations with haematinic deficiency, infections, gluten sensitive enteropathy, food sensitivities, and psychological stress have rarely been confirmed. Similar ulcers are seen in Behçet's syndrome. Local physical trauma may initiate ulcers in susceptible people. Recurrent aphthous ulcers are uncommon on keratinised oral mucosal surfaces, and the frequency of recurrent aphthous ulcers may fall if people cease any tobacco smoking habit.

PROGNOSIS About 80% of people with recurrent aphthous ulcers develop a few ulcers smaller than 1 cm in diameter that heal within 5–14 days without scarring (the pattern known as minor aphthous ulceration). The episodes recur typically after an interval of 1–4 months. One in 10 people with recurrent ulceration may have multiple minute ulcers (herpetiform ulceration). Likewise, one in 10 sufferers has a more severe form (major aphthous ulceration), with lesions larger than ▶

1 cm that may recur after a shorter interval and can cause scarring. Most of the trials in this review have focused upon the treatment of minor aphthous ulceration.

Please refer to the Clinical Evidence website for full text and references.

Burning mouth syndrome

Search date January 2004

John Buchanan and Joanna Zakrzewska

What are the effects of treatments?

LIKELY TO BE BENEFICIAL

Cognitive behavioural therapy

One small RCT found that cognitive behavioural therapy reduced symptom intensity in people with resistant burning syndrome after 6 months compared with placebo treatment.

UNKNOWN EFFECTIVENESS

Antidepressants; benzydamine hydrochloride

We found insufficient evidence on the effects of these interventions.

Dietary supplements

We found insufficient evidence from three small methodologically flawed RCTs to draw reliable conclusions about the effects of alphalipoic acid in people with burning mouth syndrome. We found no RCTs evaluating other vitamin or coenzyme supplements.

Hormone replacement therapy in postmenopausal women

We found limited evidence from one small methodologically flawed RCT that tibolone improved symptoms compared with oryzanol plus vitamin E at 6 months.

DEFINITION Burning mouth syndrome is a psychogenic or idiopathic burning discomfort or pain affecting people with clinically normal oral mucosa in whom a medical or dental cause has been excluded.[1-3] Terms previously used to describe what is now called burning mouth syndrome include glossodynia, glossopyrosis, stomatodynia, stomatopyrosis, sore tongue, and oral dysaesthesia.[4] A survey of 669 men and 758 women randomly selected from 48 500 people aged between 20 and 69 years found that people with burning mouth also have subjective dryness (66%), take some form of medication (64%), report other systemic illnesses (57%), and have altered taste (11%).[5] Many studies of people with symptoms of burning mouth do not distinguish those with burning mouth syndrome (i.e. idiopathic disease) from those with other conditions (such as vitamin B deficiency), making results unreliable. Local and systemic factors (such as infections, allergies, ill fitting dentures,[6] hypersensitivity reactions,[7] and hormone and vitamin deficiencies[8-10]) may cause the symptom of burning mouth and should be excluded before diagnosing burning mouth syndrome.

INCIDENCE/ Burning mouth syndrome mainly affects women,[11-13] particularly after the
PREVALENCE menopause, when its prevalence may be 18–33%.[14] One recent study in Sweden found a prevalence of 4% for the symptom of burning mouth without clinical abnormality of the oral mucosa (11/669 [2%] men, mean age 59 years; 42/758 [6%] women, mean age 57 years), with the highest prevalence (12%) in women aged 60–69 years.[5] Reported prevalence in general populations varies from 1%[15] to 15%.[11] Incidence and prevalence vary according to diagnostic criteria,[4] and many studies included people with the symptom of burning mouth rather than with burning mouth syndrome as defined above.

AETIOLOGY/ The cause is unknown, and we found no good aetiological studies. Possible
RISK FACTORS causal factors include hormonal disturbances associated with the menopause,[12-14] psychogenic factors (including anxiety, depression, stress, life events, personality disorders, and phobia of cancer),[6,16,17] and neuropathy in so-called supertasters.[18]

▶

PROGNOSIS   We found no prospective cohort studies or other reliable evidence describing the natural history of burning mouth syndrome.[19] We found anecdotal reports of at least partial spontaneous remission in about half of people with burning mouth syndrome within 6–7 years.[16]

Please refer to the Clinical Evidence website for full text and references.

Candidiasis (oropharyngeal)

Search date June 2004

Caroline Pankhurst

What are the effects of interventions to prevent and treat oropharyngeal candidiasis in adults receiving treatment causing immunosuppression?

BENEFICIAL

Antifungal prophylaxis with absorbed or partially absorbed antifungal drugs in people undergoing cancer treatments

One systematic review and one subsequent RCT found that absorbed antifungal drugs (ketoconazole, itraconazole, fluconazole) reduced the risk of oropharyngeal candidiasis compared with placebo or no drug treatment, or compared with unabsorbed antifungals (nystatin alone, nystatin plus chlorhexidine, amphotericin B alone, or amphotericin B combined with nystatin, norfloxacin, natamycin, thymostimulin, or chlorhexidine). The review also found that partially absorbed antifungal drugs (miconazole, clotrimazole) reduced the risk of oropharyngeal candidiasis compared with placebo or no drug treatment. The review found no significant difference in the risk of oropharyngeal candidiasis between unabsorbed drugs and placebo. However, there was significant heterogeneity among studies. The review found no significant difference in adverse events between absorbed antifungal drugs and placebo.

UNKNOWN EFFECTIVENESS

Antifungal prophylaxis in people receiving tissue transplants

Two small RCTs in people with liver transplant found no significant difference in the risk of oropharyngeal candidiasis between nystatin and fluconazole or clotrimazole. However, the trials may have lacked power to detect clinically important differences. We found insufficient evidence from two RCTs about the effects of prophylactic chlorhexidine mouth rinse with or without nystatin compared with placebo in people receiving bone marrow transplant.

Antifungal treatment in people undergoing chemotherapy, radiotherapy, or both treatments for cancer

One systematic review and one subsequent RCT found insufficient evidence about the clinical effects of antifungals compared with placebo for treating oropharyngeal candidiasis in people undergoing chemotherapy or radiotherapy, or about the effects of different antifungal agents or doses in people with oropharyngeal candidiasis receiving radiotherapy or chemotherapy.

What are the effects of interventions to prevent and treat oropharyngeal candidiasis in infants and children?

BENEFICIAL

Antifungal treatment with miconazole or fluconazole in immunocompetent and immunocompromised infants and children (more effective than nystatin)

RCTs found that miconazole and fluconazole increased clinical cure of oropharyngeal candidiasis compared with nystatin in immunocompetent and immunocompromised infants and children.

▶

LIKELY TO BE BENEFICIAL

Antifungal prophylaxis with fluconazole in immunocompromised infants and children (more effective than oral nystatin or amphotericin B)

One large RCT in immunocompromised infants and children found that fluconazole reduced the incidence of oropharyngeal candidiasis compared with oral nystatin, amphotericin B, or both.

What are the effects of interventions to prevent and treat oropharyngeal candidiasis in people with diabetes?

UNKNOWN EFFECTIVENESS

Treatments in people with diabetes mellitus

We found no systematic review or RCTs assessing preventive interventions or treatments for oropharyngeal candidiasis in people with diabetes.

What are the effects of interventions for oropharyngeal candidiasis in people with dentures?

UNKNOWN EFFECTIVENESS

Antifungal treatment for denture stomatitis

We found insufficient evidence from small RCTs to compare effects of antifungal agents versus placebo or versus each other for treating oropharyngeal candidiasis in people who wear dentures.

Denture hygiene

We found insufficient evidence from three RCTs, two of which were underpowered, to assess clinical effects on oropharyngeal candidiasis of mouth rinses, disinfectants, denture soaks, denture scrubbing, and microwave irradiation of dentures. Microwave treatment is not suitable for all dentures.

What are the effects of interventions to prevent and treat oropharyngeal candidiasis in people with HIV infection?

BENEFICIAL

Antifungal prophylaxis with fluconazole, itraconazole or nystatin in people with advanced HIV disease

RCTs in people with HIV infection found that daily or weekly antifungal prophylaxis with fluconazole, itraconazole, or nystatin reduced incidence and relapse of oropharyngeal candidiasis compared with placebo. One large RCT found that fluconazole reduced recurrence of oropharyngeal candidiasis compared with clotrimazole.

Oral suspension of systemically absorbed azoles in people with HIV infection

RCTs found that topical preparations of itraconazole, fluconazole, miconazole nitrate, and clotrimazole effectively treated oropharyngeal candidiasis in people with HIV infection. One RCT found that fluconazole reduced symptoms and signs of oropharyngeal candidiasis compared with topical nystatin.

▶

Candidiasis (oropharyngeal)

Which treatments reduce the risk of acquiring resistance to antifungal drugs?

UNKNOWN EFFECTIVENESS

Continuous prophylaxis versus intermittent treatment in people with HIV infection and acute episodes of oropharyngeal candidiasis (in preventing antifungal resistance)

One RCT in people with HIV infection and acute episodes of oropharyngeal candidiasis found no significant difference between continuous antifungal prophylaxis with fluconazole and intermittent antifungal treatment with fluconazole in terms of the emergence of antifungal resistance.

DEFINITION Oropharyngeal candidiasis is an opportunistic mucosal infection caused, in most cases, by *Candida albicans*. The four main types of oropharyngeal candidiasis are: (1) pseudomembranous (thrush), consisting of white discrete plaques on an erythematous background, on the buccal mucosa, throat, tongue, or gingivae; (2) erythematous, consisting of smooth red patches on the hard or soft palate, dorsum of tongue, or buccal mucosa; (3) hyperplastic, consisting of white, firmly adherent patches or plaques, usually bilaterally distributed on the buccal mucosa; and (4) denture induced stomatitis, presenting as either a smooth or granular erythema confined to the denture bearing area of the hard palate and often associated with an angular cheilitis.[1] Symptoms vary, ranging from none to a sore and painful mouth with a burning tongue and altered taste. Oropharyngeal candidiasis can impair speech, nutritional intake, and quality of life.

INCIDENCE/ PREVALENCE *Candida* species are commensals in the gastrointestinal tract. Transmission occurs directly between infected people or on fomites (objects that can harbour pathogenic organisms). *Candida* is found in the mouth of 31–60% of healthy people.[2] Denture stomatitis associated with *Candida* is prevalent in 65% of denture wearers.[2] Oropharyngeal candidiasis affects 15–60% of people with haematological or oncological malignancies during periods of immunosuppression.[3] Oropharyngeal candidiasis occurs in 7–48% of people with HIV infection and in over 90% of those with advanced disease. In severely immunosuppressed people, relapse rates are high (30–50%) and relapse usually occurs within 14 days of stopping treatment.[4]

AETIOLOGY/ RISK FACTORS Risk factors associated with symptomatic oropharyngeal candidiasis include local or systemic immunosuppression, haematological disorders, broad spectrum antibiotic use, inhaled or systemic steroids, xerostomia, diabetes, and wearing dentures, obturators, or orthodontic appliances.[1,5] The same strain may persist for months or years in the absence of infection. In people with HIV infection, there is no direct correlation between the number of organisms and the presence of clinical disease. Symptomatic oropharyngeal candidiasis associated with *in vitro* resistance to fluconazole occurs in 5% of people with advanced HIV disease.[6] Resistance to azole antifungals is associated with severe immunosuppression ($\leq$ 50 CD4 cells/mm^3), more episodes treated with antifungal drugs, and longer median duration of systemic azole treatment.[7]

PROGNOSIS In most people, untreated candidiasis persists for months or years unless associated risk factors are treated or eliminated. In neonates, spontaneous cure of oropharyngeal candidiasis usually occurs after 3–8 weeks.

Please refer to the Clinical Evidence website for full text and references.

What are the effects of treatments in people with physiological halitosis?

LIKELY TO BE BENEFICIAL

Regular-use mouthwash

Two RCTs found that regular use of a mouthwash (one mouthwash containing cetylpyridinium chloride plus chlorhexidine plus zinc lactate; the other mouthwash containing cetylpyridinium chloride) reduced breath odour at 2–4 weeks compared with placebo.

Single-use mouthwash (short term benefit only)

Four small RCTs found limited evidence that single-use mouthwash reduced odour unpleasantness and odour intensity between 1–8 hours after use compared with distilled water, saline rinse, or no treatment. One of these RCTs found no significant difference between single-use mouthwash and distilled water in odour unpleasantness or odour intensity after 24 hours.

UNKNOWN EFFECTIVENESS

Artificial saliva; sugar free chewing gums; tongue cleaning, brushing, or scraping; zinc toothpastes

We found no RCTs on the effects of these interventions.

DEFINITION
Halitosis is an unpleasant odour emitted from the mouth. It may be caused by oral conditions including poor oral hygiene and periodontal disease or extra oral conditions such as chronic sinusitis and bronchiectasis.[1,2] In this chapter, we deal only with physiological halitosis, that is, confirmed persistent bad breath in the absence of systemic, periodontal, or gum disease. We have excluded halitosis due to underlying disease, which would require disease specific treatment, pseudo-halitosis (in people who believe they have bad breath but whose breath is not considered malodourous by others), and artificially induced halitosis (e.g. in studies requiring people to stop brushing their teeth). This topic is only applicable, therefore, to people in whom underlying causes have been ruled out, and in whom pseudo-halitosis has been excluded. There is no consensus regarding duration of bad breath for diagnosis of halitosis, although the standard organoleptic test for bad breath involves smelling the breath on at least two or three different days.[1]

INCIDENCE/ PREVALENCE
We found no reliable estimate of prevalence, although several studies report the population prevalence of halitosis (physiological or because of underlying disease) to be about 50%.[1,3–5] One cross-sectional study of 491 people found that about 5% of people with halitosis have pseudo-halitosis and about 40% of people with halitosis have physiological bad breath not due to underlying disease.[6] We found no reliable data about age or sex distribution of physiological halitosis.

AETIOLOGY/ RISK FACTORS
We found no reliable data about risk factors for physiological bad breath. Mass spectrometric and gas chromatographic analysis of expelled air from the mouth of people with any type of halitosis have shown that the main malodourants are volatile sulphur compounds including hydrogen sulphide, methyl mercaptan, and dimethyl suphide.[7,8]

▶

Halitosis

PROGNOSIS   We found no evidence on the prognosis of halitosis.

Please refer to the Clinical Evidence website for full text and references.

Search date August 2004

Marco Esposito

Should asymptomatic and disease-free impacted wisdom teeth be removed prophylactically?

LIKELY TO BE INEFFECTIVE OR HARMFUL

Prophylactic extraction

One RCT identified by a systematic review found no evidence that prophylactic extraction of asymptomatic impacted wisdom teeth improved outcomes compared with no extraction. Removal of lower wisdom teeth causes permanent numbness of the lower lip or tongue in about 2% of people.

DEFINITION Wisdom teeth are third molars that develop in almost all adults and generally erupt between the ages of 18 and 24 years, although there is a wide variation in the age of eruption. In some people, the teeth become partially or completely impacted below the gum line because of lack of space, obstruction, or abnormal position. Impacted wisdom teeth may be diagnosed because of pain and swelling or incidentally by routine dental radiography.

INCIDENCE/ Third molar impaction is common. Over 72% of Swedish people aged 20–30
PREVALENCE years have at least one impacted lower third molar.[1] The surgical removal of impacted third molars (symptomatic and asymptomatic) is the most common procedure performed by oral and maxillofacial surgeons. It is performed on about 4/1000 people a year in England and Wales, making it one of the top 10 inpatient and day case procedures.[2–4] Up to 90% of people on oral and maxillofacial surgery hospital waiting lists are awaiting removal of wisdom teeth.[3]

AETIOLOGY/ Retention and impaction of wisdom teeth may be more common than it was
RISK FACTORS previously because the modern diet tends to be softer than in the past.[5]

PROGNOSIS Impacted wisdom teeth can cause pain, swelling, and infection, and may destroy adjacent teeth and bone. The removal of diseased and symptomatic wisdom teeth alleviates pain and suffering and improves oral health and function. We found no good evidence on untreated prognosis in people with asymptomatic impacted wisdom teeth.

Please refer to the Clinical Evidence website for full text and references.

Postoperative pulmonary infections

Search date March 2004

Andrew Smith

What are the effects of preventive interventions?

BENEFICIAL

Regional anaesthesia

One systematic review found that spinal or epidural anaesthesia (alone or in combination with general anaesthesia) reduced postoperative pneumonia compared with general anaesthesia alone.

Postoperative chest physiotherapy (deep breathing exercises)

One systematic review and one subsequent RCT found that deep breathing exercises reduced postoperative pulmonary infections compared with control. One RCT found no significant difference between physiotherapy plus deep breathing exercises and physiotherapy alone in postoperative pulmonary complications. We were unable to draw conclusions from one small RCT comparing deep breathing and coughing exercises (with or without intensive physiotherapy) versus no physiotherapy.

LIKELY TO BE BENEFICIAL

Postoperative chest physiotherapy (incentive spirometry and intermittent positive pressure breathing)

Two RCTs found that incentive spirometry reduced pulmonary complications compared with control. One RCT found that intermittent positive pressure breathing reduced postoperative pulmonary complications compared with control.

UNKNOWN EFFECTIVENESS

Advice to stop smoking preoperatively

We found no RCTs about the effects of preoperative advice to stop cigarette smoking on postoperative pulmonary infections. Two observational studies found that people who smoked were more likely to develop postoperative pulmonary complications of all kinds than those who did not. One study suggested that people who had stopped smoking 6 months prior to surgery reverted to the risk of those who had never smoked.

DEFINITION
A working diagnosis of postoperative pulmonary infection may be based on three or more new findings from: cough, phlegm, shortness of breath, chest pain, temperature above 38 °C, and pulse rate above 100 a minute.[1] In this chapter, we are dealing strictly with pneumonia that is regarded to be a complication of the operation. We examine a selection of pre-, intra-, and postoperative techniques to reduce the risk of this complication. In this chapter, the diagnosis of pneumonia implies consolidation observed in a chest radiograph.[2]

INCIDENCE/ PREVALENCE
Reported morbidity for chest complications depends on how carefully they are investigated. One study found blood gas and chest radiograph abnormalities in about 50% of people after open cholecystectomy.[3] However, fewer than 20% of these had abnormal clinical signs and only 10% had a clinically significant chest infection. Another study estimated the incidence of pneumonia as 20%.[4] Another used a similarly strict definition and found the incidence to be 23%.[5]

AETIOLOGY/ RISK FACTORS
Risk factors include increasing age (> 50 years), cigarette smoking, obesity, thoracic or upper abdominal operations, and pre-existing lung disease.[6] One ▶

multivariate analysis did not confirm the association with cigarette smoking, but suggested that longer preoperative hospital stay and higher grading on the American Society of Anesthesiologists' physical status scale (> 2) increased the risk of postoperative pulmonary complications.[5] Depression of the immune system may also contribute.[7]

PROGNOSIS In one large systematic review (search date 1997, 141 RCTs, 9559 people), 10% of people with postoperative pneumonia died.[8] If systemic sepsis ensues, mortality is likely to be substantial.[9] Pneumonia delays recovery from surgery and poor tissue oxygenation may contribute to delayed wound healing.

Please refer to the Clinical Evidence website for full text and references.

Carbon monoxide poisoning (acute)

Search date August 2004

Nicholas Phin

Many cases of mild to moderate carbon monoxide poisoning are probably misdiagnosed. A history of known exposure to carbon monoxide and the presence of clinical signs and symptoms should not be ignored even if the percentage carboxyhaemoglobin is low or within the normal range.

In cases of suspected carbon monoxide poisoning, the immediate and essential actions are to remove the person from the source of carbon monoxide and to give oxygen, preferably 100%, through a non-re-breather mask.

In a hospital setting, any decision to use hyperbaric oxygen needs to be based on the clinical history, percentage carboxyhaemoglobin, condition of the person, and feasibility of safe transportation to a hyperbaric facility.

What are the effects of oxygen treatments for acute carbon monoxide poisoning? New

BENEFICIAL

Oxygen 100% via non-re-breather mask (compared with air)* New

We found no systematic review, RCTs, or analytical observational studies comparing oxygen 100% by non-re-breather mask versus air for clinically relevant outcomes of interest. Such an RCT in people with suspected acute carbon monoxide poisoning would be considered unethical. One retrospective chart review in people with various levels of severity of acute carbon monoxide poisoning receiving oxygen 100% either by non-re-breather mask or by ventilation if intubated in a tertiary teaching hospital setting found that oxygen 100% reduced carboxyhaemoglobin half life. We found no systematic review or RCTs for other clinical outcomes of interest in people with acute carbon monoxide poisoning. Based on physiological studies, the benefits of oxygen 100% by non-re-breather mask in the emergency situation are universally accepted but there is still considerable debate about the optimum duration of treatment in secondary or tertiary care settings.

*Categorisation is based on consensus and physiological studies

LIKELY TO BE BENEFICIAL

Hyperbaric oxygen 100% at 2-3 ATA (compared with normobaric oxygen 100% in moderate to severe poisoning) New

One RCT in people with moderate to severe acute carbon monoxide poisoning found limited evidence that, compared with normobaric oxygen 100%, hyperbaric oxygen 100% delivered within 24 hours of presentation at pressures of 2–3 atmospheres reduced cognitive sequelae at 6 weeks. However, it is unclear which the types of people will benefit, the optimum treatment regime, and how long after exposure the treatment has an effect. The size of the effect derived from hyperbaric oxygen treatment may be highly sensitive to the pressure at which the oxygen is delivered, the number of treatment sessions, and the oxygen content of control treatments.

Oxygen 28% (compared with air)* New

We found no systematic review, RCTs, or analytical observational studies comparing 28% normobaric oxygen versus air in people with carbon monoxide poisoning for clinically relevant outcomes of interest. It may be considered unethical to conduct analytical studies. Oxygen 28% will affect carboxyhaemoglobin levels but ▶

may not be as effective as higher concentrations of oxygen for reducing carboxy-haemoglobin half life. UK paramedics routinely use oxygen 28% so that individuals who may be dependent on their hypoxic drive are not adversely affected.
*Categorisation is based on consensus and physiological studies

Hyperbaric oxygen 100% (compared with oxygen 100% in mild poisoning) *New*

We found no systematic review or RCTs only in people with mild carbon monoxide poisoning. Two RCTs in people with mild to moderate acute carbon monoxide poisoning found insufficient evidence to draw conclusions about the effects of hyperbaric oxygen versus oxygen 100% via non-re-breather mask for prevention of delayed neurological complications. We found no systematic review or RCTs for other clinical outcomes of interest.

DEFINITION Carbon monoxide is an odourless, colourless gas and poisoning causes hypoxia, cell damage, and death.[1,2] **Diagnosis of carbon monoxide poisoning:** Exposure to carbon monoxide is measured either directly from blood samples and expressed as a percentage of carboxyhaemoglobin or indirectly using the carbon monoxide in expired breath. Percentage carboxyhaemoglobin is the most frequently used biomarker of carbon monoxide exposure. Although the diagnosis of carbon monoxide poisoning can be confirmed by detecting elevated levels of blood carboxyhaemoglobin levels, the presence of clinical signs and symptoms after known exposure to carbon monoxide should not be ignored. The signs and symptoms of carbon monoxide poisoning are mainly associated with the brain and heart which are most sensitive to hypoxia. The symptoms of carbon monoxide poisoning are non-specific and varied and include headache, fatigue,[3] malaise, "trouble thinking", confusion, nausea, dizziness, visual disturbances, chest pain, shortness of breath, loss of consciousness, and seizures.[4-6] In people suffering from coexisting morbidities, symptoms such as shortness of breath or chest pain may be more evident. The classical signs of carbon monoxide, described as cherry-red lips, peripheral cyanosis, and retinal haemorrhages, are in reality rarely seen.[7] **Interpretation of carboxyhaemoglobin levels:** Non-smokers living away from urban areas have carboxyhaemoglobin levels of between 0.4% and 1.0% reflecting endogenous carbon monoxide production whereas levels of up to 5% may be considered normal in a busy urban or industrial setting.[8] Smokers are exposed to increased levels of carbon monoxide in cigarettes and otherwise healthy heavy smokers can tolerate levels of carboxyhaemoglobin of up 15%.[9] The use of percentage carboxyhaemoglobin as a measure of severity of carbon monoxide poisoning or to predict treatment options is limited because carboxyhaemoglobin levels are affected by the removal from the source of carbon monoxide and any oxygen treatment given before measurement of percentage carboxyhaemoglobin. In addition, people with co-morbidities that make them more sensitive to the hypoxia associated with carbon monoxide can present with symptoms of poisoning at carboxyhaemoglobin levels that are either low or within the normal range.[10] Attempts have been made in the literature to equate symptoms and signs to different carboxyhaemoglobin levels[11] but it is accepted that carboxyhaemoglobin levels in an acutely poisoned person only roughly correlate with the clinical signs and symptoms, especially those relating to neurological function.[12] Earlier studies attempted to differentiate between smokers and non-smokers. Attempts have also been made in the literature to divide carbon monoxide poisoning into mild, moderate, and severe based on percentage carboxyhaemoglobin levels and clinical symptoms,[13] but there is no clear clinical consensus or agreement on this issue. The degree of poisoning has been described in the literature as *mild carbon monoxide poisoning:* a carboxyhaemoglobin level of greater than 10% without clinical signs or symptoms of ▶

Carbon monoxide poisoning (acute)

carbon monoxide poisoning; *moderate carbon monoxide poisoning*: a carboxyhaemoglobin level of greater than 10% and less than 20–25% with minor clinical signs and symptoms of poisoning such as headache, lethargy or fatigue; and *severe carbon monoxide poisoning*: a carboxyhaemoglobin level of greater than 20–25%, loss of consciousness and confusion or signs of cardiac ischaemia, or both. **Population:** For the purpose of this review, we have included adults presenting to health care professionals with suspected carbon monoxide poisoning. Although there is as yet no clear consensus on this issue, most studies examining carbon monoxide poisoning and its management use a carboxyhaemoglobin level of 10% or more or the presence of clinical signs and symptoms after known exposure to carbon monoxide to be indicative of acute carbon monoxide poisoning. Unless otherwise stated this is the definition of acute carbon monoxide poisoning that has been used throughout this chapter. Where appropriate, the terms mild, moderate, or severe have been used to reflect the descriptions of populations in individual studies.

INCIDENCE/ PREVALENCE

Carbon monoxide poisoning is considered to be one of the leading causes of death and injury worldwide and a major public health problem.[14] In 2000, there were 521 deaths where carbon monoxide was the recorded cause of death (ICD 9 – E986) in England and Wales[15] compared with 1363 deaths recorded in 1985;[16] a trend that has also been observed in the US.[17] Of the 521 deaths attributed to carbon monoxide poisoning, 148 were accidental and the remaining 373 the result of suicide or self inflicted injury. Poisoning by carbon monoxide is almost certainly underdiagnosed because of the varied ways in which it can present and it has been estimated in the US that there are over 40 000 emergency department visits a year; many presenting with a flu-like illness.[18] In 2003, there were 534 recorded medical episodes in English hospitals involving people suffering from the toxic effects of carbon monoxide.[19] This may be a substantial underestimate if the US experience reflects the true morbidity associated with carbon monoxide poisoning. Studies in the US have shown that the incidence of accidental carbon monoxide poisoning peaks during the winter months,[20,21] and is associated with increased use of indoor heating and petrol powered generators and reduced external ventilation. This seasonal rise in numbers coincides with the annual increase in influenza notifications and given the similarity in symptoms many cases of mild carbon monoxide poisoning are probably misdiagnosed.

AETIOLOGY/ RISK FACTORS

People at high risk: People who are most at risk from carbon monoxide poisoning include those with coronary heart disease, vascular disease, or anaemia; pregnant women and their fetus; infants; and the elderly. In people with coronary heart disease, experimentally induced blood carboxyhaemoglobin levels of 4.5% shorten the period of exercise before the onset of anginal pain and the duration of pain is prolonged.[22–24] In people with anaemia the oxygen carrying capacity of the blood is already compromised and therefore they will be more sensitive to carbon monoxide.[25] The elderly are at risk because of existing co-morbidities such as heart disease or respiratory disease and because of a reduced compensatory response to hypoxic situations. During pregnancy, a woman's oxygen carrying capacity is reduced because of an increased endogenous carbon monoxide production and additional endogenous carbon monoxide from the developing fetus leading to an increased carboxyhaemoglobin concentration.[26] A higher ventilation rate during pregnancy will lead to increased uptake of carbon monoxide at any given carbon monoxide concentration.[27] The fetus is also at risk and there have been occasional fetal deaths in non-fatal maternal exposures.[26,28,29] In the developing fetus, oxygen is released at a lower oxygen partial pressure and fetal haemoglobin binds with carbon monoxide more quickly compared with adults. Carbon monoxide may be a teratogen where there is a significant increase in maternal carboxyhaemoglobin or where there is moderate to severe maternal toxicity.[30] Infants may be more susceptible to the effect of carbon monoxide because of their greater oxygen consumption in relation to adults and their response and symptoms are more variable. There are recorded instances of children travelling in the same car and having varying symptoms with similar carboxyhaemoglobin levels or widely varying carboxyhaemoglobin levels with similar carbon monoxide exposure.[31] **Sources of carbon monoxide:** Carbon monoxide is produced by the incomplete combustion of carbon containing fuel, such as gas (domestic or bottled), charcoal, coke, oil, and wood. Gas stoves, fires, and boilers; gas powered water heaters; car exhaust fumes; charcoal barbeques; paraffin heaters; solid fuel powered stoves; boilers; and room heaters that are faulty or inadequately ventilated are all potential sources. A sometimes overlooked source of carbon monoxide is methylene chloride in some paint strippers and sprays. Methylene chloride is readily absorbed through the skin and lungs and once in the liver, is converted to carbon monoxide. Methylene chloride is stored in body tissues and released gradually; the carbon monoxide elimination half life in people exposed to methylene chloride is more than twice that of inhaled carbon monoxide. Natural background levels of carbon monoxide in the outdoor environment range from $0.01–0.23$ mg/m^3 ($0.009 .0.2$ ppm)[32] but in urban traffic in the UK the 8 hour mean concentrations are higher at about 20 mg/m^3 (17.5 ppm);[33] exposure to this level for prolonged periods could result in a carboxyhaemoglobin level of about 3%.

PROGNOSIS The data regarding prognosis in carbon monoxide poisoning are inconclusive and contradictory. However, there is general agreement that outcome and prognosis are related to the level of carbon monoxide that a person is exposed to, the duration of exposure, and the presence of underlying risk factors.[33] A poor outcome is predicted by lengthy carbon monoxide exposure, loss of consciousness, and advancing age. In addition, hypotension and cardiac arrest independently predict permanent disability and death. After acute carbon monoxide poisoning the organs most sensitive to hypoxia will be most affected; i.e. the brain and the heart. Pre-existing co-morbidities that affect these organs will to an extent influence the clinical presentation and the prognosis; an individual with pre-existing heart disease may present with myocardial ischaemia that could lead to infarction and death. The prognosis for people resuscitated after experiencing cardiac arrest with carbon monoxide poisoning is poor. In a small retrospective study,[34] 18 people with carboxyhaemoglobin levels of $31.7 \pm 11.0\%$ given hyperbaric oxygen after resuscitation after cardiac arrest all died. The effects on the brain are more subtle given that different sections of the brain are more sensitive to hypoxic insults either as a consequence of reduced oxygen delivery or by direct effects on intracellular metabolism.[35] Therefore, in addition to the acute neurological sequelae leading to loss of consciousness, coma and death, neurological sequelae such as poor concentration and memory problems may be apparent in people recovering from carbon monoxide poisoning (persistent neurological sequelae) or develop after a period of apparent normality (delayed neurological sequelae). Delayed neurological sequelae develop between 2 days to 240 days after exposure and are reported to affect 10–32% of people recovering from carbon monoxide poisoning.[36,37] Symptoms include cognitive changes, personality changes, incontinence, psychosis, and Parkinsonism.[38] Fortunately 50–75% of people recover within 1 year.[39]

Please refer to the Clinical Evidence website for full text and references.

Organophosphorus poisoning (acute)

Search date September 2004

Michael Eddleston, Surjit Singh, and Nick Buckley

What are the effects of treatments for acute organophosphorus poisoning?

LIKELY TO BE BENEFICIAL

Atropine*

Atropine is considered the mainstay of treatment, and many case series have found that it reverses the early muscarinic effects of acute organophosphorus poisoning. We found no RCTs comparing atropine versus placebo but it would now be considered unethical to perform such an RCT. One small RCT found no significant difference in mortality or ventilation rates between atropine and glycopyrronium bromide, but it may have lacked power to detect clinically important differences.

Benzodiazepines to control organophosphorus induced seizures*

Diazepam is considered standard treatment for organophosphorus induced seizures. We found no RCTs comparing diazepam or other benzodiazepines versus placebo or another anticonvulsant. It would now be considered unethical to perform an RCT comparing benzodiazepines versus placebo in people with seizures.

Glycopyrronium bromide (glycopyrrolate)*

We found no RCTs comparing glycopyrronium bromide (glycopyrrolate) versus placebo, but it is unlikely that such a trial would be considered ethical unless glycopyrronium bromide and placebo were administered in addition to atropine. One small RCT found no significant difference in mortality or ventilation rates between glycopyrronium bromide and atropine, but it may have lacked power to detect clinically important differences. Glycopyrronium bromide has been used instead of atropine because it is thought to have fewer adverse effects on the central nervous system.

Washing the poisoned person and removing contaminated clothes*

We found no RCTs or observational studies of sufficient quality that evaluated washing the poisoned person and removing contaminated clothes. However, this appears to be an obvious way to reduce further dermal and mucocutaneous exposure and is widely recommended. An RCT would therefore be considered unethical. Healthcare workers should ensure that washing does not distract them from other treatment priorities and they should also protect themselves through the use of gloves, aprons, and eye protection, with careful disposal of contaminated equipment and clothes.

UNKNOWN EFFECTIVENESS

Activated charcoal (single or multiple dose)

We found no systematic review, RCTs, or observational studies of sufficient quality evaluating activated charcoal, in either single or multiple dose regimens, in people with acute organophosphorus poisoning.

Gastric lavage

We found no RCTs or observational studies of sufficient quality evaluating gastric lavage in people with acute organophosphorus poisoning. Adverse effects are common when gastric lavage is performed in physically restrained, non-consenting patients without careful control of the airway. If the patient cannot be sedated and intubated, the risk of harm due to aspiration is likely to outweigh its potential benefits.

Milk or other home remedy immediately after ingestion

We found no RCTs or observational studies of sufficient quality that assessed giving a "home remedy" soon after the ingestion.

N-methyl-D-aspartate receptor antagonists

We found no RCTs or observational studies of sufficient quality evaluating n-methyl-D-aspartate receptor antagonists in people with acute organophosphorus poisoning.

Organophosphorus hydrolases

We found no RCTs or observational studies of sufficient quality evaluating organophosphorus hydrolases in people with acute organophosphorus poisoning.

Oximes

One systematic review provided insufficient evidence to assess oximes in people with acute organophosphorus poisoning.

Sodium bicarbonate

We found no RCTs or observational studies of sufficient quality evaluating sodium bicarbonate in acute organophosphorus poisoning.

α_2 Adrenergic receptor agonists (clonidine)

We found no RCTs or observational studies of sufficient quality evaluating clonidine in people with acute organophosphorus poisoning.

LIKELY TO BE INEFFECTIVE OR HARMFUL

Cathartics

We found no RCTs or observational studies of sufficient quality evaluating cathartics in people with acute organophosphorus poisoning. Organophosphorus poisoning itself causes diarrhoea, which may lead to electrolyte imbalance. This may be exacerbated by cathartics, suggesting that the risk of harm may outweigh its potential benefits.

Ipecacuanha (ipecac)

We found no RCTs or observational studies of sufficient quality evaluating ipecacuanha (ipecac) in people with acute organophosphorus poisoning. Clinical consensus suggests that the risk of harm, although not quantified, probably outweighs any potential benefits.

*Based on consensus, RCTs would be considered unethical

DEFINITION   Acute organophosphorus poisoning occurs after dermal, respiratory, or oral exposure to either low volatility pesticides (e.g. chlorpyrifos, dimethoate) or high volatility nerve gases (e.g. sarin, tabun). Inhibition of acetylcholinesterase at synapses results in accumulation of acetylcholine and over-activation of acetylcholine receptors at the neuromuscular junction and in the autonomic and central nervous systems.[1] Early clinical features reflect involvement of the parasympathetic system: bronchorrhoea, miosis, salivation, lachrymation, defecation, urination, and hypotension. Features indicating involvement of the neuromuscular junction (muscle weakness and fasciculations) and central nervous system (seizures [with nerve gases], coma,

Organophosphorus poisoning (acute)

respiratory failure) are also common at this stage. An intermediate syndrome has been described (cranial nerve palsies and proximal muscle weakness with preserved distal muscle power after resolution of early cholinergic symptoms), but its definition, pathophysiology, and incidence are still unclear. A late motor or motor/sensory peripheral neuropathy may also develop after recovery from acute poisoning with some organophosphorus compounds.[1]

INCIDENCE/ PREVALENCE
Most cases occur in the developing world following occupational or deliberate exposure to organophosphorus pesticides.[2] Although data are sparse, organophosphates appear to be the most important cause of death from deliberate self poisoning worldwide.[3] For example, in Sri Lanka, about 10 000 to 20 000 admissions to hospital for organophosphorus poisoning occur each year. Of these, about 10% die. In most cases, the poisoning is intentional.[4] Case fatality rates across the developing world are commonly greater than 20%.[3] In Central America, occupational poisoning is more common than intentional poisoning, and deaths are fewer.[5] Extrapolating from limited data, the World Health Organization has estimated that each year more than 200 000 people worldwide die from pesticide poisoning,[6] but these figures are old and widely contested.[2] Most deaths occur in Asia, and organophosphorus pesticides probably cause at least 50% of cases.[3] Deaths from organophosphorus nerve gases occurred during the Iran–Iraq war.[7] Military or terrorist action with these chemical weapons remains possible. Twelve people died in a terrorist attack in Tokyo and probably thousands died in Iran after military use.

AETIOLOGY/ RISK FACTORS
The widespread accessibility of pesticides in rural parts of the developing world makes them easy options for acts of self harm.[3] Occupational exposure is usually due to insufficient or inappropriate protective equipment.[2]

PROGNOSIS
There are no validated scoring systems for categorising severity or predicting outcome, although many have been proposed. The highly variable natural history and difficulty in determining ingested dose make predicting outcome for an individual inaccurate and potentially hazardous, because people admitted in good condition can deteriorate rapidly and require intubation and mechanical ventilation. Prognosis in acute self poisoning is likely to depend on dose and toxicity of the ingested organophosphorus (e.g. neurotoxicity potential, half life, rate of ageing, whether activation to the toxic compound is required [pro-poison], and whether dimethylated or diethylated).[8] Prognosis in occupational exposure is better because the dose is normally smaller and the route is dermal.

Please refer to the Clinical Evidence website for full text and references.

Paracetamol (acetaminophen) poisoning

Search date March 2004

Nick Buckley and Michael Eddleston

What are the effects of treatments?

Acetylcysteine

One systematic review found one RCT in people with established paracetamol induced liver failure. It found that acetylcysteine reduced mortality after 21 days compared with placebo. One observational study found that people given early treatment with acetylcysteine were less likely to develop liver damage than untreated historical controls. We found no RCTs comparing acetylcysteine versus methionine.

Methionine

One small RCT identified by a systematic review found no significant difference in mortality between methionine and supportive care, although it lacked power to detect a clinically important difference. It found limited evidence that methionine reduced hepatotoxicity compared with supportive care. We found no RCTs comparing methionine versus acetylcysteine.

Activated charcoal (single or multiple dose)

One systematic review found no evidence on the effects of activated charcoal, whether in single or multiple dose regimens, in people poisoned by paracetamol. One large case series found that clinically significant complications of multiple dose activated charcoal were rare.

Gastric lavage

One systematic review found no RCTs examining the effects of gastric lavage in paracetamol poisoning.

Ipecacuanha

One systematic review found no RCTs examining the effects of ipecacuanha in paracetamol poisoning.

DEFINITION Paracetamol poisoning occurs as a result of either accidental or intentional overdose with paracetamol (acetaminophen).

INCIDENCE/ Paracetamol is the most common drug used for self poisoning in the UK.[1] It
PREVALENCE is also a common means of self poisoning in the rest of Europe, North America, and Australasia. An estimated 41 200 cases of poisoning with products containing paracetamol occurred in 1989–1990 in England and Wales, with a mortality of 0.40% (95% CI 0.38% to 0.46%). Overdoses owing to paracetamol alone result in an estimated 150–200 deaths and 15–20 liver transplants each year in England and Wales. More recent studies suggest that paracetamol poisoning is at least as common now in the UK, although there is limited evidence that there have been modest reductions in large overdoses, liver transplants, and deaths since packaging restrictions were instituted in 1998.[2]

Paracetamol (acetaminophen) poisoning

AETIOLOGY/ RISK FACTORS Most cases in the UK are impulsive acts of self harm in young people.[1,3] In one study of 80 people who had overdosed with paracetamol, 42 had obtained the tablets for the specific purpose of taking an overdose and 33 had obtained them less than 1 hour before the act.[3]

PROGNOSIS People with blood paracetamol concentrations above the standard treatment line (defined in the UK as a line joining 200 mg/L at 4 hours and 30 mg/L at 15 hours on a semilogarithmic plot) have a poor prognosis without treatment**⑤**.[4-6] In one study of 57 untreated people with blood concentrations above this line, 33 developed severe liver damage and three died.[5] People with a history of chronic alcohol misuse, use of enzyme inducing drugs, eating disorders, or multiple paracetamol overdoses may be at risk of liver damage with blood concentrations below this line.[7] In the USA, a lower line is used as an indication for treatment but we found no data relating this line to prognostic outcomes.[8] **Dose effect:** The dose ingested also indicates the risk of hepatotoxicity. People ingesting less than 125 mg/kg had no significant hepatotoxicity, with a sharp dose dependent rise for higher doses.[9] The threshold for toxicity after acute ingestion may be higher in children, where a single dose of less than 200 mg/kg has not been reported to lead to death and rarely causes hepatotoxicity.[10] For people who present later than 24 hours or an unknown time after ingestion, several other prognostic indicators have been proposed, including prothrombin time and abnormal liver function tests.[11,12] These have not been validated prospectively.

Please refer to the Clinical Evidence website for full text and references.

What are the effects of treatments for non-ruptured tubal pregnancy?

TRADE OFF BETWEEN BENEFITS AND HARMS

Choice between open and laparoscopic salpingostomy

One systematic review found that, compared with laparoscopic salpingostomy open salpingostomy increased rates of elimination of tubal pregnancy. It found no significant difference in rates of subsequent intrauterine pregnancy or repeat ectopic pregnancy, but perioperative blood loss was higher with open salpingostomy.

UNKNOWN EFFECTIVENESS

Methotrexate (oral)

One small RCT identified by a systematic review found no significant difference between oral methotrexate 2.5 mg daily for 5 days and expectant management in the need for laparoscopy for persistent adnexal mass within 3 months.

Salpingostomy

We found no RCTs comparing salpingostomy with expectant management. One RCT identified by a systematic review found no significant difference in rates of elimination of tubal pregnancy plus tubal preservation, spontaneous intrauterine pregnancy, or repeat ectopic pregnancy at 18 months between multiple dose intramuscular methotrexate (1 mg/kg on days 1, 2, 4, and 6) plus folic acid compared with laparoscopic salpingostomy. The same RCT found that multiple dose methotrexate decreased health related quality of life compared with laparoscopic salpingostomy. One systematic review found higher rates of persistent ectopic pregnancy and lower rates of elimination of tubal pregnancy with single dose intramuscular methotrexate 1 mg/kg or 50 mg/m^2 compared with laparoscopic salpingostomy.

Fimbrial expression, salpingectomy, and salpingo-oophorectomy

We found no systematic review or RCTs that evaluated these interventions.

UNLIKELY TO BE BENEFICIAL

Methotrexate (intramuscular, multiple or single dose

One RCT identified by a systematic review found no significant difference in rates of elimination of tubal pregnancy plus tubal preservation, spontaneous intrauterine pregnancy, or repeat ectopic pregnancy at 18 months between multiple dose intramuscular methotrexate (1 mg/kg on days 1, 2, 4, and 6) plus folic acid compared with laparoscopic salpingostomy. The same RCT found that multiple dose methotrexate decreased health related quality of life compared with laparoscopic salpingostomy. One systematic review found higher rates of persistent ectopic pregnancy and lower rates of elimination of tubal pregnancy with single dose intramuscular methotrexate 1 mg/kg or 50 mg/m^2 compared with laparoscopic salpingostomy.

DEFINITION   In ectopic pregnancy, the fertilised ovum implants on a surface other than the uterine endometrium. Almost all ectopic pregnancies implant in the fallopian tubes. Ectopic pregnancies are detected by clinical suspicion and serial measurement of serum human chorionic gonadotrophin (hCG) or ultrasound.[1] Spontaneous resolution occurs only in selected cases: in women with ▶

Ectopic pregnancy

a small adnexal mass on transvaginal sonography, decreasing hCG levels, and only minor symptoms.[2,3] **Population:** This chapter covers management in women with non-ruptured, tubal ectopic pregnancy only. Typically, this group would consist of women with small tubal pregnancies confirmed ultrasonographically or based on serial hCG levels. We have excluded women with an acute presentation of ectopic pregnancy (such as peritonism, or with evidence of rupture or bleeding).

INCIDENCE/ PREVALENCE
Small studies suggest that 1–2% of reported pregnancies are ectopic.[4,5] A recent large study attempted to estimate the proportion of ectopic pregnancies in the USA using national data sets, but found that data were too flawed to provide an accurate estimate of the incidence.[6]

AETIOLOGY/ RISK FACTORS
A recent large case-control study suggested that the main risk factors for ectopic pregnancy were history of pelvic infection (OR 3.4, 95% CI 2.4 to 5.0) and smoking (OR 3.9, 95% CI 2.6 to 5.9).[7] Other risk factors were age, previous spontaneous abortion, history of infertility, and previous use of an intrauterine contraceptive device.[7] Earlier studies have found that previous ectopic pregnancy, previous tubal surgery including tubal sterilisation, documented tubal pathology, intrauterine contraceptive device, previous genital infections, smoking and *in utero* diethylstilbestrol exposure were associated with ectopic pregnancy.[8–10] The risk of ectopic pregnancy varies with method of tubal sterilisation. Women sterilised by bipolar tubal coagulation before the age of 30 years were found to have a risk of ectopic pregnancy 27 times greater than women who had postpartum partial salpingectomy.[9]

PROGNOSIS
Risks of ectopic pregnancy include tubal rupture, life-threatening bleeding, and subsequent infertility. The combination of transvaginal ultrasound and hCG measurements allow the condition to be diagnosed earlier now than previously. Consequently, mortality has fallen over time in the developed world from 35.5 deaths per 10 000 cases to 3.8 deaths per 10 000 cases between 1970 and 1989 in the USA and from 16 deaths per 10 000 cases to three deaths per 10 000 pregnancies between 1973 and 1993 in the UK.[3] However, mortality remains high in poorer countries: 100–300 deaths per 10 000 cases in one African survey.[11] Evaluating expectant management to assess prognosis is difficult because of ethical concerns about exposing women to undue risk of acute complications, which may also have medico-legal implications.[12] However, expectant management has been suggested as a feasible option in women at low risk of acute complications (such as asymptomatic women and women with small adnexal masses and decreasing hCG levels), and in the presence of close monitoring. A recent non-systematic review found rates of spontaneous resolution with expectant management to range from 46–65%.[3] One prospective cohort study (118 women) found that rates of spontaneous resolution varied with hCG level from 98% where hCG concentrations were less than 200 mIU/mL to 25% for hCG concentration greater than 2000 mIU/mL.[2] However, no factors have yet been found that reliably predict tubal rupture or bleeding.[3]

Please refer to the Clinical Evidence website for full text and references.

What are the effects of treatment for nausea and vomiting in early pregnancy?

BENEFICIAL

Ginger

Three RCTs and one randomised crossover trial found that ginger reduced nausea and vomiting in early pregnancy. One further RCT found that ginger reduced nausea and dry retching, but had no effect on episodes of vomiting.

LIKELY TO BE BENEFICIAL

Acupressure

One systematic review of small RCTs found limited evidence that P6 acupressure reduced self reported morning sickness compared with sham acupressure or no intervention. Three subsequent RCTs and two randomized trials found that P6 acupressure reduced the duration, but not necessarily the intensity, of nausea and vomiting.

Antihistamines (H1 antagonists)

Two systematic reviews found limited evidence that antihistamines reduced nausea and vomiting, with no evidence of teratogenicity.

Cyanocobalamin (vitamin B_{12})

One systematic review has found that cyanocobalamin reduces vomiting episodes compared with placebo.

Pyridoxine (vitamin B_6)

Two systematic reviews found limited evidence that pyridoxine reduced nausea but found no evidence of an effect on vomiting.

UNKNOWN EFFECTIVENESS

Acupuncture

One RCT found that acupuncture reduced nausea and retching compared with no acupuncture, with no evidence of adverse effects. However, an improvement was also found with sham acupuncture compared with no treatment. A second smaller RCT found no significant difference in nausea between acupuncture and sham acupuncture.

Dietary interventions (other than ginger)

We found no RCTS of dietary interventions (other than ginger).

Phenothiazines

One systematic review found limited evidence that phenothiazines reduced the proportion of women with nausea and vomiting. However, results were not conclusive. The review found no evidence of teratogenicity.

Nausea and vomiting in early pregnancy

What are the effects of treatments for hyperemesis gravidarum?

UNKNOWN EFFECTIVENESS

Acupuncture

One small randomised, crossover RCT found a faster reduction in nausea, as measured on a visual analogue scale, after active PC6 acupuncture compared with sham acupuncture. Episodes of vomiting were also reduced. However, we were unable to draw reliable conclusions from this study.

Corticosteroids

One small RCT found no significant improvement in persistent vomiting or readmission to hospital after 1 week of treatment with prednisolone compared with placebo. One small RCT found no significant improvement in persistence of vomiting but found that prednisolone reduced admission to hospital compared with promethazine.

Corticotropins

One small RCT found no significant difference in nausea and vomiting between intramuscular corticotropin (adrenocorticotrophic hormone [ACTH]) and placebo.

Diazepam

One RCT provided insufficient evidence to assess the effects of diazepam in women with hyperemesis gravidarum.

Dietary interventions (other than ginger)

One small crossover RCT found no significant difference in nausea and vomiting after 3 weeks of dietary supplementation with carob seed flour compared with placebo.

Ginger

One small RCT provided insufficient evidence to assess the effects of ginger in hyperemesis gravidarum.

Ondansetron

One small RCT provided insufficient evidence to assess the effects of ondansetron in hyperemesis gravidarum.

DEFINITION **Nausea and vomiting** are both common in early pregnancy. Although often called "morning sickness", nausea and vomiting can occur at any time of the day and may be constant.[1] Symptoms usually start between 4 and 7 weeks' gestation (one study found this to be the case in 70% of affected women)[2] and stop by 16 weeks in about 90% of women.[1–3] One study found that fewer than 10% of affected women suffer nausea and/or vomiting before the first missed period.[3] Most women do not require treatment. However, persistent vomiting and severe nausea can progress to hyperemesis if the woman is unable to maintain adequate hydration, fluid and electrolyte balance, and nutrition. **Hyperemesis gravidarum** is a diagnosis of exclusion, characterised by prolonged and severe nausea and vomiting, dehydration, and weight loss.[1] Laboratory investigation may show elevated plasma ketone levels in the absence of acidosis (ketosis), low serum levels of sodium (hyponatraemia), potassium (hypokalaemia), and urea (hypouricaemia), metabolic hypochloraemic alkalosis (excess base alkali in the body fluids caused by chloride loss), and excess ketones in the urine (ketonuria).

INCIDENCE/ PREVALENCE	Nausea affects about 70% and vomiting about 60% of pregnant women.[1] The true incidence of hyperemesis gravidarum is not known. It has been documented to range from 3 to 20 per thousand pregnancies. However, most authors report an incidence of 1 in 200.[2]
AETIOLOGY/ RISK FACTORS	The causes of nausea and vomiting in pregnancy are unknown. One theory, that they are caused by the rise in human chorionic gonadotrophin concentration, is compatible with the natural history of the condition, its severity in pregnancies affected by hydatidiform mole, and its good prognosis (see prognosis below).[4] The aetiology of hyperemesis gravidarum is also uncertain. Again, endocrine and psychological factors are suspected, but evidence is inconclusive.[4]
PROGNOSIS	One systematic review (search date 1988) found that nausea and vomiting were associated with a reduced risk of miscarriage (6 studies, 14 564 women; OR 0.36, 95% CI 0.32 to 0.42) but found no association with perinatal mortality.[5] Nausea and vomiting and hyperemesis usually improve over the course of pregnancy, but in one cross sectional observational study 13% of women reported that nausea and vomiting persisted beyond 20 weeks' gestation.[6]

Please refer to the Clinical Evidence website for full text and references.

Perineal care

Search date April 2004

Chris Kettle

What are the effects of intrapartum surgical interventions on rates of perineal trauma?

BENEFICIAL

Restrictive use of episiotomy (reduces risk of posterior trauma compared with routine use)

One systematic review found that restricting episiotomy to specific fetal and maternal indications reduced the rates of posterior perineal trauma, need for suturing, and healing complications compared with routine use, but increased the rates of anterior vaginal and labial trauma, which carries minimal morbidity.

TRADE OFF BETWEEN BENEFITS AND HARMS

Vacuum extraction (less perineal trauma than with forceps but newborns have increased risk of cephalhaematoma)

One systematic review and subsequent RCTs found that vacuum extraction reduced the rate of severe perineal trauma compared with forceps delivery, but increased the incidence of neonatal cephalhaematoma and retinal haemorrhage.

UNLIKELY TO BE BENEFICIAL

Midline episiotomy incision (associated with higher risk of third or fourth degree tears compared with mediolateral incision)

We found no evidence that midline episiotomy incision improved perineal pain or wound dehiscence compared with mediolateral incision. Limited evidence from one quasi-randomised trial suggested that midline incision may increase the risk of third and fourth degree tears compared with mediolateral incision.

LIKELY TO BE INEFFECTIVE OR HARMFUL

Epidural anaesthesia (increases instrumental delivery, which is associated with increased rates of perineal trauma)

One systematic review found no direct evidence about the effects of epidural compared with other forms of anaesthesia on rates of perineal trauma. However, RCTs identified by the review found that epidural anaesthesia maintained beyond the first stage of labour compared with epidural restricted to the first stage of labour increased the risk of instrumental delivery, which in turn is associated with an increased risk of perineal trauma.

What are the effects of intrapartum non-surgical interventions on the rates of perineal trauma?

BENEFICIAL

Continuous support during labour (reduces operative vaginal birth compared with usual care)

One systematic review found that providing continuous support for women during childbirth reduced the rate of operative vaginal birth (vacuum extraction or forceps) compared with usual care. It found no significant difference in the overall rates of episiotomy or perineal trauma (defined as episiotomy or laceration requiring suturing).

▶

◀ **TRADE OFF BETWEEN BENEFITS AND HARMS**

Upright versus supine or lithotomy position during delivery (fewer episiotomies but more second degree tears than supine or lithotomy positions)

One systematic review found that any upright position for delivery marginally reduced episiotomies compared with supine or lithotomy positions but this was offset by an increase in second degree tears. Rates of assisted vaginal delivery were slightly reduced in the upright group.

"Hands poised" versus "hands on" method of delivery (increases pain and need for manual delivery of placenta, no significant difference in rate of perineal trauma, and reduces episiotomy rate)

One multicentre RCT and one quasi-randomised trial found that the "hands poised" method (not touching the baby's head or supporting the mother's perineum) reduced episiotomy rates compared with the conventional "hands on" method (applying pressure to the baby's head during delivery and supporting the mother's perineum). The RCT found no evidence of an effect on the risk of perineal trauma, but found that the "hands poised" group had an increased risk of requiring manual removal of the placenta and higher rates of short term perineal pain.

UNKNOWN EFFECTIVENESS

Passive descent in the second stage of labour

One RCT comparing passive fetal descent versus immediate active pushing found no significant difference in perineal trauma.

Sustained breath holding (Valsalva) method of pushing

One systematic review of two poor quality controlled clinical trials found no significant difference in the extent or rate of perineal trauma between sustained breath holding (Valsalva) and spontaneous exhalatory methods of pushing during the second stage of labour.

What are the effects of different methods and materials for primary repair of first and second degree tears and episiotomies?

BENEFICIAL

Absorbable synthetic sutures for perineal repair of first and second degree tears and episiotomies (reduced short term pain compared with catgut sutures)

One systematic review found that absorbable synthetic sutures reduced pain at up to 10 days after birth compared with catgut sutures. One subsequent RCT, however, found no significant difference in perineal pain at 3 days, although it may have lacked power to detect a clinically important effect. The systematic review and the subsequent RCT found no significant difference between absorbable synthetic sutures and catgut sutures in pain or dyspareunia at 3 months, but one RCT with 12 months' follow up, which was included in the review, found lower rates of dyspareunia with absorbable synthetic sutures. RCTs found no significant difference between rapidly absorbed and standard synthetic sutures in overall perineal pain, pain on sitting, or dyspareunia. RCTs also found reduced perineal pain on walking and a reduction in suture material removal with rapidly absorbed synthetic sutures.

▶

Perineal care

Continuous subcutaneous technique of perineal skin closure of first and second degree tears and episiotomies (reduced short term pain compared with interrupted sutures)

One systematic review found that continuous subcuticular sutures for perineal skin reduced short term pain compared with interrupted sutures, but found no significant difference in perineal pain or dyspareunia at 3 months postpartum. One RCT found that a loose continuous technique for repair of all layers reduced short term perineal pain and suture removal compared with interrupted sutures up to 3 months postpartum.

LIKELY TO BE BENEFICIAL

Non-suturing of perineal skin in first and second degree tears and episiotomies (reduces dyspareunia)

One large RCT found no significant difference between leaving the perineal skin unsutured compared with conventional suturing in pain at 10 days after birth. A second RCT found that non-suturing reduced pain for up to 3 months after delivery. Both RCTs found that non-suturing of the perineal skin reduced dyspareunia at 3 months after birth.

LIKELY TO BE INEFFECTIVE OR HARMFUL

Non-suturing of muscle and skin in first and second degree perineal tears (poorer wound healing than with suturing)

Two small RCTs found no significant difference in short term perineal pain between non-suturing and suturing of first and second degree tears. One of the RCTs found no significant difference in healing between groups but the second RCT found that a greater proportion of women in the non-sutured group had poorer wound healing at 6 weeks after birth.

What are the effects of different methods and materials for primary repair of third and fourth degree tears?

UNKNOWN EFFECTIVENESS

Different methods and materials for repair of third and fourth degree tears

One small RCT comparing the overlap method versus the end-to-end method for primary repair of third degree obstetric tears found no significant difference in perineal discomfort and a non-significant reduction in the rate of reported faecal urgency and anal incontinence with the overlap technique compared with the end-to-end method.

DEFINITION   Perineal trauma is any damage to the genitalia during childbirth that occurs spontaneously or intentionally by surgical incision (episiotomy). Anterior perineal trauma is injury to the labia, anterior vagina, urethra, or clitoris, and is usually associated with little morbidity. Posterior perineal trauma is any injury to the posterior vaginal wall, perineal muscles, or anal sphincter. First degree spontaneous tears involve only skin; second degree tears involve perineal muscles; third degree tears partially or completely disrupt the anal sphincter; and fourth degree tears completely disrupt the external and internal anal sphincter and epithelium.[1]

INCIDENCE/   Over 85% of women having a vaginal birth sustain some form of perineal
PREVALENCE trauma,[2] and 60–70% receive stitches — equivalent to 400 000 women a year in the UK in 1997.[2,3] There are wide variations in rates of episiotomy: 8% in the Netherlands, 14% in England, 50% in the USA, and 99% in east European countries.[4–6] Sutured spontaneous tears are reported in about a third of women in the USA[6] and the UK,[7] but this is probably an underestimate ▶

because of inconsistency of reporting and classification of perineal trauma. The incidence of anal sphincter tears varies between 0.5% in the UK, 2.5% in Denmark, and 7% in Canada.[9]

AETIOLOGY/ RISK FACTORS
Perineal trauma occurs during spontaneous or assisted vaginal delivery and is usually more extensive after the first vaginal delivery.[1] Associated risk factors also include increased fetal size, mode of delivery, and malpresentation and malposition of the fetus. Other maternal factors that may increase the extent and degree of trauma are ethnicity (white people are probably at greater risk than black people), older age, abnormal collagen synthesis, and poor nutritional state.[9] Clinicians' practices or preferences in terms of intrapartum interventions may influence the severity and rate of perineal trauma (e.g. use of ventouse v forceps).

PROGNOSIS
Perineal trauma affects women's physical, psychological, and social wellbeing in the immediate postnatal period as well as the long term. It can also disrupt breast feeding, family life, and sexual relations. In the UK, about 23–42% of women will continue to have pain and discomfort for 10–12 days postpartum, and 7–10% of women will continue to have long term pain (3–18 months after delivery);[2,3,10] 23% of women will experience superficial dyspareunia at 3 months; 3–10% will report faecal incontinence;[11,12] and up to 24% will have urinary problems.[2,3] Complications depend on the severity of perineal trauma and on the effectiveness of treatment.

Please refer to the Clinical Evidence website for full text and references.

Postnatal depression

Search date January 2004

Louise Howard

What are the effects of treatments?

LIKELY TO BE BENEFICIAL

Antidepressants (fluoxetine)

Limited evidence from one small RCT suggested that fluoxetine may improve postnatal depression at 4 and 12 weeks compared with placebo. The RCT had problems with recruitment and a high drop out rate, and it excluded breastfeeding women. We found no RCTs that satisfactorily compared fluoxetine with psychological treatment. We found no RCTs on the effects of other antidepressants in women with postnatal depression, and no RCTs that satisfactorily compared other antidepressants with psychological treatments.

Cognitive behavioural therapy (individual)

One RCT provided limited evidence that individual cognitive behavioural therapy and ideal standard care both improved depressive symptoms, but that there was no significant difference between the two interventions. Limited evidence from one RCT suggested that individual cognitive behavioural therapy may improve postnatal depression in the short term (immediately after treatment) compared with routine primary care. The RCT found no clear longer term benefits (9 months to 5 years postpartum) from individual cognitive behavioural therapy compared with routine primary care, non-directive counselling, or psychodynamic therapy.

Interpersonal psychotherapy

One RCT found that interpersonal psychotherapy improved postnatal depression compared with waiting list controls at 12 weeks.

Non-directive counselling

Limited evidence from two RCTs suggests that, in the short term (immediately after treatment), non-directive counselling may improve postnatal depression compared with routine primary care. The one RCT with follow up beyond 12 weeks found no clear longer term benefits (from 9 months to 5 years postpartum) from non-directive counselling compared with routine primary care, individual cognitive behavioural therapy, or psychodynamic therapy.

Psychodynamic therapy

Limited evidence from one RCT suggests that psychodynamic therapy may improve postnatal depression in the short term (immediately after treatment) compared with routine primary care. The RCT found no clear longer term benefits (9 months to 5 years postpartum) from psychodynamic therapy compared with routine primary care, non-directive counselling, or cognitive behavioural therapy.

UNKNOWN EFFECTIVENESS

Antidepressants other than fluoxetine

We found no RCTs on the effects of antidepressants in women with postnatal depression, and no RCTs that satisfactorily compared antidepressants other than fluoxetine versus psychological treatments.

Cognitive behavioural therapy (group)

One small RCT in women with a high level of depressive symptoms on screening found that group cognitive behavioural therapy improved symptoms at 6 months compared with routine primary care.

▶

Hormones

Limited evidence from one small RCT in women with severe postnatal depression suggests that oestrogen treatment may improve postnatal depression at 3 and 6 months compared with placebo.

Light therapy

We found no RCTs evaluating light therapy.

Mother–infant interaction coaching

One small RCT found that mother–infant interaction coaching had no significant effect on maternal depression scores compared with usual treatment, but it improved maternal responsiveness to the infant within 10 weeks of starting treatment.

Psychoeducation with partner

One small RCT found that psychoeducation with partner reduced patients' depression scores and partners' psychiatric morbidity at 10 weeks compared with psychoeducation without partner.

Telephone based peer support (mother to mother)

One small RCT found that telephone based peer support reduced depression scores after 8 weeks compared with usual treatment.

DEFINITION Postnatal depression (PND) is broadly defined as non-psychotic depression occurring during the first 6 months postpartum. Puerperal mental disorders have only recently been categorised separately in psychiatric classifications, but both the International Classification of Diseases (ICD-10)[1] and the Diagnostic and Statistical Manual of mental disorders, fourth edition (DSM-IV) ❶ require certain qualifications to be met that limit their use: ICD-10 categorises mental disorders that occur postpartum as puerperal, but only if they cannot otherwise be classified, and DSM-IV allows "postpartum onset" to be specified for mood disorders starting within 4 weeks' postpartum.[2] In clinical practice and research, the broader definition above is often used, because whether or not PND is truly distinct from depression in general, depression in the postpartum period raises treatment issues for the nursing mother and has implications for the developing infant (see prognosis below). The symptoms are similar to symptoms of depression at other times of life, but in addition to low mood, sleep disturbance, change in appetite, diurnal variation in mood, poor concentration, and irritability, women with PND also experience guilt about their inability to look after their new baby. In many countries, health visitors screen for PND using the Edinburgh Postnatal Depression Scale,[3,4] which elicits depressive symptoms.

INCIDENCE/ PREVALENCE The prevalence of depression in women postpartum is similar to that found in women generally. However, the incidence of depression in the first month after childbirth is three times the average monthly incidence in non-childbearing women.[5] Studies across different cultures have shown a consistent incidence of postnatal depression (PND) (10–15%),[6] with higher rates in teenage mothers. A meta-analysis of studies mainly based in the developed world found the incidence of postnatal depression to be 12–13%.[7]

AETIOLOGY/ RISK FACTORS Three systematic reviews have identified the following risk factors for postnatal depression: past history of any psychopathology (including history of previous postnatal depression), low social support, poor marital relationship, and recent life events.[7–9]

PROGNOSIS Most episodes of PND resolve spontaneously within 3–6 months,[10] but about one in four affected mothers are still depressed on the child's first birthday.[11] In the developed world, suicide is now the main cause of maternal deaths in the first year postpartum,[12] but the suicide rate is lower at this time than in age ▶

Postnatal depression

matched non-postpartum women.[13] PND is also associated with reduced likelihood of secure attachment,[14] deficits in maternal–infant interactions,[15] and impaired cognitive and emotional development of the child, particularly in boys living in areas of socioeconomic deprivation.[15–17] These associations remain significant even after controlling for subsequent episodes of depression in the mother.

Please refer to the Clinical Evidence website for full text and references.

What are the effects of preventive interventions in women at risk of pre-eclampsia?

BENEFICIAL

Antiplatelet drugs

One systematic review and one subsequent RCT found that, in women considered at risk of pre-eclampsia, antiplatelet drugs (mainly aspirin) reduced the risk of pre-eclampsia, death of the baby, and delivery before 37 weeks compared with placebo or no treatment. The RCTs found no significant difference in other important outcomes. The systematic review found no evidence that aspirin increased the risk of bleeding in mother or baby compared with placebo.

Calcium supplementation

One systematic review found that calcium supplementation (mainly 2 g/day) reduced the risk of pre-eclampsia and reduced the risk of having a baby with birth weight under 2500 g compared with placebo. It found no significant difference between calcium supplements and placebo on the risk of caesarean section, preterm delivery, or stillbirth or death of the baby before discharge from hospital.

UNKNOWN EFFECTIVENESS

Antioxidants

Two RCTs found limited evidence that antioxidants (vitamins C plus E or lycopene) reduced the risk of pre-eclampsia compared with placebo. The RCTs provided insufficient evidence on other clinically important outcomes.

Magnesium supplementation

One systematic review found insufficient evidence about the effects of magnesium supplements on the risk of pre-eclampsia or its complications.

Other pharmacological agents (atenolol or nitrates)

We found two small RCTs; one compared atenolol versus placebo and the other compared glyceryl trinitrate patches versus placebo. Both RCTs were too small to allow any reliable conclusions to be drawn.

Salt restriction

Limited evidence from one systematic review found no significant difference in the risk of pre-eclampsia with a low salt diet compared with a normal diet.

Fish oil and/or evening primrose oil

We found six RCTs of fish oil and/or evening primrose oil, which were too small to allow reliable conclusions to be drawn.

What are the effects of interventions in women who develop mild–moderate hypertension during pregnancy?

UNKNOWN EFFECTIVENESS

Antihypertensive drugs for mild to moderate hypertension

Two systematic reviews have found that antihypertensive agents may halve the risk of severe hypertension but the effects of antihypertensive agents on other important outcomes are unclear. Systematic reviews found that angiotensin converting enzyme inhibitors used in pregnancy were associated with fetal renal

Pre-eclampsia and hypertension

failure, and found that ß blockers increased the risk of the baby being small for its gestational age. It remains unclear whether treatment of mild to moderate hypertension during pregnancy is worthwhile with any antihypertensive agent compared with no treatment.

Bed rest/hospital admission

We found insufficient evidence about hospital admission or bed rest compared with outpatient or day care or normal activities in hospital.

What are the effects of interventions in women who develop severe pre-eclampsia or very high blood pressure during pregnancy?

BENEFICIAL

Prophylactic magnesium sulphate in severe pre-eclampsia

One systematic review found that prophylactic magnesium sulphate halved the risk of eclampsia compared with placebo in women with severe pre-eclampsia. It found that magnesium sulphate reduced maternal mortality compared with placebo, although differences between groups did not reach significance. The review found no significant difference between magnesium sulphate and placebo on the risk of stillbirth or neonatal death in babies born to women with severe pre-eclampsia. The review also found that magnesium sulphate reduced the risk of eclampsia compared with phenytoin or nimodipine. A quarter of women given magnesium sulphate reported side effects (mainly flushing) compared with 5% of those given placebo. The review found insufficient evidence about the effects of diazepam compared with magnesium sulphate in women with severe pre-eclampsia.

LIKELY TO BE BENEFICIAL

Antihypertensive drugs for very high blood pressure*

Consensus opinion is that women with severe hypertension during pregnancy should have antihypertensive treatment. Placebo trials would therefore be unethical. One systematic review and one subsequent RCT in women with blood pressures high enough to merit immediate treatment found that all of the included antihypertensives reduced blood pressure, but found no evidence of a difference in the control of blood pressure by various antihypertensive drugs. The studies were too small to draw any further conclusions about the relative effects of different agents. Ketanserin and diazoxide may be associated with more adverse effects than hydralazine and labetalol, respectively.

*Consensus opinion is that women with severe hypertension during pregnancy should have antihypertensive treatment. Placebo controlled trials would therefore be unethical.

UNKNOWN EFFECTIVENESS

Interventionist obstetric management for severe early onset pre-eclampsia

One systematic review based on two small RCTs found no evidence that interventionist obstetric management reduced stillbirth or perinatal death rates compared with expectant management in babies born to mothers with severe early onset pre-eclampsia. However, it found that interventionist management increased rates of admission to neonatal intensive care and increased the risk of necrotising enterocolitis and respiratory distress in the baby compared with expectant management. The review found insufficient evidence about effects of interventionist compared with expectant management in the mother.

◀ **Antioxidants in severe pre-eclampsia**

One RCT found insufficient evidence about the effects of a combination of vitamin E plus vitamin C plus allopurinol compared with placebo.

Choice of analgesia during labour with severe pre-eclampsia

One RCT in women with severe pre-eclampsia found that epidural analgesia during labour reduced mean pain scores compared with patient controlled analgesia given intravenously, but the clinical importance of the difference was unclear.

Plasma volume expansion in severe pre-eclampsia

One systematic review comparing plasma volume expansion versus no expansion found insufficient evidence to draw reliable conclusions.

What is the best choice of anticonvulsant for women with eclampsia?

BENEFICIAL

Magnesium sulphate for eclampsia (better and safer than other anticonvulsants)

Systematic reviews have found that magnesium sulphate reduces the risk of further fits in women with eclampsia compared with phenytoin, diazepam, or lytic cocktail. One systematic review found that magnesium sulphate reduced the risk of maternal death compared with diazepam. Two other systematic reviews found lower maternal death rates with magnesium sulphate compared with phenytoin or lytic cocktail, although differences between groups did not reach significance.

DEFINITION Hypertension during pregnancy may be associated with one of several conditions. **Pregnancy induced hypertension** is a rise in blood pressure, without proteinuria, during the second half of pregnancy. **Pre-eclampsia** is a multisystem disorder, unique to pregnancy, which is usually associated with raised blood pressure and proteinuria. It rarely presents before 20 weeks' gestation. **Eclampsia** is one or more convulsions in association with the syndrome of pre-eclampsia. **Pre-existing hypertension** (not covered in this chapter) is known hypertension before pregnancy or raised blood pressure before 20 weeks' gestation. It may be essential hypertension or, less commonly, secondary to underlying disease.[1]

INCIDENCE/ PREVALENCE Pregnancy induced hypertension affects 10% of pregnancies, and pre-eclampsia complicates 2–8% of pregnancies.[2] Eclampsia occurs in about 1/2000 deliveries in developed countries.[3] In developing countries, estimates of the incidence of eclampsia vary from 1/100–1/1700.[4,5]

AETIOLOGY/ RISK FACTORS The cause of pre-eclampsia is unknown. It is likely to be multifactorial, and may result from deficient placental implantation during the first half of pregnancy.[6] Pre-eclampsia is more common among women likely to have a large placenta, such as those with multiple pregnancy, and among women with medical conditions associated with microvascular disease, such as diabetes, hypertension, and collagen vascular disease.[7,8] Other risk factors include genetic susceptibility, increased parity, and older maternal age.[9] Cigarette smoking seems to be associated with a lower risk of pre-eclampsia, but this potential benefit is outweighed by an increase in adverse outcomes such as low birth weight, placental abruption, and perinatal death.[10]

PROGNOSIS The outcome of pregnancy in women with pregnancy induced hypertension alone is at least as good as that for normotensive pregnancies.[7,11] However, once pre-eclampsia develops, morbidity and mortality rise for both mother and child. For example, perinatal mortality for women with severe pre-eclampsia is ▶

double that for normotensive women.[7] Perinatal outcome is worse with early gestational hypertension.[7,9,11] Perinatal mortality also increases in women with severe essential hypertension.[12]

Please refer to the Clinical Evidence website for full text and references.

What are the effects of preventive interventions in women at high risk of preterm delivery?

LIKELY TO BE BENEFICIAL

Prophylactic cervical cerclage for women at risk of cervical incompetence where cervical changes have not been identified

Systematic reviews identified five RCTs that found different results for women where cervical changes have not been identified. One large RCT found that cervical cerclage at 9–29 weeks reduced delivery before 33 weeks' gestation in women with a previous preterm delivery or previous cervical surgery, but doubled the risk of puerperal pyrexia compared with no cerclage. The other four smaller RCTs found no significant difference in preterm delivery before 34 weeks between cerclage at 10–30 weeks and no cerclage in women with a variety of risk factors for preterm delivery.

UNKNOWN EFFECTIVENESS

Prophylactic cervical cerclage for women at risk of cervical incompetence where cervical changes have been identified

Two RCTs identified by a systematic review found different results for women where cervical changes were present. One RCT found no significant difference in delivery before 34 weeks. The other small RCT found that cerclage plus bed rest reduced delivery before 34 weeks compared with bed rest alone. Neither RCT found a significant difference in perinatal death between cerclage plus bed rest and bed rest alone.

UNLIKELY TO BE BENEFICIAL

Enhanced antenatal care programmes for socially deprived population groups/high risk groups

RCTs carried out in a range of countries found no significant difference between enhanced antenatal care and usual care in reducing the risk of preterm delivery.

What are the effects of interventions to improve outcome after preterm rupture of the membranes?

LIKELY TO BE BENEFICIAL

Antibiotic treatment for premature rupture of the membranes (prolongs gestation and may reduce infection, but unknown effect on perinatal mortality)

One systematic review in women with premature rupture of membranes has found that antibiotics prolong pregnancy and reduce the risk of neonatal morbidity, such as neonatal infection, requirement for treatment with oxygen, and abnormal cerebral ultrasound, compared with placebo. It found that co-amoxiclav (amoxycillin plus clavulanic acid) increased the risk of neonatal necrotising enterocolitis compared with placebo.

▶

Preterm birth

UNKNOWN EFFECTIVENESS

Amnioinfusion for preterm rupture of the membranes

One systematic review found insufficient evidence from one RCT about the effects of amnioinfusion compared with no amnioinfusion in improving neonatal outcomes after preterm rupture of the membranes.

What are the effects of treatments to stop contractions in preterm labour?

LIKELY TO BE BENEFICIAL

Calcium channel blockers

We found no systematic review or RCTs comparing calcium channel blockers versus placebo. One systematic review has found that calcium channel blockers significantly reduce deliveries within 48 hours, neonatal morbidity, and withdrawals caused by maternal adverse effects compared with other tocolytics (mainly β agonists).

UNKNOWN EFFECTIVENESS

Oxytocin receptor antagonists (atosiban)

One systematic review identified two RCTs that compared atosiban with placebo and found different results. The larger RCT found that atosiban prolonged pregnancy compared with placebo but found that atosiban appeared to increase fetal deaths below 28 weeks' gestation. The other RCT found that atosiban increased delivery within 48 hours.

Prostaglandin inhibitors (indometacin)

One systematic review found limited evidence that indometacin reduced delivery within 48 hours and 7 days and delivery before 37 weeks' gestation compared with placebo. However, it found no significant difference between indometacin and placebo or no treatment in perinatal mortality, respiratory distress syndrome, bronchopulmonary dysplasia, necrotising enterocolitis, neonatal sepsis, or low birth weight. The review may have lacked power to detect a clinically important effect.

UNLIKELY TO BE BENEFICIAL

Magnesium sulphate

One systematic review found no significant difference between magnesium sulphate and placebo in delivery before 36 weeks; perinatal mortality or respiratory distress syndrome. A second systematic review found no significant difference between magnesium sulphate and other tocolytics (betamimetics, calcium channel blockers, prostaglandin synthetase inhibitors, nitroglycerine, alcohol and dextrose infusion) in delivery within 48 hours, although results were heterogeneous.

LIKELY TO BE INEFFECTIVE OR HARMFUL

Betamimetics

One systematic review has found no significant difference between β2 agonists and placebo or no treatment in perinatal mortality, respiratory distress syndrome or birth weight less than 2500 g. It found that β2 agonists increased maternal adverse effects such as chest pain, palpitations, dyspnoea, tremor, nausea, vomiting, headache, hyperglycaemia, hypokalaemia compared with placebo or no treatment.

What are the effects of elective compared with selective caesarean delivery for women in preterm labour?

UNLIKELY TO BE BENEFICIAL

Elective rather than selective caesarean delivery in preterm labour

One systematic review has found that elective caesarean delivery increases maternal morbidity compared with selective caesarean delivery, and found no significant difference in neonatal morbidity or mortality. The RCTs may have been underpowered to detect a clinically important neonatal benefit.

What are the effects of interventions to improve outcome in preterm delivery?

BENEFICIAL

Antenatal corticosteroids

One systematic review found that antenatal corticosteroids significantly reduced respiratory distress syndrome, intraventricular haemorrhage, and neonatal mortality compared with placebo or no treatment.

LIKELY TO BE INEFFECTIVE OR HARMFUL

Antibiotic treatment for preterm labour with intact membranes

One systematic review found that antibiotics do not prolong pregnancy and do not reduce perinatal mortality compared with placebo, but they do reduce the incidence of maternal infection.

Thyrotropin releasing hormone plus corticosteroids before preterm delivery

One systematic review in women at risk of preterm birth has found no significant difference between thyrotropin releasing hormone plus corticosteroids and corticosteroids alone in improving neonatal outcomes. Thyrotropin releasing hormone plus corticosteroids increased maternal and fetal adverse events compared with corticosteroids alone.

DEFINITION Preterm or premature birth is defined by the World Health Organization as delivery of an infant before 37 completed weeks of gestation.[1] There is no set lower limit to this definition, but 23–24 weeks' gestation is widely accepted,[1] which approximates to an average fetal weight of 500g.

INCIDENCE/ PREVALENCE Preterm birth occurs in about 5–10% of all births in developed countries,[2–4] but in recent years the incidence seems to have increased in some countries, particularly the USA.[5] We found little reliable evidence for incidence (using the definition of premature birth given above) in less developed countries. The rate in northwestern Ethiopia has been reported to vary between 11–22% depending on the age group of mothers studied, and is highest in teenage mothers.[6]

AETIOLOGY/ RISK FACTORS About 30% of preterm births are unexplained and spontaneous.[4,7,8] The two strongest risk factors for idiopathic preterm labour are low socioeconomic status and previous preterm delivery. Multiple pregnancy accounts for about another 30% of cases.[4,7] Other known risk factors include genital tract infection, preterm rupture of the membranes, antepartum haemorrhage, cervical incompetence, and congenital uterine abnormalities, which collectively account for about 20–25% of cases. The remaining cases (15–20%) are attributed to elective preterm delivery secondary to hypertensive disorders of pregnancy, intrauterine fetal growth restriction, congenital abnormalities, trauma and medical disorders of pregnancy.[4,5,7,8]

Preterm birth

PROGNOSIS   Preterm labour usually results in preterm birth. One systematic review (search date not reported), which compared tocolysis versus placebo, found that about 27% of preterm labours resolved spontaneously and about 70% progressed to preterm delivery.[9] Observational studies have found that one preterm birth significantly raises the risk of another in a subsequent pregnancy.[10]

Please refer to the Clinical Evidence website for full text and references.

What are the effects of treatments for acute bronchitis in people without chronic respiratory disease?

TRADE OFF BETWEEN BENEFITS AND HARMS

Antibiotics

One systematic review and one subsequent RCT found that antibiotics (doxycycline, erythromycin and sulphamethoxazole-trimethoprim) modestly reduced cough at 1–2 weeks compared with placebo. However, they found no significant difference in quality of life or impairment in normal activity compared with placebo. We found no RCTs comparing amoxicillin (amoxycillin) versus placebo. RCTs found no significant difference in clinical improvement or cure between amoxicillin and roxithromycin or cefuroxime. RCTs found no significant difference between azithromycin and clarithromycin, among different cephalosporins, or between cefuroxime and amoxicillin plus clavulanic acid. Antibiotics increased the risk of adverse events such as nausea, vomiting, rash, headache, and vaginitis compared with placebo. Two RCTs found that adverse effects were less common with cefuroxime than with amoxicillin plus clavulanic acid. Widespread antibiotic use may lead to bacterial resistance to antibiotics.

UNKNOWN EFFECTIVENESS

Antihistamines

One RCT found insufficient evidence about the effects of antihistamines compared with placebo in people with acute bronchitis.

Antitussives

RCTs found no significant difference in cough severity between codeine or dextromethorphan and placebo in children or adults with acute bronchitis. The RCTs may have been too small to detect a clinically important difference. We found limited evidence from one RCT that moguisteine modestly reduced cough severity compared with placebo in adults, but was associated with more adverse gastrointestinal effects.

Expectorants

We found no RCTs about the effects of expectorants in people with acute bronchitis.

β_2 agonists

One systematic review found no significant difference in cough or ability to return to work between β_2 agonists (inhaled or oral) and placebo in people with acute bronchitis. It found limited evidence from one small RCT that β_2 agonists reduced cough compared with erythromycin. The review found that β_2 agonists were more frequently associated with shaking and tremor in adults than placebo.

DEFINITION Acute bronchitis is transient inflammation of the trachea and major bronchi. Clinically, it is diagnosed on the basis of cough and occasionally sputum, dyspnoea, and wheeze. This review is limited to episodes of acute bronchitis in people (smokers and non-smokers) with no pre-existing respiratory disease ▶

Bronchitis (acute)

such as a pre-existing diagnosis of asthma or chronic bronchitis, evidence of fixed airflow obstruction, or both, and excluding those with clinical or radiographic evidence of pneumonia. However, using a clinical definition for acute bronchitis implies that people with conditions such as transient/mild asthma or mild chronic obstructive pulmonary disease may have been recruited to some of the reported studies.

INCIDENCE/ PREVALENCE Acute bronchitis affects 44/1000 adults (> 16 years old) a year, with 82% of episodes occurring in autumn or winter.[1] One survey found that acute bronchitis was the fifth most common reason to present to a general practitioner in Australia.[2]

AETIOLOGY/ RISK FACTORS Infection is believed to be the trigger for acute bronchitis. However, pathogens have been identified in fewer than 55% of people.[1] Community studies that attempted to isolate pathogens from the sputum of people with acute bronchitis found viruses in 8–23%, typical bacteria (*Streptococcus pneumoniae*, *Haemophilus influenzae*, *Moraxella catarrhalis*) in 45%, and atypical bacteria (*Mycobacterium pneumoniae*, *Chlamydia pneumoniae*, *Bordetella pertussis*) in 0–25%.[1,3,4] It is unclear whether smoking affects the risk for developing acute bronchitis.

PROGNOSIS Acute bronchitis is regarded as a mild self limiting illness but there are few data on prognosis and rates of complications such as chronic cough or progression to chronic bronchitis or pneumonia. One prospective longitudinal study reviewed 653 previously well adults who presented to suburban general practices over a 12 month period with symptoms of acute lower respiratory tract infection.[1] It found that within the first month of the illness 20% of people re-presented to their general practitioner with persistent or recurrent symptoms. One prospective study of 138 previously well adults found that 34% had symptoms consistent with either chronic bronchitis or asthma 3 years after initial presentation with acute bronchitis.[5] It is also unclear whether acute bronchitis plays a causal role in the progression to chronic bronchitis or is simply a marker of predisposition to chronic lung disease. Although smoking has been identified as the most important risk factor for chronic bronchitis,[6,7] it is unclear whether the inflammatory effects of cigarette smoke and infection causing acute bronchitis have additive effects in leading to chronic inflammatory airway changes.

Please refer to the Clinical Evidence website for full text and references.

What are the effects of treatments?

LIKELY TO BE BENEFICIAL

Antihistamines (may improve runny nose and sneezing, no significant difference in overall symptoms)

One systematic review found that chlorpheniramine or doxylaminine reduced runny nose and sneezing after 2 days compared with placebo in people with common cold, but the clinical benefit was small. Another review, that assessed a wide variety of antihistamines, found no significant difference in overall cold symptoms at 1–10 days between antihistamines and placebo and found that first generation antihistamines increased adverse effects, including sedation.

Decongestants (norephedrine, oxymetazoline, or pseudoephedrine) provided short term (3–10 hour) relief of congestive symptoms

One systematic review found that, compared with placebo, decongestants (norephedrine, oxymetazoline, or pseudoephedrine) reduced nasal congestion over 3–10 hours after a single dose in people with common cold. The review identified no RCTs of other decongestants. One case control study found weak evidence that phenylpropanolamine may increase the risk of haemorrhagic stroke.

UNKNOWN EFFECTIVENESS

Analgesics or anti-inflammatory drugs

We found no RCTs of analgesics or anti-inflammatory drugs in people with common cold.

Decongestants (insufficient evidence to assess longer term [> 10 hours] effects on congestive symptoms)

One systematic review provided insufficient evidence to assess the effects of longer use of decongestants in people with colds.

Echinacea

Systematic reviews found limited evidence that some preparations of echinacea may improve cold symptoms compared with placebo, but we found insufficient evidence about the effects of any specific product. Two subsequent RCTs, one in adults and one in children, found no significant difference between echinacea and placebo in severity or duration of cold symptoms.

Steam inhalation

One systematic review provided insufficient evidence to assess steam inhalation in people with common cold.

Vitamin C

One systematic review found limited evidence from quasi-randomised and controlled trials that vitamin C slightly reduced the duration of cold symptoms compared with placebo. However, the beneficial effect was small.

Zinc (intranasal gel or lozenges)

One systematic review found limited evidence that zinc gluconate or acetate lozenges may reduce duration of cold symptoms at 7 days compared with placebo. Another review found no significant difference in duration of symptoms. Both reviews found that symptoms were unchanged at 3 or 5 days. Two RCTs found that ▶

Common cold

zinc intranasal gel reduced the mean duration of cold symptoms compared with placebo. A third RCT found no significant difference in overall symptom duration between intranasal zinc and placebo.

LIKELY TO BE INEFFECTIVE OR HARMFUL

Antibiotics

Systematic reviews and one additional RCT found no significant difference between antibiotics and placebo in cure or general improvement at 6–14 days in people with colds. The additional RCT found that, in a subgroup of people (20%) with nasopharyngeal culture positive *H influenzae*, *M catarrhalis*, or *S pneumonia*, antibiotics increased recovery at 5 days compared with placebo. However, we have no methods currently of easily identifying such people at first consultation.

DEFINITION   Common colds are defined as upper respiratory tract infections that affect the predominantly nasal part of the respiratory mucosa. Since upper respiratory tract infections can affect any part of the mucosa, it is often arbitrary whether an upper respiratory tract infection is called a "cold" or "sore throat" ("pharyngitis" or "tonsillitis"), "sinusitis", "acute otitis media", or "bronchitis" (see figure 1 in sore throat, p 429). Sometimes all areas (simultaneously or at different times) are affected in one illness. Symptoms include sneezing, rhinorrhoea (runny nose), headache, and general malaise. In addition to nasal symptoms, half of sufferers experience sore throat and 40% experience cough.[1] This review does not include treatments for people with acute sinusitis (see acute sinusitis, p 142), acute bronchitis, (see acute bronchitis, p 421), or sore throat (see sore throat, p 428).

INCIDENCE/   Upper respiratory tract infections, nasal congestion, throat complaints, and
PREVALENCE   cough are responsible for 11% of general practice consultations in Australia.[2] Each year, children suffer about five such infections and adults two to three infections.[2–4] One cross-sectional study in Norwegian children aged 4–5 years found that 48% experienced more than two common colds annually.[5]

AETIOLOGY/   Transmission of common cold infection is mostly through hand to hand contact
RISK FACTORS with subsequent passage to the nostrils or eyes rather than, as commonly perceived, through droplets in the air.[1] The organisms for common colds are mainly viruses (typically rhinovirus, but also coronavirus and respiratory syncytial virus, or metapneumovirus and others). For many colds, no infecting organism can be identified.

PROGNOSIS   Common colds are usually short-lived, lasting a few days, with a few lingering symptoms lasting longer, especially cough. Symptoms peak within 1–3 days and generally clear by 1 week, although cough often persists.[1] Although they cause no mortality or serious morbidity, common colds are responsible for considerable discomfort, lost work, and medical costs.

Please refer to the Clinical Evidence website for full text and references.

What are the effects of preventive interventions?

LIKELY TO BE BENEFICIAL

Influenza vaccine (in elderly people)

We found no RCTs that assessed the effects of influenza vaccine in preventing community acquired pneumonia. Observational studies suggest that influenza vaccine may reduce the incidence of pneumonia and may reduce mortality in the elderly.

UNLIKELY TO BE BENEFICIAL

Pneumococcal vaccine (for all cause pneumonia and mortality in immunocompetent adults)

One systematic review found no significant difference in pneumonia rates or all cause mortality between pneumococcal vaccination and no pneumococcal vaccination in immunocompetent adults. The review found some evidence that pneumococcal vaccine may reduce definitive pneumococcal infection compared with no vaccination in immunocompetent adults.

What are the effects of interventions in outpatient settings?

BENEFICIAL

Antibiotics (amoxicillin, cephalosporins, macrolides, penicillin, quinolones) in outpatient settings

One systematic review that evaluated different oral antibiotics in outpatient settings has found clinical cure or improvement in over 90% of people regardless of antibiotic taken. Another systematic review found limited evidence that azithromycin reduced clinical failures over 6–21 days compared with other macrolides, cephalosporins, or penicillin. A third systematic review and a subsequent RCT found no significant difference in clinical cure or improvement between quinolones and amoxicillin, cephalosporins, or macrolides. One RCT found no significant difference between oral telithromycin and oral clarithromycin in clinical cure rates. Most trials were designed to show equivalence between treatments rather than superiority of one antibiotic over another.

What are the effects of treatments in people admitted to hospital?

BENEFICIAL

Antibiotics (amoxicillin, cephalosporins, macrolides, penicillin, quinolones) in hospital

RCTs that compared different oral or intravenous antibiotics in people admitted to hospital found clinical cure or improvement in 73–96% of people. Four RCTs found no significant difference in clinical cure or improvement among different antibiotics. Two RCTs found that quinolones may increase clinical cure compared with co-amoxiclav (amoxicillin plus clavulanic acid) or cephalosporins. However, most trials were small and were designed to show equivalence between treatments rather than superiority of one antibiotic over another.

Community acquired pneumonia

LIKELY TO BE BENEFICIAL

Early mobilisation

One RCT in people receiving antibiotics and usual medical care found that early mobilisation plus bottle blowing physiotherapy plus encouragement to sit up regularly and take deep breaths reduced mean hospital stay compared with early mobilisation alone. It found no significant difference in duration of fever. One RCT found that early mobilisation reduced hospital stay compared with usual care.

UNLIKELY TO BE BENEFICIAL

Intravenous antibiotics in immunocompetent people in hospital without life threatening illness (compared with oral antibiotics)

One systematic review found no significant difference for clinical cure rates or mortality between oral and intravenous antibiotics in people hospitalised with non-severe community acquired pneumonia. One RCT found that inpatient regimens consisting of staged intravenous and oral antibiotic therapy reduced hospital stay compared with regimens consisting of intravenous antibiotics alone.

What are the effects of treatments in people with community acquired pneumonia receiving intensive care?

LIKELY TO BE BENEFICIAL

Prompt administration of antibiotics in people admitted to intensive care with community acquired pneumonia (improved outcomes compared with delayed antibiotic treatment)

We found no systematic review and no RCTs comparing prompt versus delayed antibiotic treatment. Two retrospective studies found that prompt administration of antibiotics improved survival. It would probably be unethical to perform an RCT of delayed antibiotic treatment.

UNKNOWN EFFECTIVENESS

Different combinations of antibiotics in intensive care settings

We found no RCTs that compared one combination of antibiotics versus another in intensive care units.

What are the effects of guidelines on the treatment of community acquired pneumonia?

UNKNOWN EFFECTIVENESS

Guidelines for treating pneumonia (for clinical outcomes)

One systematic review found no significant difference in clinical outcomes between usual care and a guideline based management strategy that incorporated early switch from intravenous to oral antibiotics and early discharge (or both). One subsequent RCT found no significant difference in clinical outcomes between a guideline plus a multifaceted implementation strategy and the issued guideline alone.

DEFINITION   Community acquired pneumonia is pneumonia contracted in the community rather than in hospital. It is defined by clinical symptoms (such as cough, sputum production, and pleuritic chest pain) and signs (such as fever, tachypnoea, and rales), with radiological confirmation.

INCIDENCE/ PREVALENCE In the northern hemisphere, community acquired pneumonia affects about 12/1000 people a year, particularly during winter and at the extremes of age (incidence: < 1 year old 30–50/1000 per year; 15–45 years 1–5/1000 per year; 60–70 years 10–20/1000 per year; 71–85 years 50/1000 per year).[1-6]

AETIOLOGY/ RISK FACTORS More than 100 microorganisms have been implicated in community acquired pneumonia, but most cases are caused by *Streptococcus pneumoniae*).[4-7] Smoking is probably an important risk factor.[8] One large cohort study conducted in Finland (4175 people aged ≥ 60 years) suggested that risk factors for pneumonia in the elderly included alcoholism (RR 9.0, 95% CI 5.1 to 16.2), bronchial asthma (RR 4.2, 95% CI 3.3 to 5.4), immunosuppression (RR 3.1, 95% CI 1.9 to 5.1), lung disease (RR 3.0, 95% CI 2.3 to 3.9), heart disease (RR 1.9, 95% CI 1.7 to 2.3), institutionalisation (RR 1.8, 95% CI 1.4 to 2.4), and increasing age (≥ 70 years v 60–69 years; RR 1.5, 95% CI 1.3 to 1.7).[9]

PROGNOSIS Severity varies from mild to life threatening illness within days of the onset of symptoms. One systematic review of prognosis studies for community acquired pneumonia (search date 1995, 33 148 people) found overall mortality to be 13.7%, ranging from 5.1% for ambulant people to 36.5% for people who required intensive care.[10] The following prognostic factors were significantly associated with mortality: male sex (OR 1.3, 95% CI 1.2 to 1.4); pleuritic chest pain (OR 0.5, 95% CI 0.3 to 0.8, i.e. lower mortality); hypothermia (OR 5.0, 95% CI 2.4 to 10.4); systolic hypotension (OR 4.8, 95% CI 2.8 to 8.3); tachypnoea (OR 2.9, 95% CI 1.7 to 4.9); diabetes mellitus (OR 1.3, 95% CI 1.1 to 1.5); neoplastic disease (OR 2.8, 95% CI 2.4 to 3.1); neurological disease (OR 4.6, 95% CI 2.3 to 8.9); bacteraemia (OR 2.8, 95% CI 2.3 to 3.6); leucopenia (OR 2.5, 95% CI 1.6 to 3.7); and multilobar radiographic pulmonary infiltrates (OR 3.1, 95% CI 1.9 to 5.1).

Please refer to the Clinical Evidence website for full text and references.

Sore throat

Search date May 2004

Chris Del Mar and Paul Glasziou

What are the effects of interventions to reduce symptoms of acute infective sore throat?

LIKELY TO BE BENEFICIAL

Non-steroidal anti-inflammatory drugs

RCTs identified by a systematic review found that non-steroidal anti-inflammatory drugs reduced sore throat symptoms both over ≤ 24 hours and at 2–5 days compared with placebo. The range of benefit was 25–75% over ≤ 24 hours, and 33–93% at 2–5 days. Non-steroidal anti-inflammatory drugs are associated with gastrointestinal and renal adverse effects.

Paracetamol

Two RCTs identified by a systematic review found that a single dose of paracetamol reduced acute sore throat pain at 2–3 hours compared with placebo. Another RCT identified by the review found that paracetamol three times daily reduced sore throat pain at 2 days compared with placebo. We found no RCTs of other analgesics in people with sore throat.

TRADE OFF BETWEEN BENEFITS AND HARMS

Antibiotics

One systematic review found that antibiotics reduced the proportion of people with sore throat, fever, and headache at 3 days compared with placebo. The review found limited evidence from indirect comparisons that the absolute and relative reduction in sore throat symptoms at 3 days was greater in people with positive throat swabs for *Streptococcus* than in people with negative swabs. It gave no information on adverse effects. We found no RCTs that assessed the effects of antibiotics in reducing the severity of sore throat symptoms. Antibiotics may increase the risk of nausea, vomiting, rash, headache, and vaginitis. Widespread antibiotic use may lead to bacterial resistance to antibiotics.

Corticosteroids

One RCT in children and adolescents with moderate to severe sore throat infection found that oral dexamethasone reduced throat pain at 24 hours compared with placebo, and reduced the duration of pain. Another RCT in people with severe sore throat infection identified by a systematic review found that adding corticosteroids to antibiotics reduced the proportion of people with sore throat pain at 24 hours compared with adding placebo. It found more limited evidence that adding corticosteroids to antibiotics also reduced the duration of pain. The RCTs provided insufficient evidence to assess adverse effects of corticosteroids in people with sore throat. However, data from systematic reviews in people with other disorders suggest that corticosteroids may be associated with serious adverse effects, although this may be only after long term use.

UNKNOWN EFFECTIVENESS

Probiotics

RCTs suggested that super-colonisation with *Streptococcus* isolated from healthy individuals apparently resistant to infections from *Streptococcus* may reduce recurrent sore throat over 2–3 months compared with placebo. However, at present, super-colonisation with *Streptococcus* is available only experimentally. We found no RCTs of other probiotics.

▶

What are the effects of interventions to prevent complications of acute infective sore throat?

TRADE OFF BETWEEN BENEFITS AND HARMS

Antibiotics

One systematic review found that antibiotics reduced suppurative and non-suppurative complications of β haemolytic streptococcal pharyngitis compared with placebo. However, in industrialised countries, non-suppurative complications are extremely rare. Widespread antibiotic use may lead to bacterial resistance to antibiotics.

DEFINITION Sore throat is an acute upper respiratory tract infection that affects the respiratory mucosa of the throat. Since infections can affect any part of the mucosa, it is often arbitrary whether an acute upper respiratory tract infection is called "sore throat" "pharyngitis" or "tonsillitis", "common cold", "sinusitis", "otitis media", or "bronchitis" **❻**. Sometimes, all areas are affected (simultaneously or at different times) in one illness. In this chapter, we aim to cover people whose principal presenting symptom is sore throat. This may be associated with headache, fever, and general malaise. Suppurative complications include acute otitis media (most commonly), acute sinusitis, and peritonsillar abscess (quinsy). Non-suppurative complications include acute rheumatic fever and acute glomerulonephritis

INCIDENCE/ There is little seasonal fluctuation in sore throat. About 10% of the Australian
PREVALENCE population present to primary healthcare services annually with an upper respiratory tract infection consisting predominantly of sore throat.[1] This reflects about one fifth of the overall annual incidence.[1] However, it is difficult to distinguish between the different types of upper respiratory tract infection.[2]

AETIOLOGY/ The causative organisms of sore throat may be bacteria (*Streptococcus*, most
RISK FACTORS commonly Group A β haemolytic, although sometimes others: *Haemophilus influenzae, Moraxella catarrhalis,* and others) or viruses (typically rhinovirus, but also coronavirus, respiratory syncytial virus, metapneumovirus, Ebstein–Barr, and others). It is difficult to distinguish bacterial from viral infections clinically. Some features are thought to predict the probability of the infection being caused by *Streptococcus* (fever above 38.5 °C; exudate on the tonsils; anterior neck lymphadenopathy; absence of cough).[3] Sore throat can be caused by processes other than primary infections, including gastro-oesophageal reflux, physical or chemical irritation (from nasogastric tubes or smoke, for example), and occasionally hay fever. However, we do not consider causes other than primary infections here.

PROGNOSIS Sore throat infections usually last a few days, with a few symptoms lasting longer, especially cough.[3] The untreated symptoms of sore throat disappear by 3 days in about 40% of people and untreated fevers in about 85%. By 1 week, 85% of people are symptom free. This natural history is similar in *Streptococcus* positive, negative, and untested patients.

Please refer to the Clinical Evidence website for full text and references.

Spontaneous pneumothorax

Search date April 2004

Abel Wakai

We found insufficient evidence to determine whether any intervention is more effective than no intervention for spontaneous pneumothorax.

What are the effects of treatments?

UNKNOWN EFFECTIVENESS

Chest tube drainage
We found no RCTs comparing chest tube drainage versus observation. RCTs provided insufficient evidence to compare chest tube drainage versus needle aspiration or chest tube drainage plus suction.

Chest tube drainage plus suction
One RCT and one controlled clinical trial found no significant difference in rate of resolution of pneumothorax whether chest tube drainage bottles were connected to suction or not. However, both trials were too small to rule out a clinically important difference.

Needle aspiration
Four RCTs provided insufficient evidence to compare needle aspiration versus observation or chest tube drainage.

One way valves on chest tubes
One RCT found no significant difference in rate of resolution between one way valves and drainage bottles with underwater seals, but it is likely to have been too small to detect a clinically important difference. It found that people treated with one way valves used less analgesia and were less likely to be admitted to hospital than people treated with drainage bottles.

Small versus standard sized chest tubes
We found no RCTs assessing small or standard sized tubes for chest drainage.

What are the effects of interventions to prevent recurrence?

TRADE OFF BETWEEN BENEFITS AND HARMS

Pleurodesis
Two RCTs found that adding chemical pleurodesis to chest tube drainage reduced the rate of recurrence of spontaneous pneumothorax compared with chest tube drainage alone. One of the RCTs found that chemical pleurodesis injection was intensely painful. The RCTs found no significant difference in length of hospital stay. One RCT found that thoracoscopic surgery with talcum powder instillation reduced the rate of recurrence at 5 years compared with chest tube drainage. Two RCTs provided insufficient evidence to compare video assisted thorascopic surgery versus thoracotomy. We found no RCTs comparing chemical versus surgical pleurodesis.

UNKNOWN EFFECTIVENESS

Optimal timing of pleurodesis (after first, second, or subsequent episodes)
We found no RCTs or high quality cohort studies assessing whether pleurodesis should take place after the first, second, or subsequent episodes of spontaneous pneumothorax.

DEFINITION   A pneumothorax is air in the pleural space. A spontaneous pneumothorax occurs when there is no provoking factor, such as trauma, surgery, or diagnostic intervention. It implies a leak of air from the lung parenchyma through the visceral pleura into the pleural space. This review does not include people with tension pneumothorax.

INCIDENCE/   In a survey in Minnesota, USA, the incidence of spontaneous pneumothorax
PREVALENCE   was 7/100 000 for men and 1/100 000 for women.[1] In England and Wales, the overall rate of people consulting with pneumothorax (in both primary and secondary care combined) is 24/100 000 a year for men and 9.8/100 000 a year for women.[2] The overall annual incidence of emergency hospital admissions for pneumothorax in England and Wales is 16.7/100 000 for men and 5.8/100 000 for women.[2] Smoking increases the likelihood of spontaneous pneumothorax by 22 times for men and eight times for women.[3] A dose–response relationship was observed.[3]

AETIOLOGY/   Spontaneous pneumothorax can be primary (typically in young fit people and
RISK FACTORS   thought to be because of a congenital abnormality of the visceral pleura) or secondary (caused by underlying lung disease, typically occurring in older people with emphysema or pulmonary fibrosis).

PROGNOSIS   Death from spontaneous pneumothorax is rare. Morbidity with pain and shortness of breath is common. Published recurrence rates vary. One cohort study in Denmark found that, after a first episode of primary spontaneous pneumothorax, 23% of people suffered a recurrence within 5 years, most within 1 year.[4] Recurrence rates had been thought to increase substantially after the first recurrence, but one retrospective case control study (147 military personnel) found that 28% of men with a first primary spontaneous pneumothorax had a recurrence; 23% of the 28% had a second recurrence; and 14% of that 23% had a third recurrence, giving a total recurrence rate of 35%.[5]

Please refer to the Clinical Evidence website for full text and references.

Asthma

Search date May 2003

J Mark FitzGerald, Rodolfo J Dennis, and Ivan Solarte

What are the effects of treatments for chronic asthma?

BENEFICIAL

Adding long acting inhaled β_2 agonists in people with mild, persistent asthma that is poorly controlled by inhaled corticosteroids

One systematic review and three additional RCTs have found that adding regular doses of long acting inhaled β_2 agonists improves lung function and symptoms and reduces rescue medication compared with increasing the dose of inhaled corticosteroids. However, one further RCT found that increasing inhaled corticosteroid dose reduced exacerbations compared with adding long acting inhaled β_2 agonists. We found insufficient evidence about effects of adding long acting inhaled β_2 agonists on mortality.

Adding long acting inhaled β_2 agonists to inhaled corticosteroids in poorly controlled mild to moderate, persistent asthma (for symptom control)

RCTs have found that, in people with asthma that is poorly controlled with inhaled corticosteroids, adding regular long acting inhaled β_2 agonists improves symptoms and lung function compared with adding placebo or a leukotriene antagonist. We found insufficient evidence about effects of adding long acting inhaled β_2 agonists on mortality.

Low dose, inhaled corticosteroids in mild, persistent asthma

Systematic reviews and RCTs have found that, in people with mild, persistent asthma, low doses of inhaled corticosteroids improve symptoms and lung function compared with placebo or regular inhaled β_2 agonists.

Short acting inhaled β_2 agonists as needed for symptom relief (as effective as regular use) in adults with mild to moderate, persistent asthma

One systematic review and one subsequent RCT found no significant difference between regular and as needed short acting inhaled β_2 agonists for clinically important outcomes.

LIKELY TO BE BENEFICIAL

Adding leukotriene antagonists in people with mild to moderate, persistent asthma (likely to be better than adding no treatment, but no clear evidence of benefit over adding inhaled corticosteroids)

RCTs in people taking β_2 agonists alone have found that leukotriene antagonists reduce asthma symptoms and β_2 agonist use compared with placebo. One systematic review and three out of nine subsequent RCTs have found that adding leukotriene antagonists increases exacerbations, reduces lung function, and are less effective for symptom control compared with inhaled corticosteroids. The other six RCTs found no significant difference between adding leukotriene antagonists and adding corticosteroids. Two RCTs have found that an inhaled corticosteroid plus a long acting β_2 agonist improved symptoms, lung function, and exacerbations compared with a leukotriene antagonist at 12 weeks.

Adding theophylline in people with mild to moderate, persistent asthma poorly controlled by inhaled corticosteroids

One RCT has found that adding theophylline improves peak expiratory flow rate compared with continuing low dose corticosteroids plus placebo after 6 months in people with mild to moderate, persistent asthma that was poorly controlled with ▶

inhaled corticosteroids alone. One small RCT found no significant difference in lung function or symptoms between theophylline and formoterol (a long acting β agonist) or between theophylline and zafirlukast (a leukotriene antagonist) after 3 months.

UNKNOWN EFFECTIVENESS

Adding leukotriene antagonists plus inhaled corticosteroids in people with mild to moderate, persistent asthma

One systematic review in people taking inhaled corticosteroids found no significant difference between leukotriene antagonists and placebo for exacerbation rates at 4–16 weeks. However, one subsequent RCT in people taking a stable dose of budesonide found that adding montelukast increased asthma free days and decreased nocturnal waking compared with placebo at 16 weeks. One RCT in people taking inhaled corticosteroids found no significant difference between adding montelukast and doubling budesonide in peak expiratory flow rate, daytime symptoms, nocturnal wakening, days with asthma exacerbations, and quality of life.

What are the effects of treatments for acute asthma?

BENEFICIAL

Inhaled corticosteroids for acute asthma (better than placebo)

One systematic review has found that inhaled corticosteroids given in the emergency department reduced hospital admission rates in adults compared with placebo. One systematic review and one subsequent RCT found no significant difference in relapse rates following emergency department discharge between oral and inhaled steroids at 7–10 days. One systematic review found no significant difference in relapse rates between inhaled plus oral corticosteroids and oral corticosteroids alone up to 24 days.

Inhaled plus oral corticosteroids for acute asthma (as effective as oral corticosteroid alone)

One systematic review found no significant difference in relapse rates for inhaled plus oral corticosteroid compared with oral corticosteroids up to 24 days.

Ipratropium bromide added to β_2 agonists for acute exacerbations

Two systematic reviews and one subsequent RCT have found that ipratropium bromide plus salbutamol improves lung function compared with salbutamol alone and is likely to reduce hospital admission in people with severe acute asthma.

Short courses of systemic corticosteroids for acute exacerbations

Two systematic reviews and one subsequent RCT have found that early treatment with systemic corticosteroids reduce admission and relapse rates compared with placebo in people with acute asthma. One systematic review and one small subsequent RCT found no significant difference between oral and inhaled steroids after emergency department discharge in relapse rates at 7–10 days in adults with acute asthma.

Spacer devices for delivering inhaled medications from pressurised metered dose inhalers in acute asthma (as good as nebulisers)

One systematic review in people with acute, but not life threatening exacerbations of asthma found no significant difference between β_2 agonists delivered by spacer device compared with nebulisers in rates of hospital admission, time spent in the emergency department, peak expiratory flow rate, or forced expiratory volume in 1 second.

Asthma

LIKELY TO BE BENEFICIAL

Education about acute asthma

One systematic review and one subsequent RCT provided evidence that education to facilitate self management of asthma in adults reduced hospital admission, unscheduled visits to the doctor, and days off work compared with usual care. One subsequent RCT provided insufficient evidence about effects of asthma education on quality of life or social functioning at 6 months.

Magnesium sulphate for people with severe acute asthma

We found limited evidence from one systematic review and two subsequent RCTs that intravenous magnesium improved lung function compared with placebo in people with severe acute asthma. One systematic review and three subsequent RCTs found no significant difference between intravenous magnesium sulphate and placebo for hospital admission rates.

Mechanical ventilation for people with severe acute asthma*

We found no RCTs comparing mechanical ventilation with or without inhaled β_2 agonists versus no mechanical ventilation in people with severe acute asthma. Evidence from cohort studies support its use, although observational studies suggest that ventilation is associated with a high level of morbidity.

Oxygen supplementation for acute asthma*

We found no systematic review or RCTs of oxygen in acute asthma. However, consensus opinion and pathophysiology suggest that its role is vital in acute asthma.

Specialist care for acute exacerbations (more effective than generalist care)

One systematic review found limited evidence that specialist care improved outcomes in people with acute asthma compared with generalist care.

*Highly likely to be effective. RCTs unlikely to be conducted.

UNLIKELY TO BE BENEFICIAL

Continuous nebulised short acting β_2 agonists for acute asthma (no more effective than intermittent nebulised short acting β_2 agonists)

One systematic review and one subsequent RCT found no significant difference in admission rate between continuous and intermittent nebulised short acting β_2 agonists for hospital admission rates in adults. The subsequent RCT also found no significant difference between continuous and intermittent nebulised short acting β_2 agonists in lung function.

Helium–oxygen mixture for acute asthma

One systematic review found no significant difference between helium–oxygen mixture and air or oxygen in pulmonary function tests at 60 minutes for adults and children.

Intravenous short acting β_2 agonists for acute asthma (no more effective than nebulised short acting β_2 agonists)

One systematic review found that intravenous delivery of short acting β_2 agonists was no more effective than nebulised delivery in improving peak expiratory flow rate at 60 minutes.

DEFINITION
Asthma is characterised by variable airflow obstruction and airway hyperresponsiveness. Symptoms include dyspnoea, cough, chest tightness, and wheezing. The normal diurnal variation of peak expiratory flow rate is increased in people with asthma🅣. Chronic asthma is defined here as asthma requiring maintenance treatment. Asthma is classified differently in the USA and UK🅣. Where necessary, the text specifies the system of classification used.[1,2] Acute asthma is defined here as an exacerbation of underlying asthma requiring urgent treatment.

INCIDENCE/ PREVALENCE
Reported prevalence of asthma is increasing worldwide. About 10% of people have suffered an attack of asthma.[3-5] Epidemiological studies have also found marked variations in prevalence in different countries.[6,7]

AETIOLOGY/ RISK FACTORS
Most people with asthma are atopic. Exposure to certain stimuli initiates inflammation and structural changes in airways causing airway hyperresponsiveness and variable airflow obstruction, which in turn cause most asthma symptoms. There are a large number of such stimuli; the more important include environmental allergens, occupational sensitising agents, and respiratory viral infections.[8,9]

PROGNOSIS
Chronic asthma: In people with mild asthma, prognosis is good and progression to severe disease is rare. However, as a group, people with asthma lose lung function faster than those without asthma, although less quickly than people without asthma who smoke.[10] People with chronic asthma can improve with treatment. However, some people (possibly up to 5%) have severe disease that responds poorly to treatment. These people are most at risk of morbidity and death from asthma. **Acute asthma:** About 10–20% of people presenting to the emergency department with asthma are admitted to hospital. Of these, fewer than 10% receive mechanical ventilation.[11,12] Those who are ventilated are at 19-fold increased risk of ventilation for a subsequent episode.[13] It is unusual for people to die unless they have suffered respiratory arrest before reaching hospital.[14] One prospective study of 939 people discharged from emergency care found that 17% (95% CI 14% to 20%) relapsed by 2 weeks.[15]

Please refer to the Clinical Evidence website for full text and references.

Bronchiectasis

Search date June 2004

Nick ten Hacken, Huib Kerstjens, and Dirkje Postma

What are the effects of treatments in people with bronchiectasis but without cystic fibrosis?

LIKELY TO BE BENEFICIAL

Exercise or physical training

One systematic review found that inspiratory muscle training improved quality of life and exercise endurance compared with no intervention or sham training in people with non-cystic fibrosis bronchiectasis.

UNKNOWN EFFECTIVENESS

Inhaled steroids

One systematic review found insufficient evidence from two small RCTs to compare inhaled steroids versus placebo in people with bronchiectasis not due to a specific congenital disease.

Long acting β_2 agonists

One systematic review identified no RCTs comparing long acting β_2 agonists versus placebo or other treatments in people with non-cystic fibrosis bronchiectasis.

Mucolytics (bromhexine or deoxyribonuclease)

One systematic review found insufficient evidence from three RCTs to compare the effects of bromhexine or recombinant human deoxyribonuclease versus placebo in people with non-cystic fibrosis bronchiectasis.

Oral steroids

One systematic review found no RCTs comparing steroids versus placebo, no treatment, or any other pharmacological or non-pharmacological treatment in people with non-cystic fibrosis bronchiectasis.

DEFINITION Bronchiectasis is defined as irreversible widening of medium sized airways (bronchi) in the lung. It is characterised by inflammation, destruction of bronchial walls, and chronic bacterial infection. The condition may be limited to a single lobe or lung segment, or it may affect one or both lungs more diffusely. Clinically, the condition manifests as chronic cough and chronic overproduction of sputum (up to about 500 ml daily), which is often purulent.[1] People with severe bronchiectasis may have life threatening haemoptysis and may develop features of chronic obstructive airways disease, such as wheezing, chronic respiratory failure, pulmonary hypertension, and right sided heart failure.

INCIDENCE/ PREVALENCE We found few reliable data. Incidence has declined over the past 50 years and prevalence is low in higher income countries. Prevalence is much higher in poorer countries and is a major cause of morbidity and mortality.

AETIOLOGY/ RISK FACTORS Bronchiectasis is most commonly a long term complication of previous lower respiratory infections such as measles pneumonitis, pertussis, and tuberculosis. Foreign body inhalation and allergic, autoimmune, and chemical lung damage also predispose to the condition.[2] Underlying congenital disorders such as cystic fibrosis, ciliary dysmotility syndromes, α_1 antitrypsin deficiency, and congenital immunodeficiencies may also predispose to bronchiectasis and may be of greater aetiological importance than respiratory infection in higher income countries. Cystic fibrosis is the most common congenital cause.

PROGNOSIS   Bronchiectasis is a chronic condition with frequent relapses of varying severity. Long term prognosis is variable. Data on morbidity and mortality are sparse.[3] Bronchiectasis frequently coexists with other respiratory disease, making it difficult to distinguish prognosis for bronchiectasis alone.

Please refer to the Clinical Evidence website for full text and references.

Chronic obstructive pulmonary disease

Search date February 2004

Huib Kerstjens, Dirkje Postma, and Nick ten Hacken

We found no evidence about effects of most interventions on progression of chronic obstructive pulmonary disease (measured by decline in lung function).

What are the effects of maintenance drug treatment in stable chronic obstructive pulmonary disorder?

BENEFICIAL

Inhaled anticholinergics (improve exacerbation rate, symptoms, and FEV_1 compared with placebo)

RCTs found that inhaled anticholinergics improved forced expiratory volume in 1 second (FEV_1), exercise capacity, and symptoms compared with placebo. One large RCT found that adding ipratropium to a smoking cessation programme had no significant impact compared with the smoking cessation programme alone on decline in FEV_1 over 5 years. RCTs found that inhaled tiotropium (a long acting anticholinergic drug) reduced exacerbation rates compared with placebo or ipratropium.

Inhaled anticholinergics plus β_2 agonists (improve FEV_1 compared with either drug alone)

RCTs found that combining a long or short acting β_2 agonist with an anticholinergic drug for 2–12 weeks modestly improved FEV_1 compared with either drug alone. One RCT found that, when combined with an anticholinergic drug, a long acting β_2 agonist improved FEV_1 and peak expiratory flow rate more than a short acting β_2 agonist. We found no RCTs of long term treatment comparing anticholinergics plus β_2 agonists with placebo.

Inhaled corticosteroids plus long acting β_2 agonists (improve exacerbation rate, symptoms, quality of life, FEV_1 compared with placebo)

RCTs found that the combination of an inhaled corticosteroid plus a long acting β_2 agonist reduced exacerbation rates and improved lung function, symptoms, and health related quality of life compared with placebo. In general, the combination was more effective than inhaled corticosteroid alone or long acting β_2 agonist alone, although this difference was not significant for all outcomes.

Inhaled β_2 agonists (improve FEV_1 compared with placebo)

RCTs found that treatment with inhaled β_2 agonists for 1 week to 12 months improved FEV_1 compared with placebo. RCTs provided insufficient direct evidence about effects of short or long acting β_2 agonists on quality of life or symptoms. RCTs provided insufficient evidence about effects of long acting inhaled β_2 agonists on exacerbation rates.

LIKELY TO BE BENEFICIAL

Inhaled anticholinergics compared with β_2 agonists (improve FEV_1 compared with β_2 agonists in long term)

RCTs found inconsistent evidence about the effects of short acting inhaled anticholinergics compared with long acting β_2 agonists for up to 3 months. Two RCTs found that 6 months of a long acting inhaled anticholinergic improved FEV_1 compared with a long acting inhaled β_2 agonist. One RCT found no significant difference between a long acting inhaled anticholinergic and a long acting inhaled β_2 agonist in quality of life or exacerbation rates at 6 months.

◄ **Long term domiciliary oxygen (beneficial in people with severe hypoxaemia)**

One RCT in people with severe daytime hypoxaemia found that domiciliary oxygen improved survival compared with no domiciliary oxygen. A second RCT in people with severe hypoxaemia found that continuous oxygen reduced mortality compared with nocturnal oxygen. Three RCTs in people with milder hypoxaemia or with nocturnal hypoxaemia only, found no significant difference in mortality between long term domiciliary oxygen and no oxygen.

Mucolytics (improve exacerbation rates)*

Two systematic reviews found limited evidence that mucolytics for 3–24 months reduced the frequency and duration of exacerbations compared with placebo.

TRADE OFF BETWEEN BENEFITS AND HARMS

Theophyllines

One systematic review found that theophyllines slightly improved FEV_1 compared with placebo after 3 months. One large RCT found that theophyllines improved FEV_1 compared with placebo after 12 months' treatment. The usefulness of these drugs is limited by adverse effects and the need for frequent monitoring of blood concentrations.

Inhaled corticosteroids (improve exacerbation rates, but may have long term harms)

RCTs found no significant difference between inhaled corticosteroids and placebo in lung function (FEV_1) over 10 days to 10 weeks. One systematic review and one subsequent RCT found no significant difference in decline in FEV_1 between inhaled corticosteroids and placebo after 24 months. However, a second systematic review that examined effects of high dose inhaled corticosteroids and four subsequent RCTs found that inhaled corticosteroids slightly reduced the decline in FEV_1 compared with placebo after 12–24 months. One systematic review and one subsequent RCT found that long term inhaled steroids reduced the frequency of exacerbations compared with placebo. Two subsequent RCTs found no significant difference in exacerbation rates. Long term inhaled steroids may predispose to adverse effects, including skin bruising, and oral candidiasis.

UNKNOWN EFFECTIVENESS

Deoxyribonuclease

We found no RCTs comparing the long term effects of deoxyribonuclease versus placebo.

Prophylactic antibiotics

One systematic review found limited evidence of a small reduction in exacerbation rates and days with disability with prophylactic antibiotics. These benefits probably do not outweigh the harms of antibiotics, especially the development of antibiotic resistance. All the identified RCTs were conducted more than 30 years ago, and the results are unlikely to apply to current practice.

α_1 Antitrypsin

One RCT in people with α_1 antitrypsin deficiency and moderate emphysema found no significant difference between α_1 antitrypsin infusion and placebo in the decline in FEV_1 after 1 year.

Chronic obstructive pulmonary disease

Oral corticosteroids (evidence of harm but no evidence of long term benefits)

We found no RCTs on long term benefits. One systematic review found that treatment with oral corticosteroids for 2–4 weeks improved FEV_1 compared with placebo. Long term systemic corticosteroids are associated with serious adverse effects, including osteoporosis and diabetes.

Oral versus inhaled corticosteroids (evidence of harm but no evidence of long term benefits)

Two RCTs provided insufficient evidence about effects of oral compared with inhaled corticosteroids over 2 weeks. We found no RCTs of long term treatment with oral compared with inhaled corticosteroids. Long term oral corticosteroids are associated with serious adverse effects, including osteoporosis and diabetes.

What are the effects of smoking cessation interventions in stable chronic obstructive pulmonary disease?

Psychosocial plus pharmacological interventions

One large RCT in people with mild chronic obstructive pulmonary disease found that nicotine gum plus a psychosocial smoking cessation and abstinence maintenance programme (with or without ipratropium) slowed the decline of FEV_1, and reduced respiratory symptoms and lower respiratory illnesses, but increased weight gain compared with usual care (without psychosocial intervention). The RCT found no significant difference between treatments in all cause mortality at 5 years.

Pharmacological interventions alone

One systematic review found no RCTs in people with chronic obstructive pulmonary disease.

Psychosocial interventions alone

We found no systematic review or RCTs in people with chronic obstructive pulmonary disease.

*Extrapolated from studies of different types of pulmonary disease, including chronic obstructive pulmonary disease

DEFINITION	Chronic obstructive pulmonary disease (COPD) is a disease state characterised by airflow limitation that is not fully reversible. The airflow limitation is usually both progressive and associated with an abnormal inflammatory response of the lungs to noxious particles or gases.[1] Classically, it has been thought to be a combination of emphysema and chronic bronchitis, although only one of these may be present in some people with COPD. Emphysema is abnormal permanent enlargement of the air spaces distal to the terminal bronchioles, accompanied by destruction of their walls and without obvious fibrosis. Chronic bronchitis is chronic cough or mucus production for at least 3 months in at least 2 successive years when other causes of chronic cough have been excluded.[2]
INCIDENCE/ PREVALENCE	COPD mainly affects middle aged and elderly people. In 1998, the World Health Organization estimated that COPD was the fifth most common cause of death worldwide, responsible for 4.2% of all mortality (estimated ▶

2 249 000 deaths in 1998)[3] and morbidity is increasing. Estimated prevalence in the USA rose by 41% between 1982 and 1994 and age adjusted death rates rose by 71% between 1966 and 1985. All cause age adjusted mortality declined over the same period by 22% and mortality from cardiovascular diseases by 45%.[2] In the UK, physician diagnosed prevalence was 2% in men and 1% in women between 1990 and 1997.[4]

AETIOLOGY/ RISK FACTORS   COPD is largely preventable. The main cause in developed countries is exposure to tobacco smoke. The disease is rare in lifelong non-smokers (estimated prevalence 5% in 3 large representative US surveys of non-smokers from 1971–1984), in whom "passive" exposure to environmental tobacco smoke has been proposed as a cause.[5,6] Other proposed causes include bronchial hyperresponsiveness, indoor and outdoor air pollution, and allergy.[7–9]

PROGNOSIS   Airway obstruction is usually progressive in those who continue to smoke, resulting in early disability and shortened survival. Smoking cessation reverts the rate of decline in lung function to that of non-smokers.[10] Many people will need medication for the rest of their lives, with increased doses and additional drugs during exacerbations.

Please refer to the Clinical Evidence website for full text and references.

Lung cancer

Search date September 2003

Alan Neville

What are the effects of treatments for non-small cell lung cancer?

Palliative chemotherapy in stage 4 non-small cell lung cancer

Systematic reviews in people with stage 4 non-small cell lung cancer have found that adding chemotherapy regimens containing cisplatin to best supportive care increases survival at 1 year compared with supportive care alone. Limited evidence from RCTs suggests that adding chemotherapy to best supportive care may improve quality of life compared with best supportive care alone.

Thoracic irradiation plus chemotherapy in unresectable stage 3 non-small cell lung cancer (compared with thoracic irradiation alone)

Systematic reviews and two RCTs in people with unresectable stage 3 non-small cell lung cancer have found that adding chemotherapy to irradiation improves survival at 2–5 years compared with irradiation alone. One RCT found no significant difference in median survival between radical radiotherapy plus chemotherapy and radiotherapy alone. Observational evidence suggests that, in people aged over 70 years with unresectable stage 3 non-small cell lung cancer, chemotherapy plus radiotherapy may reduce quality adjusted survival compared with radiotherapy alone. We found insufficient evidence about effects on quality of life.

Hyperfractionated radiation treatment in unresectable stage 3 non-small cell lung cancer

One systematic review found no clear evidence that altered fractionation regimens, accelerated, hyperfractionated, or hyperfractionated split course regimens are any more effective than conventional radiotherapy. One RCT identified by the review has found that continuous, hyperfractionated, accelerated radiotherapy reduces mortality at 2 years compared with conventional radiotherapy in people with stage 3A, 3B, 1, or 2 non-small cell lung cancer.

Palliative single drug chemotherapy regimens in stage 4 non-small cell lung cancer (not clearly better that combination chemotherapy)

One systematic review and subsequent RCTs in people with stage 3 and 4 non-small cell lung cancer found inconclusive evidence on the effects of single agent chemotherapy compared with combined chemotherapy. One systematic review and subsequent RCTs provided insufficient evidence to compare first line platinum based versus non-platinum based chemotherapy.

Preoperative chemotherapy in people with resectable stage 3 non-small cell lung cancer

One systematic review of small, weak RCTs and one subsequent RCT provided inconclusive evidence about the effects of preoperative chemotherapy in people with resectable stage 3 non-small cell lung cancer.

Postoperative chemotherapy in people with resected stage 1–3 non-small cell lung cancer

Systematic reviews and subsequent RCTs in people with completely resected stage 1–3 non-small cell lung cancer found no significant difference in survival at 5 years ▶

between postoperative cisplatin based chemotherapy and surgery with or without concomitant radiotherapy, although subgroup analysis in one RCT suggests that postoperative chemotherapy may increase survival in people with stage 3 disease. One systematic review has found that postoperative alkylating agents increase mortality compared with no postoperative chemotherapy.

What are the effects of treatments for small cell lung cancer?

BENEFICIAL

Chemotherapy plus thoracic irradiation in limited stage small cell lung cancer (improves survival compared with chemotherapy alone)

Two systematic reviews in people with limited stage small cell lung cancer have found that adding thoracic irradiation to chemotherapy improves survival at 3 years and local control. However, one of these reviews has found that chemotherapy plus thoracic irradiation increases deaths related to treatment.

LIKELY TO BE BENEFICIAL

Prophylactic cranial irradiation for people in complete remission from limited or extensive stage small cell lung cancer

One systematic review in people with small cell lung cancer in complete remission has found that prophylactic cranial irradiation improves survival at 3 years and reduces the risk of developing brain metastases compared with no irradiation. While long term cognitive dysfunction after cranial irradiation has been described in non-randomised studies, RCTs have not found a cumulative increase in neuropsychological dysfunction.

UNKNOWN EFFECTIVENESS

Dose intensification of chemotherapy (insufficient evidence compared with chemotherapy alone)

One systematic review found limited evidence that intensifying chemotherapy dose by either increasing the number of chemotherapy cycles, increasing chemotherapy dose, or increasing dose intensity per cycle may modestly improve survival compared with standard chemotherapy. However, additional RCTs have found inconclusive evidence about the effects of dose intensification on survival.

LIKELY TO BE INEFFECTIVE OR HARMFUL

Oral etoposide in extensive stage small cell lung cancer (likely to reduce survival compared with combination chemotherapy)

Two RCTs in people with extensive stage small cell lung cancer found that oral etoposide reduced survival compared with combination chemotherapy at 1 year. One RCT, in people with extensive stage small cell lung cancer who had not responded to induction combination chemotherapy, found no significant difference between oral etoposide and no further treatment in mortality at 3 years, although overall mortality was lower in people taking etoposide. RCTs found that etoposide may reduce nausea, alopecia, and numbness in the short term compared with combination chemotherapy. They found no evidence that it offered better quality of life overall.

DEFINITION   Lung cancer (bronchogenic carcinoma) is an epithelial cancer arising from the bronchial surface epithelium or bronchial mucous glands. It is broadly divided into small cell and non-small cell lung cancer. For a description of the stages of lung cancer see table 1.❶

Lung cancer

**INCIDENCE/
PREVALENCE**
Lung cancer is the leading cause of cancer death in both men and women annually, affecting about 100 000 men and 80 000 women in the USA, and about 40 000 men and women in the UK. Small cell lung cancer constitutes about 20–25% of all lung cancers, the remainder being non-small cell lung cancers of which adenocarcinoma is now the most prevalent form.[1]

**AETIOLOGY/
RISK FACTORS**
Smoking remains the major preventable risk factor, accounting for about 80–90% of all cases.[2] Other respiratory tract carcinogens have been identified that may enhance the carcinogenic effects of tobacco smoke, either in the workplace (e.g. asbestos and polycyclic aromatic hydrocarbons) or in the home (e.g. indoor radon).[3]

PROGNOSIS
Lung cancer has an overall 5 year survival rate of 10–12%.[4] At the time of diagnosis, 10–15% of people with lung cancer have localised disease. Of these, half will have died at 5 years despite potentially curative surgery. Over half of people have metastatic disease at the time of diagnosis. People with non-small cell cancer who have surgery have a 5 year survival of 60–80% for stage 1 disease and 25–50% for stage 2 disease.[4] In people with small cell cancer, those with limited stage disease who have combined chemotherapy and mediastinal irradiation have a median survival of 18–24 months, whereas those with extensive stage disease who are given palliative chemotherapy have a median survival of 10–12 months.[4] About 5–10% of people with small cell lung cancer present with central nervous system involvement, and half develop symptomatic brain metastases by 2 years. Of these, only half respond to palliative radiation, and their median survival is less than 3 months.[4]

Please refer to the Clinical Evidence website for full text and references.

Bacterial vaginosis may resolve spontaneously.

What are the effects of different antibacterial regimens in non-pregnant women with symptomatic bacterial vaginosis on cure rates and symptom relief?

BENEFICIAL

Antibacterial treatment with metronidazole or clindamycin (short term benefit)

One systematic review found that more women having antibacterial treatment (intravaginal clindamycin cream or intravaginal metronidazole gel) achieved cure than women using placebo. One systematic review found no significant difference in cure rates or adverse effects at 5–10 days or 4 weeks between intravaginal clindamycin and oral metronidazole. However, comparison of results across RCTs found that yeast vulvovaginitis may be less common with intravaginal clindamycin than with oral metronidazole. Intravaginal clindamycin has been associated, rarely, with mild to severe colitis and vaginal candidiasis in non-pregnant women. Another systematic review found that a 7 day course of twice daily oral metronidazole increased cure rates compared with a single 2 g dose; it gave no information on adverse effects. Limited evidence from RCTs found no significant difference in cure rates between oral clindamycin and oral metronidazole, and found that both treatments were associated with nausea and metallic taste. One RCT found no significant difference in cure rates at 35 days between 3 day treatment with intravaginal clindamycin ovules and 7 day treatment with intravaginal clindamycin cream. It found that the proportion of people who had adverse effects was similar in both groups, but ovules were associated with a higher incidence of vaginal pain and headache, and cream with a higher incidence of flu syndrome. Another RCT found no significant difference in cure rates or adverse effects between once and twice daily dosing with intravaginal metronidazole gel. We found no evidence on long term outcomes. One small RCT suggested that more than 50% of women had recurrent bacterial vaginosis 2 months after antibacterial treatment.

What are the effects of antibacterial treatments in pregnant women to reduce adverse outcomes of pregnancy and prevent neonatal complications?

LIKELY TO BE BENEFICIAL

Antibacterial treatment (except intravaginal clindamycin) in pregnant women who have had a previous preterm birth

One systematic review found that antibiotics reduced the risk of low birth weight in women with bacterial vaginosis who had a previous preterm delivery, although results for preterm delivery varied widely between trials. One subsequent RCT found that oral clindamycin given early in the second trimester reduced miscarriages or preterm deliveries compared with placebo in women with previous late miscarriage or preterm delivery.

Bacterial vaginosis

UNKNOWN EFFECTIVENESS

Antibacterial treatment in low risk pregnancy

One systematic review in general populations of pregnant women found no significant difference between antibiotics (oral or vaginal) and placebo or no treatment in the risk of preterm delivery, low birth weight, neonatal sepsis, or perinatal death. However, subsequent RCTs in women with bacterial vaginosis or abnormal genital tract flora (may or may not have included bacterial vaginosis) found that oral or intravaginal clindamycin given early in the second trimester reduced miscarriages or preterm deliveries compared with placebo.

LIKELY TO BE INEFFECTIVE OR HARMFUL

Intravaginal clindamycin cream

In studies that assessed women regardless of previous preterm delivery, three RCTs found a non-significant increase in preterm birth and low birth weight in women with bacterial vaginosis treated with clindamycin cream compared with placebo. However, one subsequent RCT found limited evidence in women with abnormal genital tract flora (may or may not have included bacterial vaginosis) that intravaginal clindamycin cream given early in the second trimester reduced preterm birth compared with placebo.

Does treating male partners prevent recurrence?

LIKELY TO BE INEFFECTIVE OR HARMFUL

Treating a woman's male sexual partner with metronidazole or clindamycin (did not reduce the woman's risk of recurrence)

One systematic review found that in women receiving antibacterial agents, and who have one steady male sexual partner, treating the partner with an oral antibacterial agent did not reduce the woman's risk of recurrence.

What are the effects of treatment before gynaecological procedures?

LIKELY TO BE BENEFICIAL

Oral or intravaginal antibacterial treatment before surgical abortion

Three RCTs found a lower rate of post operative pelvic inflammatory disease with oral or intravaginal antibacterial treatment compared with placebo given to women with bacterial vaginosis who were about to have surgical abortion, but the difference was significant only in the largest RCT. The RCTs gave no information on adverse effects. In RCTs in non-pregnant women with bacterial vaginosis, intravaginal clindamycin was associated, rarely, with mild to severe colitis and vaginal candidiasis. Oral metronidazole was associated with nausea and metallic taste.

UNKNOWN EFFECTIVENESS

Antibacterial treatment before gynaecological procedures other than abortion

We found no RCTs on the effects of antibacterial treatment in women with bacterial vaginosis about to have gynaecological procedures other than abortion.

DEFINITION

Bacterial vaginosis is a microbial disease characterised by an change in the bacterial flora of the vagina from mainly *Lactobacillus* species to high concentrations of anaerobic bacteria. The condition is asymptomatic in 50% of infected women. Women with symptoms have an excessive white to grey, or malodorous vaginal discharge, or both; the odour may be particularly noticeable during sexual intercourse. Commonly practiced clinical diagnosis requires three out of four features: the presence of clue cells on microscopy; a homogenous discharge adherent to the vaginal walls; pH of vaginal fluid greater than 4.5; and a "fishy" amine odour of the vaginal discharge before or after addition of 10% potassium hydroxide. Some experts prefer other methods of diagnosis, (e.g. Gram stain of vaginal secretions), particularly in a research setting. Gram stain using Nugent's criteria[1] categorise the flora of vagina into three categories – normal, intermediate, and flora consistent with bacterial vaginosis. Abnormal vaginal flora includes intermediate flora and bacterial vaginosis.

INCIDENCE/ PREVALENCE

Bacterial vaginosis is the most common infectious cause of vaginitis, being about twice as common as candidiasis.[2] Prevalences of 10–61% have been reported among unselected women from a range of settings.[3] Data on incidence are limited but one study found that, over a 2 year period, 50% of women using an intrauterine contraceptive device had at least one episode, as did 20% of women using oral contraceptives.[4] Bacterial vaginosis is particularly prevalent among lesbians.[5]

AETIOLOGY/ RISK FACTORS

The cause of bacterial vaginosis is not fully understood. Risk factors include new or multiple sexual partners[2,4,6] and early age of sexual intercourse,[7] but no causative microorganism has been shown to be transmitted between partners. Use of an intrauterine contraceptive device[4] and douching[6] have also been reported as risk factors. Infection seems to be most common around the time of menstruation.[8]

PROGNOSIS

The course of bacterial vaginosis varies and is poorly understood. Without treatment, symptoms may persist or resolve in both pregnant and non-pregnant women. Recurrence after treatment occurs in about a third of women. A history of bacterial vaginosis is associated with increased rates of complications in pregnancy: low birth weight;[7] preterm birth (pooled OR from 10 cohort studies: 1.8, 95% CI 1.5 to 2.6);[9] preterm labour; premature rupture of membranes;[7] late miscarriage; chorioamnionitis;[10] endometritis after normal delivery (8.2% v 1.5%; OR 5.6, 95% CI 1.8 to 17.2);[11] endometritis after caesarean section (55% v 17%; OR 5.8, 95% CI 3.0 to 10.9);[12] and surgery to the genital tract.[13,14] Women who have had a previous preterm delivery are especially at risk of complications in pregnancy, with a sevenfold increased risk of preterm birth (24/428 [5.6%] in all women v 10/24 [41.7%] in women with a previous preterm birth).[15] Bacterial vaginosis can also increase the risk of HIV acquisition and transmission.[16]

Please refer to the Clinical Evidence website for full text and references.

Chlamydia (uncomplicated, genital)

Search date March 2004

Nicola Low

Short term microbiological cure is the outcome used in most RCTs, but this may not mean eradication of *Chlamydia trachomatis*. Long term cure rates have not been studied extensively because of high default rates and difficulty in distinguishing persistent infection from reinfection due to re-exposure.

What are the effects of antibiotic treatment for men and non-pregnant women with uncomplicated genital chlamydial infection?

BENEFICIAL

Azithromycin (single dose)

A systematic review of 12 blinded and unblinded RCTs found no significant difference in microbiological cure of *C trachomatis* between a single dose of azithromycin and a 7 day course of doxycycline. Rates of adverse effects were similar.

Doxycycline, teracycline (multiple dose regimens)

Small RCTs with short term follow up and high withdrawal rates found that multiple dose regimens of tetracyclines (doxycycline, tetracycline) achieve microbiological cure in at least 95% of people with genital chlamydia. A systematic review of 12 blinded and unblinded RCTs found no significant difference in microbiological cure of *C trachomatis* between a 7 day course of doxycycline and a single dose of azithromycin. Rates of adverse effects were similar. Meta-analysis of two RCTs found that doxycycline reduced microbiological failure compared with ciprofloxacin.

LIKELY TO BE BENEFICIAL

Erythromycin (multiple dose regimens)

Three small RCTs found that erythromycin achieved microbiological cure in 77–100% of people, with the highest cure rate with a 2g compared with a 1g daily dose.

UNKNOWN EFFECTIVENESS

Amoxicillin, ampicillin, clarithromycin, lymecycline, minocycline, ofloxacin, pivampicillin, rifampicin, roxithromycin, sparfloxacin, trovafloxacin (multiple dose regimens)

We found limited evidence on the effects of these regimens.

UNLIKELY TO BE BENEFICIAL

Ciprofloxacin (multiple dose regimens)

Two RCTs found that ciprofloxacin cured 63–92% of people. Meta-analysis of these two RCTs found that ciprofloxacin increased microbiological failure compared with doxycycline.

What are the effects of antibiotic treatment for pregnant women with uncomplicated genital chlamydial infection?

LIKELY TO BE BENEFICIAL

Azithromycin (single dose)

One systematic review found that a single dose of azithromycin increased microbiological cure and decreased the risk of an adverse effect, sufficient to stop treatment, when compared with a 7 day course of erythromycin. Two subsequent unblinded RCTs found no significant difference in cure rate between single dose azithromycin and multiple dose amoxicillin.

Erythromycin, amoxicillin (multiple dose regimens)

One small RCT identified in a systematic review found that erythromycin versus placebo increased microbiological cure. The review found that a 7 day course of erythromycin reduced microbiological cure and increased the risk of an adverse event sufficient to stop treatment, compared with a single dose of azithromycin. Two subsequent unblinded RCTs found no significant difference in cure rates between multiple dose amoxicillin and single dose azithromycin. Other RCTs in the review found high cure rates with erythromycin and amoxicillin and no significant difference in microbiological cure between the two drugs.

UNKNOWN EFFECTIVENESS

Clindamycin (multiple dose regimens)

One small RCT found no significant difference in cure rates between clindamycin and erythromycin.

DEFINITION Genital chlamydia is a sexually transmitted infection of the urethra in men, and of the endocervix or urethra (or both) in women. It is defined as **uncomplicated** if it has not ascended to the upper genital tract. Infection is asymptomatic in up to 80% of cases, but may cause non-specific symptoms, including vaginal discharge and intermenstrual bleeding. Infection in men causes urethral discharge and urethral irritation or dysuria, but may also be asymptomatic in up to half of cases.[1] **Complicated** chlamydial infection includes spread to the upper genital tract (causing pelvic inflammatory disease in women [see pelvic inflammatory disease, p 463] and epididymoorchitis in men) and extragenital sites, such as the eye. Interventions for complicated chlamydial infection are not included in this chapter.

INCIDENCE/ Genital chlamydia is the most commonly reported bacterial sexually transmit-
PREVALENCE ted infection in developed countries [1] and reported rates increased by around 20% in the UK and USA between 2000 and 2002.[2,3] In women, infection occurs most commonly between the ages of 16 and 19 years. In this age group, about 1300/100 000 new infections are reported each year in the UK,[2] compared with 1900/100 000 in Sweden,[4] and 2536 per 100 000 in the USA.[3] The peak age group for men is 20–24 years, with about 965/100 000 new infections per year in the UK and USA and 1200/100 000 in Sweden.[2–4] Rates decline markedly with increasing age. Reported rates are highly dependent on the level of testing. The population prevalence of uncomplicated genital chlamydia in 18–44 year olds in the UK in 1999 was 2.2% (95% CI 1.5% to 3.2%) in men and 1.5% (95% CI 1.1% to 2.1%) in women.[5]

AETIOLOGY/ Infection is caused by the bacterium *C trachomatis* serotypes D–K. It is
RISK FACTORS transmitted primarily through sexual intercourse, but also perinatally and through direct or indirect oculogenital contact.[1]

Chlamydia (uncomplicated, genital)

PROGNOSIS In women, untreated chlamydial infection that ascends to the upper genital tract causes pelvic inflammatory disease (see pelvic inflammatory disease, p 463) in an estimated 30–40% of cases.[6] Tubal infertility has been found to occur in about 11% of women after a single episode of pelvic inflammatory disease, and the risk of ectopic pregnancy is increased six- to sevenfold.[7] Ascending infection in men causes epididymitis, but evidence that this causes male infertility is limited.[8] Maternal to infant transmission can lead to neonatal conjunctivitis and pneumonitis in 30–40% of cases.[1] Chlamydia may coexist with other genital infections and may facilitate transmission and acquisition of HIV infection.[1] Untreated chlamydial infection persists in most women for at least 60 days and for a shorter period in men.[9] Spontaneous remission also occurs at an estimated rate of 5% per month.[10]

Please refer to the Clinical Evidence website for full text and references.

What are the effects of interventions to prevent sexual transmission of herpes simplex virus?

LIKELY TO BE BENEFICIAL

Antiviral treatment of infected sexual partner (reduced transmission to uninfected partner)

One RCT found that daily use of valaciclovir reduced the risk of transmission of herpes simplex virus-2 to a previously uninfected sexual partner compared with placebo.

Male condom use to prevent sexual transmission from infected men to uninfected sexual partners*

One prospective cohort study found limited evidence that condom use by men infected with genital herpes reduced transmission of herpes simplex virus-2 to their uninfected sexual partners.

UNKNOWN EFFECTIVENESS

Female condoms

We found no systematic review or RCTs on the effects of female condoms to prevent sexual transmission.

Male condom use to prevent sexual transmission from infected women to uninfected men

Subgroup analysis of one prospective cohort study found no significant difference between male condom use and no male condom use in transmission of herpes simplex virus-2 to uninfected men from their infected female partners.

Vaccines other than recombinant glycoprotein vaccines

We found no systematic review or RCTs.

UNLIKELY TO BE BENEFICIAL

Recombinant glycoprotein vaccines (gB2 and gD2) in people at high risk of infection (unless known to be HSV-1 and HSV-2 negative before vaccination)

One RCT found no significant difference between recombinant glycoprotein vaccine (gB2 plus gD2) and placebo in preventing genital herpes simplex virus-2 infection in people at high risk of infection. Subgroup analysis in a second RCT found that recombinant herpes simplex virus-2 glycoprotein-D-adjuvant vaccine reduced the risk of genital herpes infection compared with placebo in women who had been seronegative for herpes simplex virus-1 and herpes simplex virus-2 at baseline and who had regular sexual partners with clinically confirmed genital herpes. Subgroup analyses also found no significant difference between the vaccine and placebo in infection rate for men or in women who had been seropositive for herpes simplex virus-1 and who had regular sexual partners with genital herpes.

▶

Genital herpes

What are the effects of interventions to prevent transmission of herpes simplex virus from mother to neonate?

UNKNOWN EFFECTIVENESS

Caesarean delivery in women with genital lesions at term

We found no systematic review or RCTs on the effects of caesarean delivery on mother to baby transmission of genital herpes in mothers with genital lesions at term. The procedure carries the risk of increased maternal morbidity and mortality.

Oral antiviral maintenance treatment in late pregnancy (36 or more weeks of gestation) in women with a history of genital herpes

One systematic review provided insufficient evidence to assess the effects of oral antiviral agents during pregnancy on transmission of infection to neonates. The review found that aciclovir reduced the recurrence of infection at term in women with first or recurrent episodes of genital herpes simplex virus during pregnancy, and reduced the need for caesarean delivery because of genital herpes.

Serological screening and counselling in late pregnancy

We found no systematic review or RCTs on the effects of either serological screening or counselling to prevent maternal infection in late pregnancy.

What are the effects of antiviral treatment in people with a first episode of genital herpes?

BENEFICIAL

Oral antiviral treatment in first episodes of genital herpes

Three RCTs found that oral aciclovir treatment decreased the duration of lesions, symptoms, and viral shedding compared with placebo.

UNKNOWN EFFECTIVENESS

Different types of oral antiviral treatment for first episodes of genital herpes

One RCT found no difference in clinical outcomes between oral aciclovir and valaciclovir.

What are the effects of interventions to reduce the impact of recurrence?

BENEFICIAL

Oral antiviral maintenance treatment in people with high rates of recurrence

RCTs found that daily maintenance treatment with oral antiviral agents (valaciclovir, aciclovir or famciclovir) reduced the frequency of recurrences, and that oral aciclovir and oral valaciclovir improved quality of life compared with placebo.

Oral antiviral treatment taken at the start of recurrence

One systematic review, one non-systematic review, and one RCT found that oral antiviral treatment (aciclovir, famciclovir or valaciclovir) taken at the start of recurrence reduced the duration of lesions and viral shedding and increased the rate of aborted recurrences compared with placebo, in people with recurrent genital herpes. RCTs found that aciclovir, famciclovir, and valaciclovir were similarly ▶

effective in reducing symptom duration, lesion healing time, and viral shedding compared with placebo. Two RCTs found no difference between valaciclovir taken for 3 days or 5 days.

UNKNOWN EFFECTIVENESS

Psychotherapy to reduce recurrence

One systematic review of poor quality studies provided insufficient evidence about the effects of psychosocial interventions to prevent recurrence of genital herpes.

What are the effects of treatments in people with genital herpes and HIV?

LIKELY TO BE BENEFICIAL

Oral antiviral maintenance treatment for preventing recurrence of genital herpes in people with HIV

One RCT found that valaciclovir was more effective than placebo in preventing herpes simplex virus infection. One RCT found no significant difference between valaciclovir and aciclovir in preventing recurrent herpes simplex virus infections over 48 weeks.

UNKNOWN EFFECTIVENESS

Oral antiviral treatment for an acute recurrent episode of genital herpes in people with HIV

Two RCTs found no significant differences in duration of lesions and symptoms between famciclovir or valaciclovir or aciclovir.

Oral antiviral treatment for first episode genital herpes in people with HIV

We found no RCTs on the treatment of first episode genital herpes in people with HIV.

*Categorisation based on observational or non-randomised evidence in the context of practical and ethical problems of performing RCTs.

DEFINITION   Genital herpes is an infection with herpes simplex virus type 1 (HSV-1) or type 2 (HSV-2). The typical clinical features include painful shallow anogenital ulceration. Herpes simplex virus infections can be confirmed on the basis of virological and serological findings. Types of infection include **first episode primary infection**, which is defined as herpes simplex virus confirmed in a person without prior findings of HSV-1 or HSV-2 antibodies; **first episode non-primary infection**, which is HSV-2 confirmed in a person with prior findings of HSV-1 antibodies or vice versa; **first recognised recurrence**, which is HSV-1 (or HSV-2) confirmed in a person with prior findings of HSV-1 (or HSV-2) antibodies; and **recurrent genital herpes**, which is caused by reactivation of latent herpes simplex virus. HSV-1 can also cause gingivosto-matitis and orolabial ulcers; HSV-2 can also cause other types of herpes infections, such as ocular herpes; and both virus types can cause infection of the central nervous system (e.g. encephalitis).

INCIDENCE/   Genital herpes infections are among the most common sexually transmitted
PREVALENCE   diseases. Seroprevalence studies showed that 22% of adults in the USA had HSV-2 antibodies.[1] A UK study found that 23% of adults attending sexual medicine clinics and 7.6% of blood donors in London had antibodies to HSV-2.[2] Seroprevalence of HSV-2 increased by 30.0% (95% CI 15.8% to 45.8%) between the periods 1976–1980 and 1988–1994.[1] However, it should be noted that although antibody levels prove the existence of present ▶

or past infections, they do not differentiate between possible manifestations of HSV-2 infections (e.g. genital/ocular). Thus, the figures have to be treated with caution when applied to genital herpes only.

AETIOLOGY/ RISK FACTORS Both HSV-1 and HSV-2 can cause a first episode of genital infection, but HSV-2 is more likely to cause recurrent disease.[3] Most people with HSV-2 infection have only mild symptoms and remain unaware that they have genital herpes. However, these people can still pass on the infection to sexual partners and newborns.[4,5]

PROGNOSIS Sequelae of herpes simplex virus infection include neonatal herpes simplex virus infection, opportunistic infection in immunocompromised people, recurrent genital ulceration, and psychosocial morbidity. HSV-2 infection is associated with an increased risk of HIV transmission and acquisition.[6] The most common neurological complications are aseptic meningitis (reported in about 25% of women during primary infection) and urinary retention (reported in up to 15% of women during primary infection).[5] The absolute risk of neonatal infection is high (41%, 95% CI 26% to 56%) in babies born to women who acquire infection near the time of labour and low (< 3%) in women with established infection, even in those who have a recurrence at term.[7,8] About 15% of neonatal infections result from postnatal transmission from oral lesions of relatives or hospital personnel.[5]

Please refer to the Clinical Evidence website for full text and references.

What are the effects of treatments for external genital warts?

BENEFICIAL

Cryotherapy (as effective in clearing warts as trichloroacetic acid and more effective than podophyllin)

We found no RCTs comparing cryotherapy versus placebo or no treatment. Two RCTs found no significant difference between cryotherapy and trichloroacetic acid in clearance of warts after 6–10 weeks' treatment. One of the RCTs found no significant difference in recurrence of warts 2 months after the end of treatment. One RCT found limited evidence that cryotherapy was less effective for clearance than electrosurgery after 6 weeks' treatment. However, follow up of the people with successful wart clearance revealed no significant difference in the proportion of people who had warts at 3–5 months. Another RCT found no significant difference in wart clearance at 3 months between cryotherapy and electrosurgery. One RCT found that cryotherapy increased clearance after 6 weeks' treatment compared with podophyllin, and follow up of the people with successful wart clearance found that fewer people receiving cryotherapy had warts at 3–5 months.

Electrosurgery (at least as effective as cryotherapy and more effective than podophyllin in clearing warts)

One RCT found that electrosurgery increased clearance of warts at 6 months compared with no treatment. One RCT found that electrosurgery increased clearance of warts at 6 months compared with systemic interferon but the increase was not significant. One RCT found that electrosurgery improved clearance after 6 weeks' treatment compared with cryotherapy. However, follow up of the people with successful wart clearance revealed no significant difference in the proportion of people who had warts at 3–5 months after treatment. It also found that electrosurgery improved clearance after 6 weeks' treatment compared with podophyllin, and follow up of the people with successful wart clearance revealed that the difference was maintained at 3–5 months after treatment. Another RCT found no significant difference in wart clearance at 3 months between electrosurgery and cryotherapy.

Imiquimod in people without HIV

One systematic review and one subsequent RCT found that 5% or 1% imiquimod cream increased wart clearance and reduced recurrence compared with placebo in people without HIV. One RCT in women without HIV found that twice daily doses of imiquimod 5% did not increase wart clearance over 20 weeks compared with once daily or three times weekly doses, but found that it increased skin erythema. One RCT in people without HIV found that imiquimod 5% increased moderate to severe erythema, erosion, excoriation, oedema, and scabbing compared with imiquimod 1% or placebo.

Interferon, topical

Three RCTs found that topical interferon increased wart clearance at 4 weeks after treatment compared with placebo. One of the RCTs also found that topical interferon increased wart clearance at 4 weeks after treatment compared with podophyllotoxin.

▶

Genital warts

Laser surgery (as effective as surgical excision in clearing warts)

We found no RCTs comparing laser surgery versus no treatment. One RCT found no significant difference in wart clearance or recurrence rates over 36 weeks between laser and surgical excision.

Podophyllin (as effective as podophyllotoxin or surgical excision in clearing warts but less effective than cryotherapy and electrosurgery; less effective than surgical excision in preventing recurrence)*

We found no RCTs comparing podophyllin versus placebo, but there is consensus that podophyllin is effective for clearing genital warts. Six RCTs provided no consistent evidence of a difference between podophyllotoxin and podophyllin in wart clearance or recurrence. RCTs found no significant difference between surgical (scissor) excision and podophyllin in wart clearance. However, they found that surgical excision was more effective than podophyllin in preventing recurrence at 6–12 months. One RCT found that podophyllin was less effective than cryotherapy or electrosurgery in clearing warts at 6 weeks, and follow up of the people with successful wart clearance revealed that more people receiving podophyllin had warts at 3–5 months. One RCT found no significant difference in wart clearance at 3 months between podophyllin plus trichloroacetic acid and podophyllin alone. One RCT found that podophyllin was more effective than systemic interferon in clearing warts at 3 months.

Podophyllotoxin

RCTs found that podophyllotoxin increased wart clearance within 16 weeks compared with placebo. Six RCTs provided no consistent evidence of a difference between podophyllotoxin and podophyllin in wart clearance or recurrence. One RCT found that podophyllotoxin was less effective than topical interferon in clearing warts at 4 weeks.

Surgical excision (as effective as laser surgery or podophyllin in clearing warts; more effective than podophyllin in preventing recurrence)

We found no RCTs comparing surgical excision versus no treatment. RCTs found no significant difference between surgical (scissor) excision and laser surgery or podophyllin in wart clearance. However, they found that surgical excision was more effective than podophyllin in preventing recurrence at 6–12 months.

LIKELY TO BE BENEFICIAL

Bi- and trichloroacetic acid (as effective as cryotherapy in clearing warts)

We found no RCTs comparing bi- and trichloroacetic acid versus placebo. Two RCTs found no significant difference between trichloroacetic acid and cryotherapy in clearance of warts after 6–10 weeks' treatment, and one of the RCTs found no significant difference in recurrence of warts 2 months after the end of treatment. One RCT found no significant difference in wart clearance at 3 months between trichloroacetic acid plus podophyllin and podophyllin alone.

UNKNOWN EFFECTIVENESS

Imiquimod in people with HIV

One RCT in people with HIV found no significant difference in wart clearance over 16 weeks between imiquimod cream and placebo. One RCT in people without HIV found that imiquimod 5% increased moderate to severe erythema, erosion, excoriation, oedema, and scabbing compared with imiquimod 1% or placebo.

Interferon, systemic

We found five RCTs comparing different formulations of systemic interferon versus placebo or no treatment. Two of the RCTs found that systemic interferon improved wart clearance compared with placebo or no treatment, whereas three of the RCTs found no significant difference between interferon and placebo in complete or partial wart clearance. Systemic interferon was associated with important adverse effects, including anaphylaxis, blood disorders, flu-like symptoms, headache, fatigue, myalgia, fever, and weight loss. One RCT found no significant difference in wart clearance at 6 months between electrosurgery and systemic interferon. One RCT found that systemic interferon was less effective than podophyllin in clearing warts at 3 months.

What are the effects of interventions to prevent transmission of human papillomavirus or external genital warts?

Condoms

Observational studies provided insufficient evidence to assess the effects of condom use on transmission of human papillomavirus. Penetrative intercourse is not required for spread because this can occur with external genital–genital or hand–genital touching. One case control and one cross-sectional study suggested that people who always used condoms were less likely to have genital warts than people who never or occasionally used them.

*No placebo controlled RCTs found; categorisation based on consensus opinion.

DEFINITION External genital warts are benign epidermal growths on the external perigenital and perianal regions. There are four morphological types: condylomatous, keratotic, papular, and flat warts.

INCIDENCE/ PREVALENCE In 1996, external and internal genital warts accounted for more than 180 000 initial visits to private physicians' offices in the USA, which is about 60 000 fewer than were reported for 1995.[1] In the USA, 1% of sexually active men and women aged 18–49 years are estimated to have external genital warts.[2] It is believed that external and cervical lesions caused by the human papillomavirus (HPV) are the most prevalent sexually transmitted disease among persons 18–25 years of age. In the USA, 50–60% of women aged 18–25 years test positive for HPV DNA, but no more than 10–15% ever have genital warts.[3]

AETIOLOGY/ RISK FACTORS External genital warts are caused by HPV and are sexually transmitted. They are more common in people with impaired immune function.[3] Although more than 100 types of HPV have been identified, most external genital warts in immunocompetent people are caused by HPV types 6 and 11.[4,5]

PROGNOSIS The ability to clear and remain free of external genital warts is a function of cellular immunity.[6] In immunocompetent people, the prognosis in terms of clearance and avoiding recurrence is good,[7] but people with impaired cellular immunity (e.g. people with HIV and AIDS) have great difficulty in achieving and maintaining wart clearance.[3] Without treatment, external genital warts may remain unchanged, may increase in size or number, or may resolve completely. Clinical trials have found that recurrences may occur and may necessitate repeated treatment. External genital warts rarely, if ever, progress to cancer.[8] ▶

Genital warts

Juvenile laryngeal papillomatosis, a rare and sometimes life threatening condition, occurs in children of women with a history of genital warts. Its rarity makes it difficult to design studies that can evaluate whether treatment in pregnant women alters the risk.[9,10]

Please refer to the Clinical Evidence website for full text and references.

What are the effects of treatments for uncomplicated infections in men and non-pregnant women?

BENEFICIAL

Single dose antibiotic regimens*

One systematic review found limited evidence that single dose regimens (ceftriaxone, ciprofloxacin, gatifloxacin, spectinomycin, azithromycin, ofloxacin, cefixime) achieve cure rates of 95% or higher in urogenital or rectal infection. Cure rates were lower (about 80%) for pharyngeal infection. Resistance to penicillins, tetracyclines, and sulphonamides is now widespread, and resistance to fluoroquinolones has become common in some geographic areas.

What are the effects of treatments for uncomplicated infections in pregnant women?

BENEFICIAL

Single dose antibiotic regimens

One systematic review found that antibiotic treatment (amoxicillin plus probenecid, spectinomycin, ceftriaxone, cefixime) was effective for curing gonorrhoea in pregnant women. We found no reports of serious adverse effects.

What are the effects of treatments for disseminated gonococcal infection?

LIKELY TO BE BENEFICIAL

Multidose antibiotic regimens†

We found no RCTs assessing treatments for disseminated gonococcal infection, but there is consensus that multidose regimens using injectable cephalosporins or quinolones (except where quinolone-resistant *Neisseria gonorrhoeae* have been reported) are the most effective treatments. We found no reports of treatment failures with these regimens.

What are the effects of dual treatment for gonorrhoea and chlamydia infection?

UNKNOWN EFFECTIVENESS

Dual antibiotic treatment

Dual treatment with an antimicrobial effective against gonorrhoea and chlamydia infections is based on theory and expert opinion rather than on evidence from RCTs. The balance between benefits and harms will vary with the prevalence of co-infection in each population.

*Based on comparisons of results across arms of different trials.
†Based on non-RCT evidence and consensus.

Gonorrhoea

DEFINITION   Gonorrhoea is caused by infection with *Neisseria gonorrhoeae*. In men, uncomplicated urethritis is the most common manifestation, with dysuria and urethral discharge. Less typically, signs and symptoms are mild and indistinguishable from those of chlamydial urethritis. In women, the most common site of infection is the uterine cervix where infection results in symptoms such as vaginal discharge, lower abdominal discomfort, and dyspareunia in only half of cases. Co-infection with *Chlamydia trachomatis* is reported in 20–40% of people.[1–3]

INCIDENCE/   Between 1975 and 1997, the reported incidence of gonorrhoea in the USA
PREVALENCE   fell by 74%, reaching a nadir of 122/100 000 people. Since 1997, 125–133 cases have been reported per 100 000 people each year.[4] Rates are highest in younger people. In 2002, the incidence was highest in women aged 15–19 years (676/100 000) and men aged 20–24 years (538/100 000). In England, Wales, and Northern Ireland, diagnoses of gonorrhoea have increased from 1994 to 2002 reaching 296/100 000 for 20–24 year old men and 214/100 000 for 16–19 year old women in 2002.[5] Rates in 2004 were similar to those in 2003.

AETIOLOGY/   Most infections result from penile–vaginal, penile–rectal, or penile–pharyngeal
RISK FACTORS   contact. An important minority of infections are transmitted from mother to child during birth, which can cause a sight-threatening purulent conjunctivitis (ophthalmia neonatorum). Less common are ocular infections in older children and adults as a result of sexual exposure, poor hygiene, or the medicinal use of urine.

PROGNOSIS   The natural history of untreated gonococcal infection is spontaneous resolution and microbiological clearance after weeks or months of unpleasant symptoms.[6] During this time, there is a substantial likelihood of transmission to others and of complications developing in the infected individual.[6] In many women, the lack of readily discernible signs or symptoms of cervicitis means that infections go unrecognised and untreated. An unknown proportion of untreated infections causes local complications, including lymphangitis, periurethral abscess, bartholinitis, and urethral stricture; epididymitis in men; and in women involvement of the uterus, fallopian tubes, or ovaries causing pelvic inflammatory disease (see pelvic inflammatory disease, p 463). One review found *N gonorrhoeae* was cultured from 8–32% of women with acute pelvic inflammatory disease in 11 European studies and from 27–80% of women in eight US studies.[7] The proportion of *N gonorrhoeae* infections in women that lead to pelvic inflammatory disease has not been well studied. However, one study of 26 women exposed to men with gonorrhoea found that 19 women were culture positive and of these, five women had pelvic inflammatory disease and another four had uterine adnexal tenderness.[8] Pelvic inflammatory disease may lead to infertility (see pelvic inflammatory disease, p 463). In some people, localised gonococcal infection may disseminate. A US study estimated the risk of dissemination to be 0.6–1.1% among women, whereas a European study estimated it to be 2.3–3.0%.[9,10] The same European study found a lower risk in men, estimated to be 0.4–0.7%.[10] When gonococci disseminate, they cause petechial or pustular skin lesions; asymmetrical arthropathies, tenosynovitis, or septic arthritis; and rarely, meningitis or endocarditis.

Please refer to the Clinical Evidence website for full text and references.

We found no good evidence on the effects of partner notification on relationships between patients and partners and, in particular, on the rate of violence, abuse, and abandonment of patient or partner. We also found no studies comparing the effects of an intervention across different groups, such as people with different diseases or combinations of diseases, or people from different settings.

What are the effects of different partner notification strategies in different groups of people and what are the effects of interventions to improve patient referral?

LIKELY TO BE BENEFICIAL

Contract referral (as effective as provider referral in people with syphilis)

One systematic review of one large RCT comparing different partner notification strategies in people with syphilis found no significant difference in the proportion of partners notified between provider referral and contract referral, when people receiving the contract referral option were given 2 days to notify their partners.

Offering a choice between provider and patient referral (v patient referral) in people with HIV

One systematic review of one RCT comparing different partner notification strategies found that in people with HIV, offering a choice between provider referral (where the identity of the index patient was not revealed) and patient referral was improved notification rates compared with offering patient referral alone.

Provider referral or contract referral (v patient referral) in people with gonorrhoea or non-gonococcal urethritis (mainly chlamydia)

One systematic review, has found that, for people with gonorrhoea, contract referral compared with patient referral increased the rate of partners presenting for treatment. For people with non-gonococcal urethritis, one systematic review found that provider versus patient referral increased the proportion of partners notified and of positive partners detected per patient.

UNKNOWN EFFECTIVENESS

Adding telephone reminders and contact cards to patient referral; educational videos; information pamphlets; patient referral by different types of healthcare professionals; patient referral in HIV

We found insufficient evidence about the effects of these interventions in improving partner notification.

DEFINITION   Partner notification is a process whereby the sexual partners of people with a diagnosis of sexually transmitted infection are informed of their exposure to infection. The main methods are patient referral, provider referral, contract referral, and outreach assistance.

INCIDENCE/ PREVALENCE   A large proportion of people with sexually transmitted infections will have neither symptoms nor signs of infection. For example, 22–68% of men with gonorrhoea who were identified through partner notification were asymptomatic.[1] Partner notification is one of the two strategies to reach such ▶

individuals, the other strategy being screening. Managing infection in people with more than one current sexual partner is likely to have the greatest impact on the spread of sexually transmitted infections.[2]

PROGNOSIS   We found no studies showing that partner notification results in a health benefit, either to the partner or to future partners of infected people. Obtaining such evidence would be technically and ethically difficult. One RCT in asymptomatic women compared identifying, testing, and treating women at increased risk for cervical chlamydial infection versus usual care. It found these reduced incidence of pelvic inflammatory disease (RR 0.44, 95% CI 0.2 to 0.9).[3] This evidence suggests that partner notification, which also aims to identify and treat people who are largely unaware of infection, would provide a direct health benefit to partners who are infected.

Please refer to the Clinical Evidence website for full text and references.

Search date April 2004

Jonathan Ross

What are the effects of empirical treatment compared with treatment delayed until the results of microbiological investigations are known?

UNKNOWN EFFECTIVENESS

Empirical antibiotic treatment versus treatment guided by test results

We found no RCTs comparing empirical antibiotic treatment (before receiving results of microbiological tests) versus treatment that is guided by test result in women with suspected pelvic inflammatory disease.

How do different antimicrobial regimens compare?

LIKELY TO BE BENEFICIAL

Antibiotics (for symptoms and microbiological clearance in women with confirmed pelvic inflammatory disease)

There is consensus that antibiotic treatment is more effective than no treatment for women with confirmed pelvic inflammatory disease. One systematic review of observational studies and RCTs found that several different antibiotic regimens (including parenteral clindamycin plus parenteral aminoglycoside; parenteral cephalosporin with or without probenecid plus oral doxycycline; and oral ofloxacin) were similarly effective in relieving the symptoms of pelvic inflammatory disease, and achieve high rates of clinical and microbiological cure.

Oral antibiotics (versus parenteral antibiotics)

Two RCTs found no significant difference between oral ofloxacin and parenteral cefoxitin plus doxycycline.

Outpatient (versus inpatient) antibiotic treatment

One RCT found no significant difference between outpatient treatment with intramuscular cefoxitin plus probenecid plus oral doxycycline and inpatient treatment with parenteral antibiotics in recurrence of pelvic inflammatory disease, infertility, or ectopic pregnancy at 35 months.

UNKNOWN EFFECTIVENESS

Different durations of antibiotic treatment

We found no good evidence on the optimal duration of treatment.

What are the effects of routine antibiotic prophylaxis to prevent pelvic inflammatory disease before intrauterine contraceptive device insertion?

UNKNOWN EFFECTIVENESS

Routine antibiotic prophylaxis before intrauterine device insertion in women at high risk

We found no good evidence about antibiotic prophylaxis before intrauterine device insertion in women at high risk of pelvic inflammatory disease.

Pelvic inflammatory disease

◄ UNLIKELY TO BE BENEFICIAL

Routine antibiotic prophylaxis before intrauterine device insertion in women at low risk

One systematic review found no significant difference in the incidence of pelvic inflammatory disease between routine prophylaxis with doxycycline and placebo before intrauterine contraceptive device insertion in women at low risk of pelvic inflammatory disease.

DEFINITION Pelvic inflammatory disease (PID) is inflammation and infection of the upper genital tract in women, typically involving the fallopian tubes, ovaries, and surrounding structures.

INCIDENCE/ PREVALENCE The exact incidence of pelvic inflammatory disease (PID) is unknown because the disease cannot be diagnosed reliably from clinical symptoms and signs.[1–3] Direct visualisation of the fallopian tubes by laparoscopy is the best single diagnostic test, but it is invasive and not used routinely in clinical practice. PID is the most common gynaecological reason for admission to hospital in the USA, accounting for 49/10 000 recorded hospital discharges. A diagnosis of PID is made in 1/62 (1.6%) women aged 16–45 years attending their primary care physician in England and Wales.[4] However, because most PID is asymptomatic, this figure underestimates the true prevalence.[1,5] A crude marker of PID in developing countries can be obtained from reported hospital admission rates, where it accounts for 17–40% of gynaecological admissions in sub-Saharan Africa, 15–37% in Southeast Asia, and 3–10% in India.[6]

AETIOLOGY/ RISK FACTORS Factors associated with pelvic inflammatory disease (PID) mirror those for sexually transmitted infections: young age, reduced socioeconomic circumstances, lower educational attainment, and recent new sexual partner.[2,7,8] Infection ascends from the cervix, and initial epithelial damage caused by bacteria (especially *Chlamydia trachomatis* and *Neisseria gonorrhoeae*) allows the opportunistic entry of other organisms. Many different microbes, including *Mycoplasma hominis* and anaerobes, may be isolated from the upper genital tract.[9] The spread of infection to the upper genital tract may be increased by instrumentation of the cervix, but reduced by the barrier method, levonorgestrel implants, and oral contraceptives compared with other forms of contraception.[10–14]

PROGNOSIS Pelvic inflammatory disease (PID) has a high morbidity; about 20% of affected women become infertile, 20% develop chronic pelvic pain, and 10% of those who conceive have an ectopic pregnancy.[2] Uncontrolled observations suggest that clinical symptoms and signs resolve in a significant proportion of untreated women.[15] Repeated episodes of PID are associated with a four to six times increase in the risk of permanent tubal damage.[16] One case control study (76 cases and 367 controls) found that delaying treatment by even a few days is associated with impaired fertility (OR 2.6, 95% CI 1.2 to 5.9).[17]

Please refer to the Clinical Evidence website for full text and references.

What are the effects of topical treatments in people with acne vulgaris? *New*

BENEFICIAL

Benzoyl peroxide *New*

One systematic review identified four RCTs, primarily in people with moderate acne, which found that topical benzoyl peroxide reduced either total lesion count or the number of inflammatory and non-inflammatory lesions at 4, 11, or 12 weeks compared with vehicle; these results were supported by more limited evidence from a fifth RCT with weak methods of analysis. None of the RCTs assessed patient perception of improvement. One of the RCTs found that benzoyl peroxide increased the proportion of people who had adverse effects, including dryness, scaling, burning, tingling, and redness, compared with vehicle. Another RCT found that more people using benzoyl peroxide had peeling compared with people using vehicle. A third RCT found similar rates of local adverse effects between benzoyl peroxide and vehicle.

Clindamycin (reduced the number of inflammatory lesions) *New*

RCTs in people with mild, moderate, or severe acne identified by a systematic review found that topical clindamycin reduced the number of inflammatory lesions compared with placebo or vehicle. However, it found inconclusive evidence about the effects of clindamycin on non-inflammatory lesions. Three RCTs found that clindamycin increased the proportion of people who perceived that their acne was "markedly improved" or "improved"; in two of these RCTs the difference between groups was significant. The RCTs gave little information on adverse effects.

Erythromycin (reduced the number of inflammatory lesions) *New*

RCTs in people with mild, moderate, or severe acne identified by a systematic review found that topical erythromycin reduced the number of inflammatory lesions at 12 weeks compared with vehicle. One RCT found that a similar proportion of people using erythromycin compared with vehicle perceived that their acne had improved from baseline at 12 weeks; the other RCTs did not assess patient perception of improvement. The RCTs found no significant difference in adverse effects between erythromycin and vehicle.

Tretinoin *New*

Four large RCTs, primarily in people with mild to moderate acne, identified by a systematic review found that topical tretinoin reduced the number of inflammatory and non-inflammatory lesions at 8–12 weeks compared with vehicle but increased erythema, peeling, burning, and pruritus. One RCT found that more people taking tretinoin compared with vehicle perceived that their acne had improved; the other RCTs did not assess patient perception of improvement. In the absence of data regarding the risk of birth defects, it is recommended that topical retinoids are not used in pregnancy or by women of childbearing age who are not taking adequate contraceptive precautions.

LIKELY TO BE BENEFICIAL

Adapalene *New*

One large RCT in people with moderate acne found that topical adapalene reduced the number of non-inflammatory and inflammatory lesions at 12 weeks compared with vehicle. It found similar quality of life scores in people using adapalene or ▶

Acne vulgaris

vehicle. It found that adapalene increased erythema, dryness, scaling, stinging/ burning, and pruritus at 2 weeks compared with vehicle, but found no significant difference between groups in these outcomes at 12 weeks. In the absence of data regarding the risk of birth defects, it is recommended that topical retinoids are not used in pregnancy or by women of childbearing age who are not taking adequate contraceptive precautions.

Azelaic acid New

Two RCTs, primarily in people with moderate acne, identified by a systematic review found limited evidence that topical azelaic acid reduced the number of inflammatory and non-inflammatory lesions after 8–12 weeks compared with placebo or vehicle. Neither of the RCTs assessed patient perception of improvement. The RCTs, and controlled and uncontrolled studies, found that azelaic acid was associated with itching, stinging, burning, and erythema.

Erythromycin plus zinc New

Two RCTs identified by a systematic review found that topical erythromycin plus zinc reduced acne severity compared with placebo. One RCT found that topical erythromycin plus zinc reduced both inflammatory and non-inflammatory lesions; the other found that it reduced papules but not pustules. Neither RCT assessed patient perception of improvement. The RCTs give little information on adverse effects.

Isotretinoin New

Two RCTs in people with mild to moderate acne identified by a systematic review found that topical isotretinoin reduced the number of inflammatory and non-inflammatory lesions compared with placebo. These results were supported by more limited evidence from two other RCTs with weak methods of analysis. One of the RCTs found limited evidence from within group comparisons from baseline that a similar proportion of people using isotretinoin compared with vehicle perceived that their acne had improved from baseline at 12 weeks; the other RCTs did not assess patient perception of improvement. The RCTs found that topical isotretinoin was associated with severe erythema, dryness, soreness, and burning. In the absence of data regarding the risk of birth defects, it is recommended that topical retinoids are not used in pregnancy or by women of childbearing age who are not taking adequate contraceptive precautions.

Tetracycline New

Three RCTs in people with moderate to severe acne identified by a systematic review found that topical tetracycline reduced acne severity at 12–16 weeks compared with placebo. This was supported by more limited evidence from a fourth RCT with weak methods of analysis. One of the RCTs found that a similar proportion of people taking topical tetracycline compared with placebo "considered that their condition was better than before treatment", the other RCTs did not assess participant perception of improvement. Three of the RCTs found that topical tetracycline was associated with skin discolouration.

UNKNOWN EFFECTIVENESS

Meclocycline New

We found no RCTs comparing topical meclocycline versus vehicle in people with acne vulgaris. One large multicentre non-randomised controlled trial found that meclocycline reduced the number of inflammatory lesions at 11 weeks compared with vehicle but did not reduce comedones. The trial did not assess patient perception of improvement. It found that meclocycline was associated with follicular staining.

◀ *What are the effects of oral treatments in people with acne vulgaris?* New

LIKELY TO BE BENEFICIAL

Erythromycin New

One systematic review identified no RCTs comparing oral erythromycin versus placebo in people with acne vulgaris. One RCT found that both oral erythromycin and oral doxycycline reduced the number of papules and pustules after 6 weeks with no significant difference between groups. The RCT did not assess patient perception of improvement. Two RCTs in people with mild, moderate, or severe acne found that both erythromycin and oral tetracycline improved acne but found no significant difference in the number of lesions or total inflammation scores between the drugs at 3–6 months. A third RCT did not compare oral erythromycin versus oral tetracycline directly but found that fewer people within the group taking erythromycin had a "good" or "very good" response as assessed by their physician than people within the group taking tetracycline although high proportions in both groups responded well. One of the RCTs found no significant difference between oral erythromycin and oral tetracycline in the proportion of people who perceived that their acne had improved; the other RCTs did not assess patient perception of improvement.

TRADE OFF BETWEEN BENEFITS AND HARMS

Doxycycline New

One RCT identified by a systematic review provided insufficient evidence to assess oral doxycycline compared with placebo in people with acne vulgaris. One subsequent RCT found that doxycycline reduced inflammatory lesions and comedones after 6 months compared with placebo. It found no significant difference in patient perception of improvement. One systematic review found no significant difference in inflammatory lesions, total lesion count, overall efficacy, or patient perception of improvement between oral doxycycline and oral minocycline. One RCT found that both oral doxycycline and oral erythromycin reduced the number of papules and pustules after 6 weeks with no significant difference between groups and another small RCT found no significant difference in mean lesion count at 8 weeks between oral doxycycline and oral oxytetracycline. The RCTs did not assess patient perception of improvement. Tetracyclines may harm bones and teeth and should not be taken by pregnant or breastfeeding women. They may cause contraceptive failure during the initial weeks of treatment.

Lymecycline New

One systematic review identified no RCTs comparing oral lymecycline versus placebo in people with acne vulgaris. One RCT in people with moderate to severe acne identified by another systematic review found no significant difference between oral lymecycline and oral minocycline in inflammatory or non-inflammatory lesions or patient perception of improvement at 12 weeks. Tetracyclines may harm bones and teeth and should not be taken by pregnant or breastfeeding women. They may cause contraceptive failure during the initial weeks of treatment.

Minocycline New

Two RCTs identified by a systematic review provided insufficient evidence to compare oral minocycline versus placebo or oral oxytetracycline. The review found no significant difference in inflammatory lesions, non-inflammatory lesions, total lesion count, overall efficacy, or patient perception of improvement between oral minocycline and oral doxycycline, lymecycline, or tetracycline. Two systematic ▶

Acne vulgaris

reviews of one case control study and case reports suggested that oral minocycline was associated with an increased risk of developing the rare but serious condition systemic lupus erythematosus and one review of case reports suggested that it may increase the risk of developing severe hepatic dysfunction. The evidence about adverse effects should be interpreted with caution because of wide variation between studies in numbers of reported adverse events. Tetracyclines may harm bones and teeth and should not be taken by pregnant or breastfeeding women. They may cause contraceptive failure during the initial weeks of treatment.

Oxytetracycline New

One systematic review identified no RCTs comparing oral oxytetracycline versus placebo in people with acne vulgaris. One small RCT found no significant difference in mean lesion count at 8 weeks between oral doxycycline and oral oxytetracycline. The RCT did not assess patient perception of improvement. Another RCT identified by a systematic review provided insufficient evidence to compare oral oxytetracycline versus oral minocycline. Tetracyclines may harm bones and teeth and should not be taken by pregnant or breastfeeding women. They may cause contraceptive failure during the initial weeks of treatment.

Tetracycline New

Four RCTs identified by a systematic review found that oral tetracycline reduced acne severity compared with placebo; these results were supported by more limited evidence from two further RCTs with weak methods of analysis. A seventh RCT identified by the review found no significant difference in the number of inflammatory lesions between oral tetracycline and placebo, but may have lacked power to detect a clinically important difference. One of the RCTs found that oral tetracycline increased the proportion of people who perceived that their acne was "markedly improved" or "improved" compared with vehicle; this was supported by weaker evidence from an RCT that compared changes from baseline within groups. RCTs in people with mild, moderate, or severe acne identified by systematic reviews found no significant difference in acne severity between oral tetracycline and oral erythromycin or oral minocycline and that all reduced acne severity. One of the RCTs found no significant difference between oral tetracycline and oral erythromycin in the proportion of people who perceived that their acne had improved; the other RCTs did not assess patient perception of improvement. The RCTs and controlled trials identified by the reviews found few adverse effects associated with oral tetracycline. Tetracyclines may harm bones and teeth and should not be taken by pregnant or breastfeeding women. They may cause contraceptive failure during the initial weeks of treatment.

DEFINITION Acne vulgaris is a common inflammatory pilosebaceous disease characterised by comedones, papules, pustules, inflamed nodules, superficial pus filled cysts, and (in extreme cases) canalising and deep, inflamed, sometimes purulent sacs.[1] Lesions are most common on the face, but the neck, chest, upper back, and shoulders may also be affected. Acne can cause scarring and considerable psychological distress.[2] It is classified as mild, moderate, or severe.[1] Mild acne is defined as non-inflammatory lesions (comedones), a few inflammatory (papulopustular) lesions, or both. Moderate acne is defined as more inflammatory lesions, occasional nodules, or both, and mild scarring. Severe acne is defined as widespread inflammatory lesions; nodules, or both, and scarring; moderate acne which has not settled with 6 months of treatment; or acne of any "severity" with serious psychological upset. This review excludes acne rosacea, acne secondary to industrial occupations, and treatment of acne in people under 13 years of age.

INCIDENCE/ Acne is the most common skin disease of adolescence, affecting over 80% of
PREVALENCE teenagers (aged 13–18 years) at some point.[3] Estimates of prevalence vary ▶

depending on study populations and the method of assessment used. Prevalence of acne in a community sample of 14–16 year olds in the UK has been recorded as 50%.[4] In a sample of adolescents from schools in New Zealand, acne was present in 91% of males and 79% of females.[5] It has been estimated that up to 30% of teenagers have acne of sufficient severity to require medical treatment.[6] Acne was the presenting complaint in 3.1% of people aged 13–25 years attending primary care in a UK population.[7] Overall incidence is similar in both men and women and peaks at 17 years of age.[6] The number of adults with acne, including people over 25 years, is increasing; the reasons for this increase are uncertain.[8]

AETIOLOGY/
RISK FACTORS
The exact cause of acne is unknown. Four factors contribute to the development of acne: increased sebum secretion rate, abnormal follicular differentiation causing obstruction of the pilosebaceous duct, bacteriology of the pilosebaceous duct, and inflammation.[9] The anaerobic bacterium *Proprionibacterium acnes* plays an important role in the pathogenesis of acne. Androgen secretion is the major trigger for adolescent acne.[10]

PROGNOSIS
In the absence of treatment, acne persists in most sufferers for an average of 8–12 years.[11]

Please refer to the Clinical Evidence website for full text and references.

Athlete's foot

Search date December 2003

Fay Crawford

What are the effects of topical treatments for athlete's foot?

BENEFICIAL

Topical allylamines

One systematic review and four subsequent RCTs have found that allylamines are more effective than placebo for curing fungal skin infections. The review found insufficient evidence comparing different allylamines versus one another. It found that topical allylamines increased cure rates at 3–12 weeks compared with topical azoles. We found no evidence on recurrence rates after clinical cure.

Topical azoles

One systematic review has found that azole creams administered for 4–6 weeks increase cure rates compared with placebo. We found no RCTs evaluating differences between individual azoles. It found that topical azoles were less effective than topical allylamines in increasing cure rates at 3–12 weeks. We found no evidence on recurrence rates after clinical cure.

UNKNOWN EFFECTIVENESS

Improved foot hygiene, including socks and hosiery

We found no systematic review or RCTs on the effects of foot hygiene and hosiery in the treatment of athlete's foot.

DEFINITION	Athlete's foot is a cutaneous fungal infection caused by dermatophyte infection. It is characterised by itching, flaking, and fissuring of the skin. It may manifest in three ways: the skin between the toes may appear mascerated (white) and soggy; the soles of the feet may become dry and scaly; and the skin all over the foot may become red, and vesicular eruptions may appear.[1] It is conventional in dermatology to refer to fungal skin infections as superficial in order to distinguish them from systemic fungal infections.
INCIDENCE/ PREVALENCE	Epidemiological studies have produced various estimates of the prevalence of athlete's foot. Studies are usually conducted in populations of people who attend dermatology clinics, sports centres or swimming pools, or who are in the military. UK estimates suggest that athlete's foot is present in about 15% of the general population.[2] Studies conducted in dermatology clinics in Italy[3] and China (1014 people)[4] found prevalences of 25% and 27%, respectively. A population based study conducted in Israel found the prevalence among children to be 30%.[5]
AETIOLOGY/ RISK FACTORS	Swimming pool users and industrial workers may be at increased risk of fungal foot infection. However, one survey identified fungal foot infection in only 9% of swimmers, with the highest prevalence (20%) being in men aged 16 years and older.[2]
PROGNOSIS	Fungal infections of the foot are not life threatening in people with normal immune status, but in some people they cause persistent itching and, ultimately, fissuring. Other patients are apparently unaware of persistent infection. The infection can spread to other parts of the body and to other individuals.

Please refer to the Clinical Evidence website for full text and references.

Search date May 2004

Andrew Morris

What are the effects of treatments?

LIKELY TO BE BENEFICIAL

Antibiotics

We found no RCTs comparing antibiotics versus placebo. RCTs comparing different single antibiotic regimens found clinical cure in 50–100% of people.

UNKNOWN EFFECTIVENESS

Comparative effects of different antibiotic regimens

RCTs provided insufficient information on differences between regimens. However, most of the RCTs included only a small number of people with cellulitis or erysipelas, and were designed to test equivalence rather than to detect a clinically significant difference in cure rates between antibiotics.

Oral versus intravenous antibiotics

We found no satisfactory RCTs comparing oral antibiotics versus intravenous antibiotics.

Short versus long courses of antibiotics

We found no RCTs comparing different durations of antibiotics.

Treatment of predisposing factors to prevent recurrence

We found no RCTs or observational studies on the effects of treating predisposing factors for recurrence of cellulitis or erysipelas.

DEFINITION **Cellulitis** is a spreading bacterial infection of the dermis and subcutaneous tissues. It causes local signs of inflammation such as warmth, erythema, pain, lymphangitis, and frequently systemic upset with fever and raised white blood cell count. **Erysipelas** is a form of cellulitis and is characterised by pronounced superficial inflammation. The lower limbs are by far the most common sites, but any area can be affected. The term erysipelas is commonly used when the face is affected.

INCIDENCE/ We found no specific data on the incidence of cellulitis, but cellulitis and
PREVALENCE abscess infections were responsible for 158 consultations per 10 000 person years at risk in the UK in 1991.[1] In 1985 in the UK, skin and subcutaneous tissue infections resulted in 29 820 hospital admissions and a mean occupancy of 664 hospital beds each day.[2]

AETIOLOGY/ The most common infective organisms for cellulitis and erysipelas in adults are
RISK FACTORS streptococci (particularly *Streptococcus pyogenes*) and *Staphylococcus aureus*.[3] In children, *Haemophilus influenzae* was a frequent cause prior to the introduction of the HiB vaccination. Several risk factors for cellulitis and erysipelas have been identified in a case control study (167 cases and 294 controls): lymphoedema (OR 71.2, 95% CI 5.6 to 908.0), leg ulcer (OR 62.5, 95% CI 7.0 to 556.0), toe web intertrigo (OR 13.9, 95% CI 7.2 to 27.0), and traumatic wounds (OR 10.7, 95% CI 4.8 to 23.8).[4]

PROGNOSIS Cellulitis can spread through the bloodstream and lymphatic system. A retrospective case study of people admitted to hospital with cellulitis found that systemic symptoms such as fever and raised white blood cell count were present in up to 42% of cases at presentation.[5] Lymphatic involvement can lead to obstruction and damage the lymphatic system that predisposes to recurrent cellulitis. Recurrence can occur rapidly or after months or years. One ▶

Cellulitis and erysipelas

study found that 29% of people with erysipelas had a recurrent episode within 3 years.[6] Local necrosis and abscess formation can also occur. It is not known whether the prognosis of erysipelas differs from that of cellulitis. We found no evidence about factors that predict recurrence, or a better or worse outcome. We found no good evidence on the prognosis of untreated cellulitis.

Please refer to the Clinical Evidence website for full text and references.

RCTs provided insufficient evidence on the effects of non-drug treatments for chronic plaque psoriasis.

What are the effects of non-drug treatments?

UNKNOWN EFFECTIVENESS

Acupuncture

One RCT provided insufficient evidence on the effects of acupuncture for chronic plaque psoriasis.

Balneotherapy

RCTs provided insufficient evidence on the effects of balneotherapy for chronic plaque psoriasis.

Fish oil supplementation

RCTs provided insufficient evidence on the effects of fish oil supplementation for chronic plaque psoriasis.

Heliotherapy

One RCT provided insufficient evidence on the effects of heliotherapy for chronic plaque psoriasis.

Psychotherapy

One RCT provided insufficient evidence on the effects of psychotherapy for chronic plaque psoriasis.

Sunbeds

One RCT provided insufficient evidence on the effects of sunbeds for chronic plaque psoriasis.

What are the effects of topical drug treatments?

BENEFICIAL

Vitamin D derivatives

One systematic review found that topical vitamin D derivatives improved plaque psoriasis compared with placebo. Systematic reviews found no significant difference in effectiveness between topical vitamin D derivatives and "potent" topical steroids, but found that calcipotriol caused more perilesional and lesional irritation. One systematic review and one subsequent RCT found that topical vitamin D derivatives improved psoriasis at 4–12 weeks compared with dithranol, and caused fewer adverse effects. One systematic review found that calcipotriol improved psoriasis compared with coal tar, alone or in combination with allantoin and hydrocortisone. RCTs found that combination treatment with vitamin D derivatives plus "potent" topical steroids improved psoriasis compared with either treatment alone or with placebo. In the short term, the combination of vitamin D derivates plus topical steroids decreased irritation compared with monotherapy. RCTs provided insufficient evidence to assess other combination treatments containing topical vitamin D derivatives.

Chronic plaque psoriasis

Dithranol

One systematic review of small RCTs found that dithranol improved chronic plaque psoriasis after 4–8 weeks compared with placebo. One systematic review of small RCTs found no significant difference between conventional and short contact dithranol treatment, but the RCTs may have lacked power to detect clinically relevant differences. One systematic review and one subsequent RCT found that dithranol was less effective than topical vitamin D derivatives and caused more adverse effects.

Topical retinoids (tazarotene)

RCTs found that tazarotene improved chronic plaque psoriasis in the short term compared with placebo. One RCT found no significant difference between tazarotene and fluocinonide in the reduction of lesion severity at 12 weeks. Three RCTs found that adding topical steroids to tazarotene treatment improved response rate compared with tazarotene treatment alone. One RCT found that combined topical steroid and tazarotene treatment increased the proportion of people with marked improvement compared with calcipotriol.

Topical steroids

One systematic review found that topical steroids, especially "potent" and "very potent" ones, improved psoriasis in the short term compared with placebo. Systematic reviews found no significant difference in effectiveness between "potent" topical steroids and vitamin D derivatives, but found that vitamin D derivatives caused more perilesional and lesional irritation. One RCT found no significant difference between fluocinomide and tazarotene in the reduction of lesion severity at 12 weeks. Topical steroids may cause striae and atrophy, which increase with potency and use of occlusive dressings. Continuous use may lead to adrenocortical suppression, and case reports suggest that severe flares of the disease may occur on withdrawal.

Emollients and keratolytics

RCTs provided insufficient evidence on the effects of emollients and keratolytics.

Tars

One small RCT identified by a systematic review provided insufficient evidence on the effects of coal tar compared with placebo. Small RCTs found conflicting results on the effects of tars in combination with ultraviolet B exposure or dithranol. One systematic review found that coal tar, alone or in combination with allantoin and hydrocortisone, was less effective than topical vitamin D derivatives (calcipotriol).

What are the effects of treatments with ultraviolet light?

Psoralen plus ultraviolet A*

We found no systematic review or RCTs that compared psoriasis clearance with psoralen plus ultraviolet A versus no treatment. However, there is consensus that psoralen plus ultraviolet A is effective for clearance of psoriasis. One RCT found that psoralen plus ultraviolet A was more effective than the Ingram regimen in clearing psoriasis. One systematic review found that higher doses of psoralen improved psoriasis clearance more than lower doses of psoralen. One large RCT ▶

◄ found that maintenance treatment with psoralen plus ultraviolet A reduced relapse compared with no maintenance treatment. Long term adverse effects of psoralen plus ultraviolet A treatment include photoaging and skin cancer (mainly squamous cell carcinoma).

LIKELY TO BE BENEFICIAL

Ingram regimen*

We found no RCTs comparing the Ingram regimen with placebo or no treatment. However, there is consensus that the Ingram regimen is likely to be beneficial for the clearance of psoriasis. One RCT found that the Ingram regimen was less effective than psoralen plus ultraviolet A in clearing psoriasis.

Ultraviolet B*

We found no RCTs comparing ultraviolet B with placebo or no treatment. However, there is consensus that ultraviolet B is effective in people with plaque psoriasis. RCTs provided insufficient evidence on the effects of ultraviolet B compared with other treatments, or on the effects of narrow band compared with broad band ultraviolet B for either clearance or maintenance treatment. One RCT found limited evidence that ultraviolet B given three times weekly cleared psoriasis faster than twice weekly treatment.

UNKNOWN EFFECTIVENESS

Goeckerman treatment

We found no good evidence on the effects of the Goeckerman treatment.

What are the effects of systemic drug treatments?

LIKELY TO BE BENEFICIAL

Etanercept

Two RCTs found that etanercept increased the proportion of responders at 12–24 weeks compared with placebo. One of the RCTs found that quality of life improved more with etanercept than with placebo at 12 weeks. Etanercept is a relatively new drug for the treatment of psoriasis, and there is limited evidence regarding the possibility of long term or rare adverse events.

TRADE OFF BETWEEN BENEFITS AND HARMS

Oral retinoids (etretinate, acitretin)

One systematic review found limited evidence that oral retinoids improved clearance compared with placebo in people with chronic plaque psoriasis. RCTs provided insufficient evidence on the effects of oral retinoids as maintenance treatment. Adverse effects led to discontinuation of oral retinoid treatment in 10–20% of people. Teratogenicity renders oral retinoids less acceptable. Etretinate is no longer available in many countries.

Methotrexate*

One small RCT provided insufficient evidence about effects of methotrexate compared with placebo. However, there is consensus that methotrexate is effective for the treatment of psoriasis. One RCT found no significant difference between methotrexate and cyclosporin in complete or partial remission, or in duration of remission of psoriasis. Methotrexate can induce acute myelosuppression. Long term methotrexate carries the risk of hepatic fibrosis and cirrhosis, which is related to the dose regimen employed.

Chronic plaque psoriasis

Cyclosporin

One systematic review found that cyclosporin improved clearance compared with placebo. One RCT found no significant difference between cyclosporin and methotrexate in complete or partial remission, or in duration of remission. Two RCTs found that cyclosporin was more effective than etretinate for reducing psoriasis severity. Two RCTs found that a cyclosporin dose of 5.0 mg/kg daily increased response compared with a cyclosporin dose of 2.5 mg/kg daily. Any advantage of doses greater than 5.0 mg/kg daily may be offset by an increase in dose related adverse effects, particularly increased renal toxicity. The review found that a cyclosporin dose of 3.0 mg/kg daily was more effective than lower doses or than placebo for maintenance.

Tacrolimus

One RCT found limited evidence that tacrolimus improved psoriasis compared with placebo. The adverse effects of tacrolimus are reported to be similar to those of cyclosporin.

Fumaric acid derivatives

One systematic review of four small RCTs found limited evidence that oral fumaric acid esters improved chronic plaque psoriasis after 16 weeks compared with placebo. However, acute adverse effects were common and included flushing and gastrointestinal symptoms. We found no RCTs on the effects of fumaric acid derivatives as maintenance treatment.

UNKNOWN EFFECTIVENESS

Anti-CD4 monoclonal antibodies

Two small RCTs provided insufficient evidence on the effects of anti-CD4 mono-clonal antibodies.

Infliximab

One RCT found that infliximab improved response rates at 10 weeks compared with placebo. Infliximab is a relatively new drug for the treatment of psoriasis, and there is limited evidence regarding the possibility of long term or rare adverse events.

*Based on consensus.

DEFINITION Chronic plaque psoriasis, or psoriasis vulgaris, is a chronic inflammatory skin disease that is characterised by well demarcated erythematous scaly patches on the extensor surfaces of the body and scalp. The lesions may itch, sting, and occasionally bleed. Dystrophic nail changes are found in more than a third of people with chronic plaque psoriasis, and psoriatic arthropathy occurs in 1–3%. The condition waxes and wanes, with wide variations in course and severity among individuals. Other varieties of psoriasis include guttate, inverse, pustular, and erythrodermic psoriasis. This review deals with treatments for chronic plaque psoriasis.

INCIDENCE/ Psoriasis affects 1–2% of the general population. It is believed to be less
PREVALENCE frequent in people from Africa and Asia, but we found no reliable epidemiological data.[1]

AETIOLOGY/ About a third of people with psoriasis have a family history of psoriasis, but
RISK FACTORS physical trauma, acute infection, and some medications (e.g. lithium salts and β blockers) are believed to trigger the condition. A few observational studies have linked the onset or relapse of psoriasis with stressful life events and personal habits, including cigarette smoking and, less consistently, alcohol consumption. Others have found an association of psoriasis with body mass index and an inverse association with intake of fruit and vegetables.

◄ **PROGNOSIS** We found no long term prognostic studies. With the exceptions of erythrodermic and acute generalised pustular psoriasis (severe conditions which affect < 1% of people with psoriasis and require intensive hospital care), psoriasis is not known to affect mortality. Psoriasis may substantially affect quality of life, by influencing a negative body image and self image, and limiting daily activities, social contacts, and work. More severe psoriasis is associated with lower levels of quality of life than milder psoriasis.[2] At present, there is no cure for psoriasis.

Please refer to the Clinical Evidence website for full text and references.

Head lice

Search date October 2003

Ian Burgess

What are the effects of treatments?

LIKELY TO BE BENEFICIAL

Insecticide based pharmaceutical products

Two RCTs identified by a systematic review found that permethrin and malathion both increased lice eradication rates compared with placebo. Limited evidence from an earlier systematic review suggested that permethrin increased eradication rates compared with lindane. We found inconclusive evidence from three RCTs about the comparative efficacy of insecticides and combing. One RCT found no significant difference between a herbal product and insecticide.

UNKNOWN EFFECTIVENESS

Herbal and essential oils

We found no RCTs that compared herbal treatment with placebo. One RCT found no significant difference in eradication rates between a herbal product (coconut, anise, and ylang ylang) and insecticide (permethrin, malathion, and piperonyl butoxide). However, results may not generalise to different concentrations of these components or to different herbal preparations.

Mechanical removal of lice or viable eggs by combing

We found inconclusive evidence from three RCTs about effects of combing instead of or in addition to insecticides.

Repellents

We found insufficient evidence on the effects of these interventions.

DEFINITION   Head lice are obligate ectoparasites of socially active humans. They infest the scalp and attach their eggs to the hair shafts. Itching, resulting from multiple bites, is not diagnostic but may increase the index of suspicion. Eggs glued to hairs, whether hatched (nits) or unhatched, are not proof of active infection, because eggs may retain a viable appearance for weeks after death. A conclusive diagnosis can only be made by finding live lice.

INCIDENCE/   We found no studies on incidence and no recent published prevalence results
PREVALENCE   from any developed country. Anecdotal reports suggest that prevalence has increased in the past few years in most communities in the UK and USA.

AETIOLOGY/   Observational studies indicate that infections occur most frequently in school
RISK FACTORS   children, although there is no proof of a link with school attendance.[1,2] We found no evidence that lice prefer clean hair to dirty hair.

PROGNOSIS   The infection is almost harmless. Sensitisation reactions to louse saliva and faeces may result in localised irritation and erythema. Secondary infection of scratches may occur. Lice have been identified as primary mechanical vectors of scalp pyoderma caused by streptococci and staphylococci usually found on the skin.[3]

Please refer to the Clinical Evidence website for full text and references.

What are the effects of interventions aimed at preventing attacks?

LIKELY TO BE BENEFICIAL

Oral antiviral agents (aciclovir)

Six RCTs found limited evidence suggesting that prophylactic oral antiviral agents may reduce the frequency and severity of attacks compared with placebo, but the optimal timing and duration of treatment is uncertain.

Sunscreen

Two small crossover RCTs found limited evidence that ultraviolet sunscreen may reduce herpes recurrence compared with placebo.

UNKNOWN EFFECTIVENESS

Topical antiviral agents

We found no RCTs on the effects of topical antiviral agents used as prophylaxis.

What are the effects of antiviral treatments for the first attack?

LIKELY TO BE BENEFICIAL

Oral antiviral agents (aciclovir)

One small RCT in children found that oral aciclovir reduced the mean duration of pain compared with placebo. Another small RCT in children found that oral aciclovir reduced the median time to healing compared with placebo.

UNKNOWN EFFECTIVENESS

Topical antiviral agents

We found no RCTs on the effects of topical antiviral agents.

What are the effects of treatments for recurrent attack?

LIKELY TO BE BENEFICIAL

Oral antiviral agents (aciclovir and valciclovir)

Four RCTs found that oral aciclovir and valaciclovir (if taken early in the attack) marginally reduced the duration of symptoms and pain compared with placebo. Two large RCTs found no significant difference between a 1 day and a two course regimen of valaciclovir, and found that a higher proportion of people experienced headaches with valaciclovir compared with placebo.

Topical antiviral agents (aciclovir and penciclovir)

Twelve RCTs found limited evidence that topical penciclovir or aciclovir reduced the duration of pain and symptoms compared with placebo, but stronger evidence that healing time is reduced.

▶

Herpes labialis

UNKNOWN EFFECTIVENESS

Topical anaesthetic agents

One small RCT found limited evidence that topical tetracaine reduced the mean time to scab loss and increased the proportion of people who subjectively rated the treatment as effective compared with placebo. However, the clinical importance of these results is unclear.

Zinc oxide cream

One small RCT found limited evidence that zinc oxide cream reduced time to healing compared with placebo, but found that it increased the risk of skin irritation.

DEFINITION   Herpes labialis is a mild self limiting infection with herpes simplex virus type 1. It causes pain and blistering on the lips and perioral area (cold sores); fever and constitutional symptoms are rare. Most people have no warning of an attack, but some experience a recognisable prodrome.

INCIDENCE/
PREVALENCE   Herpes labialis accounts for about 1% of primary care consultations in the UK each year; 20–40% of people have experienced cold sores at some time.[1]

AETIOLOGY/
RISK FACTORS   Herpes labialis is caused by herpes simplex virus type 1. After the primary infection, which usually occurs in childhood, the virus is thought to remain latent in the trigeminal ganglion.[2] A variety of factors, including exposure to bright sunlight, fatigue, or psychological stress, can precipitate a recurrence.

PROGNOSIS   In most people, herpes labialis is a mild, self limiting illness. Recurrences are usually shorter and less severe than the initial attack. Healing is usually complete in 7–10 days without scarring.[3] Rates of reactivation are unknown. Herpes labialis can cause serious illness in immunocompromised people.

Please refer to the Clinical Evidence website for full text and references.

Search date October 2003

Philip Savage, Thomas Crosby, and Malcolm Mason

What are the effects of preventive interventions?

UNKNOWN EFFECTIVENESS

Sunscreens

We found no RCTs about the preventive effects of sunscreens. Systematic reviews of case control studies found inconclusive evidence about the effects of sunscreen in preventing malignant melanoma.

What is the optimal excision margin for different Breslow thicknesses?

UNLIKELY TO BE BENEFICIAL

Wide excision (no better than narrower excision in people with tumours of < 2 mm Breslow thickness)

One systematic review and one subsequent RCT found no significant difference in overall survival over 4–10 years between more radical local surgery (4–5 cm excision margins) and less radical surgery (1–2 cm excision margins). The RCTs also found no significant difference in local recurrence rates between wider and narrower excision margins. One of the RCTs found that wider excision increased the need for skin grafting and the duration of hospital stay compared with narrower excision. Only 8.9% of people in the RCTs had tumours of > 2 mm Breslow thickness, therefore we were unable to draw conclusions about the optimum excision margin in these people)

What are the effects of sentinel lymph node biopsy?

UNKNOWN EFFECTIVENESS

Sentinel lymph node biopsy

We found no RCTs of sentinel lymph node biopsy that assessed survival in people with malignant melanoma.

What are the effects of elective lymph node dissection?

UNLIKELY TO BE BENEFICIAL

Elective lymph node dissection

One systematic review found no significant difference in survival at 5 years between elective lymph node dissection and delayed or no lymph node dissection in people with malignant melanoma without clinically detectable lymph node metastases.

What are the effects of adjuvant treatment?

TRADE OFF BETWEEN BENEFITS AND HARMS

High dose adjuvant alfa interferon

Two RCTs have found that high dose alfa interferon extends the time to relapse at median follow up of 6.9 years compared with no adjuvant treatment. One of them ▶

Malignant melanoma (non-metastatic)

also found that high dose alfa interferon may improve overall survival. However, a third RCT found no significant difference in relapse rates or overall survival between high dose interferon and no adjuvant treatment. One RCT found that high dose alfa interferon improved both relapse free and overall survival compared with ganglioside GM2 vaccine. Toxicity (myelosuppression, hepatotoxicity, and neurotoxicity) and withdrawal rates were high; in one RCT toxicity occurred in 15–28% of people.

UNKNOWN EFFECTIVENESS

Adjuvant vaccines in people with malignant melanoma

Four RCTs found no significant difference in survival between adjuvant vaccines and surgery alone or surgery plus placebo vaccine in people with malignant melanoma. A different vaccine preparation was used in each RCT, making the results difficult to generalise.

Low dose adjuvant alfa interferon

RCTs found inconsistent evidence on the effects of low dose alfa interferon compared with no adjuvant treatment on relapse free and overall survival. In one RCT, toxicity occurred in 10% of people.

Surveillance for early treatment of recurrence

We found no RCTs of surveillance for early treatment of recurrent melanoma.

DEFINITION   Cutaneous malignant melanoma is a tumour derived from melanocytes in the basal layer of the epidermis. After undergoing malignant transformation, the tumour becomes invasive by penetrating into and beyond the dermis.

INCIDENCE/   Incidence in developed countries has increased by 50% in the past 20 years.
PREVALENCE   Incidence varies in different populations (see table 1❶) and is about 10-fold higher in white than in non-white populations. Despite the rise in incidence, death rates have flattened and even fallen in some populations (e.g. in women and young men in Australia).[1,2] During the same period there has been a sixfold increase in the incidence of melanoma *in situ*, suggesting earlier detection.

AETIOLOGY/   The number of common, atypical, and dysplastic naevi on a person's body
RISK FACTORS correlates closely with the risk of developing malignant melanoma. A genetic predisposition probably accounts for 5–10% of all cases. Although the risk of developing malignant melanoma is higher in fair skinned populations living close to the equator, the relationship between sun exposure, sunscreen use, and skin type and risk is not clear. Exposure to excessive sunlight and severe sunburn in childhood are associated with an increased risk of developing malignant melanoma in adult life. However, people do not necessarily develop tumours at sites of maximum exposure to the sun.

PROGNOSIS   The prognosis of early malignant melanoma (stages I–III) (see table 2❶) relates to the depth of invasion of the primary lesion, the presence of ulceration, and involvement of the regional lymph nodes, with the prognosis worsening with the number of nodes involved.[3] A person with a thin lesion (Breslow thickness < 0.75 mm) and without lymph node involvement has a 3% risk of developing metastases and a 95% chance of surviving 5 years.[4] If regional lymph nodes are macroscopically involved, then there is a 20–50% chance of surviving 5 years. Most studies have shown a better prognosis in women and in people with lesions on the extremities than in those with lesions on the trunk.

Please refer to the Clinical Evidence website for full text and references.

What are the effects of treatments?

BENEFICIAL

Permethrin

One systematic review has found that permethrin increases clinical and parasitic cure after 28 days compared with crotamiton. The systematic review found conflicting results with permethrin versus lindane. One subsequent RCT found limited evidence that permethrin increased clinical cure at 14 days compared with ivermectin.

LIKELY TO BE BENEFICIAL

Crotamiton

One systematic review found that crotamiton was less successful in terms of clinical and parasite cure after 28 days compared with permethrin. One systematic review identified one RCT that found no significant difference between crotamiton and lindane in clinical cure rates at 28 days.

Oral ivermectin

One systematic review identified one RCT that found that ivermectin increased clinical cure rates after 7 days compared with placebo. Another small RCT identified by the review found no significant difference between ivermectin and benzyl benzoate in clinical cure rates at 30 days. One subsequent RCT found that, compared with benzyl benzoate, ivermectin increased clinical cure rates at 30 days. One systematic review identified one small RCT that found no significant difference between ivermectin and lindane in cure rates at 15 days. One subsequent RCT found no significant difference between ivermectin and lindane in failed clinical cure rates at 2 weeks, but it found that ivermectin decreased failed cure rates at 4 weeks. One RCT found limited evidence that ivermectin reduced clinical cure rates at 14 days compared with permethrin. Experience suggests oral ivermectin is safe in younger adults being treated for onchocerciasis, but no such experience exists for children, and there have been reports of increased risk of death in elderly people.

TRADE OFF BETWEEN BENEFITS AND HARMS

Lindane

One systematic review identified one RCT that found no significant difference between lindane and crotamiton in clinical cure rates at 28 days. The systematic review found conflicting results between lindane and permethrin after 28 days. Another small RCT identified by the review found no significant difference between lindane and ivermectin in cure rates at 15 days. One subsequent RCT found no significant difference between lindane and ivermectin in failed clinical cure rates at 2 weeks, but it found a higher proportion of people with failed clinical cure between lindane and ivermectin at 4 weeks. We found reports of rare, serious adverse effects such as convulsions.

UNKNOWN EFFECTIVENESS

Benzyl benzoate

One systematic review identified one small RCT that found no significant difference between benzyl benzoate and ivermectin in clinical cure rates at 30 days. One subsequent RCT found that benzyl benzoate reduced clinical cure at 30 days ▶

Scabies

compared with ivermectin. One systematic review identified one RCT that found no significant difference with benzyl benzoate versus sulphur ointment in clinical cure at 8 or 14 days.

Malathion

One systematic review found no RCTs on the effects of malathion. Case series have reported cure rates in scabies of over 80%.

Sulphur compounds

One systematic review identified one RCT that found no significant difference with sulphur ointment versus benzyl benzoate in clinical cure at 8 or 14 days.

DEFINITION Scabies is an infestation of the skin by the mite *Sarcoptes scabiei*.[1] Typical sites of infestation are skin folds and flexor surfaces. In adults, the most common sites are between the fingers and on the wrists, although infection may manifest in elderly people as a diffuse truncal eruption. In infants and children, the face, scalp, palms, and soles are also often affected.

INCIDENCE/ PREVALENCE Scabies is a common public health problem with an estimated prevalence of 300 million cases worldwide, mostly affecting people in developing countries where prevalence can exceed 50%.[2] In industrialised countries, it is most common in institutionalised communities. Case studies suggest that epidemic cycles occur every 7–15 years and that these partly reflect the population's immune status.

AETIOLOGY/ RISK FACTORS Scabies is particularly common where there is social disruption, overcrowding with close body contact, and limited access to water.[3] Young children, immobilised elderly people, people with HIV/AIDS, and other medically and immunologically compromised people are predisposed to infestation and have particularly high mite counts.[4]

PROGNOSIS Scabies is not life threatening, but the severe, persistent itch and secondary infections may be debilitating. Occasionally, crusted scabies develops. This form of the disease is resistant to routine treatment and can be a source of continued reinfestation and spread to others.

Please refer to the Clinical Evidence website for full text and references.

Search date November 2003

Bruce C. Gee

What are the effects of topical treatments for seborrhoeic dermatitis of the scalp in adults?

BENEFICIAL

Ketoconazole

Five RCTs found that ketoconazole 2% shampoo improved scalp symptoms (including scaling, itching, redness, and dandruff) compared with placebo over 4 weeks.

Selenium sulphide

One RCT found that selenium sulphide shampoo reduced dandruff compared with placebo.

Tar shampoo

One RCT found that tar shampoo was more effective at reducing scalp dandruff and redness than placebo.

LIKELY TO BE BENEFICIAL

Bifonazole

One small RCT found that bifonazole shampoo improved scalp symptoms compared with placebo.

Topical steroids

We found no RCTs comparing topical steroids (hydrocortisone, betamethasone valerate, clobetasone butyrate, mometasone furate, or clobetasol propionate) versus placebo. There is consensus that topical steroids are effective in treating seborrhoeic dermatitis of the scalp in adults.

UNKNOWN EFFECTIVENESS

Emollients; terbinafine

We found no RCTs comparing these interventions versus placebo in adults with seborrhoeic dermatitis of the scalp.

What are the effects of topical treatments for seborrhoeic dermatitis of the face and body in adults?

LIKELY TO BE BENEFICIAL

Bifonazole

One RCT found that bifonazole improved symptoms compared with placebo after 4 weeks.

Ketoconazole

Two small RCTs found that ketoconazole 2% cream improved symptoms (erythema, scaling, papules, and pruritus) compared with placebo after 4 weeks.

Topical steroids (short term episodic treatment)

We found no RCTs comparing topical steroids (hydrocortisone, betamethasone valerate, clobetasone butyrate, mometasone furate, or clobetasol propionate) versus placebo. There is consensus that short courses of topical steroids used episodically are effective in treating seborrhoeic dermatitis of the face and body in adults.

Seborrhoeic dermatitis

UNKNOWN EFFECTIVENESS

Emollients; lithium succinate; selenium sulphide; terbinafine

We found no RCTs of sufficient quality comparing these interventions versus placebo in adults with seborrhoeic dermatitis of the face and body.

DEFINITION   Seborrhoeic dermatitis occurs in areas of skin with a rich supply of sebaceous glands and manifests as red, sharply marginated lesions with greasy looking scales. On the face it mainly affects the medial aspect of the eyebrows, the area between the eyebrows, and the nasolabial folds. It also affects skin on the chest (commonly presternal) and the flexures. On the scalp it manifests as dry, flaking desquamation (dandruff) or yellow, greasy scaling with erythema. Dandruff is a lay term commonly used in the context of mild seborrhoeic dermatitis of the scalp. However, any scalp condition that produces scales could be labelled dandruff. Common differential diagnoses for seborrhoeic dermatitis of the scalp are psoriasis, eczema (see atopic eczema, [Web only]), and tinea capitis (see table 1❶).

INCIDENCE/   Seborrhoeic dermatitis is estimated to affect around 1–3% of the general
PREVALENCE   population.[1] However, this is likely to be an underestimate because people do not tend to seek medical advice for mild dandruff.

AETIOLOGY/   *Malassezia (Pityrosporum) ovale* is considered to be the causative organism of
RISK FACTORS   seborrhoeic dermatitis and is responsible for producing an inflammatory reaction involving T cells and complement. Conditions that have been reported to predispose to seborrhoeic dermatitis include HIV,[2] neurological conditions such as Parkinson's disease, neuronal damage such as facial nerve palsy,[3] spinal injury,[4] ischaemic heart disease,[5] and alcoholic pancreatitis.[6] In this chapter we deal with treatment in immunocompetent adults who have no known predisposing conditions.

PROGNOSIS   Seborrhoeic dermatitis is a chronic condition that tends to flare and remit spontaneously, and is prone to recurrence after treatment.[1,7]

Please refer to the Clinical Evidence website for full text and references.

Squamous cell carcinoma of the skin (non-metastatic)

Search date January 2004

Adèle Green and Robin Marks

What are the effects of preventive interventions?

LIKELY TO BE BENEFICIAL

Sunscreens in prevention of squamous cell carcinoma (daily compared with discretionary use)

One RCT in adults in a subtropical community in Queensland, Australia found that daily compared with discretionary use of sunscreen on the head, neck, arms, and hands reduced the incidence of squamous cell carcinoma after 4.5 years.

Sunscreens to prevent development of new solar keratoses (compared with placebo or daily compared with discretionary use)

One RCT in people aged over 40 years living in Victoria, Australia who had previous solar keratoses (a risk factor for squamous cell carcinoma) found that daily sunscreen reduced the incidence of new solar keratoses after 7 months compared with placebo. One RCT in adults in a subtropical community in Queensland, Australia found that daily compared with discretionary use of sunscreen reduced the increase of solar keratoses over the whole body after 2.5 years.

What are the effects of treatments?

UNKNOWN EFFECTIVENESS

Micrographically controlled surgery (compared with standard surgical excision)

We found no RCTs or observational studies of sufficient quality comparing the effects of micrographically controlled surgery versus standard primary surgical excision on local recurrence rates.

Optimal primary excision margin

We found no RCTs or observational studies of sufficient quality relating size of primary excision margin to local recurrence rate.

Radiotherapy after surgery (compared with surgery alone)

We found no RCTs or observational studies of sufficient quality comparing the effects of radiotherapy after surgery versus surgery alone on local recurrence rates.

DEFINITION Cutaneous squamous cell carcinoma is a malignant tumour of keratinocytes arising in the epidermis, showing histological evidence of dermal invasion.

INCIDENCE/ PREVALENCE Incidence rates are often derived from surveys because few cancer registries routinely collect notifications of squamous cell carcinoma of the skin. Incidence rates on exposed skin vary markedly around the world according to skin colour and latitude, and range from negligible rates in black populations and white populations living at high latitudes to rates of about 1/100 in white residents of tropical Australia.[1]

AETIOLOGY/ RISK FACTORS People with fair skin colour who sunburn easily without tanning, people with xeroderma pigmentosum,[2–4] and those who are immunosuppressed[5] are susceptible to squamous cell carcinoma. The strongest environmental risk factor for squamous cell carcinoma is chronic sun exposure. Cohort and case control studies have found that the risk of squamous cell carcinoma is three times greater in people with fair skin colour, a propensity to burn on initial ▶

Skin disorders

Squamous cell carcinoma of the skin (non-metastatic)

exposure to sunlight, or a history of multiple sunburns. Clinical signs of chronic skin damage, especially solar keratoses, are also risk factors for cutaneous squamous cell carcinoma.[2,3] In people with multiple solar keratoses (> 15), the risk of squamous cell carcinoma is 10–15 times greater than in people with no solar keratoses.[2,3]

PROGNOSIS Prognosis is related to the location and size of tumour, histological pattern, depth of invasion, perineural involvement, and immunosuppression.[6,7] A world-wide review of 95 case series, each consisting of at least 20 people, found that the overall metastasis rate for squamous cell carcinoma on the ear was 11% and on the lip 14%, compared with an average for all sites of 5%.[7] A review of 71 case series found that lesions less than 2 cm in diameter have less than half the local recurrence rate compared with lesions greater than 2 cm (7% v 15%), and less than a third of the rate of metastasis (9% v 30%).[7]

Please refer to the Clinical Evidence website for full text and references.

Search date September 2003

Mike Bigby, Sam Gibbs, Ian Harvey, and Jane Sterling

What are the effects of treatments?

BENEFICIAL

Topical treatments containing salicylic acid

One systematic review has found that simple topical treatments containing salicylic acid increase complete wart clearance, successful treatment, or loss of one or more warts after 6–12 weeks compared with placebo. The review identified two RCTs comparing salicylic acid versus cryotherapy. These found no significant difference in the proportion of people with wart clearance at 3–6 months.

LIKELY TO BE BENEFICIAL

Cryotherapy

One systematic review of two small RCTs found no significant difference between cryotherapy and placebo or no treatment in the proportion of people with wart clearance after 2–4 months. However, the RCTs may have been too small to detect a clinically important difference. The review identified two RCTs that found no significant difference between cryotherapy and salicylic acid in the proportion of people with wart clearance at 3–6 months. The review found that aggressive cryotherapy increased the proportion of people with wart clearance after 1–3 months compared with cryotherapy.

Contact immunotherapy (dinitrochlorobenzene)

One systematic review found that contact immunotherapy using dinitrochlorobenzene increased wart clearance compared with placebo.

UNKNOWN EFFECTIVENESS

Carbon dioxide laser

One systematic review identified no RCTs on the effects of carbon dioxide laser.

Cimetidine

Three small RCTs provided insufficient evidence to compare cimetidine versus placebo, and one small RCT provided insufficient evidence to compare cimetidine versus local treatments. One small RCT found that cimetidine plus levamisole increased wart clearance at 12 weeks compared with cimetidine alone.

Distant healing

One RCT provided insufficient evidence to compare distant healing versus no treatment.

Hypnotic suggestion

We found no RCTs on the effects of hypnotic suggestion in the clearance of warts.

Inosine pranobex

One RCT provided insufficient evidence about the effects of inosine pranobex on wart clearance.

Intralesional bleomycin

RCTs found conflicting evidence on the effects of intralesional bleomycin. Two RCTs found that intralesional bleomycin increased the number of warts cured after 6 weeks compared with placebo. One RCT found no significant difference between bleomycin and placebo in the proportion of people with wart clearance after 30 days, and another RCT found weak evidence that bleomycin cured fewer warts ▶

Warts

than placebo after 3 months. A fifth RCT found no significant difference between different concentrations of bleomycin in the proportion of warts cured after 3 months.

Levamisole

Two RCTs and one CCT provided insufficient evidence on the effects of levamisole compared with placebo on the clearance of warts. One RCT found that levamisole plus cimetidine increased wart clearance at 12 weeks compared with cimetidine alone.

Photodynamic treatment

RCTs provided insufficient evidence on the effects of photodynamic treatment on wart clearance.

Pulsed dye laser

One RCT provided insufficient evidence on the effects of pulsed dye laser.

Surgical procedures

One systematic review identified no RCTs on the effects of surgical procedures on wart clearance.

Systemic interferon α

We found no RCTs of sufficient quality on the effects of systemic interferon α.

UNLIKELY TO BE BENEFICIAL

Homeopathy

Two RCTs found no significant difference between homeopathy and placebo in the proportion of people with wart clearance after 8–18 weeks.

DEFINITION   Non-genital warts (verrucas) are an extremely common, benign, and usually self limiting skin disease. Infection of epidermal cells with the human papillomavirus results in cell proliferation and a thickened, warty papule on the skin. Any area of skin can be infected, but the most common sites involved are the hands and feet. Genital warts are not covered in this review (see chapter on genital warts, p 455).

INCIDENCE/   There are few reliable, population based data on the incidence and preva-
PREVALENCE   lence of non-genital warts. Prevalence probably varies widely between different age groups, populations, and periods of time. Two large population based studies found prevalence rates of 0.84% in the USA[1] and 12.9% in Russia.[2] Prevalence is highest in children and young adults, and two studies in school populations have shown prevalence rates of 12% in 4–6 year olds in the UK[3] and 24% in 16–18 year olds in Australia.[4]

AETIOLOGY/   Warts are caused by human papillomavirus, of which there are over 70 different
RISK FACTORS   types. They are most common at sites of trauma, such as the hands and feet, and probably result from inoculation of virus into minimally damaged areas of epithelium. Warts on the feet can be acquired from walking barefoot in communal areas where other people walk barefoot. One observational study (146 adolescents) found that the prevalence of warts on the feet was 27% in those that used a communal shower room compared with 1.3% in those that used the locker room.[5] Warts on the hand are also an occupational risk for butchers and meat handlers. One cross-sectional survey (1086 people) found that the prevalence of warts on the hand was 33% in abattoir workers, 34% in retail butchers, 20% in engineering fitters, and 15% in office workers.[6] Immunosuppression is another important risk factor. One observational study in immunosuppressed renal transplant recipients found that at 5 years or longer after transplantation 90% had warts.[7]

◀ **PROGNOSIS** Non-genital warts in immunocompetent people are harmless and usually resolve spontaneously as a result of natural immunity within months or years. The rate of resolution is highly variable and probably depends on several factors, including host immunity, age, human papillomavirus type, and site of infection. One cohort study (1000 children in long stay accommodation) found that two thirds of warts resolved without treatment within a 2 year period.[8] One systematic review (search date 2000, 17 RCTs) comparing local treatments versus placebo found that about 30% of people using placebo (range 0–73%) had no warts after about 10 weeks (range 4–24 weeks).[9]

Please refer to the Clinical Evidence website for full text and references.

Wrinkles

Search date December 2003

Miny Samuel, Rebecca Brooke, and Christopher Griffiths

What are the effects of preventive interventions?

UNKNOWN EFFECTIVENESS

Sunscreens; vitamins C or E (topical)

We found no RCTs on the effects of these interventions in preventing wrinkles.

What are the effects of treatments?

BENEFICIAL

Tazarotene (improves fine wrinkles)

Two RCTs in people with moderately photodamaged skin found that tazarotene cream improved fine wrinkling compared with placebo at 24 weeks. One RCT found no significant difference between tazarotene and tretinoin cream in fine wrinkling at 24 weeks.

Tretinoin (improves fine wrinkles)

RCTs in people with mild to moderate photodamage found that topical tretinoin applied for up to 12 months improved fine wrinkles compared with vehicle cream but the effect on coarse wrinkles differed among studies. Four RCTs in people with moderate to severe photodamage found that topical tretinoin applied for 6 months improved fine and coarse wrinkles on the face compared with vehicle cream. Common short term adverse effects with tretinoin included itching, burning, and erythema. Skin peeling was the most common persistent adverse effect, which was most frequent and severe at 12–16 weeks. One RCT found no significant difference in fine wrinkling.

TRADE OFF BETWEEN BENEFITS AND HARMS

Isotretinoin

In people with mild to severe photodamage, two RCTs found that isotretinoin cream improved fine and coarse wrinkles after 36 weeks compared with vehicle cream. Severe facial irritation occurred in 5–10% of people using isotretinoin.

UNKNOWN EFFECTIVENESS

Carbon dioxide laser

We found no RCTs comparing carbon dioxide laser versus placebo or no treatment. Two small RCTs in women with perioral wrinkles found no significant difference between carbon dioxide laser and dermabrasion in improvement in wrinkles at 4–6 months, but a third RCT found that laser was slightly more effective than dermabrasion in improving wrinkles. Adverse effects were commonly reported. Erythema was reported in all three RCTs, two of which found that erythema was more common with laser than with dermabrasion. Small RCTs provided insufficient evidence about carbon dioxide laser compared with chemical peel, or other laser treatments.

Dermabrasion

We found no RCTs comparing dermabrasion versus placebo or no treatment. Two small RCTs in women with perioral wrinkles found no significant difference between dermabrasion and carbon dioxide laser in improvement in wrinkles at 4–6 months, but a third RCT found that dermabrasion was slightly less effective than laser in ▶

improving wrinkles. Adverse effects were commonly reported. Erythema was reported in all three RCTs, two of which found that erythema was more common with laser than with dermabrasion.

Facelift

We found no RCTs on the effects of facelifts in people with wrinkles.

Oral natural cartilage polysaccharides

One RCT found no significant difference between an oral preparation of cartilage polysaccharide and placebo in wrinkle appearance at 3 months. Smaller RCTs found that oral cartilage polysaccharide reduced fine, moderate, or severe wrinkles compared with placebo. However, these studies were small and of limited reliability. We found limited evidence that some preparations may be more effective than others.

Retinyl esters

We found no systematic review or RCTs of retinyl esters that evaluated clinical outcomes in people with wrinkles.

Vitamin C or E (topical)

One poor quality RCT found limited evidence that an ascorbic acid formulation applied daily to the face for 3 months improved fine and coarse wrinkles compared with a vehicle cream. Stinging and erythema were common but were not analysed by treatment group. We were unable to draw reliable conclusions from this study because of deficiencies in its methodology.

Topical natural cartilage polysaccharides

One small RCT found that a topical commercial preparation of natural cartilage polysaccharide reduced the number of fine and coarse wrinkles at 120 days compared with placebo. However, we were unable to draw reliable conclusions from this study.

DEFINITION Wrinkles, also known as rhytides, are visible creases or folds in the skin. Wrinkles less than 1 mm in width and depth are defined as fine wrinkles and those greater than 1 mm as coarse wrinkles. Most RCTs have studied wrinkles on the face, forearms, and hands.

INCIDENCE/ We found no information on the incidence of wrinkles alone, only on the
PREVALENCE incidence of skin photodamage, which includes a spectrum of features such as wrinkles, hyperpigmentation, tactile roughness, and telangiectasia. The incidence of skin disorders associated with ultraviolet light increases with age and develops over several decades. One Australian study (1539 people aged 20–55 years living in Queensland) found moderate to severe photodamage in 72% of men and 47% of women under 30 years of age.[1] Severity of photodamage was significantly greater with increasing age, and was independently associated with solar keratoses ($P < 0.01$) and skin cancer ($P < 0.05$). Wrinkling was more common in people with white skin, especially skin phototypes I and II. One study reported that the incidence of photodamage in European and North American populations with Fitzpatrick skin types I, II, and III is about 80–90%.[2] We found few reports of photodamage in black skin (phototypes V and VI).

AETIOLOGY/ Wrinkles may be caused by intrinsic factors (e.g. aging, hormonal status, and
RISK FACTORS intercurrent diseases) and by extrinsic factors (e.g. exposure to ultraviolet radiation and cigarette smoke). These factors contribute to epidermal thinning, loss of elasticity, skin fragility, and creases and lines in the skin. The severity of photodamage varies with skin type, which includes skin colour and the capacity to tan.[3] One review of five observational studies found that facial wrinkles in

men and women were more common in smokers than in non-smokers.[4] It also found that the risk of moderate to severe wrinkles in lifelong smokers was more than twice that in current smokers (RR 2.57, 95% CI 1.83 to 3.06). Oestrogen deficiency may contribute to wrinkles in postmenopausal women.[5]

PROGNOSIS   Although wrinkles cannot be considered to be a medical illness requiring intervention, concerns about aging may affect quality of life. Such concerns are likely to be influenced by geographical differences, culture, and personal values. In some cases concerns about physical appearance can lead to difficulties with interpersonal interactions, occupational functioning, and self esteem.[6] In societies in which the aging population is growing and a high value is placed on the maintenance of a youthful appearance, there is a growing preference for interventions that ameliorate the visible signs of aging.

Please refer to the Clinical Evidence website for full text and references.

What are the effects of non-drug treatments in older people?

UNKNOWN EFFECTIVENESS

Cognitive behavioural therapy

One systematic review identified one small RCT, which found that individual or group cognitive behavioural therapy improved sleep quality both immediately after the end of treatment and at 3 months compared with no treatment, although mean sleep quality scores were consistent with continuing insomnia both with and without treatment.

Exercise programmes

One systematic review identified one small RCT. It found that sleep quality improved after a 16 week programme of regular, moderate intensity exercise four times a week compared with no treatment. However, mean sleep quality scores were consistent with persisting insomnia both with and without exercise.

Timed exposure to bright light

One systematic review found no RCTs comparing the effects of timed bright light exposure with other treatments or no treatment.

DEFINITION	Insomnia is defined by the US National Institutes of Health as experience of poor quality sleep, with difficulty in initiating or maintaining sleep, waking too early in the morning, or failing to feel refreshed. Chronic insomnia is defined as insomnia occurring for at least three nights a week for 1 month or more.[1] Primary insomnia is defined as chronic insomnia without specific underlying medical or psychiatric disorders such as sleep apnoea, depression, or dementia. This chapter only covers primary insomnia.
INCIDENCE/ PREVALENCE	Across all adult age groups, up to 40% of people have insomnia.[2] However, prevalence increases with age, with estimates ranging from 31–38% in people aged 18–64 years to 45% in people aged 65–79 years.[3]
AETIOLOGY/ RISK FACTORS	The cause of insomnia is uncertain. The risk of primary insomnia increases with age and may be related to changes in circadian rhythms associated with age. Psychological factors and lifestyle changes may exacerbate perceived effects of changes in sleep patterns associated with age, leading to reduced satisfaction with sleep.[4] Other risk factors in all age groups include hyperarousal, chronic stress, and daytime napping.[1,5]
PROGNOSIS	We found few reliable data on long term morbidity and mortality in people with primary insomnia. Primary insomnia is a chronic and relapsing condition.[6] Likely consequences include reduced quality of life and increased risk of accidents owing to daytime sleepiness. People with primary insomnia may be at greater risk of dependence on hypnotic medication, depression, dementia, and falls, and may be more likely to require residential care.[6,7]

Please refer to the Clinical Evidence website for full text and references.

Jet lag

Search date November 2004

Andrew Herxheimer

What are the effects of interventions to prevent or minimise jet lag?

Melatonin*

One systematic review found that melatonin reduced mean jet lag scores on eastward and westward flights compared with placebo. The review found case reports of possible adverse effects, and suggested that people with epilepsy or taking warfarin (or other oral anticoagulants) should not use melatonin without medical supervision. It concluded that the pharmacology and toxicology of melatonin needs systematic study, and routine pharmaceutical quality control of melatonin products is necessary.

*The adverse effects of melatonin have not yet been adequately investigated.

Hypnotics

Three small RCTs found limited evidence that hypnotics (zopiclone, zolpidem) improved sleep duration or sleep quality or jet lag compared with placebo. Adverse effects reported with hypnotics include headache, dizziness, nausea, confusion, and amnesia. Short term benefits of hypnotics must be considered in the light of potential adverse effects.

Lifestyle and environmental adaptations (eating, avoiding alcohol or caffeine, sleeping, daylight exposure, arousal)

We found no RCTs on the effects of eating, avoiding alcohol or caffeine, sleeping, daylight exposure, or arousal. Such RCTs are unlikely to be carried out.

DEFINITION   Jet lag is a syndrome associated with rapid long haul flights across several time zones, characterised by sleep disturbances, daytime fatigue, reduced performance, gastrointestinal problems, and generalised malaise.[1] As with most syndromes, not all of the components must be present in any one case. It is due to the "body clock" continuing to function in the day–night rhythm of the place of departure. The rhythm adapts gradually under the influence of light and dark, mediated by melatonin secreted by the pineal gland: darkness switches on melatonin secretion, exposure to strong light switches it off.

INCIDENCE/ PREVALENCE   Jet lag affects most air travellers crossing five or more time zones. The incidence and severity of jet lag increases with the number of time zones crossed.

AETIOLOGY/ RISK FACTORS   Someone who has previously experienced jet lag is liable to do so again. Jet lag is worse the more time zones crossed in one flight, or series of flights, within a few days. Westward travel generally causes less disruption than eastward travel as it is easier to lengthen, rather than to shorten, the natural circadian cycle.[2]

PROGNOSIS   Jet lag is worst immediately after travel and gradually resolves over 4–6 days as the person adjusts to the new local time.[2] The more time zones that are crossed, the longer it takes to wear off.

Please refer to the Clinical Evidence website for full text and references.

Search date August 2003

Michael Hensley and Cheryl Ray

What are the effects of treatment of severe obstructive sleep apnoea-hypopnoea syndrome (OSAHS)?

BENEFICIAL

Nasal continuous positive airway pressure

One systematic review found that nasal continuous positive airway pressure (CPAP) reduced daytime sleepiness compared with placebo, no treatment, or conservative treatment in people with severe obstructive sleep apnoea-hypopnoea syndrome.

LIKELY TO BE BENEFICIAL

Oral appliance

Two small RCTs found that oral appliances that produced anterior advancement of the mandible improved sleep disordered breathing and daytime sleepiness in people with severe OSAHS compared with appliances that did not advance the mandible.

UNKNOWN EFFECTIVENESS

Weight loss

One systematic review found no RCTs on the effects of weight loss in people with severe OSAHS.

What are the effects of treatment of non-severe OSAHS?

LIKELY TO BE BENEFICIAL

Nasal continuous positive airway pressure

Two systematic reviews found no significant difference in daytime sleepiness between nasal CPAP and conservative treatment, placebo pill, or sham/subtherapeutic nasal CPAP in people with non-severe OSAHS but found that CPAP improved some measures of cognitive performance, functional outcomes, symptoms, energy and vitality, and depression. One systematic review and one small RCT found that nasal CPAP improved apnoea/hypopnoea index compared with an oral appliance.

Oral appliance

Two small RCTs found that an oral appliance that produced mandibular advancement reduced daytime sleepiness and sleep disordered breathing compared with no treatment or a control appliance. One systematic review and one small RCT found that nasal CPAP improved apnoea/hypopnoea index compared with an oral appliance.

UNKNOWN EFFECTIVENESS

Weight loss

One systematic review found no RCTs on the effect of weight loss in people with non-severe OSAHS.

Sleep apnoea

DEFINITION

Sleep apnoea is the popular term for obstructive sleep apnoea-hypopnoea syndrome (OSAHS). OSAHS is abnormal breathing during sleep that causes recurrent arousals, sleep fragmentation, and nocturnal hypoxaemia. The syndrome includes daytime sleepiness, impaired vigilance and cognitive functioning, and reduced quality of life.[1,2] Apnoea is the absence of airflow at the nose and mouth for at least 10 seconds, and hypopnoea is a major reduction (>50%) in airflow also for at least 10 seconds. Apnoeas may be "central", in which there is cessation of inspiratory effort, or "obstructive", in which inspiratory efforts continue but are ineffective, because of upper airway obstruction. The diagnosis of OSAHS is made when a person with daytime symptoms has significant sleep disordered breathing revealed by polysomnography (study of sleep state, breathing and oxygenation) or by more limited studies. Criteria for the diagnosis of significant sleep disordered breathing have not been rigorously assessed, but they have been set by consensus and convention.[3,4] Diagnostic criteria have variable sensitivity and specificity. For example, an apnoea/hypopnoea index (AHI) of less than five episodes of apnoea or hypopnoea per hour of sleep is considered normal;[5] however, people with upper airway resistance syndrome have an index below five episodes per hour,[6] and many healthy elderly people have an index greater than five episodes per hour.[7] In an effort to obtain an international consensus, new criteria have been proposed and are becoming more widely used.[8] The severity of OSAHS can be classified by the severity of two factors: daytime sleepiness (see table 1❶) and AHI (see table 2❶). Severe OSAHS is defined as severe sleep disordered breathing (AHI >35 episodes per hour) plus symptoms of excessive daytime sleepiness (Epworth Sleepiness Scale >10 or Multiple Sleep Latency Test <5 minutes [see table 2❶]). Central sleep apnoea and sleep associated hypoventilation syndromes are not covered in this chapter.

INCIDENCE/ PREVALENCE

The Wisconsin Sleep Cohort Study of over 1000 people (mean age 47 years) in North America found a prevalence of AHI greater than five episodes per hour of 24% in men and 9% in women, and of OSAHS with an index greater than five episodes per hour plus excessive sleepiness of 4% in men and 2% in women.[9] There are international differences in the occurrence of OSAHS, for which obesity is considered to be an important determinant.[10] Ethnic differences in prevalence have also been found after adjustment for other risk factors.[7,10] Little is known about the burden of illness in developing countries.

AETIOLOGY/ RISK FACTORS

The site of upper airway obstruction in the OSAHS is around the level of the tongue, soft palate, or epiglottis. Disorders that predispose to either narrowing of the upper airway or reduction in its stability (e.g. obesity, certain craniofacial abnormalities, vocal cord abnormalities, and enlarged tonsils) have been associated with an increased risk of OSAHS. It has been estimated that a 1 kg/m^2 increase in body mass index (3.2 kg for a person 1.8 m tall) leads to a 30% increase (95% CI 13% to 50%) in the relative risk of developing abnormal sleep disordered breathing (AHI ≥ 5 episodes/hour) over a period of 4 years.[10] Other strong associations include increasing age and sex (male to female ratio is 2 : 1). Weaker associations include menopause, family history, smoking, and night time nasal congestion.[10]

PROGNOSIS

The long term prognosis of people with untreated severe OSAHS is poor with respect to quality of life, likelihood of motor vehicle accidents, hypertension, and possibly cardiovascular disease and premature mortality.[11] Unfortunately, the prognosis of both treated and untreated OSAHS is unclear.[7] The limitations in the evidence include bias in the selection of participants, short duration of follow up, and variation in the measurement of confounders (e.g. smoking, alcohol use, and other cardiovascular risk factors). Treatment is widespread, making it difficult to find evidence on prognosis for untreated OSAHS. Observational studies support a causal association between OSAHS and systemic hypertension, which increases with the severity of OSAHS (OR 1.21 for ▶

non-severe OSAHS to 3.07 for severe OSAHS).[11] OSAHS increases the risk of motor vehicle accidents three- to sevenfold.[11,12] It is associated with increased risk of premature mortality, cardiovascular disease, and impaired neurocognitive functioning.[11]

Please refer to the Clinical Evidence website for full text and references.

Breast cancer (metastatic)

Search date June 2004

Justin Stebbing and Robert Glassman

What are the effects of first line hormonal treatment?

First line hormonal treatment with antioestrogens (tamoxifen) or progestins (no significant difference in survival compared with non-taxane combination chemotherapy so may be preferable in women with oestrogen receptor positive disease)

One systematic review found no significant difference in survival at 12 or 24 months between first line hormonal treatment with tamoxifen or progestins and non-taxane combination chemotherapy. The review suggested that hormonal treatment may be preferable to chemotherapy as first line treatment in women with oestrogen receptor positive disease unless disease is rapidly progressing. It found that response rates were lower with hormonal treatment than with chemotherapy but it was associated with less nausea, vomiting, and alopecia.

Selective aromatase inhibitors in postmenopausal women (at least as effective as tamoxifen in delaying disease progression)

Two RCTs found that the aromatase inhibitor anastrozole as first line treatment in metastatic postmenopausal breast cancer was at least as effective as tamoxifen in delaying disease progression and may cause fewer thromboembolic adverse events and vaginal bleeding. One RCT found that the aromatase inhibitor letrozole increased time to disease progression compared with tamoxifen.

Tamoxifen in oestrogen receptor positive women

RCTs have found that antioestrogens (primarily tamoxifen) resulted in tumour responses in a substantial proportion of women with metastatic breast cancer. The likelihood of benefit with antioestrogen treatment was greatest in postmenopausal women with oestrogen receptor positive tumours. RCTs found no significant difference in response rates, remission rates or overall survival between tamoxifen and progestins or ovarian ablation, but tamoxifen was associated with fewer adverse effects. One RCT found that tamoxifen was less effective than medroxyprogesterone in improving bone pain. Two RCTs in women with metastatic postmenopausal breast cancer found that tamoxifen and the aromatase inhibitor anastrozole were similarly effective in delaying disease progression but that tamoxifen may cause more thromboembolic adverse effects and vaginal bleeding. One RCT found that tamoxifen was less effective than the aromatase inhibitor letrozole in increasing time to disease progression.

Combined gonadorelin analogues plus tamoxifen in premenopausal women

RCTs in premenopausal women with oestrogen receptor positive metastatic breast cancer found that first line treatment with gonadorelin analogues plus tamoxifen improved response rates, overall survival, and progression free survival compared with gonadorelin analogues alone.

▶

TRADE OFF BETWEEN BENEFITS AND HARMS

Progestins (beneficial in women with bone metastases or anorexia compared with tamoxifen; higher doses associated with adverse effects)

RCTs found no significant difference in response rates, remission rates, or survival between medroxyprogesterone and tamoxifen as first line treatment. One non-systematic review found that higher doses of medroxyprogesterone increased nausea, vaginal bleeding, and exacerbations of hypertension. One RCT found that medroxyprogesterone improved bone pain compared with tamoxifen. Observational evidence suggested that progestins may increase appetite, weight gain, and wellbeing. One systematic review found no significant difference in survival at 12 or 24 months between first line hormonal treatment (with progestins or tamoxifen) and non-taxane combination chemotherapy. The review suggested that hormonal treatment may be preferable to chemotherapy as first line treatment in women with oestrogen receptor positive disease unless disease is rapidly progressing. It found that response rates were lower with hormonal treatment than with chemo-therapy but it was associated with less nausea, vomiting, and alopecia.

Ovarian ablation in premenopausal women (no significant difference in response rates or survival compared with tamoxifen but associated with substantial adverse effects)

One systematic review and one subsequent RCT in premenopausal women found no significant difference in response rate, duration of response, or survival between ovarian ablation (surgery or irradiation) and tamoxifen as first line treatment. Ovarian ablation is associated with substantial adverse effects such as hot flushes and "tumour flare".

What are the effects of second line hormonal treatment in women who have not responded to tamoxifen?

BENEFICIAL

Selective aromatase inhibitors in postmenopausal women (prolonged survival compared with progestins, as effective in delaying progression as antioestrogens)

RCTs found that, in postmenopausal women with metastatic breast cancer who had relapsed on adjuvant tamoxifen or progressed during first line treatment with tamoxifen, the selective aromatase inhibitors anastrozole, letrozole, and exemes-tane prolonged survival compared with progestins (megestrol) or non-selective aromatase inhibitors (aminoglutethimide), with fewer adverse effects. Two RCTs found no significant difference between anastrozole and fulvestrant in time to progression. The evidence suggests that selective aromatase inhibitors are most effective in oestrogen receptor positive women.

LIKELY TO BE INEFFECTIVE OR HARMFUL

Progestins (less effective in prolonging survival than selective aromatase inhibitors and have more adverse effects)

RCTs found that, in postmenopausal women with metastatic breast cancer who had relapsed on adjuvant tamoxifen or progressed during first line treatment with tamoxifen, progestins were less effective in prolonging survival as second line treatment than selective aromatase inhibitors and were associated with more adverse effects.

Breast cancer (metastatic)

What are the effects of first line chemotherapy?

BENEFICIAL

Anthracycline based non-taxane combination chemotherapy regimens (CAF) containing doxorubicin (increased response rates and survival compared with other regimens)

RCTs found that combination chemotherapy regimens containing an anthracycline, such as doxorubicin (CAF) as first line treatment increased response rates, time to progression, and survival compared with other regimens.

Classical non-taxane combination chemotherapy (CMF) (increases response rates and survival compared with modified CMF)

One systematic review found that classical CMF as first line treatment increased response rate and survival compared with modified CMF regimens.

LIKELY TO BE BENEFICIAL

Taxane based combination chemotherapy (may increase response rates compared with non-taxane combination chemotherapy)

One systematic review found that taxane based combination chemotherapy as first or second line treatment increased overall survival, time to progression, and overall response compared with non-taxane combination chemotherapy. It found no significant difference in overall survival if the analysis was restricted to RCTs of first line chemotherapy.

LIKELY TO BE INEFFECTIVE OR HARMFUL

High dose chemotherapy (no significant difference in overall survival compared with standard chemotherapy and increased adverse effects)

One systematic review found no significant difference in overall survival over 1–5 years between high dose chemotherapy (requiring haematopoietic transplant) and standard dose chemotherapy. It found that high dose chemotherapy increased treatment related morbidity and mortality compared with standard chemotherapy.

What are the effects of first line chemotherapy in combination with a monoclonal antibody?

BENEFICIAL

Chemotherapy plus monoclonal antibody (trastuzumab) in women with overexpressed *HER2/neu* oncogene

One RCT found that, in women whose tumours overexpress the *HER2/neu* oncogene, standard chemotherapy plus the monoclonal antibody trastuzumab as first line treatment increased the time to disease progression, objective response, and overall survival compared with standard chemotherapy alone. The most serious adverse effect observed was cardiac dysfunction in women who received an anthracycline plus trastuzumab.

◀ *What are the effects of second line chemotherapy?*

LIKELY TO BE BENEFICIAL

Taxane based combination chemotherapy (increases response rate in women with anthracycline resistant disease compared with non-taxane combination chemotherapy)

One systematic review has found that taxane based combination chemotherapy as first or second line treatment increased overall survival, time to progression, and overall response compared with non-taxane combination chemotherapy. The difference remained significant if the analysis was limited to women who had previously received anthracyclines. One RCT found no significant difference in progression or overall survival between docetaxel and 5-fluorouracil plus vinorelbine or between paclitaxel and capecitabine given as second line chemotherapy.

UNKNOWN EFFECTIVENESS

Capecitabine for anthracycline resistant disease

One RCT found similar response rates and time to disease progression between capecitabine and paclitaxel after anthracycline failure.

Semisynthetic vinca alkaloids for anthracycline resistant disease

One RCT found no significant difference in progression or overall survival between 5-fluorouracil plus vinorelbine and docetaxel given as second line chemotherapy. Another RCT found that second line vinorelbine improved survival and reduced progression compared with melphalan. A third RCT found no significant difference in survival or quality of life between vinorelbine plus doxorubicin and doxorubicin alone.

What are the effects of treatments for bone metastases?

BENEFICIAL

Radiotherapy plus appropriate analgesia*

We found no RCTs. We found limited evidence from non-randomised studies that persistent and localised bone pain can be treated successfully in over 80% of women with radiotherapy plus concomitant appropriate analgesia (from non-steroidal anti-inflammatory drugs to morphine and its derivatives) and that cranial nerve compression can be treated successfully with radiotherapy in 50–80% of people. RCTs found no evidence that short courses were less effective for pain relief than long courses of radiotherapy. One RCT found that different fractionation schedules can be used to treat neuropathic bone pain effectively.

LIKELY TO BE BENEFICIAL

Bisphosphonates

RCTs in women receiving standard chemotherapy or hormonal treatment for bone metastases secondary to metastatic breast cancer found that bisphosphonates reduced and delayed skeletal complications compared with placebo. They found no significant difference in survival. ▶

Breast cancer (metastatic)

What are the effects of treatments for spinal cord metastases?

BENEFICIAL

Radiotherapy plus high dose steroids in women with spinal cord compression

One small RCT in women with spinal cord compression found that adding high dose steroids to radiotherapy improved the chance of walking 6 months after treatment compared with radiotherapy alone.

Radiotherapy*

We found no RCTs. Spinal cord compression is an emergency. Retrospective studies suggested that early radiotherapy improved outcomes. However, fewer than 10% of people walked again if severe deterioration of motor function occurred before radiotherapy.

What are the effects of treatments for cerebral metastases?

LIKELY TO BE BENEFICIAL

Radiotherapy*

We found no RCTs. Retrospective studies suggested that whole brain irradiation improved neurological function in some women with brain metastases secondary to breast cancer.

UNKNOWN EFFECTIVENESS

Intrathecal chemotherapy

We found no RCTs or observational studies of intrathecal chemotherapy in people with cerebral metastases.

Radiation sensitisers

We found no RCTs of radiation sensitisers. One open label case control study found limited evidence that adding intravenous RSR13, a radiation sensitiser, during whole brain radiotherapy may prolong survival.

Surgical resection

We found no RCTs. One retrospective cohort study provided insufficient evidence to assess surgical resection in people with cerebral metastases.

What are the effects of treatments for choroidal metastases?

LIKELY TO BE BENEFICIAL

Radiotherapy*

We found no RCTs. Retrospective studies suggested that radiotherapy benefited some women with choroidal metastases.

*Not based on RCT evidence

DEFINITION Metastatic or advanced breast cancer is the presence of disease at distant sites such as the bone, liver, or lung. It is not treatable by primary surgery and is currently considered incurable. However, young people with good performance status may survive for 15–20 years.[1] Symptoms may include pain from bone metastases, breathlessness from spread to the lung, and nausea or abdominal discomfort from liver involvement.

▶

INCIDENCE/ PREVALENCE
Breast cancer is the second most frequent cancer in the world (1.05 million people) and is by far the most common malignant disease in women (22% of all new cancer cases). Worldwide, the ratio of mortality to incidence is about 36%. It ranks fifth as a cause of death from cancer overall (although it is the leading cause of cancer mortality in women — the 370 000 annual deaths represent 13.9% of cancer deaths in women). In the USA, metastatic breast cancer causes 46 000 deaths annually, and in the UK causes 15 000 deaths annually.[2] It is the most prevalent cancer in the world today and there are an estimated 3.9 million women alive who have had breast cancer diagnosed in the past 5 years (compared, for example, with lung cancer, where there are 1.4 million alive). The true prevalence of metastatic disease is high because some women live with the disease for many years. Since 1990, there has been an overall increase in incidence rates of about 1.5% annually.[3]

AETIOLOGY/ RISK FACTORS
The risk of metastatic disease relates to known adverse prognostic factors in the original primary tumour. These factors include oestrogen receptor negative disease, primary tumours 3 cm or more in diameter, and axillary node involvement — recurrence occurred within 10 years of adjuvant chemotherapy for early breast cancer in 60–70% of node positive women and 25–30% of node negative women in one large systematic review.[4]

PROGNOSIS
Prognosis depends on age, extent of disease, and oestrogen receptor status. There is also evidence that overexpression of the product of the *HER2/neu* oncogene, which occurs in about a third of women with metastatic breast cancer, is associated with a worse prognosis.[5] A short disease free interval (e.g. < 1 year) between surgery for early breast cancer and developing metastases suggests that the recurrent disease is likely to be resistant to adjuvant treatment.[6] In women who receive no treatment for metastatic disease, the median survival from diagnosis of metastases is 12 months.[7] The choice of first line treatment (hormonal or chemotherapy) is based on a variety of clinical factors).[8–11] In many countries, such as the USA, Canada, and some countries in Europe, there is evidence of a decrease in death rates in recent years. This probably reflects improvements in treatment (and therefore improved survival) as well as earlier diagnosis.[2,12]

Please refer to the Clinical Evidence website for full text and references.

Breast cancer (non-metastatic)

Search date February 2004

J Michael Dixon, Alan Rodger, and Justin Stebbing

What are the effects of interventions after breast conserving surgery for ductal carcinoma in situ?

LIKELY TO BE BENEFICIAL

Radiotherapy (reduced recurrence)

Two RCTs identified by a systematic review found that radiotherapy after breast conserving surgery for ductal carcinoma *in situ* reduced local recurrence and invasive carcinoma compared with no radiotherapy after 4 and 8 years. However, they found no evidence of an effect on survival. One RCT in women having local excision found no significant difference between tamoxifen plus radiotherapy and radiotherapy alone in total invasive or ductal carcinoma *in situ* events after median follow up of 1 year.

Tamoxifen plus radiotherapy (reduced recurrence in women with oestrogen receptor positive tumours)

One RCT found that adjuvant tamoxifen reduced breast cancer events in women who had undergone wide excision and radiotherapy after median follow up of 6 years, although subgroup analysis suggested that benefit may be limited to women with oestrogen receptor positive tumours. It found no evidence of an effect on survival. One RCT in women having local excision found no significant difference between tamoxifen plus radiotherapy and radiotherapy alone in invasive or ductal carcinoma *in situ* events after median follow up of 1 year.

What are the effects of treatments for primary operable breast cancer?

BENEFICIAL

Adjuvant combination chemotherapy

One systematic review found that adjuvant combination chemotherapy reduced recurrence and improved survival at 10 years compared with no chemotherapy. The benefit seemed to be independent of nodal or menopausal status, although the absolute improvements were greater in women with node positive disease, and probably greater in younger women. Adverse effects of chemotherapy include fatigue, nausea and vomiting, hair loss, bone marrow suppression, neuropathy, and gastrointestinal disturbance. Chemotherapy may impair fertility and ovarian function.

Adjuvant tamoxifen (in women with oestrogen receptor positive tumours)

One systematic review found that adjuvant tamoxifen taken for up to 5 years reduced the risk of recurrence and death in women with oestrogen receptor positive tumours irrespective of age, menopausal status, nodal involvement, or the addition of chemotherapy. Five years of treatment was more effective than shorter durations, but available evidence did not find benefit associated with prolongation of treatment beyond 5 years. Tamoxifen slightly increased the risk of endometrial cancer and thrombotic complications, but we found no evidence of an overall adverse effect on non-breast cancer mortality.

Anthracycline regimens as adjuvant chemotherapy

One systematic review found that adjuvant regimens containing an anthracycline reduced recurrence, and improved survival compared with a standard multidrug ▶

chemotherapy (CMF) regimen at 5 years. Adverse effects of chemotherapy include nausea and vomiting, hair loss, bone marrow suppression, fatigue, and gastrointestinal disturbance. Chemotherapy may impair fertility and ovarian function.

Combined chemotherapy plus tamoxifen

One RCT found that adding chemotherapy to tamoxifen improved survival at 5 years in women with lymph node negative, oestrogen receptor positive early breast cancer. It found that adding combined chemotherapy to tamoxifen was associated with increased adverse effects such as nausea, neutropenia, alopecia, thromboembolism, and phlebitis.

Less extensive surgery (similar survival to more extensive surgery, and better cosmetic outcome)

Two systematic reviews and long term follow up of included RCTs found that more extensive surgery did not improve outcomes compared with less extensive surgery in women with early invasive breast cancer, providing that all local disease was excised. Cosmetic appearance is worse with more extensive surgery.

Ovarian ablation in premenopausal women

One systematic review found that in premenopausal women with early breast cancer, ovarian ablation improved survival compared with no ablation after 15 years follow up.

Radiotherapy after breast conserving surgery (reduced local recurrence and had similar survival rates to breast conserving surgery alone)

One systematic review and one subsequent RCT found that adding radiotherapy to breast conserving surgery reduced the risk of local recurrence compared with breast conserving surgery alone. They found no significant difference in survival between breast conserving surgery plus radiotherapy and breast conserving surgery alone. One systematic review and one additional RCT found no significant difference in survival and local recurrence with breast conserving surgery plus radiotherapy compared with mastectomy. One RCT found that radiotherapy (with or without tamoxifen) reduced ipsilateral breast cancer recurrence compared with tamoxifen alone after median follow up of 87 months. It found no significant difference in survival. Radiotherapy may be associated with late adverse effects, which are rare, including pneumonitis, pericarditis, arm oedema, brachial plexopathy, and radionecrotic rib fracture.

Radiotherapy after mastectomy in women at high risk of local recurrence

One systematic review found that radiotherapy to the chest wall after mastectomy reduced the risk of local recurrence by about two thirds compared with no postoperative radiotherapy. It found that radiotherapy did not reduce all cause mortality and breast cancer mortality after mastectomy alone or mastectomy plus axillary clearance. However, radiotherapy did reduce all cause mortality and breast cancer mortality after mastectomy plus axillary sampling. Radiotherapy may be associated with late adverse effects, which are rare, including pneumonitis, pericarditis, arm oedema, brachial plexopathy, and radionecrotic rib fracture.

LIKELY TO BE BENEFICIAL

Neoadjuvant chemotherapy (reduced mastectomy rates and had similar survival rates to adjuvant chemotherapy)

Five RCTs found no significant difference in survival with neoadjuvant chemotherapy compared with adjuvant chemotherapy. Three RCTs found that neoadjuvant chemotherapy reduced mastectomy rate compared with adjuvant chemotherapy. Adverse effects of chemotherapy include fatigue, nausea and vomiting, hair loss, bone marrow suppression, neuropathy, and gastrointestinal disturbance. Chemotherapy may impair fertility and ovarian function.

Women's health

Breast cancer (non-metastatic)

Total nodal radiotherapy

One systematic review found that postmastectomy radiotherapy, including total nodal irradiation, reduced locoregional recurrence. It found that postmastectomy radiotherapy improved survival in women receiving mastectomy plus axillary sampling, but not in women receiving mastectomy alone or mastectomy plus axillary clearance.

TRADE OFF BETWEEN BENEFITS AND HARMS

Radiotherapy after mastectomy in women not at high risk of local recurrence

One systematic review found that radiotherapy to the chest wall after mastectomy reduced the risk of local recurrence by about two thirds compared with no postoperative radiotherapy. It found that radiotherapy did not reduce all cause mortality or breast cancer mortality after mastectomy alone or mastectomy plus axillary clearance. However, radiotherapy did reduce all cause mortality and breast cancer mortality after mastectomy plus axillary sampling. Radiotherapy may be associated with late adverse effects, which are rare, including pneumonitis, pericarditis, arm oedema, brachial plexopathy, and radionecrotic rib fracture. There is, therefore, a trade off between absolute benefits and harms in women not at high risk of local recurrence.

Axillary clearance

There is consensus that axillary clearance reduces regional recurrence compared with no axillary management. RCTs found no significant difference in survival at 5–10 years between axillary clearance and axillary sampling (followed by axillary radiotherapy in women found to be node positive) or axillary radiotherapy (regardless of axillary nodal status). One systematic review found that axillary radiotherapy reduced isolated local recurrence compared with axillary clearance, but this difference was not significant. One systematic review of mainly poor quality evidence found that the risk of arm lymphoedema was highest with axillary clearance plus radiotherapy, lower with axillary sampling plus radiotherapy, and lowest with sampling alone.

Axillary radiotherapy

One systematic review found that axillary radiotherapy reduced isolated local recurrence compared with axillary clearance, but this difference was not significant. The review found no significant difference in survival at 10 years between axillary radiotherapy and axillary clearance. One systematic review of mainly poor quality evidence found that the risk of arm lymphoedema was highest with axillary clearance plus radiotherapy, lower with axillary sampling plus radiotherapy, and lowest with sampling alone.

Axillary sampling

One RCT found no significant difference in survival at 5 years between axillary clearance and axillary sampling (followed by axillary radiotherapy in women found to be node positive). One systematic review of mainly poor quality evidence found that the risk of arm lymphoedema was highest with axillary clearance plus radiotherapy, lower with axillary sampling plus radiotherapy, and lowest with sampling alone.

UNKNOWN EFFECTIVENESS

Different neoadjuvant chemotherapy regimens (insufficient evidence regarding which regimen is most effective)

We found insufficient evidence of any difference between the common neoadjuvant chemotherapy regimens in survival, recurrence, or quality of life.

Radiotherapy to the internal mammary chain

One RCT found no significant difference in relapse or survival at 2–3 years between radiotherapy and no radiotherapy to the internal mammary chain. Treatment may increase radiation induced cardiac morbidity.

Radiotherapy to the ipsilateral supraclavicular fossa

We found insufficient evidence about the effects of irradiation of the ipsilateral supraclavicular fossa on survival. RCTs have found that radiotherapy to the chest wall and lymph nodes is associated with reduced risk of locoregional recurrence, including supraclavicular fossa nodal recurrence. Morbidity associated with irradiation of the supraclavicular fossa is rare and, where it occurs, is mild and temporary.

UNLIKELY TO BE BENEFICIAL

Enhanced dose regimens of adjuvant combination chemotherapy

RCTs did not find additional survival advantage from enhanced dose regimens of adjuvant combination chemotherapy. Adverse effects of chemotherapy include nausea and vomiting, hair loss, bone marrow suppression, fatigue, and gastrointestinal disturbance. Chemotherapy may impair fertility and ovarian function.

Prolonged adjuvant combination chemotherapy (8–12 months v 4–6 months)

One systematic review found no additional survival benefit from prolonging adjuvant chemotherapy from 4–6 to 8–12 months. Adverse effects of chemotherapy include nausea and vomiting, hair loss, bone marrow suppression, fatigue, and gastrointestinal disturbance. Chemotherapy may impair fertility and ovarian function.

LIKELY TO BE INEFFECTIVE OR HARMFUL

High dose chemotherapy

One systematic review found no significant difference between high dose chemotherapy plus autograft and conventional chemotherapy in 5 year survival for women with early, poor prognosis breast cancer. The review found that high dose chemotherapy plus autograft increased treatment related and non-cancer related deaths compared with conventional chemotherapy.

What are the effects of interventions in locally advanced breast cancer (stage III B)?

LIKELY TO BE BENEFICIAL

Hormonal treatment plus radiotherapy (improves survival compared with radiotherapy alone)

One RCT found that hormonal treatment (tamoxifen or ovarian ablation) plus radiotherapy delayed locoregional recurrence and improved survival at 8 years in locally advanced breast cancer compared with radiotherapy alone.

Radiotherapy

Two small RCTs including women with locally advanced disease (stage III B) found that radiotherapy or surgery as sole local treatments have similar effects on response rates, duration of response, and overall survival for locally advanced breast cancer that is rendered operable by prior chemotherapy. Local skin toxicity (acute and late) after radiotherapy is greater in locally advanced breast cancer than after treatment for less advanced disease, because of the need for a higher radiation dose to skin.

▶

Breast cancer (non-metastatic)

Radiotherapy after attempted curative surgery

One RCT found limited evidence that radiotherapy after attempted curative surgery reduced local and regional recurrence compared with no further local treatment, but did not improve time to relapse or overall survival. Local skin toxicity (acute and late) after radiotherapy is greater in locally advanced breast cancer than after treatment for less advanced disease, because of the need for a higher radiation dose to skin.

Surgery

Two small RCTs including women with locally advanced disease (stage III B) found that surgery or radiotherapy as sole local treatments have similar effects on response rates, duration of response, and overall survival for locally advanced breast cancer that is rendered operable by prior chemotherapy.

UNLIKELY TO BE BENEFICIAL

Adding chemotherapy (cyclophosphamide/methotrexate/fluorouracil or anthracycline based regimens) to radiotherapy

RCTs found insufficient evidence that radiotherapy plus cytotoxic chemotherapy using cyclophosphamide plus methotrexate plus fluorouracil, or an anthracycline based multidrug regimen improved survival, disease free survival, or long term locoregional control compared with radiotherapy alone in locally advanced breast cancer.

DEFINITION This chapter examines the effects of treatment for non-metastatic, primary breast cancer. **Ductal carcinoma** *in situ* is a non-invasive tumour characterised by the presence of malignant cells in the breast ducts but with no evidence that they breach the basement membrane and invade into periductal connective tissues. **Invasive breast cancer** can be separated into three main groups: early invasive breast cancer, locally advanced breast cancer, and metastatic breast cancer (see breast cancer [metastatic], p 506). **Operable breast cancer** is apparently restricted to the breast and sometimes to local lymph nodes and can be removed surgically. Although these women do not have overt metastases at the time of staging, they remain at risk of local recurrence and of metastatic spread. They can be divided into those with tumours greater than 4 cm with multifocal cancers that are usually treated by mastectomy, and those with tumours less than 4 cm with unifocal cancers that can be treated by breast conserving surgery. **Locally advanced breast cancer** is defined according to the TNM staging system of the UICC[1] as stage III B (includes T4 a–d; N2 disease, but absence of metastases). It is a disease presentation with evidence (clinical or histopathological) of skin, or chest wall involvement, or axillary nodes matted together by tumour extension, or a combination of these features. **Metastatic breast cancer** is presented in a separate chapter (see breast cancer [metastatic], p 506).

INCIDENCE/ PREVALENCE Breast cancer affects 1/10–1/11 women in the UK and causes about 21 000 deaths a year. Prevalence is about five times higher, with over 100 000 women in the UK living with breast cancer at any one time. Of the 15 000 new cases of breast cancer a year in the UK, most will present with primary operable disease.[2]

AETIOLOGY/ RISK FACTORS The risk of breast cancer increases with age, doubling every 10 years up to the menopause. Risk factors include an early age at menarche, older age at menopause, older age at birth of first child, family history, atypical hyperplasia, excess alcohol intake, radiation exposure to developing breast tissue, oral contraceptive use, postmenopausal hormone replacement therapy, and obesity. Risk in different countries varies fivefold. The cause of breast cancer in most women is unknown. About 5% of breast cancers can be attributed to mutations in the genes *BRCA1* and *BRCA2*.[3]

PROGNOSIS   **Primary carcinoma** of the breast is potentially curable. The risk of relapse depends on various clinicopathological features, of which axillary node involvement, tumour grade, tumour size, and oestrogen receptor status are the most prognostically important. Of women with operable disease 70% are alive 5 years after diagnosis and treatment (adjuvant treatment is given to most women after surgery). Risk of recurrence is highest during the first 5 years, but the risk remains even 15–20 years after surgery. Those with node positive disease have a 50–60% chance of recurrence within 5 years, compared with 30–35% for node negative disease. Recurrence at 10 years, according to one large systematic review,[4] is 60–70% compared with 25–30% of node negative women. The prognosis for a disease free survival at 5 years is worse for stage III B (33%) than that for stage III A (71%). Five year overall survival is 44% for stage III B and 84% for stage III A.[5] Poor survival and high rates of local recurrence characterise locally advanced breast cancer.

Please refer to the Clinical Evidence website for full text and references.

Breast pain

Search date March 2004

Nigel Bundred

What are the effects of treatments for breast pain?

TRADE OFF BETWEEN BENEFITS AND HARMS

Danazol

One RCT found that danazol reduced cyclical breast pain after 12 months compared with placebo, but increased adverse effects (weight gain, deepening of the voice, menorrhagia, and muscle cramps). It found no significant difference in pain relief between danazol and tamoxifen.

Tamoxifen

Three RCTs found limited evidence that tamoxifen was more effective than placebo at reducing breast pain. The two RCTs which reported on adverse effects found more hot flushes and vaginal discharge with tamoxifen compared with placebo, although differences between groups did not reach significance. One RCT found similar efficacy but fewer adverse effects with a lower dose of 10 mg compared with 20 mg. One RCT found no significant difference in pain relief between tamoxifen and danazol. One meta-analysis of four large breast cancer prevention trials found that tamoxifen used long term was associated with an increased risk of venous thromboembolism. Tamoxifen is not licensed for mastalgia in the UK or USA.

Gestrinone

One RCT found that gestrinone reduced breast pain after 3 months compared with placebo, but increased adverse effects (greasy skin, hirsutism, acne, reduction in breast size, headache, and depression).

UNKNOWN EFFECTIVENESS

Antibiotics

We found no systematic review or RCTs of sufficient quality on the effects of antibiotics.

Diet (low fat, high carbohydrate)

One small RCT found limited evidence that advice to follow a low fat, high carbohydrate diet reduced self reported premenstrual breast swelling and breast tenderness at 6 months compared with general dietary advice. However, it found no significant difference between groups in the combined outcome of breast swelling, tenderness, and nodularity on physical examination at 6 months.

Diuretics

We found no systematic review or RCTs of sufficient quality on the effects of diuretics.

Evening primrose oil

One RCT found no significant difference between evening primrose oil and placebo in frequency of pain at 6 months.

Gonadorelin analogues (luteinising hormone releasing hormone analogues)

We found no systematic review or RCTs of sufficient quality on the effects of gonadorelin analogues.

Lisuride

One RCT with weak methods found limited evidence that lisuride maleate (a dopamine agonist) reduced breast pain over 2 months compared with placebo. ▶

Pyridoxine
We found no systematic review or RCTs of sufficient quality on the effects of pyridoxine.

Tibolone
One RCT found no significant difference between tibolone and placebo in breast pain and tenderness at 12 months.

Vitamin E
We found no systematic review or RCTs of sufficient quality on the effects of vitamin E.

UNLIKELY TO BE BENEFICIAL

Bromocriptine
One RCT with high withdrawal rates and one small crossover RCT reporting results after crossover found limited evidence that bromocriptine (a dopamine agonist) reduced breast pain compared with placebo. However, both RCTs found a higher incidence of adverse effects with bromocriptine compared with placebo. Adverse events included nausea, dizziness, postural hypotension, and constipation. One of the RCTs found that withdrawals related to adverse effects were more frequent with bromocriptine compared with placebo, although differences between groups did not reach significance. Bromocriptine is now used rarely because of frequent and intolerable adverse effects and the US Food and Drug Administration has withdrawn its licence for this indication.

Hormone replacement therapy (oestrogen)
We found no placebo controlled RCTs of hormone replacement therapy for breast pain. Hormone replacement therapy is associated with an increased risk of breast cancer, venous thromboembolism, and gall bladder disease.

Progestogens
Two small crossover RCTs found no significant difference between either progesterone cream or medroxyprogesterone acetate tablets and placebo in breast pain.

DEFINITION Breast pain can be differentiated into cyclical mastalgia (worse before a menstrual period) or non-cyclical mastalgia (unrelated to the menstrual cycle).[1,2] Cyclical pain is often bilateral, usually most severe in the upper outer quadrants of the breast, and may be referred to the medial aspect of the upper arm.[1-3] Non-cyclical pain may be caused by true breast pain or chest wall pain located over the costal cartilages.[1,2,4] Specific breast pathology and referred pain unrelated to the breasts are not included in this chapter.

INCIDENCE/ PREVALENCE Up to 70% of women develop breast pain in their lifetime.[1,2] Of 1171 US women attending a gynaecology clinic, 69% suffered regular discomfort, which was judged as severe in 11% of women, and 36% had consulted a doctor about breast pain.[2]

AETIOLOGY/ RISK FACTORS Breast pain is most common in women aged 30–50 years.[1,2]

PROGNOSIS Cyclical breast pain resolves spontaneously within 3 months of onset in 20–30% of women.[5] The pain tends to relapse and remit, and up to 60% of women develop recurrent symptoms 2 years after treatment.[1] Non-cyclical pain responds poorly to treatment but may resolve spontaneously in about 50% of women.[1]

Please refer to the Clinical Evidence website for full text and references.

Candidiasis (vulvovaginal)

Search date November 2003

Des Spence

What are the effects of treatments for acute vulvovaginal candidiasis in non-pregnant women?

Intravaginal imidazoles

RCTs found that intravaginal imidazoles (butoconazole, clotrimazole, miconazole, or terconazole) reduced persistent symptoms of vulvovaginal candidiasis after 9–38 days compared with placebo. They found no clear evidence that clinical effects differ among the various intravaginal imidazoles. RCTs found no clear evidence of any difference in persistent symptoms between shorter and longer durations of treatment (1–14 days). RCTs found no significant difference in symptoms between intravaginal imidazoles and oral fluconazole, itraconazole, or ketoconazole. RCTs found that intravaginal imidazoles were associated with less nausea, headache, and abdominal pain but more vulval irritation and vaginal discharge than oral fluconazole or oral ketoconazole. Two RCTs provided insufficient evidence to compare intravaginal imidazoles versus intravaginal nystatin.

Oral fluconazole

We found no RCTs comparing oral fluconazole versus placebo or no treatment. One systematic review found no significant difference in persistent symptoms of vulvovaginal candidiasis over 1–12 weeks between oral fluconazole or oral itraconazole and intravaginal imidazoles, and found that oral fluconazole was associated with more nausea, headache, and abdominal pain but less vulval irritation and vaginal discharge than intravaginal imidazoles. One weak RCT provided insufficient evidence to compare oral fluconazole versus oral itraconazole. One systematic review found no significant difference in persistent symptoms of vulvovaginal candidiasis or in adverse effects between oral fluconazole and oral ketoconazole.

Oral itraconazole

One RCT found that oral itraconazole reduced persistent symptoms of vulvovaginal candidiasis at 1 week after treatment compared with placebo. One systematic review found no significant difference in persistent symptoms over 1–12 weeks between oral itraconazole or oral fluconazole and intravaginal imidazoles. One weak RCT provided insufficient evidence to compare oral itraconazole versus oral fluconazole.

Intravaginal nystatin

One RCT found that intravaginal nystatin reduced the proportion of women with a poor symptomatic response after 14 days' treatment compared with placebo. Two RCTs provided insufficient evidence to compare intravaginal nystatin versus intravaginal imidazoles. One RCT found that intravaginal nystatin was less effective than boric acid in increasing clinical cure rates at 4 weeks. It gave no information on the adverse effects of intravaginal nystatin compared with intravaginal boric acid. We found no RCTs comparing intravaginal nystatin versus oral fluconazole, itraconazole, or ketoconazole.

Douching

We found no RCTs of douching in women with acute vulvovaginal candidiasis. Douching is associated with serious sequelae, including pelvic inflammatory disease, endometritis, and ectopic pregnancy.

Garlic

We found no RCTs of garlic in women with acute vulvovaginal candidiasis.

Intravaginal boric acid

One RCT found that intravaginal boric acid increased clinical cure rates at 4 weeks compared with intravaginal nystatin. It gave no information on the adverse effects of intravaginal boric acid compared with intravaginal nystatin. Intravaginal boric acid can cause skin irritation.

Intravaginal tea tree oil

We found no RCTs of intravaginal tea tree oil in women with acute vulvovaginal candidiasis.

Yoghurt containing *Lactobacillus acidophilus*

We found no RCTs of lactobacillus yoghurt in women with acute vulvovaginal candidiasis.

UNLIKELY TO BE BENEFICIAL

Oral ketoconazole

We found no RCTs comparing oral ketoconazole versus placebo or no treatment. RCTs found no significant difference between oral ketoconazole and intravaginal imidazoles in persistent symptoms of vulvovaginal candidiasis, and found that oral ketoconazole may cause more nausea, fatigue, and headaches but less vulval irritation. One RCT found no significant difference in persistent symptoms or adverse effects between oral ketoconazole and oral fluconazole. Case reports have associated ketoconazole with a risk of fulminant hepatitis (1/12 000 courses of treatment with oral ketoconazole); there is consensus that the risks may outweigh the benefits in women with vulvovaginal candidiasis.

Treating a male sexual partner to resolve symptoms and prevent symptomatic recurrence in women

RCTs found no significant difference between treating and not treating a woman's male sexual partner in the resolution of the woman's symptoms of acute vulvovaginal candidiasis over 1–4 weeks or in the rate of symptomatic recurrence at 4–5 weeks after treatment.

What are the effects of treatments for recurrent vulvovaginal candidiasis in non-pregnant women?

LIKELY TO BE BENEFICIAL

Oral itraconazole

One RCT found that monthly prophylaxis with oral itraconazole reduced symptomatic recurrence of vulvovaginal candidiasis over 6 months compared with placebo. One weak, open label RCT provided insufficient evidence to compare twice weekly prophylaxis with oral itraconazole versus intravaginal clotrimazole. ►

Candidiasis (vulvovaginal)

UNKNOWN EFFECTIVENESS

Douching

We found no RCTs of douching in women with recurrent vulvovaginal candidiasis. Douching is associated with serious sequelae, including pelvic inflammatory disease, endometritis, ectopic pregnancy, gonorrhoea, and chlamydia.

Garlic

We found no RCTs of garlic in women with recurrent vulvovaginal candidiasis.

Intravaginal boric acid

We found no RCTs of intravaginal boric acid in women with recurrent vulvovaginal candidiasis.

Intravaginal imidazoles

Two RCTs provided insufficient evidence about the effects of regular prophylaxis with intravaginal clotrimazole compared with placebo in preventing symptomatic recurrence of vulvovaginal candidiasis. One RCT found no significant difference in the number of episodes of symptomatic vaginitis over 6 months between monthly prophylaxis with intravaginal clotrimazole and treatment as required, although women who took monthly prophylaxis had fewer episodes. The RCT may have been underpowered to detect a clinically important difference. More women preferred treatment as required. One RCT found insufficient evidence about the effects of regular prophylaxis with intravaginal clotrimazole compared with oral itraconazole.

Oral fluconazole

We found no RCTs about the effects of oral fluconazole in preventing symptomatic recurrence of vulvovaginal candidiasis.

Intravaginal tea tree oil

We found no RCTs of intravaginal tea tree oil in women with recurrent vulvovaginal candidiasis.

Yoghurt containing *Lactobacillus acidophilus*

Two poor quality crossover RCTs identified by a systematic review provided insufficient evidence about the effects of oral lactobacillus yoghurt in women with recurrent vulvovaginal candidiasis. Oral yoghurt may cause gastrointestinal disturbance in people with lactose intolerance. The review identified no RCTs of vaginal lactobacillus yoghurt.

UNLIKELY TO BE BENEFICIAL

Oral ketoconazole

One RCT found that oral ketoconazole, given for 5 days during the menstrual cycle at 400 mg daily or continuously at a lower dose, reduced symptomatic recurrence of vulvovaginal candidiasis over 6 months compared with placebo. This benefit is associated with an increased risk of harms, including rare cases of fulminant hepatitis (1/12 000 courses of treatment with oral ketoconazole); there is consensus that the risks may outweigh the benefits in women with vulvovaginal candidiasis.

Treating a male sexual partner to resolve symptoms and prevent symptomatic recurrence in women

One RCT found no significant difference between treating and not treating a woman's male sexual partner in the rate of symptomatic recurrence over 12 months.

DEFINITION **Vulvovaginal candidiasis** is defined as symptomatic vaginitis (inflammation of the vagina), which often involves the vulva, caused by infection with a *Candida* yeast. Predominant symptoms are vulval itching and abnormal vaginal discharge (which may be minimal, a "cheese like" material, or a watery secretion). Differentiation from other forms of vaginitis requires the presence of yeast on microscopy of vaginal fluid. **Recurrent vulvovaginal candidiasis** is commonly defined as four or more symptomatic episodes a year.[1] Studies of asymptomatic women with vaginal colonisation by *Candida* species were excluded.

INCIDENCE/ PREVALENCE Vulvovaginal candidiasis is estimated to be the second most common cause of vaginitis after bacterial vaginosis. Estimates of its incidence are limited and often derived from women who attend hospital clinics. Asymptomatic prevalence has been reported in 10% of women[2] and self-reported history of at least one episode of vulvovaginal candidiasis has been as high as 72%.[3] Recurrent symptoms are common but are caused by candidiasis in only a third of cases.[4]

AETIOLOGY/ RISK FACTORS *Candida albicans* accounts for 85–90% of cases of vulvovaginal candidiasis. Development of symptomatic vulvovaginal candidiasis probably represents increased growth of yeast that previously colonised the vagina without causing symptoms. Risk factors for vulvovaginal candidiasis include pregnancy, diabetes mellitus, and systemic antibiotics. The evidence that different types of contraceptives are risk factors is contradictory. The incidence of vulvovaginal candidiasis rises with initiation of sexual activity, but we found no direct evidence that vulvovaginal candidiasis is sexually transmitted.[5–7]

PROGNOSIS We found few descriptions of the natural history of untreated vulvovaginal candidiasis. Discomfort is the main complication and can include pain while passing urine or during sexual intercourse. Balanitis in male partners of women with vulvovaginal candidiasis can occur, but it is rare.

Please refer to the Clinical Evidence website for full text and references.

Women's health

Cervical cancer

Search date June 2003

Sudha Sundar, Amanda Horne and Sean Kehoe

What are the effects of interventions to manage early stage cervical cancer? New

LIKELY TO BE BENEFICIAL

Conisation of the cervix for microinvasive carcinoma (stage Ia1)* New

We found no systematic review or RCTs of conisation of the cervix versus simple hysterectomy for microinvasive carcinoma (stage Ia1). However, there is consensus that conisation of the cervix is effective for microinvasive carcinoma (stage Ia1), provided that excision margins are clear of cancer or cervical intraepithelial neoplasia. Conisation of the cervix can, unlike hysterectomy, preserve fertility.

Radical trachelectomy plus lymphadenectomy (preserved fertility compared with hysterectomy) New

We found no systematic review or RCTs comparing radical trachelectomy plus lymphadenectomy versus radical hysterectomy in women with early stage cervical cancer. Radical trachelectomy plus lymphadenectomy can, unlike hysterectomy, preserve fertility.

Radiotherapy or surgery* New

One RCT found no significant difference in overall survival or disease free survival between radiotherapy and radical hysterectomy plus lymphadenectomy (with or without adjuvant radiotherapy) for early stage cervical cancer. Consensus regards both surgery and radiotherapy as likely to be beneficial.

What are the effects of interventions to manage bulky early stage cervical cancer? New

BENEFICIAL

Chemoradiotherapy (increased survival compared with radiotherapy alone) New

Two RCTs found that chemoradiotherapy improved overall survival and progression free survival compared with radiotherapy, when used either before or after hysterectomy. Combined chemoradiotherapy was associated with more haematological and gastrointestinal toxicity than radiotherapy alone.

LIKELY TO BE BENEFICIAL

Neoadjuvant chemotherapy New

RCTs found limited evidence that neoadjuvant chemotherapy (before local treatment with surgery, radiotherapy, or both) improved survival and reduced local recurrence compared with local treatment alone.

*Based on consensus

DEFINITION   Cervical cancer is a malignant neoplasm arising from the uterine cervix. Approximately 80% of cervical cancers are of the squamous type; the remainder are adenocarcinomas, adenosquamous carcinomas, and other rare types.[1] Staging of cervical cancer is based on clinical evaluation (FIGO classification (see table 1 ❶). Management is determined by tumour bulk and stage. This topic deals with treatments for early stage cancer (defined as FIGO stage Ia1, Ia2, Ib1, and small IIa tumours) and bulky early stage disease (defined as FIGO stage Ib2 and larger IIa tumours).

INCIDENCE/ PREVALENCE Cervical cancer is the second most common cancer in women, with about 450 000 new cases diagnosed worldwide each year.[2] Most (80%) cases occur in less developed countries without an effective screening programme. The incidence of cervical cancer in the UK and Europe has significantly reduced since the introduction of a screening programme for detecting precancerous cervical intraepithelial neoplasia. Cervical cancer incidence fell by 42% between 1988 and 1997 (England and Wales). This fall has been reported to be related to the cervical screening programme.[3] In England and Wales, cervical cancer has an annual incidence of 3200 women, and causes about 1000 deaths each year.[4]

AETIOLOGY/ RISK FACTORS Risk factors for cervical cancer include sexual intercourse at an early age, multiple sexual partners, tobacco smoking, long term oral contraceptive use, low socioeconomic status, immunosuppressive therapy, and micronutrient deficiency. Persistent infection by oncogenic, high risk strains of human papilloma virus is strongly associated with the development of cervical cancer.[5–7] The virus is acquired mainly by sexual intercourse and has a peak prevalence of 20–30% in women aged 20–30 years,[8] although in 80% of cases the infection is transient and resolves within 12–18 months.

PROGNOSIS Overall, 5 year disease free survival is 50–70% for stages Ib2 and IIb, 30–50% for stage III, and 5–15% for stage IV.[1] In people who receive treatment, 5 year survival in stage Ia approaches 100%, falling to 70–85% for stage Ib1 and smaller IIa tumours. Survival in people with more locally advanced tumours is influenced by tumour bulk, the person's age, and coexistent medical conditions. Untreated mortality in locally advanced disease is high.

Please refer to the Clinical Evidence website for full text and references.

Domestic violence towards women

Search date March 2004

Joanne Klevens and Laura Sadowski

What are the effects of interventions initiated by healthcare professionals, aimed at female victims of domestic violence?

LIKELY TO BE BENEFICIAL

Advocacy

One RCT and one non-randomised controlled trial found that advocacy reduced reabuse compared with no treatment. The RCT also found an improvement in women's quality of life with advocacy compared with no treatment. One controlled trial in pregnant Hispanic women found no significant difference in rates of reabuse between combined counselling plus mentoring (similar to advocacy) and a resource card, but found that counselling plus mentoring slightly reduced rates of reabuse compared with unlimited counselling.

Safety planning

One RCT found that providing telephone sessions on safe behaviour in addition to usual care increased safe behaviour at 6 months compared with usual care alone. We found limited evidence from one non-randomised controlled trial in pregnant women that helping participants to make a safety plan reduced spouse abuse and increased safe behaviour at 12 months.

UNKNOWN EFFECTIVENESS

Cognitive behaviour orientated counselling

One controlled trial found that cognitive behaviour orientated therapy improved women's assertiveness and reduced their exposure to abuse compared with baseline levels, whereas non-specific support did not. However, the study did not directly compare effects of interventions.

Couple counselling

One non-randomised controlled trial found that both gender specific counselling and couple counselling reduced physical aggression, psychological aggression and depression in wives from baseline levels, but found no significant differences between treatments. One RCT found no significant difference between group and individual couple counselling on reduction in physical violence or on psychological wellbeing.

Grief resolution orientated counselling

One controlled trial found that grief resolution orientated counselling improved self esteem and self efficacy from baseline, whereas feminist orientated counselling did not. However, the study did not directly compare effects of interventions.

Peer support groups

We found no systematic reviews or controlled trials on the effect of peer support groups.

Shelters

We found no reliable controlled trials. One cohort study found a reduced incidence of violence in the weeks following shelter stay for women choosing to use the shelter when they were also engaged in other types of help seeking behaviour compared with women not choosing to stay at the shelter. Women choosing to stay at the shelter who had not sought help elsewhere experienced an increase in violence.

▶

Non-specific counselling

Two controlled trials and one comparative cohort study found no effect of counselling compared with no treatment on medical care utilisation rates, reported exposure to violence and threats of violence, or depression, anxiety, and self esteem.

DEFINITION Domestic violence, also called intimate partner violence, is actual or threatened physical or sexual violence, or emotional or psychological abuse (including coercive tactics) by a current or former spouse or dating partner (including same sex partners).[1] Other terms commonly used to describe domestic violence include domestic abuse, spouse abuse, marital violence, and battering.

INCIDENCE/ Between 10–69% of women participating in population based surveys in 48
PREVALENCE countries from around the world reported being physically assaulted by a partner during their lifetime.[2] Rates of assault by a partner are 4.3 times higher among women than men.[3] Nearly 25% of surveyed women in the USA reported being physically and/or sexually assaulted by a current or former partner at some time during their lives, and 1.5% were victimised during the previous 12 months.[3] Rates of violence against pregnant women range from 0.9–20%.[4] Between 11.7–24.5% of women in prenatal clinics[5–8] and 5.5–17% of women in primary or ambulatory care reported being abused by a partner in the past year.[9–12]

AETIOLOGY/ A recent systematic review found that physical domestic violence toward
RISK FACTORS women is associated with lower levels of education and unemployment, low family income, marital discord, and with the partner's lower level of occupation, childhood experiences of abuse, witnessing interparental violence, higher levels of anger, depression, heavy or problem drinking, drug use, jealousy, and lack of assertiveness with spouse.[13] A similar review of research on psychological aggression found that the few demographic and psychological variables assessed were either inconsistently associated with psychological domestic violence or were found to be associated with psychological domestic violence in studies with serious methodological limitations.[14]

PROGNOSIS There are few prospective studies documenting the course of domestic violence and its outcomes. Cross sectional surveys suggest that domestic violence persists for at least two thirds of women.[15,16] Among black and Hispanic people persistence of domestic violence seems to be dependent on initial severity.[17] For all ethnic groups, half of those reporting moderate domestic violence did not report occurrences of domestic violence at the 5 year follow up, but for people of black or Hispanic origin reporting severe domestic violence only a third did not report occurrences of domestic violence at the 5 year follow up. A case control study conducted in middle class working women found that, compared with non-abused women, women abused by their partners during the previous 9 years were significantly more likely to have or report headaches (48% v 35%), back pain (40% v 25%), sexually transmitted diseases (6% v 2%), vaginal bleeding (17% v 6%), vaginal infections (30% v 21%), pelvic pain (17% v 9%), painful intercourse (13% v 7%), urinary tract infections (22% v 12%), appetite loss (9% v 3%), digestive problems (35% v 19%), abdominal pain (22% v 11%), and facial injuries (8% v 1%).[18] After adjusting for age, race, insurance status, and cigarette smoking, a cross sectional survey found that women experiencing psychological abuse are also more likely to report poor physical and mental health, disability preventing work, arthritis, chronic pain, migraine and other frequent headaches, sexually transmitted infections, chronic pelvic pain, stomach ulcers, spastic colon, frequent indigestion, diarrhoea, or constipation❶.[19]

Please refer to the Clinical Evidence website for full text and references.

Dysmenorrhoea

Search date July 2004

Michelle L Proctor and Cynthia M Farquhar

What are the effects of treatments for dysmenorrhoea?

BENEFICIAL

Non-steroidal anti-inflammatory drugs (other than aspirin)

Three systematic reviews and five subsequent RCTs found that non-steroidal anti-inflammatory drugs (NSAIDs, including cyclo-oxygenase-2 inhibitors, but excluding niflumic acid) reduced pain compared with placebo. One systematic review found that NSAIDs (excluding cyclo-oxygenase-2 inhibitors) reduced restriction of daily activities, absence from work or school, and the need for additional analgesia compared with placebo. It remains unclear from direct comparisons which NSAIDs have better efficacy or safety. One small RCT identified by one systematic review found no significant difference in pain relief between an NSAID (naproxen) compared with paracetamol. One systematic review found that naproxen was associated with fewer adverse effects than co-proxamol. It also found that mefenamic acid reduced symptoms more than co-proxamol. The harms of NSAIDs including cyclo-oxygenase II inhibitor class, are considered in detail elsewhere in Clinical Evidence (see harms of non-steroidal anti-inflammatory drugs, p 348) and include gastrointestinal ulceration and haemorrhage for traditional NSAIDs and, for at least some of the COX-2 inhibitors, increased cardiovascular risk. Co-proxamol has been withdrawn in some countries due to evidence that fatal toxicity may occur with a small multiple of the normal therapeutic dose and a proportion of fatalities are caused by inadvertent overdose. Rofecoxib, an NSAID of the COX-2 inhibitor class, has been withdrawn worldwide because of cardiovascular adverse effects.

LIKELY TO BE BENEFICIAL

Aspirin, paracetamol, and compound analgesics

One systematic review found that aspirin was more effective than placebo for pain relief. Two systematic reviews found no significant difference between paracetamol compared with placebo, aspirin, or naproxen in pain relief, although some of the RCTs may have been too small to detect clinically important differences. The first review found limited evidence that co-proxamol reduced pain compared with placebo. One small RCT identified by a systematic review found no significant difference in pain relief between paracetomol and an NSAID (naproxen). One systematic review found that naproxen was associated with fewer adverse effects than co-proxamol. It also found that mefenamic acid reduced symptoms more than co-proxamol.

Magnesium

One systematic review found limited evidence from two out of three small RCTs that magnesium reduced pain after 5–6 months compared with placebo. The third RCT found no significant difference between treatments.

Thiamine

One systematic review identified one large RCT that found that thiamine reduced pain after 60 days compared with placebo.

Toki-shakuyaku-san (herbal remedy)

One systematic review found limited evidence that toki-shakuyaku-san reduced pain after 6 months and reduced the need for additional medication, compared with placebo. We found no RCTs of other herbal remedies.

Topical heat (about 39 °C)
One RCT found topical heat treatment to be as effective as ibuprofen and more effective than placebo in reducing pain.

Transcutaneous electrical nerve stimulation (high frequency stimulation only; effects of low frequency stimulation remain unclear)
One systematic review found limited evidence from small RCTs that high frequency transcutaneous electrical nerve stimulation reduced pain compared with placebo transcutaneous electrical nerve stimulation but was less effective in achieving pain relief compared with ibuprofen. Small RCTs provided insufficient evidence to assess the effects of low frequency transcutaneous electrical nerve stimulation compared with either placebo tablets, or high frequency or placebo transcutaneous electrical nerve stimulation.

Vitamin E
One systematic review identified two RCTs that found that vitamin E reduced pain compared with placebo. A second systematic review identified one RCT that found no difference in pain relief between vitamin E plus ibuprofen compared with ibuprofen alone.

UNKNOWN EFFECTIVENESS

Acupuncture
One systematic review of one small RCT provided insufficient evidence to compare clinical effects of acupuncture with placebo or no treatment.

Behavioural interventions
Two poor quality RCTs provided insufficient evidence about the effects of behavioural interventions.

Combined oral contraceptives
One systematic review and one subsequent RCT provided insufficient evidence about effects of combined oral contraceptives on pain relief compared with placebo.

Fish oil
One small crossover RCT identified by a systematic review and one additional RCT provided limited evidence that fish oil (with or without vitamin B_{12}) reduced pain and symptoms after 1–3 months compared with placebo.

Herbal remedies (other than toki-shakuyaku-san)
We found no RCTs of other herbal remedies.

Surgical interruption of pelvic nerve pathways
One small RCT found limited evidence that laparoscopic uterine nerve ablation increased pain relief compared with diagnostic laparoscopy. A second RCT found that laparoscopic uterine nerve ablation reduced pain at 12 months compared with laparoscopic presacral neurectomy, but no significant difference in pain relief between treatments at 3 months. It also found increased constipation with laparoscopic presacral neurectomy compared with laparoscopic uterine nerve ablation.

Vitamin B_{12}
We found no RCTs that compared vitamin B_{12} with placebo. One small RCT provided insufficient evidence for vitamin B_{12} compared with a low fat vegetarian diet. One RCT provided limited evidence that vitamin B_{12} plus fish oil reduced pain and symptoms after 1–3 months compared with placebo.

Dysmenorrhoea

UNLIKELY TO BE BENEFICIAL

Spinal manipulation

One systematic review found that one good quality RCT found no significant difference between spinal manipulation and placebo manipulation in pain after 1 month. The review found two small poorer quality RCTs which had conflicting results regarding the effectiveness of spinal manipulation versus placebo or no treatment.

DEFINITION   Dysmenorrhoea is painful menstrual cramps of uterine origin. It is commonly divided into primary dysmenorrhoea (pain without organic pathology) and secondary dysmenorrhoea (pelvic pain associated with an identifiable pathological condition, such as endometriosis [see endometriosis, p 526] or ovarian cysts). The initial onset of primary dysmenorrhoea is usually shortly after menarche (6–12 months), when ovulatory cycles are established. Pain duration is commonly 8–72 hours and is usually associated with the onset of menstrual flow. Secondary dysmenorrhoea can also occur at any time after menarche, but may arise as a new symptom during a woman's fourth and fifth decade, after the onset of an underlying causative condition.[1] This chapter deals with both primary and secondary dysmenorrhoea. Endometriosis, which can cause secondary dysmenorrhoea, is covered in a separate chapter (see endometriosis, p 526).

INCIDENCE/   Variations in the definition of dysmenorrhoea make it difficult to determine
PREVALENCE   prevalence precisely. Studies tend to report on prevalence in adolescent girls, and the type of dysmenorrhoea is not always specified. Adolescent girls tend to have a higher prevalence of primary dysmenorrhoea than older women, as primary dysmenorrhoea can improve with age (see Prognosis). Secondary dysmenorrhoea rates may be lower in adolescents, as onset of causative conditions may not yet have occurred. Therefore, the results from prevalence studies of adolescents may not always be extrapolated to older women, or be accurate estimates of the prevalence of secondary dysmenorrhoea. However, various types of studies have found a consistently high prevalence in women of different ages and nationalities. One systematic review (search date 1996) of the prevalence of chronic pelvic pain, summarising both community and hospital surveys from developed countries, estimated prevalence to be 45–95%.[2] A second systematic review of studies in developing countries (search date 2002) found that 25–50% of adult women and about 75% of adolescents experience pain with menstruation, with 5–20% reporting severe dysmenorrhoea or pain that prevents them from participating in their usual activities.[3] Additional studies of prevalence are summarised in Table 1 (see table 1❶).

AETIOLOGY/   A longitudinal study of a representative sample of women born in 1962 found
RISK FACTORS that the severity of dysmenorrhoea was significantly associated with the duration of menstrual flow (average duration of menstrual flow was 5.0 days for women with no dysmenorrhoea and 5.8 days for women with severe dysmenorrhoea, where severe dysmenorrhoea was defined as pain that did not respond well to analgesics and clearly inhibited daily activity; $P < 0.001$; WMD –0.80, 95% CI –1.36 to –0.24); younger menarche (13.1 years in women without dysmenorrhoea v 12.6 years in women with severe dysmenorrhoea; $P < 0.01$; WMD 0.50, 95% CI 0.09 to 0.91); and cigarette smoking (41% of smokers and 26% of non-smokers experienced moderate or severe dysmenorrhoea).[9] There is also some evidence of a dose–response relationship between exposure to environmental tobacco smoke and increased incidence of dysmenorrhoea.[10]

PROGNOSIS   Primary dysmenorrhoea is a chronic recurring condition that affects most young women. Studies of the natural history of this condition are sparse. One longitudinal study in Scandinavia found that primary dysmenorrhoea often improves in the third decade of a woman's reproductive life, and is also reduced after childbirth.[9] We found no studies that reliably examined the relationship between the prognosis of secondary dysmenorrhoea and the severity of the underlying pathology, such as endometriosis.

Please refer to the Clinical Evidence website for full text and references.

Endometriosis

Search date March 2004

Neil Johnson and Cynthia Farquhar

We found no RCTs comparing medical with surgical treatments.

What are the effects of hormonal treatments given at diagnosis?

BENEFICIAL

Combined oral contraceptives or medroxyprogesterone

RCTs found that hormonal treatments at diagnosis (combined oral contraceptives, danazol, gestrinone, gonadorelin analogues, or medroxyprogesterone acetate) reduced pain attributed to endometriosis over 3–6 months of treatment, and were all similarly effective. One small RCT identified by a systematic review found that low dose combined oral contraceptive reduced dysmenorrhoea compared with goserelin during 6 months of treatment, but all women improved 6 months after stopping treatment. One additional, larger RCT found no significant difference in relief of menstrual or non-menstrual pain between combined oral contraceptives and combined oral contraceptives plus gonadorelin analogues. Adverse effects of hormonal treatments are common. One RCT found that combined oral contraceptives reduced hot flushes, insomnia, and vaginal dryness compared with gonadorelin analogues.

TRADE OFF BETWEEN BENEFITS AND HARMS

Danazol, gestrinone, or gonadorelin analogues

RCTs found that hormonal treatments at diagnosis (combined oral contraceptives, danazol, gestrinone, gonadorelin analogues, or medroxyprogesterone acetate) reduced pain attributed to endometriosis over 3–6 months of treatment, and were all similarly effective. One small RCT identified by a systematic review found that low dose combined oral contraceptive reduced dysmenorrhoea compared with goserelin during 6 months of treatment, but all women improved 6 months after stopping treatment. One additional, larger RCT found no significant difference in relief of menstrual or non-menstrual pain between combined oral contraceptives and combined oral contraceptives plus gonadorelin analogues. Adverse effects of hormonal treatments are common, and include hot flushes and bone loss with gonadorelin analogues or gestrinone and androgenic adverse effects with danazol. One RCT found that combined oral contraceptives reduced hot flushes, insomnia, and vaginal dryness compared with gonadorelin analogues.

UNKNOWN EFFECTIVENESS

Dydrogesterone

One small RCT provided insufficient evidence to compare dydrogesterone with placebo.

What are the effects of hormonal treatments before surgery?

UNKNOWN EFFECTIVENESS

Hormonal treatment before surgery

Two RCTs provided insufficient evidence on the effects of hormonal treatment before surgery in women with pain attributed to endometriosis.

◄ *What are the effects of surgical treatments?*

Combined laparoscopic ablation of endometrial deposits and uterine nerve

One RCT found limited evidence that laparoscopic ablation of endometrial deposits plus laparoscopic uterine nerve ablation reduced pain at 6 months compared with diagnostic laparoscopy, and that pain reduction persisted for up to 5 years in more than 50% of the women. Two small RCTs identified by a systematic review and one larger subsequent RCT found no significant difference between laparoscopic ablation of endometrial deposits plus laparoscopic uterine nerve ablation and laparoscopic ablation alone in rates of recurrent dysmenorrhoea at 6 months to 3 years. The subsequent RCT found no significant difference between treatments in treatment satisfaction at 1 year. However, the RCTs may have been too small to detect clinically important differences.

Laparoscopic ablation of endometrial deposits alone

We found no RCTs comparing laparoscopic ablation of endometrial deposits alone in women with pain attributed to endometriosis. Two small RCTs identified by a systematic review and one larger subsequent RCT found no significant difference between laparoscopic ablation alone and laparoscopic ablation of endometrial deposits plus laparoscopic uterine nerve ablation alone in rates of recurrent dysmenorrhoea at 6 months to 3 years. The subsequent RCT found no significant difference between treatments in treatment satisfaction at 1 year. However, the RCTs may have been too small to detect clinically important differences. We found no RCTs comparing laser versus diathermy ablation of endometrial deposits.

Laparoscopic uterine nerve ablation alone

We found no RCTs evaluating laparoscopic uterine nerve ablation alone in women with pain attributed to endometriosis.

What are the effects of hormonal treatment after conservative surgery?

Hormonal treatment after conservative surgery

RCTs found that, compared with placebo or expectant management, 6 months of hormonal treatment with danazol or gonadorelin analogues after surgery reduced pain and delayed the recurrence of pain at 12 and 24 months. Treatment for 3 months with danazol or gonadorelin analogues or treatment with combined oral contraceptives for 6 months did not seem to be effective. One RCT found that cyproterone acetate and combined oral contraceptives were similarly effective in women with modest and severe pain. One small RCT found that a levonorgestrel releasing intrauterine device inserted after surgery reduced dysmenorrhoea compared with surgery alone at 1 year. Adverse effects of hormonal treatment are common and include hot flushes and bone loss with gonadorelin analogues and androgenic adverse effects with danazol.

▶

Endometriosis

What are the effects of hormonal treatment after oophorectomy (with or without hysterectomy)?

UNKNOWN EFFECTIVENESS

Hormonal treatment after oophorectomy

One RCT in women who previously had an oophorectomy found insufficient evidence on the effects of hormone replacement therapy in recurrence of endometriosis compared with no treatment.

What are the effects of treatments for ovarian endometrioma?

LIKELY TO BE BENEFICIAL

Laparoscopic cystectomy for ovarian endometrioma (reduces pain compared to drainage)

One RCT found that laparoscopic cystectomy reduced pain caused by ovarian endometrioma at 2 years compared with laparoscopic drainage. Complication rates were similar.

DEFINITION   Endometriosis is characterised by ectopic endometrial tissue, which can cause dysmenorrhoea, dyspareunia, non-cyclical pelvic pain, and subfertility. Diagnosis is made by laparoscopy. Most endometrial deposits are found in the pelvis (ovaries, peritoneum, uterosacral ligaments, pouch of Douglas, and rectovaginal septum). Extrapelvic deposits, including those in the umbilicus and diaphragm, are rare. Severity of endometriosis is defined by the American Fertility Society: this review uses the terms mild (stage I and II), moderate (stage III), and severe (stage IV).[1] Endometriomas are cysts of endometriosis within the ovary. This review assesses dysmenorrhoea, dyspareunia, and non-cyclical pelvic pain associated with endometriosis. For subfertility associated with endometriosis see infertility and subfertility, p 535.

INCIDENCE/   In asymptomatic women, the prevalence of endometriosis is 2–22%.[2–5]
PREVALENCE   Variations in estimates of prevalence are thought to be mostly due to differences in diagnostic thresholds and criteria between studies, and in variations in childbearing age between populations, rather than underlying genetic differences. In women with dysmenorrhoea, the incidence of endometriosis is 40–60%, and in women with subfertility is 20–30%.[3,6,7] The severity of symptoms and the probability of diagnosis increase with age.[8] Incidence peaks at about 40 years of age.[9] Symptoms and laparoscopic appearance do not always correlate.[10]

AETIOLOGY/   The cause of endometriosis is unknown. Risk factors include early menarche
RISK FACTORS and late menopause. Embryonic cells may give rise to deposits in the umbilicus, whereas retrograde menstruation may deposit endometrial cells in the diaphragm.[11,12] Use of oral contraceptives reduces the risk of endometriosis, and this protective effect persists for up to 1 year after their discontinuation.[9]

PROGNOSIS   We found two RCTs in which laparoscopy was repeated after treatment in women given placebo.[13,14] Over 6–12 months, endometrial deposits resolved spontaneously in up to a third of women, deteriorated in nearly half, and were unchanged in the remainder.

Please refer to the Clinical Evidence website for full text and references.

Search date December 2003

Anne Lethaby and Beverley Vollenhoven

What are the effects of medical treatment alone?

LIKELY TO BE BENEFICIAL

Gonadorelin analogues (GnRHa) plus progestogen (no significant difference in heavy bleeding compared with GnRHa alone, but adding progestogen reduces vasomotor symptoms and hot flushes associated with GnRHa)

One small RCT found no significant difference between leuprorelin (leuprolide) acetate plus progestogen and leuprorelin acetate alone in the proportion of women who had heavy bleeding at 12 months. One small RCT found that GnRHa plus medroxyprogesterone acetate significantly reduced vasomotor symptoms over 12 months compared with GnRHa alone. One small RCT found that leuprorelin acetate plus progestogen significantly reduced the proportion of women with hot flushes over 24 weeks compared with leuprorelin acetate alone.

Gonadorelin analogues plus tibolone (no significant difference in fibroid symptoms compared with GnRHa alone but adding tibolone reduces hot flushes and prevents loss in bone mineral density associated with GnRHa)

Two small RCTs found no significant difference between GnRHa alone and GnRHa plus tibolone in fibroid related symptoms or uterine and fibroid size. They found that adding tibolone reduced hot flushes, vaginal dryness, and night sweats and prevented loss in bone mineral density.

TRADE OFF BETWEEN BENEFITS AND HARMS

Gonadorelin analogues alone

RCTs found that GnRHa reduced fibroid related symptoms compared with placebo, but were associated with important adverse effects. Two RCTs found that GnRHa increased amenorrhoea compared with placebo after about 3 months. One RCT provided insufficient evidence to compare nafarelin versus buserelin. One RCT found that higher doses of nafarelin increased amenorrhoea at 16 weeks compared with lower doses. Two RCTs found that nafarelin reduced bone density from baseline after 16 weeks' treatment compared with placebo, but that bone density returned to pretreatment levels 6 months after treatment was stopped. Two RCTs found that hot flushes were more common with nafarelin than with placebo or buserelin. One RCT found that hot flushes and sweating were more common with goserelin than placebo.

UNKNOWN EFFECTIVENESS

Gonadorelin analogues plus combined oestrogen–progestogen (insufficient evidence on effects compared with GnRHa plus progestogen)

One small RCT provided insufficient evidence to compare GnRHa plus combined oestrogen–progestogen hormone replacement therapy versus GnRHa plus progestogen hormone replacement therapy.

Gonadorelin analogues plus raloxifene (insufficient evidence on effects compared with GnRHa alone)

One RCT found that adding raloxifene to GnRHa reduced fibroid size compared with GnRHa alone. It found no significant difference in fibroid related symptoms or hot flushes.

Fibroids (uterine myomatosis, leiomyomas)

Non-steroidal anti-inflammatory drugs

Two small RCTs provided insufficient evidence to assess non-steroidal anti-inflammatory drugs in women with fibroids.

Gestrinone; levonorgestrel intrauterine system; mifepristone

We found no RCTs on the effects of these interventions.

In women scheduled for fibroid surgery, what are the effects of preoperative medical treatments?

LIKELY TO BE BENEFICIAL

Gonadorelin analogues

One systematic review found that GnRHa for at least 3 months before fibroid surgery improved preoperative haemoglobin concentration and haematocrit, and reduced uterine and pelvic symptoms compared with placebo or no pretreatment. Preoperative gonadorelin also reduced the rate of vertical incisions during laparotomy. Women having hysterectomy were more likely to have a vaginal rather than an abdominal procedure after GnRHa pretreatment compared with placebo or no pretreatment. Preoperative goserelin reduced intra-operative blood loss although the difference was small and the clinical importance is uncertain. One subsequent RCT found no significant difference between preoperative triptorelin and immediate surgery in intra-operative blood loss. One small RCT found that GnRHa combined with endometrial resection reduced the need for further treatment (either medical or surgical) over 1 year compared with GnRHa alone. However, preoperative GnRHa is associated with adverse hypo-oestrogenic effects, such as hot flushes, vaginal symptoms, and sweating, and women receiving GnRHa were more likely to withdraw from treatment because of adverse effects.

What are the effects of surgical treatments?

BENEFICIAL

Laparoscopic myomectomy (maintains fertility compared to hysterectomy; reduces recovery time and postoperative pain compared with abdominal myomectomy)

Two RCTs found limited evidence that laparosopic myomectomy reduced postoperative pain, fever, and recovery time compared to abdominal myomectomy. We found no RCTs comparing laparoscopic myomectomy versus total abdominal, vaginal, or laparoscopic hysterectomy, but the main benefit of myomectomy compared with hysterectomy is that it maintains fertility.

LIKELY TO BE BENEFICIAL

Laparoscopically assisted vaginal hysterectomy (reduces recovery time and postoperative pain compared with total abdominal hysterectomy, but increases operating time and blood loss compared with total vaginal hysterectomy)

Two RCTs found that women having laparoscopically assisted vaginal hysterectomy had shorter recovery times and less postoperative pain compared with women having total abdominal hysterectomy. One RCT found that women having laparoscopically assisted vaginal hysterectomy had longer operating time and more blood loss than women having total vaginal hysterectomy.

Total abdominal hysterectomy (reduces fibroid related symptoms compared with no treatment)*

We found no RCTs comparing total abdominal hysterectomy versus no treatment or sham surgery. An RCT is unlikely to be conducted. There is consensus that total abdominal hysterectomy is superior to no treatment in reducing fibroid related symptoms. RCTs found that women having total abdominal hysterectomy had longer surgery, more blood loss, pain and fever, longer hospital stay, later return to work, and less satisfaction than women having total vaginal hysterectomy. Two RCTs found that women having total abdominal hysterectomy had longer recovery times and more postoperative pain but shorter operating times and less blood loss than women having laparoscopically assisted vaginal hysterectomy. One RCT found that women having total abdominal hysterectomy had more postoperative fever, longer hospital stay, and recovery times than women having total laparoscopic hysterectomy.

Total laparoscopic hysterectomy (reduces postoperative fever, hospital stay, and recovery time compared with total abdominal hysterectomy)

One RCT found that women having total laparoscopic hysterectomy had less postoperative fever, shorter hospital stay, and shorter recovery times compared with women having total abdominal hysterectomy.

Total vaginal hysterectomy (reduces operation time, blood loss, pain, fever, and hospital stay compared with total abdominal hysterectomy and increases satisfaction with operation)

Two RCTs found that women having total vaginal hysterectomy had shorter operation time, less blood loss, pain and fever, shorter hospital stay, earlier return to work, and greater satisfaction than women having total abdominal hysterectomy. One RCT found that women having total vaginal hysterectomy had shorter operation times and less blood loss than women having laparoscopically assisted vaginal hysterectomy.

*Based on consensus. RCTs unlikely to be conducted.

UNKNOWN EFFECTIVENESS

Thermal balloon ablation

We found no RCTs comparing thermal balloon ablation versus non-surgical treatment or hysterectomy. One RCT compared thermal balloon ablation versus rollerball endometrial ablation in women with fibroids smaller than the average size of a 12 week pregnancy, all of whom had been pretreated with gonadorelin analogues. It found no significant difference between thermal balloon and rollerball ablation in amenorrhoea rates, pictorial bleeding assessment chart score, haemoglobin, or hysterectomy rates at 12 months. It found that thermal balloon ablation reduced operation time and intraoperative complication rate compared with rollerball ablation. About one third of women reported being "not very satisfied" with either operation.

DEFINITION   Fibroids (uterine leiomyomas) are benign tumours of the smooth muscle cells of the uterus. Women with fibroids can be asymptomatic or may present with menorrhagia (30%), pelvic pain with or without dysmenorrhoea or pressure symptoms (34%), infertility (27%), and recurrent pregnancy loss (3%).[1] Much of the data describing the relationship between the presence of fibroids and symptoms are based on uncontrolled studies that have assessed the effect of myomectomy on the presenting symptoms.[2] The prevalence of fibroids in infertile women can be as high as 13%, but no direct causal relationship between fibroids and infertility has been established.[3]

Fibroids (uterine myomatosis, leiomyomas)

INCIDENCE/ PREVALENCE
The reported incidence of fibroids varies from 5.4–77.0% depending on the method of diagnosis (the gold standard is histological evidence). A random sample of 335 Swedish women aged 25–40 years was reported to have an incidence of fibroids of 5.4% (95% CI 3.0% to 7.8%) based on transvaginal ultrasound examination.[4] The prevalence of these tumours increased with age (age 25–32 years: 3.3%, 95% CI 0.7% to 6.0%; 33–40 years: 7.8%, 95% CI 3.6% to 12.0%).[4] Another large case control study found that the rate of fibroids was higher in women aged less than 50 years; it found a rate of pathologically confirmed fibroids of 4.24/1000 woman years in women aged 50 years or more compared with 6.20/1000 in women aged 45–50 years, 4.63/1000 in women aged 40–45 years, 2.67/1000 in women aged 35–40 years, 0.96/1000 in women aged 30–35 years and 0.31/1000 in women aged 25–30 years.[5] Based on postmortem examination, 50% of women were found to have these tumours.[6] Gross serial sectioning at 2 mm intervals of 100 consecutive hysterectomy specimens revealed the presence of fibroids in 50/68 [73%] premenopausal women and 27/32 [84%] postmenopausal women.[7] These women were having hysterectomies for reasons other than fibroids. The incidence of fibroids in black women is three times greater than that in white women, based on ultrasound or hysterectomy diagnosis.[8] Submucosal fibroids have been diagnosed in 6–34% of women having a hysteroscopy for abnormal bleeding, and in 2–7% of women having infertility investigations.[9]

AETIOLOGY/ RISK FACTORS
The cause of fibroids is unknown. It is known that each fibroid is of monoclonal origin and arises independently.[10,11] Factors thought to be involved include the sex steroid hormones oestrogen and progesterone as well as the insulin-like growth factors, epidermal growth factor and transforming growth factor. Risk factors for fibroid growth include nulliparity and obesity. There is a risk reduction to a fifth with five term pregnancies, compared with nulliparous women (P < 0.001).[5] Obesity increases the risk of fibroid development by 21% with each 10 kg weight gain (P = 0.008).[5] The combined oral contraceptive pill also reduces the risk of fibroids with increasing duration of use (women who have taken oral contraceptives for 4–6 years compared with women who have never taken oral contraceptives: OR 0.8, 95% CI 0.5 to 1.2; women who have taken oral contraceptives for ≥ 7 years compared with women who have never taken oral contraceptives: OR 0.5, 95% CI 0.3 to 0.9).[12] Women who have had injections containing 150 mg depot medroxyprogesterone acetate also have a reduced incidence compared with women who have never had injections of this drug (OR 0.44, 95% CI 0.36 to 0.55).[13]

PROGNOSIS
There are few data on the long term untreated prognosis of these tumours, particularly in women who are asymptomatic at diagnosis. One small case control study reported that in a group of 106 women treated with observation alone over 1 year there was no significant change in symptoms and quality of life over that time.[14] Fibroids tend to shrink or fibrose after the menopause.[5]

Please refer to the Clinical Evidence website for full text and references.

What are the effects of non-surgical treatments in women with genital prolapse?

Pelvic floor muscle exercises

We found no RCTs or observational studies of sufficient quality examining the effects of pelvic floor muscle exercises on the symptoms of genital prolapse.

Vaginal oestrogen

We found no systematic review or RCTs on the effects of vaginal oestrogen.

Vaginal pessaries*

We found no RCTs or observational studies of sufficient quality examining effects of vaginal pessaries on the symptoms of genital prolapse. However, consensus opinion suggests that they are effective for short term relief of genital prolapse prior to surgery, or in the long term if surgery is contraindicated.

*Consensus regards vaginal pessaries as effective.

DEFINITION	Genital prolapse (also known as pelvic organ prolapse) refers to uterine, uterovaginal, or vaginal prolapse. Genital prolapse results from loss of muscle support in the pelvic region. In uterine prolapse the uterus descends into the vaginal canal with the cervix at its leading edge; this may in turn pull down the vagina, in which case it may be referred to as uterovaginal prolapse. In vaginal prolapse one or more regions of the vaginal wall protrude into the vaginal canal. Vaginal prolapse is classified according to the region of the vaginal wall that is affected: a cystocoele involves the anterior upper vaginal wall, urethrocoele the lower anterior vaginal wall, rectocoele the posterior vaginal wall, and enterocoele the upper posterior vaginal wall. After hysterectomy, the apex of the vagina may prolapse as a vault prolapse. This usually pulls down the anterior and posterior walls as well. The two main systems for grading the severity of genital prolapse, the Baden–Walker halfway system[1] and the Pelvic Organ Prolapse Quantification (POPQ) system,[2] are summarised in Table 1❶. Mild genital prolapse may be asymptomatic. Symptoms of genital prolapse are mainly non specific. Common symptoms include pelvic heaviness, genital bulge, and difficulties during sexual intercourse, such as pain or loss of vaginal sensation. Symptoms that may be more commonly associated with specific forms of prolapse include urinary incontinence, which is associated with cystocoele; incomplete urinary emptying, which is associated with cystocoele or uterine prolapse, or both; and need to apply digital pressure to the perineum or posterior vaginal wall for defaecation, which is associated with rectocoele.[3]
INCIDENCE/ PREVALENCE	Prevalence estimates vary widely, depending on the population and the way in which women were recruited into studies. One study conducted in the USA (497 women aged 18–82 years attending a routine general gynaecology clinic) found that 93.6% had some degree of genital prolapse (43.3% POPQ stage 1, 47.7% POPQ stage 2, 2.6% POPQ stage 3, and 0% POPQ stage 4).[4] In that study the incidence of clinically relevant prolapse (POPQ stage 2 or greater) was found to increase with advancing parity: non-parous, 14.6%; one to three births, 48%; and more than three births, 71.2%. One Swedish study (487 women) found that 30.8% of women between the ages of 20 and 59 years had some degree of genital prolapse on clinical assessment.[5] The prevalence of genital prolapse increased with age, from 6.6% in women aged 20–29 years to 55.6% in women aged 50–59 years. Prevalence of genital ▶

Genital prolapse

prolapse was also higher in parous women (44%) than in non-parous women (5.8%). A cross-sectional study (241 perimenopausal women aged 45–55 years seeking to enter a trial of hormone replacement therapy) found that 23% had POPQ stage 1 genital prolapse, 4% had POPQ stage 2 prolapse, and no women had POPQ stage 3 or 4 prolapse.[6] One cross-sectional study conducted in the UK (285 perimenopausal and postmenopausal women attending a menopause clinic with climacteric symptoms) found that 20% had some degree of uterovaginal or vault prolapse, 51% some degree of anterior wall vaginal prolapse, and 27% some degree of posterior wall vaginal prolapse.[7] Severe prolapse (equivalent to POPQ stage 3 or 4) was found in 6% of women. One prospective study (412 postmenopausal women aged 50–79 years) found that the baseline prevalence of cystocoele was 24.6% (for grades 1, 2, and 3 the prevalences were 14.4%, 9.5%, and 0.7%, respectively), the baseline prevalence of rectocoele was 12.9% (for grades 1 and 2 the prevalences were 7.8% and 5.1%, respectively), and the baseline prevalence of uterine prolapse was 3.8% (for grades 1 and 2 the prevalences were 3.3% and 0.6%, respectively).[8] Among women who entered the study the annual incidences of cystocoele, rectocoele, and uterine prolapse were 9%, 6%, and 2%, respectively.

AETIOLOGY/ RISK FACTORS One case control study found that the strongest risk factors for severe (POPQ stages 3 or 4) genital prolapse are increasing age (OR 1.12 for each additional year, 95% CI 1.09 to 1.15), increasing weight of largest baby delivered vaginally (OR 1.24 for each additional pound, 95% CI 1.06 to 1.44), previous hysterectomy (OR 2.37, 95% CI 1.16 to 4.86), and previous surgery for genital prolapse (OR 5.09, 95% CI 1.49 to 17.26).[10] The study did not find a significant association between severe genital prolapse and chronic medical conditions such as obesity, hypertension, or chronic obstructive pulmonary disease.

PROGNOSIS We found no reliable information about the natural history of untreated mild genital prolapse (POPQ stages 1 and 2, Baden–Walker grades 1 and 2). We found one prospective study on the progression of genital prolapse in women who were treated or untreated with hormone replacement therapy (oestrogen + progesterone).[8] However, the results were not reported separately by treatment group and therefore they may not apply to untreated women. In addition, the investigators used an examination technique whose reliability, reproducibility, and ability to discriminate between absence of prolapse and mild prolapse was not known. It found that, over 1 year, cystocoeles progressed from grade 1 to grades 2–3 in 9% of cases, regressed from grades 2–3 to grade 0 in 9%, and regressed from grade 1 to grade 0 in 23%. Rectocoeles progressed from grade 1 to grades 2–3 in 1%, but regressed from grades 2–3 to grade 0 in 3%, and from grade 1 to grade 0 in 2%. Uterine prolapse regressed from grade 1 to grade 0 in 48%. The incidence of morbidity associated with genital prolapse is also difficult to estimate. The annual incidence of hospital admission for prolapse in the UK has been estimated at 2.04 per 1000 women under the age of 60 years.[9] Genital prolapse is also a major cause of gynaecological surgery.

Please refer to the Clinical Evidence website for full text and references.

What are the effects of treatments for infertility caused by ovulation disorders?

LIKELY TO BE BENEFICIAL

Clomifene

One systematic review has found that clomifene (clomiphene) increases pregnancy rate compared with placebo in women who ovulate infrequently. Four other studies, including two RCTs, have found no significant difference in ovulation or pregnancy rates between clomifene and tamoxifen. One RCT found that clomifene plus metformin increased pregnancy rates after 6 months' treatment compared with clomifene alone.

TRADE OFF BETWEEN BENEFITS AND HARMS

Gonadotrophins

We found no RCTs comparing gonadotrophins versus placebo or clomifene. One systematic review found that pregnancy rates with human menopausal gonadotrophins or urofollitropin (urofollitrophin, urinary follicle stimulating hormone) ranged from 10–12%. The review found no significant difference in pregnancy rates between treatments. Two RCTs found that pregnancy rates with follitropin (recombinant follicle stimulating hormone) or urofollitropin ranged from 24–27%. It found no significant difference between treatments. The review found that urofollitropin reduced the risk of ovarian hyperstimulation syndrome compared with human menopausal gonadotrophins, although this was confined to women who were not treated with concomitant gonadotrophin releasing hormone analogues. One systematic review and one subsequent RCT found no significant difference in pregnancy rates between gonadotrophins and laparoscopic ovarian drilling, but found that gonadotrophins increased rates of multiple pregnancies. Observational evidence suggests that gonadotrophins may be associated with an increased risk of non-invasive ovarian tumours and multiple pregnancies.

UNKNOWN EFFECTIVENESS

Cyclofenil

One RCT provided insufficient evidence about the effects of cyclofenil in women with ovulatory disorders.

Laparoscopic ovarian drilling

We found no RCTs comparing laparoscopic ovarian drilling versus no treatment. One systematic review and one subsequent small RCT found no significant difference in pregnancy rates between laparoscopic ovarian drilling and gonadotrophins. They found that laparoscopic ovarian drilling reduced rates of multiple pregnancies.

Pulsatile gonadotrophin releasing hormone

One systematic review of small, weak RCTs provided insufficient evidence to assess pulsatile gonadotrophin releasing hormone treatment.

What are the effects of treatments for tubal infertility?

BENEFICIAL

In vitro fertilisation

We found no RCTs comparing in vitro fertilisation versus no treatment. RCTs are unlikely to be conducted. Observational evidence in the UK and the USA suggests an average live birth rate of 22–25% per in vitro fertilisation cycle if intracytoplasmic sperm injection is taken into account. One RCT found that immediate compared with delayed in vitro fertilisation increased pregnancy and live birth rates. Three RCTs found no significant difference in numbers of live births between in vitro fertilisation and intracytoplasmic sperm injection. Observational evidence suggests that adverse effects associated with in vitro fertilisation include multiple pregnancies and ovarian hyperstimulation syndrome.

LIKELY TO BE BENEFICIAL

Tubal flushing with oil soluble media

One systematic review found that tubal flushing with oil soluble media increased pregnancy rates compared with no intervention. It found that tubal flushing with oil soluble media increased the live birth rate compared with flushing with water soluble media.

Tubal surgery before in vitro fertilisation

One systematic review in women with hydrosalpinges undergoing in vitro fertilisation has found that tubal surgery increases pregnancy and live birth rates compared with no treatment or medical treatment. One systematic review found no significant difference in pregnancy rates among different types of tubal surgery. One systematic review found no significant difference in pregnancy rates between tubal surgery plus additional treatments to prevent adhesion formation (steroids, dextran, noxytioline) and tubal surgery alone. Another systematic review provided insufficient evidence to assess postoperative hydrotubation or second look laparoscopy.

UNKNOWN EFFECTIVENESS

Selective salpingography plus tubal catheterisation

We found no RCTs on the effects of selective salpingography plus tubal catheterisation.

Tubal flushing with water soluble media

One systematic review identified no RCTs comparing tubal flushing with water soluble media versus no intervention. It found that tubal flushing with water soluble media decreased live birth rate compared with flushing with oil soluble media.

What are the effects of treatment for infertility associated with endometriosis?

LIKELY TO BE BENEFICIAL

Intrauterine insemination plus gonadotrophins

One RCT found that intrauterine insemination plus gonadotrophins increased live birth rates compared with no treatment. A second RCT found no significant difference in birth rates between intrauterine insemination plus pituitary down regulation plus gonadotrophins and expectant management, but it is likely to have been underpowered to detect a clinically important difference. A third RCT found that intrauterine insemination plus gonadotrophins increased pregnancy rates after the first treatment cycle compared with intrauterine insemination alone.

In vitro fertilisation

We found no RCTs comparing in vitro fertilisation versus no treatment in women with endometriosis related infertility. RCTs are unlikely to be conducted. Observational evidence in the UK and the USA suggests an average live birth rate of 22–25% per in vitro fertilisation cycle if intracytoplasmic sperm injection is taken into account. Observational studies found inconclusive evidence about whether in vitro fertilisation is as effective in women with endometriosis as in women with tubal infertility.

Laparoscopic ablation of endometrial deposits

We found no RCTs comparing laparoscopic surgery versus no treatment or versus ovarian suppression. One systematic review has found that laparoscopic resection or ablation of endometrial deposits increases live birth rates and ongoing pregnancy rates compared with diagnostic laparoscopy. Operative complications were not increased with laparoscopic surgery.

LIKELY TO BE INEFFECTIVE OR HARMFUL

Drug Induced ovarian suppression

One systematic review found no significant difference in pregnancy rates between drugs that induce ovarian suppression and placebo. The review found that ovulation suppression agents (medroxyprogesterone, gestrinone, combined oral contraceptives, and gonadotrophin releasing hormone analogues) cause adverse effects, including weight gain, hot flushes, and osteoporosis, and that danazol may cause dose related weight gain and androgenic effects.

What are the effects of treatments for male factor infertility?

BENEFICIAL

Intracytoplasmic sperm injection plus in vitro fertilisation

We found no RCTs of intracytoplasmic sperm injection plus in vitro fertilisation that assessed pregnancy and live birth rates. Observational evidence in the UK suggests an average live birth rate of 22% per in vitro fertilisation cycle if intracytoplasmic sperm injection is taken into account.

Intrauterine insemination

Two systematic reviews have found that intrauterine insemination increases pregnancy rates per cycle compared with intracervical insemination or timed intercourse.

UNKNOWN EFFECTIVENESS

Donor insemination

We found no RCTs on the effects of donor insemination. Observational evidence suggests an average live birth rate of 11%, but it is sometimes unclear whether ovarian stimulation was used in addition to donor insemination.

In vitro fertilisation versus gamete intrafallopian transfer

One small RCT provided insufficient evidence to compare in vitro fertilisation versus gamete intrafallopian transfer.

Women's health

What are the effects of treatments for unexplained infertility?

BENEFICIAL

Intrauterine insemination plus gonadotrophins

Two systematic reviews and one subsequent RCT have found that intrauterine insemination plus gonadotrophins increases pregnancy rates compared with timed intercourse or intracervical insemination. One systematic review found no significant difference between intrauterine insemination and timed intercourse or intracervical insemination in pregnancy rates. However, it found that adding gonadotrophins to any of the three interventions increased pregnancy rates per cycle. One systematic review and one subsequent RCT have found that fallopian tube sperm perfusion increases pregnancy rates compared with intrauterine insemination. One systematic review found no significant difference in live birth rate between intrauterine insemination with or without ovarian stimulation and in vitro fertilisation.

LIKELY TO BE BENEFICIAL

Clomifene

One systematic review found limited evidence that clomifene (clomiphene) increased rates of pregnancy per cycle compared with placebo.

Fallopian tube sperm perfusion

One systematic review and one subsequent RCT have found that fallopian tube sperm perfusion increases pregnancy rates compared with intrauterine insemination.

UNKNOWN EFFECTIVENESS

Gamete intrafallopian transfer

We found no RCTs comparing gamete intrafallopian transfer versus no treatment. RCTs found conflicting effects on pregnancy rates of gamete intrafallopian transfer versus other treatments (intrauterine insemination, timed intercourse, and in vitro fertilisation).

In vitro fertilisation

Observational evidence in the UK and the USA suggests an average live birth rate of 22–25% per in vitro fertilisation cycle. However, one systematic review identified one RCT in couples with unexplained infertility that found no significant difference in pregnancy rates between in vitro fertilisation and expectant management. RCTs included in the review found no significant difference in live birth rate between in vitro fertilisation and either gamete intrafallopian transfer or intrauterine insemination with or without ovarian stimulation.

DEFINITION Normal fertility has been defined as achieving a pregnancy within 2 years by regular sexual intercourse.[1] However, many define infertility as the failure to conceive after 1 year of unprotected intercourse. Infertility can be primary, in couples who have never conceived, or secondary, in couples who have previously conceived. Infertile couples include those who are sterile (who will never achieve a natural pregnancy) and those who are subfertile (who could eventually achieve a natural pregnancy).

INCIDENCE/ PREVALENCE Although there is no evidence of a major change in the prevalence of infertility, many more couples are seeking help than previously. Currently, about 1/7 couples in industrialised countries will seek medical advice for infertility.[2] Rates of primary infertility vary widely between countries, ranging from 10% in Africa to about 6% in North America and Europe.[1] Reported rates of secondary infertility are less reliable.

AETIOLOGY/ RISK FACTORS   In the UK, nearly a third of infertility cases are unexplained.[3] The rest are caused by ovulatory failure (27%), low sperm count or quality (19%), tubal damage (14%), endometriosis (5%), and other causes (5%).[3]

PROGNOSIS   In developed countries, 80–90% of couples attempting to conceive are successful after 1 year and 95% after 2 years.[3] The chances of becoming pregnant vary with the cause and duration of infertility, the woman's age, the couple's previous pregnancy history, and the availability of different treatment options.[2,4] For the first 2–3 years of unexplained infertility, cumulative conception rates remain high (27–46%) but decrease with increasing age of the woman and duration of infertility.[4] The background rates of spontaneous pregnancy in infertile couples can be calculated from longitudinal studies of infertile couples who have been observed without treatment.[4]

Please refer to the Clinical Evidence website for full text and references.

Menopausal symptoms

Search date March 2004

Edward Morris and Janice Rymer

What are the effects of medical treatments?

BENEFICIAL

Progestogens alone

Five RCTs found that progestogens alone reduced vasomotor symptoms compared with placebo and one RCT found no significant difference in vasomotor symptoms between progestogens and placebo. One RCT found no significant difference in vasomotor symptoms between progesterone alone and oestrogen alone. We found no RCTs examining effects of progestogens alone on urogenital symptoms. One RCT found no significant difference in psychological symptoms or quality of life between progesterone and placebo.

Tibolone

Two RCTs found that tibolone improved vasomotor symptoms compared with placebo. One RCT found that tibolone improved sexual function compared with placebo. Two RCTs provided limited evidence that tibolone was not as effective for reducing vasomotor symptoms as oestrogen plus progestogen. Two RCTs found that tibolone improved sexual function compared with oestrogen plus progestogen. We found no RCTs assessing psychological symptoms or quality of life.

TRADE OFF BETWEEN BENEFITS AND HARMS

Oestrogens alone (improved menopausal symptoms but increased risk of breast cancer, endometrial cancer, stroke, and venous thromboembolism after long term use)

Systematic reviews and subsequent RCTs found that oestrogen improved vasomotor symptoms, urogenital symptoms, psychological symptoms, and quality of life in the short term compared with placebo. However, important adverse effects of oestrogen include increased risk of breast cancer, endometrial cancer, stroke, and venous thromboembolic disease. Adding progestogen reduces the risk of endometrial hyperplasia.

Oestrogens plus progestogens (improved menopausal symptoms but increased risk of breast cancer, stroke, and venous thromboembolism after long term use)

One systematic review and subsequent RCTs found that oestrogen plus progestogens improved vasomotor symptoms, urogenital symptoms, and psychological symptoms in the short term compared with placebo. However, important adverse effects include increased risk of breast cancer, stroke, and venous thromboembolic disease. Two RCTs provided limited evidence that oestrogen plus progestogen reduced vasomotor symptoms compared with tibolone, but that tibolone improved sexual function compared with oestrogen plus progestogen.

UNKNOWN EFFECTIVENESS

Antidepressants

We found no RCTs on the effects of antidepressants on menopausal symptoms.

Clonidine

One small RCT found that transdermal clonidine reduced the number and intensity of hot flushes after 8 weeks compared with placebo. However, we were unable to draw reliable conclusions from this study. We found no RCTs that assessed the effects of clonidine on sexual function, psychological symptoms, or quality of life. ▶

Phyto-oestrogens

Nine RCTs provided no consistent evidence that phyto-oestrogens reduced vaso-motor or other menopausal symptoms compared with placebo. We found no RCTs that assessed quality of life.

Testosterone

Small RCTs provided no consistent evidence about the effects of testosterone plus oestrogens on vasomotor symptoms or sexual function compared with oestrogen alone or placebo. We found no RCTs that assessed psychological symptoms or quality of life.

DEFINITION Menopause is defined as the end of the last menstrual period. A woman is deemed to be postmenopausal 1 year after her last period. For practical purposes, most women are diagnosed as menopausal after 1 year of amenorrhoea. Menopausal symptoms often begin in the perimenopausal years. The complex of menopausal symptomatology includes vasomotor symptoms (hot flushes), sleeplessness, mood changes, reduction in energy levels, loss of libido, vaginal dryness, and urinary symptoms.

INCIDENCE/ PREVALENCE In the UK, the mean age for the start of the menopause is 50 years and 9 months. The median onset of the perimenopause is 45.5–47.5 years. One Scottish survey (6096 women aged 45–54 years) found that 84% of women had experienced at least one of the classic menopausal symptoms, with 45% finding one or more symptoms to be a problem.[1]

AETIOLOGY/ RISK FACTORS Urogenital symptoms of menopause are caused by decreased oestrogen concentrations, but the cause of vasomotor symptoms and psychological effects is complex and remains unclear.

PROGNOSIS Menopause is a physiological event. Timing of the natural menopause in healthy women may be determined genetically. Although endocrine changes are permanent, menopausal symptoms such as hot flushes, which are experienced by about 70% of women, usually resolve with time.[2] Some symptoms, however, such as genital atrophy, may remain the same or worsen.

Please refer to the Clinical Evidence website for full text and references.

Menorrhagia

Search date October 2003

Kirsten Duckitt and Keri McCully

What are the effects of treatments?

BENEFICIAL

Endometrial thinning before hysteroscopic surgery

One systematic review has found that preoperative gonadorelin (gonadotrophin releasing hormone) analogues reduce moderate or heavy periods and increase amenorrhoea compared with placebo, no preoperative treatment, or preoperative danazol. We found insufficient evidence about effects of preoperative danazol or progestogens compared with placebo or no preoperative treatment.

Hysterectomy (v endometrial destruction) after medical failure

Systematic reviews have found that hysterectomy reduces menstrual blood loss and the number of women requiring further operations, and increases satisfaction compared with endometrial destruction. RCTs found no differences in effectiveness between different types of hysterectomy. One large cohort study reported major or minor complications in about a third of women undergoing hysterectomy.

Non-steroidal anti-inflammatory drugs

One systematic review has found that non-steroidal anti-inflammatory drugs reduce mean menstrual blood loss compared with placebo. One systematic review found no significant difference in menstrual blood loss between mefenamic acid and naproxen, or between non-steroidal anti-inflammatory drugs and oral progestogens, oral contraceptives, or progesterone releasing intrauterine devices.

Tranexamic acid

Systematic reviews have found that tranexamic acid reduces menstrual blood loss compared with placebo or other drugs (oral progestogens, mefenamic acid, etamsylate, flurbiprofen, and diclofenac). Adverse effects of tranexamic acid include leg cramps and nausea, which occur in about a third of women using this drug. One long term population based observational study found no evidence that tranexamic acid increases the risk of thromboembolism.

LIKELY TO BE BENEFICIAL

Hysteroscopic versus non-hysteroscopic destruction after medical failure

One systematic review found that hysteroscopic methods of endometrial destruction increased amenorrhoea at 12 months compared with non-hysteroscopic methods. We found no consistent evidence of a difference in amenorrhoea or satisfaction rates among different types of hysteroscopic procedure. RCTs found that complications, such as infection, haemorrhage, or uterine perforation occurred in up to 15% of women undergoing endometrial destruction.

TRADE OFF BETWEEN BENEFITS AND HARMS

Danazol

Systematic reviews found limited evidence that danazol reduced blood loss compared with placebo, luteal phase oral progestogens, mefenamic acid, naproxen, or oral contraceptives, but found that danazol increased adverse effects compared with either non-steroidal anti-inflammatory drugs or oral progestogens. ▶

◀ **UNKNOWN EFFECTIVENESS**

Combined oral contraceptives

One systematic review found insufficient evidence about effects of oral contraceptives in women with menorrhagia.

Endometrial resection versus medical treatment

One systematic review and one additional RCT found no consistent evidence of a difference in blood loss or satisfaction between transcervical endometrial resection and medical treatment. RCTs found that complications, such as infection, haemorrhage, or uterine perforation occurred in up to 15% of women undergoing endometrial destruction.

Etamsylate

We found insufficient evidence from one systematic review about effects of etamsylate compared with placebo, mefenamic acid, aminocaproic acid, or tranexamic acid.

Intrauterine progestogens

We found no systematic review or RCTs comparing intrauterine progestogens versus placebo. Two systematic reviews and three subsequent RCTs found conflicting evidence about menstrual blood loss, satisfaction rates, and quality of life scores with levonorgestrel releasing intrauterine devices compared with other treatments (endometrial resection, thermal balloon ablation, norethisterone, medical treatment, non-steroidal anti-inflammatory drugs, and hysterectomy).

Dilatation and curettage after medical failure; gonadorelin (gonadotrophin releasing hormone) analogues; myomectomy after medical failure

We found no RCTs on the effects of these interventions.

UNLIKELY TO BE BENEFICIAL

Oral progestogens (longer cycle)

We found no RCTs comparing oral progestogens versus placebo. One RCT identified by a systematic review found no significant difference in menstrual blood loss between a longer treatment cycle of oral progestogen and a levonorgestrel releasing intrauterine device.

LIKELY TO BE INEFFECTIVE OR HARMFUL

Oral progestogens in luteal phase only

We found no RCTs comparing oral progestogens versus placebo. One systematic review has found that luteal phase oral progestogens increase mean menstrual blood loss compared with danazol, tranexamic acid, or a progesterone releasing intrauterine device.

DEFINITION   Menorrhagia is defined as heavy but regular menstrual bleeding. Idiopathic ovulatory menorrhagia is regular heavy bleeding in the absence of recognisable pelvic pathology or a general bleeding disorder. Objective menorrhagia is taken to be a total menstrual blood loss of 80 mL or more in each menstruation.[1] Subjectively, menorrhagia may be defined as a complaint of regular excessive menstrual blood loss occurring over several consecutive cycles in a woman of reproductive years.

INCIDENCE/   In the UK, 5% of women (aged 30–49 years) consult their general practitioner
PREVALENCE   each year with menorrhagia.[2] In New Zealand, 2–4% of primary care consultations by premenopausal women are for menstrual problems.[3]

Menorrhagia

AETIOLOGY/ RISK FACTORS Idiopathic ovulatory menorrhagia is thought to be caused by disordered prostaglandin production within the endometrium.[4] Prostaglandins may also be implicated in menorrhagia associated with uterine fibroids, adenomyosis, or the presence of an intrauterine device. Fibroids have been reported in 10% of women with menorrhagia (80–100 mL/cycle) and 40% of those with severe menorrhagia (≥ 200 mL/cycle).[5]

PROGNOSIS Menorrhagia limits normal activities and causes iron deficiency anaemia in two thirds of women proved to have objective menorrhagia.[1,6,7] One in five of all women in the UK and one in three women in the USA have a hysterectomy before the age of 60 years; menorrhagia is the main presenting problem in at least 50% of these women.[8–10] About 50% of the women who have a hysterectomy for menorrhagia are found to have a normal uterus.[11]

Please refer to the Clinical Evidence website for full text and references.

We found insufficient evidence on the effects of any treatments on quality of life.

What are the effects of surgical treatments for ovarian cancer that is advanced at first presentation?

UNKNOWN EFFECTIVENESS

Primary surgery versus no surgery; primary surgery plus chemotherapy versus chemotherapy alone

We found no RCTs.

Routine interval debulking after primary surgery plus chemotherapy

One RCT found that interval debulking after primary surgery plus chemotherapy improved overall survival over about 3.5 years compared with chemotherapy alone. A second RCT found that interval debulking had no effect on survival, but it was probably underpowered to detect a clinically important effect.

UNLIKELY TO BE BENEFICIAL

Routine second look surgery

Two RCTs found no evidence that routine second look surgery improved overall survival compared with watchful waiting in women undergoing chemotherapy after primary surgery for advanced ovarian cancer.

What are the effects of cytotoxic chemotherapy for ovarian cancer that is advanced at first presentation?

BENEFICIAL

Adding a single platinum agent to a non-platinum combination regimen

One systematic review (4 RCTs, 1024 women) found that adding a platinum agent to a non-platinum combination regimen reduced mortality compared with the non-platinum regimen alone.

Adding a taxane (paclitaxel) to a platinum regimen

One systematic review and one additional RCT have found that adding paclitaxel to platinum based chemotherapy significantly improves progression free survival and overall survival after primary surgery for advanced ovarian cancer.

Platinum based chemotherapy (at least as effective as non-platinum regimens)

A systematic review and subsequent RCTs have found that platinum based regimens are at least as effective as non-platinum regimens, and that adding a platinum compound to a non-platinum combination regimen improves survival.

LIKELY TO BE BENEFICIAL

Single agent platinum regimens (as effective as combination platinum chemotherapy, but with fewer adverse effects and better than single agent non-platinum regimens)

One systematic review and three subsequent RCTs found that single agent platinum based regimens were at least as effective for progression free or overall ▶

Ovarian cancer

survival as combination platinum regimens, and had fewer adverse effects. One RCT found that cisplatin improved progression free survival but not overall survival compared with thiotepa.

UNKNOWN EFFECTIVENESS

Relative efficacy of different platinum agents (cisplatin versus carboplatin) added to a taxane (paclitaxel)

One RCT found no significant difference in progression free or overall survival between adding cisplatin and adding carboplatin to paclitaxel, although it may have lacked power to detect clinically important effects.

Relative efficacy of different taxanes (paclitaxel versus docetaxel) added to a platinum agent docetaxel

We found no reliable RCTs comparing the effects of carboplatin plus paclitaxel versus those of carboplatin plus docetaxel.

DEFINITION Ovarian tumours are classified according to the assumed cell type of origin (surface epithelium, stroma, or germ cells). Most malignant ovarian tumours (85–95%) are derived from the epithelium of the ovarian surface, and thus are termed epithelial.[1] These can be further grouped into histological types (serous, mucinous, endometroid, and clear cell). Epithelial ovarian cancer is staged using the FIGO classification (see table A on web extra). This review concerns only advanced epithelial ovarian cancer, which is regarded as FIGO stages II–IV.

INCIDENCE/ PREVALENCE The worldwide annual incidence of ovarian cancer exceeds 140 000.[2] Rates vary between countries. Differences in reproductive patterns, including age of menarche and menopause, gravidity, breast feeding, and use of the oral contraceptive pill, may contribute to this variation. Rates are highest in Scandinavia, northern America, and the UK; and lowest in Africa, India, China, and Japan.[3] In the UK ovarian cancer is the fourth most common malignancy in women and is the leading cause of death from gynaecological cancers, with a lifetime risk of about 2%.[4] In the UK the incidence was 5174 in 1988[5] and 6880 in 1998.[6] The incidence of ovarian cancer appears to be stabilising in some other countries, and in some affluent countries (Finland, Denmark, New Zealand, and the USA) rates are declining.

AETIOLOGY/ RISK FACTORS Risk factors include increasing age, family history of ovarian cancer, low fertility, use of fertility drugs, and low parity.[7–11] Case control studies found that using the combined oral contraceptive pill for more than 5 years was associated with a 40% reduction in the risk of ovarian cancer.[3,7,12,13]

PROGNOSIS More than 80% of women present with advanced disease, and the overall 5 year survival rates are poor (< 30%).[6] For advanced disease the major independent prognostic factors appear to be stage, and residual tumour mass after surgery.

Please refer to the Clinical Evidence website for full text and references.

What are the effects of treatments?

LIKELY TO BE BENEFICIAL

Cyproterone acetate–ethinylestradiol (co-cyprindiol; reduced hirsutism from baseline, no significant difference in hirsutism between cyproterone acetate–ethinylestradiol and other combined oral contraceptives)

We found no RCTs comparing cyproterone acetate–ethinylestradiol versus placebo. One RCT found limited evidence by assessing within group changes from baseline that cyproterone acetate–ethinylestradiol reduced hirsutism and oligomenorrhoea. Two RCTs found that cyproterone acetate–ethinylestradiol and other combined oral contraceptive regimens were effective in reducing hirsutism at 6 months. One of these RCTs also found limited evidence that cyproterone acetate–ethinylestradiol may be less effective than ketoconazole in reducing hirsutism at 6 months. A fourth RCT found that cyproterone acetate–ethinylestradiol was less effective in reducing hirsutism at 6 months than metformin. A fifth RCT found that adding finasteride to cyproterone acetate–ethinylestradiol reduced hirsutism at 6 months compared with cyproterone acetate–ethinylestradiol alone. Cyproterone acetate–ethinylestradiol is associated with an increased risk of venous thromboembolism.

Finasteride (may be equally effective in reducing hirsutism compared with flutamide and spironolactone)

Two RCTs found that finasteride reduced hirsutism after 6 months' treatment compared with placebo and three others found more limited evidence that it reduced hirsutism from baseline. Small RCTs, which included women with idiopathic hirsutism, provided insufficient evidence to compare the relative effectiveness of finasteride, flutamide, and spironolactone. Of the three RCTs that directly compared treatments, two found no significant difference in hirsutism among treatments, and the third found that finasteride was less effective than flutamide in reducing hirsutism at 12 months. A sixth RCT found that adding finasteride to cyproterone acetate–ethinylestradiol reduced hirsutism at 6 months compared with cyproterone acetate–ethinylestradiol alone. We found no RCTs that assessed effects on oligomenorrhoea.

Flutamide (may be equally effective in reducing hirsutism compared with finasteride and spironolactone)

Small RCTs, which included women with idiopathic hirsutism, provided insufficient evidence to compare the relative effectiveness of finasteride, flutamide, and spironolactone. One of the RCTs found that flutamide improved hirsutism compared with placebo, and three other RCTs found more limited evidence that it improved hirsutism from baseline. Of the three RCTs that directly compared treatments, two found no significant difference in hirsutism among treatments, and the third found that flutamide was more effective than finasteride in reducing hirsutism at 12 months. We found no RCTs that assessed effects on oligomenorrhoea.

Metformin (improved menstrual pattern compared with placebo; reduced hirsutism compared with cyproterone acetate–ethinylestradiol)

One RCT found limited evidence that metformin improved menstrual pattern over 3 months compared with placebo. Another RCT found that adding metformin to a low calorie diet reduced oligomenorrhoea at 6 months compared with placebo, ▶

Polycystic ovary syndrome

◄ and found more limited evidence by assessing within group changes from baseline that it also reduced hirsutism. A third RCT found that metformin was more effective in reducing hirsutism at 12 months than cyproterone acetate–ethinylestradiol.

Spironolactone (may be equally effective in reducing hirsutism compared with finasteride and flutamide)

One systematic review of two RCTs in women with hirsutism attributed to polycystic ovary syndrome or idiopathic hirsutism found that spironolactone reduced hirsutism at 6 months compared with placebo. One small RCT found limited evidence that spironolactone was less effective in reducing hirsuitism at 6 months than ketoconazole. One small RCT found that spironolactone, finasteride, and flutamide all reduced hirsutism at 6 months compared with placebo, and found no significant difference among groups. This RCT may have been underpowered to detect a clinically important difference among active treatments. We found no RCTs that assessed effects on oligomenorrhoea.

UNKNOWN EFFECTIVENESS

Cyproterone acetate–ethinylestradiol (co-cyprindiol; for reducing oligomenorrhoea)

We found no RCTs comparing cyproterone acetate–ethinylestradiol versus placebo. One RCT found limited evidence by assessing within group changes from baseline that cyproterone acetate–ethinylestradiol reduced oligomenorrhoea.

Interventions to achieve weight loss

We found no systematic review or RCTs comparing interventions to achieve weight loss versus no intervention that assessed clinical outcomes in women with polycystic ovary syndrome. One RCT found limited evidence by assessing within group changes from baseline that a high or a low protein diet aimed at achieving weight loss may improve menstrual pattern over 16 weeks.

Ketoconazole

One RCT found limited evidence that ketoconazole reduced hirsutism at 6 months compared with cyproterone acetate–ethinylestradiol or spironolactone. We found no RCTs that assessed effects on oligomenorrhoea.

Mechanical hair removal

We found no RCTs of the effects of mechanical hair removal in women with hirsutism attributed to polycystic ovary syndrome.

DEFINITION   Polycystic ovary syndrome (PCOS; Stein–Leventhal syndrome, sclerocystic ovarian disease) is defined as an accumulation of many incompletely developed follicles in the ovaries due to chronic anovulation with an increase in ovarian androgen production. The diagnosis excludes secondary causes such as androgen producing neoplasm, hyperprolactinaemia, and adult onset congenital adrenal hyperplasia.[1] It is characterized by irregular menstrual cycles, scanty or absent menses, multiple small cysts on the ovaries (polycystic ovaries), mild hirsutism, and infertility. Many women also have insulin resistance, acne, and weight gain.[1] Until recently, there was no overall consensus on the criteria for diagnosing PCOS. In some studies, it has been diagnosed based on the ultrasound findings of polycystic ovaries, rather than on clinical criteria. An international consensus definition of PCOS has now been published, which defines PCOS as the presence of at least 12 follicles measuring 2–9 mm in diameter and/or an ovarian volume in excess of 10 mL.[2]

▶

INCIDENCE/ PREVALENCE	PCOS is diagnosed in 4–10% of women attending gynaecology clinics in developed countries,[1,3] but this figure may not reflect the true prevalence because there have been no specific population based studies and the criteria used for diagnosis are varied. Most women present in their thirties.[3]
AETIOLOGY/ RISK FACTORS	The aetiology is unknown. Genetic factors may play a part, but the exact mechanisms are unclear. Two studies demonstrated some evidence of familial aggregation of hyperandrogenaemia (with or without oligomenorrhoea) in first degree relatives of women with PCOS.[3,4] In the first study, 22% of sisters of women with PCOS fulfilled diagnostic criteria for PCOS.[3] In the second study, of the 78 mothers and 50 sisters evaluated clinically, 19 (24%) mothers and 16 (32%) sisters had PCOS.[4]
PROGNOSIS	There is some evidence that women with PCOS are at increased risk of developing type 2 diabetes and cardiovascular disorders secondary to hyperlipidaemia compared with women who do not have PCOS.[5] Oligomenorrhoeic and amenorrhoeic women are at increased risk of developing endometrial hyperplasia and, later, endometrial carcinoma.[6]

Please refer to the Clinical Evidence website for full text and references.

Pyelonephritis in non-pregnant women

Search date July 2003

Adriana Wechsler

What are the effects of treatments?

LIKELY TO BE BENEFICIAL

Intravenous antibiotics in women admitted to hospital with uncomplicated infection*

We found no RCTs comparing intravenous antibiotics versus no antibiotics. Consensus holds that intravenous antibiotics are effective, and it is unlikely that a placebo controlled RCT would now be performed. One RCT found no significant difference between intravenous ampicillin plus intravenous gentamicin and intravenous co-trimoxazole plus intravenous gentamicin for relief of symptoms and recurrence of bacteriuria at 28 days. We found insufficient evidence to compare clinical effects of different intravenous regimens.

Oral antibiotics for women with uncomplicated infection*

We found no RCTs comparing oral antibiotics with no antibiotics. However, consensus holds that these drugs are effective, and it is unlikely that such an RCT would now be performed. One systematic review and one subsequent RCT in women with uncomplicated pyelonephritis (none of whom were admitted to hospital) have found no consistent differences between co-amoxiclav, or quinolones (ciprofloxacin, norfloxacin, levofloxacin, or lomefloxacin) in bacteriological or clinical cure rates. However, observational data suggest that broader spectrum antibiotics, such as quinolones, are more effective than narrow spectrum antibiotics such as amoxicillin and trimethoprim–sulphamethoxazole in areas with high prevalence of resistance to these drugs.

*This categorisation is not based on placebo controlled RCTs. Such studies are likely to be considered unethical.

Relative effectiveness of different oral and antibiotic regimens, inpatient versus outpatient management, intravenous versus oral antibiotics

We found no RCTs in women with acute uncomplicated pyelonephritis.

DEFINITION Acute pyelonephritis, or upper urinary tract infection, is an infection of the kidney characterised by pain when passing urine, fever, flank pain, nausea, and vomiting. White blood cells are almost always present in the urine and occasionally white blood cell casts are also seen on urine microscopy. There is no real consensus on the definitions for grades of severity. However, people with acute pyelonephritis may be divided into those able to take oral antibiotics and without signs of sepsis, who may be managed at home, and those requiring intravenous antibiotics in hospital. There is little difference in the application of treatments between men and non-pregnant women.

INCIDENCE/ In the USA, there are 250 000 cases of acute pyelonephritis a year.[1]
PREVALENCE Worldwide prevalence and incidence are unknown.

AETIOLOGY/ Pyelonephritis is most commonly caused when bacteria in the bladder ascend
RISK FACTORS the ureters and invade the kidneys. In some cases, this may result in bacteria entering and multiplying in the bloodstream. People with structural or functional urinary tract abnormalities are more prone to pyelonephritis that is refractory to oral therapy or complicated by bacteraemia. Repeated urinary tract infections also predispose them to drug resistant organisms.

PROGNOSIS   Complications include urosepsis, renal impairment, and renal abscess. Conditions such as underlying renal disease, diabetes mellitus, and immunosuppression may worsen prognosis, but we found no good long term evidence about rates of sepsis or death among people with such conditions.

Please refer to the Clinical Evidence website for full text and references.

Recurrent cystitis in non-pregnant women

Search date April 2003

Adriana Wechsler

What are the effects of interventions to prevent further recurrence of cystitis?

BENEFICIAL

Continuous antibiotic prophylaxis (trimethoprim, co-trimoxazole, nitrofurantoin, cefaclor, or a quinolone)

RCTs have found that continuous antibiotic prophylaxis for 6–12 months with trimethoprim, co-trimoxazole, nitrofurantoin, cefaclor, or a quinolone reduces rates of recurrent cystitis compared with placebo (see table 1❶), and have found no consistent difference in recurrence rates among different continuous regimens. One RCT comparing continuous daily antibiotic prophylaxis versus postcoital antibiotic prophylaxis found no significant difference in rates of positive urine culture after 1 year.

Postcoital antibiotic prophylaxis (co-trimoxazole, nitrofurantoin, or a quinolone)

Four RCTs have found that co-trimoxazole, nitrofurantoin, or a quinolone up to 2 hours after sexual intercourse reduces the rates of cystitis compared with placebo (see table 2❶). One RCT comparing continuous daily antibiotic prophylaxis versus postcoital antibiotic prophylaxis found no significant difference in rates of positive urine culture after 1 year.

UNKNOWN EFFECTIVENESS

Cranberry juice and cranberry products

One systematic review of two weak RCTs provided insufficient evidence on the effects of cranberry juice and other cranberry products in women with recurrent cystitis.

Prophylaxis with methenamine hippurate

One systematic review of weak RCTs provided insufficient evidence to assess methenamine hippurate (hexamine hippurate) in women with recurrent cystitis.

Single dose self administered co-trimoxazole

One small RCT found single dose, self administered co-trimoxazole started at the onset of cystitis symptoms was less effective in reducing recurrence rates over 1 year than continuous co-trimoxazole prophylaxis. However, evidence was too limited to draw firm conclusions.

DEFINITION   Cystitis is an infection of the lower urinary tract, which causes pain when passing urine, and causes frequency, urgency, haematuria, or suprapubic pain not associated with passing urine. White blood cells and bacteria are almost always present in the urine. The presence of fever, flank pain, nausea, or vomiting suggests pyelonephritis (upper urinary tract infection) (see pyelonephritis in non-pregnant women, p 550). Recurrent cystitis may be either a reinfection (after successful eradication of infection) or a relapse after inadequate treatment.

INCIDENCE/   The incidence of cystitis among premenopausal sexually active women is
PREVALENCE   0.5–0.7 infections per person year,[1] and 20–40% of women will experience cystitis during their lifetime. Of those, 20% will develop recurrence, almost always (90% of cases) because of reinfection rather than relapse. Rates of infection fall during the winter months.[2]

▶

AETIOLOGY/ Cystitis is caused by uropathogenic bacteria in the faecal flora that colonise the
RISK FACTORS vaginal and periurethral openings, and ascend the urethra into the bladder.
Prior infection, sexual intercourse, and exposure to vaginal spermicide are risk
factors for developing cystitis.[3,4]

PROGNOSIS We found little evidence on the long term effects of untreated cystitis. One study
found that progression to pyelonephritis was infrequent, and that most cases of
cystitis regressed spontaneously, although symptoms sometimes persisted for
several months.[5] Women with a baseline rate of more than two infections a
year, over many years, are likely to have ongoing recurrent infections.[6]

Please refer to the Clinical Evidence website for full text and references.

Stress incontinence

Search date December 2003

Joseph Onwude

What are the effects of non-surgical treatments for women with stress incontinence?

Oestrogen supplements (short term treatment only; effectiveness of long term treatment is uncertain, and may be associated with increased risk of stroke and endometrial cancer if unopposed, and breast cancer, coronary heart disease, and pulmonary embolism if combined with progestogen)

One systematic review found that short term treatment with oestrogen supplements improved cure or improvement rates compared with placebo. The review found that pelvic floor muscle exercises increased rates of cure or improvement compared with short term treatment with oestrogen supplements. It found no significant difference in rates of cure or improvement between pelvic floor electrical stimulation and short term treatment with oestrogen supplements, but it may have lacked the power to detect a clinically important difference. There are concerns about the safety of long term oestrogen use. One RCT found that combined oral oestrogen and progestogen supplements increased the risk of invasive breast cancer, coronary heart disease, stroke, and pulmonary embolism in postmenopausal women with a uterus at 5 years. One RCT found that oral oestrogen supplements increased the risk of strokes in women without a uterus at 6 years. There is limited evidence that unopposed oestrogen is associated with an increased risk of endometrial cancer in women with a uterus.

Pelvic floor electrical stimulation

RCTs found that pelvic floor electrical stimulation reduced symptoms compared with no treatment or sham pelvic floor electrical stimulation. One systematic review found no significant difference in cure or improvement rates at 12 months between pelvic floor electrical stimulation and pelvic floor muscle exercises. It found that pelvic floor electrical stimulation was associated with a small number of cases of vaginal irritation and difficulties in maintaining motivation for treatment. RCTs found no significant difference between pelvic floor electrical stimulation and vaginal cones in self reported cure or improvement rates or urinary leakage over 4 weeks to 12 months, but they may have lacked power to detect a clinically important difference. One systematic review found no significant difference in cure or improvement rates between pelvic floor electrical stimulation and oestrogen supplements, but it may have lacked the power to detect a clinically important difference.

Pelvic floor muscle exercises

One systematic review found that pelvic floor muscle exercises increased cure or improvement rates and reduced the number of leakages over 3–6 months compared with no treatment or placebo. It found no significant difference in cure or improvement rates at 12 months between pelvic floor muscle exercises and pelvic muscle electrical stimulation. It found that pelvic floor muscle exercises reduced the number of leakage episodes at 6 months compared with vaginal cones, but there was no significant difference between treatments in cure or improvement rates at 12 months. One systematic review found that pelvic floor muscle exercises increased cure or improvement rates compared with oestrogen supplements.

Vaginal cones

One systematic review found that vaginal cones improved self reported cure and improvement rates compared with control over 6–12 months. It found no significant difference in leakage episodes. RCTs found no significant difference in self reported cure or improvement rates over 12 months between vaginal cones and pelvic floor muscle exercises. It found that vaginal cones were less effective than pelvic floor muscle exercises in reducing the number of leakage episodes over 6 months. RCTs also found no significant difference between vaginal cones and pelvic floor electrical stimulation in self reported cure or improvement rates, or in urinary leakage over 4 weeks to 12 months, but they may have lacked power to detect a clinically important difference. The most common adverse effect associated with vaginal cones was difficulty maintaining motivation for use, but a small number of more serious events such as vaginitis and abdominal pain were reported.

What are the effects of surgical interventions for women with stress incontinence?

BENEFICIAL

Laparoscopic colposuspension (similar cure rates to open retropubic colposuspension and tension free vaginal tape)

We found no RCTs comparing laparoscopic colposuspension versus no treatment, sham treatment, non-surgical treatment, anterior vaginal repair, suburethral slings, or needle colposuspension. One systematic review found that open retropubic colposuspension improved objective cure rates at 1 year compared with laparoscopic colposuspension. However, it found no significant difference in objective cure rates at 5 years, or in subjective cure rates at 1 or 5 years. One RCT identified by a review found a higher cure rate with tension free vaginal tape than with laparoscopic colposuspension at 6 months to 2 years, while two subsequent RCTs found no significant difference in cure rate between treatments at 6 weeks to 1 year.

Open retropubic colposuspension (higher cure rates than non-surgical treatment, anterior vaginal repair, or needle colposuspension, but more adverse effects than non-surgical treatment)

We found no RCTs comparing open retropubic colposuspension versus no treatment or sham treatment. One systematic review found that open retropubic colposuspension increased cure rates at 1–5 years compared with non-surgical treatment, anterior vaginal repair, or needle colposuspension. Open retropubic colposuspension was associated with more adverse effects than non-surgical treatment, but fewer surgical complications than needle colposuspension. It found that open retropubic colposuspension improved objective cure rates at 1 year compared with laparoscopic colposuspension. However, it found no significant difference in objective cure rates at 5 years, or in subjective cure rates at 1 or 5 years. It found no significant difference in cure rates at 1 year between open retropubic colposuspension and suburethral slings. One systematic review found no significant difference in cure rate between tension free vaginal tape and open retropubic colposuspension at up to 2 years. However, the included trials may have lacked power to exclude a clinically important difference in cure rates. RCTs included in the review found that open retropubic colposuspension was associated with a lower incidence of bladder perforation than tension free vaginal tape, but a higher incidence of postoperative fever.

Stress incontinence

Tension free vaginal tape (similar cure rates to open retropubic colposuspension and laparoscopic colposuspension)

We found no RCTs comparing tension free vaginal tape versus no treatment, sham treatment, non-surgical treatment, anterior vaginal repair, or needle colposuspension. One RCT found no significant difference in cure rates between tension free vaginal tape and suburethral slings at 12 months. One systematic review found no significant difference in cure rate between tension free vaginal tape and open retropubic colposuspension at up to 2 years. However, the included trials may have lacked statistical power to exclude a clinically important difference in cure rates. RCTs included in the review found that tension free vaginal tape was associated with a higher incidence of bladder perforation than open retropubic colposuspension, but a lower incidence of postoperative fever. One RCT identified by a systematic review found a higher cure rate with tension free vaginal tape than with laparoscopic colposuspension at 6–24 months, while two subsequent RCTs found no significant difference in cure rate between groups at 6 weeks to 1 year.

TRADE OFF BETWEEN BENEFITS AND HARMS

Suburethral slings other than tension free vaginal tape (similar cure rates to open retropubic colposuspension and needle colposuspension, but more perioperative complications than needle colposuspension)

We found no RCTs comparing suburethral slings versus no treatment, non-surgical treatment, anterior vaginal repair, or laparoscopic colposuspension. Five RCTs identified by a systematic review found no significant difference in cure rates between suburethral slings and open retropubic colposuspension at up to 6 years, although the studies may have lacked power to detect a clinically important difference. One small RCT identified by the review found no significant difference in cure rates at 1 year between suburethral slings and needle colposuspension, but it may have lacked power to detect a clinically important difference. The RCT found that suburethral slings increased perioperative complications compared with needle colposuspension. One RCT found no significant difference in subjective cure rates between tension free vaginal tape and suburethral slings at 12 months.

UNLIKELY TO BE BENEFICIAL

Anterior vaginal repair (lower cure rates than open retropubic colposuspension)

We found no RCTs comparing anterior vaginal repair (anterior colporrhaphy) versus no treatment, suburethral slings, tension free vaginal tape, or laparoscopic colposuspension. One RCT provided insufficient evidence to compare anterior vaginal repair versus non-surgical treatment. One systematic review found that anterior vaginal repair was less effective than open retropubic colposuspension in increasing cure rates at 12 months or 5 years. It found no significant difference in overall operative complications between the two procedures. It found no significant difference in cure rates at 12 months between anterior vaginal repair and needle colposuspension.

Needle colposuspension (lower cure rates and more surgical complications than open retropubic colposuspension)

We found no RCTs comparing needle colposuspension versus no treatment, non-surgical treatment, tension free vaginal tape, or laparoscopic colposuspension. One systematic review found no significant difference in cure rates between needle colposuspension and anterior vaginal repair or suburethral slings, but found that needle colposuspension was associated with fewer perioperative complications than suburethral slings. Another systematic review found that open retropubic colposuspension improved cure rates and was associated with fewer surgical complications than needle colposuspension at 5 years.

DEFINITION Stress incontinence is involuntary leakage on effort or exertion, or on sneezing or coughing.[1] Stress incontinence predominantly affects women, and can cause social and hygiene problems. Typically, there is no anticipatory feeling of needing to pass urine. Physiologically, stress incontinence is defined as intravesical pressure that exceeds urethral pressure in the absence of a detrusor contraction.

INCIDENCE/ PREVALENCE Stress incontinence is a common problem. Prevalence has been estimated at 17–45% of adult women in the setting of a high income country.[2] One cross-sectional study (15 308 women in Norway under the age of 65 years) found that the prevalence of stress incontinence was 4.7% in women who have not borne a child, 6.9% in women who had caesarian deliveries only, and 12.2% in women who had vaginal deliveries only.[3] During 2000–2001, about 10 000 operations on the outlet of the female bladder were carried out in England.[4] About 4000 were open abdominal operations, about 3000 were vaginal, about 1500 were endoscopic, and the rest were categorised as "other".

AETIOLOGY/ RISK FACTORS Aetiological factors include pregnancy, vaginal or caesarean delivery, cigarette smoking, and obesity.[3,5–7] One cross-sectional study (15 308 women in Norway) found that when compared with women who have not borne a child, the risk of stress incontinence was increased in women who have delivered by caesarean section (age adjusted OR 1.4, 95% CI 1.0 to 2.0) or by vaginal delivery (age adjusted OR 3.0, 95% CI 2.5 to 3.5).[3] The risk of stress incontinence was also increased in women who had a vaginal delivery compared with women who had a caesarean section (adjusted OR 2.4, 95% CI 1.7 to 3.2). One case control study (606 women) found that the risk of genuine stress incontinence was increased in former smokers (adjusted OR 2.20, 95% CI 1.18 to 4.11) and in current smokers (adjusted OR 2.48, 95% CI 1.60 to 3.84).[7] We found no reliable data measuring the risks associated with obesity.

PROGNOSIS We found no reliable data about the natural history of stress incontinence. Untreated stress incontinence is believed to be a persistent, lifelong condition.

Please refer to the Clinical Evidence website for full text and references.

Bites (mammalian)

Search date November 2003

Iara Marques de Medeiros and Humberto Saconato

What are the effects of interventions to prevent mammalian bites?

LIKELY TO BE BENEFICIAL

Education

We found no RCTs of the effect of education programmes on the incidence of mammalian bites. One RCT in school children found that an educational programme increased precautionary behaviour around dogs compared with no education.

UNKNOWN EFFECTIVENESS

Education in specific occupational groups

We found no RCTs of education to prevent bites in specific occupational groups.

What are the effects of measures to prevent complications from mammalian bites?

LIKELY TO BE BENEFICIAL

Antibiotic prophylaxis

The effects of antibiotic prophylaxis in preventing complications of mammalian bites remain unclear. Limited evidence from one systematic review found that, when all causes and sites of mammalian bite were combined, there was no evidence of a difference in infection rate between antibiotics and placebo. Meta-analysis according to the site of the wound found that antibiotics reduced infections of the hand only. One small RCT in the review found that in people with human bites, antibiotics reduced the rate of infection compared with placebo.

Debridement, irrigation, and decontamination

We found no reliable studies assessing debridement, irrigation, decontamination measures, or infiltration of serum into the wound. However, there is consensus that such measures are likely to be beneficial.

UNKNOWN EFFECTIVENESS

Primary wound closure

One poor quality RCT comparing primary wound closure with no closure in people with dog bites found no significant difference in the incidence of infection, but the RCT was too small to exclude clinically important effects.

Tetanus immunisation after mammalian bites

We found no evidence on the effects of tetanus toxoid or tetanus immunoglobulin in preventing tetanus after human or animal bites.

▶

What are the effects of treatments for infected mammalian bites?

LIKELY TO BE BENEFICIAL

Antibiotics

We found no RCTs of antibiotics compared with placebo for infected mammalian bites. However, there is consensus that antibiotics are likely to be beneficial

UNKNOWN EFFECTIVENESS

Comparative effectiveness of different antibiotics

One RCT in people with infected and uninfected animal and human bites found no significant difference in failure rate (which was undefined) with penicillin, with or without dicloxacillin, compared with amoxicillin/clavulanic acid.

DEFINITION Bite wounds are mainly caused by humans, dogs, or cats. They include superficial abrasions (30–43%), lacerations (31–45%), and puncture wounds (13–34%).[1]

INCIDENCE/ PREVALENCE In areas where rabies is poorly controlled among domestic animals, dogs account for 90% of reported mammalian bites compared with less than 5% in areas where rabies is well controlled. In the USA, an estimated 3.5–4.7 million dog bites occur each year.[2] About 1 in 5 people bitten by a dog seek medical attention, and 1% of those require admission to hospital.[3,4] Between a third and half of all mammalian bites occur in children.[5]

AETIOLOGY/ RISK FACTORS In over 70% of cases, people are bitten by their own pets or by an animal known to them. Males are more likely to be bitten than females, and are more likely to be bitten by dogs, whereas females are more likely to be bitten by cats.[2] One study found that children under 5 years old were significantly more likely than older children to provoke animals before being bitten.[6] One study of infected dog and cat bites found that the most commonly isolated bacteria was *Pasteurella*, followed by *Streptococci, Staphylococci, Moraxella, Corynebacterium*, and *Neisseria*.[7] Mixed aerobic and anaerobic infection was more common than anaerobic infection alone.

PROGNOSIS In the USA, dog bites cause about 20 deaths a year.[8] In children, dog bites frequently involve the face, potentially resulting in severe lacerations and scarring.[9] Rabies, a life threatening viral encephalitis, may be contracted as a consequence of being bitten or scratched by a rabid animal. More than 99% of human rabies is in developing countries where canine rabies is endemic.[10]

Please refer to the Clinical Evidence website for full text and references.

Burns (minor thermal)

Search date December 2003

Jason Wasiak and Heather Cleland

What are the effects of treatments for minor thermal burns?

UNKNOWN EFFECTIVENESS

Antibiotics

We found no RCTs comparing the use of topical or oral antibiotics versus placebo or no treatment in the management of minor burns. Routine prophylactic use of antibiotics may promote the emergence of resistant organisms in the community.

Chlorhexidine impregnated paraffin gauze dressing

Two RCTs comparing chlorhexidine impregnated paraffin gauze versus hydrocolloid dressing found no significant difference in time to wound healing but, subjectively, both investigators and patients in one of the RCTs rated the hydrocolloid dressing more favourably. One RCT found that chlorhexidine impregnated paraffin gauze increased time to wound healing and was perceived as more painful compared with polyurethane film.

Hydrocolloid dressing

Two RCTs comparing hydrocolloid dressing versus paraffin impregnated gauze dressings found no significant difference in time to wound healing between the two treatment groups but, subjectively, both investigators and patients in one of the RCTs rated the hydrocolloid dressing more favourably. One RCT found no significant difference in time to wound healing, pain, or interference with activities of daily living between hydrocolloid dressing and a combination of chlorhexidine impregnated paraffin gauze dressing plus silver sulfadiazine cream. One RCT found that hydrocolloid dressing reduced time to healing, pain, and limitation of activity compared with silver sulfadiazine dressing. One RCT found that healing time was shorter with hydrocolloid dressing alone compared with hydrocolloid dressing plus silver sulfadiazine cream and found no difference in pathogenic bacteria growth with hydrocolloid dressing alone compared with hydrocolloid dressing plus silver sulfadiazine cream.

Paraffin gauze dressing

One RCT found no significant difference in pain or time to wound healing with paraffin gauze compared with polyurethane film.

Polyurethrane film

One RCT comparing polyurethane film versus paraffin gauze found no significant difference in pain or the number of days to wound healing. One RCT found that polyurethane film reduced time to wound healing and was perceived as less painful compared with chlorhexidine impregnated paraffin gauze.

Silicone coated nylon

One RCT found that silicone coated nylon dressing reduced time to wound healing in children compared with silver sulfadiazine dressing.

LIKELY TO BE INEFFECTIVE OR HARMFUL

Silver sulfadiazine cream

One RCT comparing a combination of chlorhexidine impregnated paraffin gauze dressing plus silver sulfadiazine cream versus hydrocolloid dressing found no significant difference in time to wound healing, pain levels, or interference with activities of daily living. One RCT found that silver sulfadiazine dressing increased time to healing, pain, and limitation of activity compared with hydrocolloid ▶

dressing. One RCT found that healing time was longer with hydrocolloid dressing plus silver sulfadiazine cream compared with hydrocolloid dressing alone and found no significant difference in pathogenic bacteria growth between the two groups. One RCT found that silver sulfadiazine dressing increased time to wound healing in children compared with silicone coated nylon dressing.

DEFINITION Minor thermal burns can be defined as being caused by exposure to heat sufficient to cause damage to the epidermis and papillary dermis of the skin. They are characterised by pain and hypersensitivity. The skin appears moist and pink or red and is perfused, as demonstrated by blanching on pressure. This type of injury will blister and heal within 2–3 weeks with minimal scarring if no infection is present.

INCIDENCE/ PREVALENCE The incidence of minor thermal burns is difficult to estimate. Generally, less than 5% of all burn injuries requiring treatment will necessitate admission to hospital.[1] Worldwide estimates surrounding all thermal burn injuries suggest that approximately two million people are burned, up to 80 000 are hospitalised and 6500 die of burn wounds every year.

AETIOLOGY/ RISK FACTORS The pattern of injury varies among different age groups. Males aged 18–25 years appear more susceptible to injury due to a variety of causes — mainly flame, electrical, and, to a lesser extent, chemicals.[2] Many burn injuries in this age group are due to the inappropriate use of flammable agents such as petrol; however, the majority of burns occur in the home. Thermal burns, in particular scalds, are common among the young as well as the elderly. The kitchen is reported to be the most common place of injury for children, as is the bathroom for the elderly. Those with concomitant conditions or complicating factors such as motor or neurological impairment are at greater risk.

PROGNOSIS Superficial thermal burns will heal spontaneously with minimal hypertrophic scarring within 2–3 weeks if the wound remains free of infection.[3] The capacity to heal is also dependent on the health and age of the individual, with the elderly and those with concomitant medical conditions prone to delayed healing. Cooling the burn significantly reduces pain and wound oedema if started within 3 hours of injury. The optimal duration of cooling may vary, but recommended periods of 20–30 minutes with tap water (at a temperature of 5–25 °C) have been suggested.[4] Use of iced water or prolonged periods of cooling can deepen tissue injury, induce hypothermia, and are best avoided. Cleaning solutions and dressings aim to prevent wound infection. The ideal dressing will establish an optimum microenvironment for wound healing. It will maintain the wound temperature and moisture level, permit respiration, allow epithelial migration,[5] and exclude environmental bacteria.

Please refer to the Clinical Evidence website for full text and references.

Pressure sores

Search date January 2004

Nicky Cullum, E Andrea Nelson, and Jane Nixon

What are the effects of preventive interventions?

BENEFICIAL

Foam alternatives (compared with standard foam mattresses)

One systematic review found that foam alternatives to the standard hospital foam mattress reduced the incidence of pressure sores over 10–14 days in people at high risk. One subsequent RCT found no significant difference in pressure sores between a standard mattress and a foam alternative. We found no clear evidence of a "best" foam alternative.

Pressure relieving overlays on operating tables

Three RCTs identified by a systematic review found that pressure relieving overlays on operating tables reduced the incidence of pressure sores.

LIKELY TO BE BENEFICIAL

Low air loss beds in intensive care (compared with standard beds)

One RCT in people in intensive care found that low air loss beds reduced the risk of new pressure sores compared with standard intensive care beds.

Medical sheepskin overlays

One RCT found that medical sheepskin overlays reduced the incidence of pressure sores compared with standard treatment in people aged 60 years or more who underwent orthopaedic surgery.

UNKNOWN EFFECTIVENESS

Alternating pressure surfaces

Two RCTs identified by a systematic review and one subsequent RCT found that alternating pressure mattresses reduced pressure sores compared with a standard foam mattress or a constant low pressure mattress, but seven other smaller RCTs identified by the review found no significant difference between alternating pressure devices and constant low pressure mattresses.

Different seat cushions

We found insufficient evidence about the effects of different seat cushions in preventing pressure sores.

Electric profiling beds

We found insufficient evidence about the effects of electric profiling beds in preventing pressure sores.

Low tech constant low pressure supports

We found insufficient evidence about the effects of low tech constant low pressure supports in preventing pressure sores.

Repositioning (regular "turning")

One systematic review found insufficient evidence about the effects of repositioning (regular "turning").

Topical lotions and dressings

One systematic review found insufficient evidence about the effects topical lotions or dressings.

© BMJ Publishing Group Ltd 2005

Air filled vinyl boots with foot cradle

One small RCT found that air filled vinyl boots with foot cradles were associated with more rapid development of pressure sores compared with hospital pillows.

Low air loss hydrotherapy beds

One RCT found that low air loss hydrotherapy beds increased the risk of developing a pressure sore compared with a range of support surfaces in people with incontinence.

What are the effects of treatments?

LIKELY TO BE BENEFICIAL

Air fluidised supports (compared with standard care)

Two RCTs found that air fluidised supports reduced pressure sores after 15 days compared with standard care. One RCT with methodological weaknesses and one very small RCT found no significant difference between air fluidised supports and standard care.

UNKNOWN EFFECTIVENESS

Alternating pressure surfaces

We found insufficient evidence on the effects of alternating pressure surfaces in healing pressure sores.

Debridement

RCTs provided insufficient evidence to compare effects of different debriding agents on healing.

Dressings other than hydrocolloid

Small, methodologically weak RCTs provided insufficient evidence about the effect of dressings other than hydrocolloid.

Electrotherapy

Three RCTs found limited evidence that electrotherapy increased healing compared with sham therapy. However, the RCTs were small and of limited quality, and their conclusions are therefore unreliable.

Hydrocolloid dressings

We found inconclusive evidence about the effects of hydrocolloid dressings.

Low air loss beds

We found insufficient evidence on the effects of low air loss beds in healing pressure sores.

Low level laser therapy

We found insufficient evidence from two RCTs about the effects of low level laser therapy on healing.

Low tech constant low pressure supports

We found insufficient evidence on the effects of low tech constant low pressure supports in healing pressure sores.

Nutritional supplements

RCTs found no significant difference in healing between nutritional supplements and control interventions (low dose or no supplements). However, studies were small and may have lacked power to detect clinically important differences between treatments.

Pressure sores

Seat cushions
We found insufficient evidence on the effects of seat cushions in healing pressure sores.

Surgery
We found no RCTs of surgical treatments for pressure sores.

Therapeutic ultrasound
Two RCTs identified by a systematic review found no significant difference in healing between ultrasound and sham ultrasound.

Topical negative pressure
We found insufficient evidence from two small RCTs about the effects of topical negative pressure on healing.

Topical phenytoin
One small RCT provided insufficient evidence about the effects of topical phenytoin on healing.

DEFINITION	Pressure sores (also known as pressure ulcers, bed sores, and decubitus ulcers) may present as persistently hyperaemic, blistered, broken, or necrotic skin and may extend to underlying structures, including muscle and bone.
INCIDENCE/ PREVALENCE	Reported prevalence rates range between 4.7–32.1% for hospital populations, between 4.4–33% for community care populations, and between 4.6–20.7% for nursing home populations.[1]
AETIOLOGY/ RISK FACTORS	Pressure sores are caused by unrelieved pressure, shear, or friction. They are most common below the waist and at bony prominences, such as the sacrum, heels, and hips. They occur in all health care settings. Increased age, reduced mobility, impaired nutrition, vascular disease, faecal incontinence, and skin condition at baseline consistently emerge as risk factors.[2,3] However, the relative importance of these and other factors is uncertain.
PROGNOSIS	The presence of pressure sores has been associated with a twofold to fourfold increased risk of death in elderly people and people in intensive care.[4,5] However, pressure sores are a marker for underlying disease severity and other comorbidities rather than an independent predictor of mortality.[4]

Please refer to the Clinical Evidence website for full text and references.

Search date July 2004

E Andrea Nelson, Nicky Cullum, and June Jones

What are the effects of treatments?

Compression bandages and stockings

One systematic review and one additional RCT found that compression bandages or stockings healed more venous leg ulcers than no compression. One systematic review and one subsequent RCT found insufficient evidence to suggest a difference between multilayer elastomeric and non-elastomeric high compression bandages. One systematic review and four subsequent RCTs found no significant difference in healing rates between multilayer elastomeric high compression bandages and short stretch bandages or Unna's boot. One systematic review found that multi-layer compression increased ulcer healing compared with single layer bandages. One systematic review and two subsequent RCTs found no significant difference in the proportion of people healed with four layer elastomeric bandages compared with other high compression multilayer bandages. We found insufficient evidence from one small RCT about the effects of compression bandages compared with intermittent pneumatic compression.

Oral pentoxifylline

One systematic review and two subsequent RCTs found that oral pentoxifylline increased the proportion of ulcers healed over 6–12 months compared with placebo.

Cultured allogenic bilayer skin replacement

One RCT found that cultured allogenic bilayer skin replacement increased the proportion of ulcers healed after 6 months compared with a non-adherent dressing.

Oral flavonoids

Two RCTs found that adding flavonoids to compression increased the proportion of ulcers healed after 2–6 months compared with compression alone.

Oral sulodexide

Two RCTs found that sulodexide plus compression increased the proportion of ulcers healed after 2–3 months' treatment compared with compression alone.

Peri-ulcer injection of granulocyte-macrophage colony stimulating factor

One RCT found that peri-ulcer injection of granulocyte-macrophage colony stimulating factor increased the proportion of ulcers healed after 13 weeks' treatment compared with placebo.

Systemic mesoglycan

One RCT found that systemic mesoglycan plus compression increased the proportion of ulcers healed after 24 weeks' treatment compared with compression alone.

Debriding agents

One systematic review of small RCTs provided insufficient evidence about the effects of debriding agents on ulcer healing.

Venous leg ulcers

Foam, film, hyaluronic acid-derived dressings, or alginate (semi-occlusive) dressings

One systematic review provided insufficient evidence to compare the effects of semi-occlusive dressings (foam, film, hyaluronic acid-derived, or alginate) versus simple low adherent dressings, in the presence of compression. One systematic review and two subsequent RCTs found no significant difference in healing rates between semi-occlusive and occlusive dressings.

Intermittent pneumatic compression

One small RCT found insufficient evidence to compare intermittent pneumatic compression with compression bandages or stockings. One RCT found that intermittent pneumatic compression plus compression stockings improved ulcer healing at 3 months compared with compression stockings alone. Two other RCTs found no significant difference in healing at 6 months between intermittent pneumatic compression plus elastic stockings, and Unna's boot, and between intermittent pneumatic compression plus Unna's boot, and Unna's boot alone.

Laser treatment (low level)

RCTs provided insufficient evidence about the effects of low level laser on ulcer healing.

Oral aspirin

One RCT provided insufficient evidence about the effects of oral aspirin on ulcer healing.

Oral rutosides

RCTs provided insufficient evidence about the effects of oral rutosides on ulcer healing.

Oral thromboxane α_2 antagonists

One RCT provided insufficient evidence about the effects of oral thromboxane α_2 antagonists on ulcer healing.

Oral zinc

RCTs provided insufficient evidence about the effects of oral zinc on ulcer healing.

Skin grafting

RCTs provided insufficient evidence about the effects of skin grafting on ulcer healing.

Superficial vein surgery

Three RCTs found no evidence of a benefit associated with superficial vein surgery for ulcer healing. One systematic review identified one RCT which compared two forms of surgery. It found no difference between open surgery and endoscopic surgery in healing rates, but it found that higher rates of infection were associated with open surgery.

Therapeutic ultrasound

RCTs provided insufficient evidence about the effects of therapeutic ultrasound on ulcer healing.

Topical antimicrobial agents

RCTs provided insufficient evidence about the effects of topical antimicrobial agents on ulcer healing.

Topical calcitonin gene related peptide plus vasoactive intestinal polypeptide

One RCT provided insufficient evidence about the effects of topical calcitonin gene related peptide plus vasoactive intestinal polypeptide on ulcer healing.

Topical mesoglycan

One RCT provided insufficient evidence about the effects of topical mesoglycan on ulcer healing.

Topical negative pressure

RCTs provided insufficient evidence about the effects of topical negative pressure on ulcer healing.

Topical recombinant keratinocyte growth factor 2

RCTs provided insufficient evidence about the effects of topical recombinant keratinocyte growth factor 2 on ulcer healing.

UNLIKELY TO BE BENEFICIAL

Hydrocolloid (occlusive) dressings in the presence of compression

One systematic review found that, in the presence of compression, hydrocolloid dressings did not heal more venous leg ulcers than simple, low adherent dressings. One systematic review and two subsequent RCTs found no significant difference in healing rates between occlusive and semi-occlusive dressings.

Topically applied autologous platelet lysate

One RCT found no significant difference in the proportion of people with healed ulcers after 9 months between topically applied autologous platelet lysate compared with placebo.

What are the effects of interventions to prevent recurrence?

BENEFICIAL

Compression stockings

RCTs found that compression stockings reduced recurrence at 6 months compared with no compression, but non-compliance with compression is a risk factor for recurrence.

LIKELY TO BE BENEFICIAL

Superficial vein surgery

Three RCTs provided evidence that superficial vein surgery with or without compression reduced recurrence compared with compression alone. One RCT identified by a systematic review compared open versus endoscopic surgery and found no recurrences in either group, but higher infection rates with open surgery. Vein surgery has the usual risks of surgery and anaesthesia.

UNKNOWN EFFECTIVENESS

Oral rutoside

One RCT identified by a systematic review provided insufficient evidence on the effects of oral rutoside versus placebo on ulcer recurrence.

Oral stanozolol

One RCT identified by a systematic review provided insufficient evidence on the effects of oral stanozolol versus placebo on ulcer recurrence.

DEFINITION Definitions of leg ulcers vary, but the following is widely used: loss of skin on the leg or foot that takes more than 6 weeks to heal. Some definitions exclude ulcers confined to the foot, whereas others include ulcers on the whole of the lower limb. This review deals with ulcers of venous origin in people without concurrent diabetes mellitus, arterial insufficiency, or rheumatoid arthritis.

Venous leg ulcers

INCIDENCE/ PREVALENCE Between 1.5 and 3.0/1000 people have active leg ulcers. Prevalence increases with age to about 20/1000 in people aged over 80 years.[1]

AETIOLOGY/ RISK FACTORS Leg ulceration is strongly associated with venous disease. However, about a fifth of people with leg ulceration have arterial disease, either alone or in combination with venous problems, which may require specialist referral.[1] Venous ulcers (also known as varicose or stasis ulcers) are caused by venous reflux or obstruction, both of which lead to poor venous return and venous hypertension.

PROGNOSIS People with leg ulcers have a poorer quality of life than age matched controls because of pain, odour, and reduced mobility.[2] In the UK, audits have found wide variation in the types of care (hospital inpatient care, hospital clinics, outpatient clinics, home visits), in the treatments used (topical agents, dressings, bandages, stockings), in healing rates, and in recurrence rates (26–69% in 1 year).[3,4]

Please refer to the Clinical Evidence website for full text and references.

INDEX

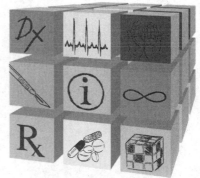

Clinical evidence
concise comments

Clinical Evidence is an evolving resource and we welcome any feedback on the content of this issue and suggestions for future issues.

Please photocopy and complete this form, then return it to us.

For UK and rest of world - Fax: + 44 (0) 20 7383 6242, mail: BMJ Clinical Evidence, BMJ Publishing Group, BMA House, Tavistock Square, London WC1H 9JR, UK

For North and South America - Fax: 1-240-646-7005, mail: BMJ Clinical Evidence, PO Box 512, Annapolis Jct, MD20701-0512, USA

Alternatively, email us at CEfeedback@bmjgroup.com

Name: ....

Address: ....

....

....Email: ....

Position

☐ GP/Primary Care Physician

☐ Hospital Doctor/ Specialist Physician

☐ Pharmacist

☐ Resident/Registrar

☐ Nurse

☐ PAM

☐ Manager

☐ Press

☐ Researcher

☐ Administrator

☐ Librarian

☐ Medical Student

☐ Member of Public/ Patient Support Group

☐ Other.......................

1. Comments concerning the selection of studies

Section..

Topic ....

Reference ....

Comment...

....

....

2. Suggestions for future issues

....

....

....

3. Other comments/questions

....

....

....

Estimating cardiovascular risk and treatment benefit

Adapted from the New Zealand guidelines on management of dyslipidaemia[1] and raised blood pressure[2] by Rod Jackson

How to use these colour charts

The charts help the estimation of a person's absolute risk of a cardiovascular event and the likely benefit of drug treatment to lower cholesterol or blood pressure. For these charts, cardiovascular events include: myocardial infarction, new angina, ischaemic stroke, transient ischaemic attack, peripheral vascular disease, congestive heart failure, and cardiovascular-related death.

There is a group of patients in whom risk can be assumed to be high (>20% in 5 years) without using the charts. They include those with symptomatic cardiovascular disease (angina, myocardial infarction, congestive heart failure, stroke, TIA, and peripheral vascular disease), or left ventricular hypertrophy on ECG.

To estimate a person's absolute 5 year risk:
■ Find the table relating to their sex, diabetic status (on insulin, oral hypoglycaemics, or fasting blood glucose over 8 mmol/L), smoking status, and age. The age shown in the charts is the mean for that category, i.e. age 60 = 55 to 65 years.
■ Within the table find the cell nearest to the person's blood pressure and total cholesterol : HDL ratio. For risk assessment it is enough to use a mean blood pressure based on two readings on each of two occasions, and cholesterol measurements based on one laboratory or two non-fasting Reflotron measurements. More readings are needed to establish the pre-treatment baseline. When the systolic and diastolic values fall in different risk levels, the higher category applies.
■ The colour of the box indicates the person's 5 year cardiovascular disease risk (see below).

RISK LEVEL
5 year CVD risk
(non-fatal and fatal)

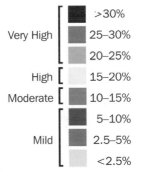

Very High	>30%
	25–30%
	20–25%
High	15–20%
Moderate	10–15%
Mild	5–10%
	2.5–5%
	<2.5%

Notes: (1) People with a strong history of CVD (first degree male relatives with CVD before 55 years, female relatives before 65 years) or obesity (body mass index above 30 kg/m^2) are likely to be at greater risk than the tables indicate. The magnitude of the independent predictive value of these risk factors remains unclear — their presence should influence treatment decisions for patients at borderline treatment levels. (2) If total cholesterol or total cholesterol : HDL ratio is greater than 8 then the risk is at least 15%. (3) Nearly all people aged 75 years or over also have an absolute cardiovascular risk over 15%.

Charts reproduced with permission from The National Heart Foundation of New Zealand. Also available on http://www.nzgg.org.nz/guidelines/0035/CVD_Risk_Full.pdf

REFERENCES

1. Dyslipidaemia Advisory Group. 1996 National Heart Foundation clinical guidelines for the assessment and management of dyslipidaemia. *NZ Med J* 1996;109:224–232.
2. National Health Committee. Guidelines for the management of mildly raised blood pressure in New Zealand: Ministry of Health National Health Committee Report, Wellington, 1995.

Estimating cardiovascular risk and treatment benefit

RISK LEVEL: MEN

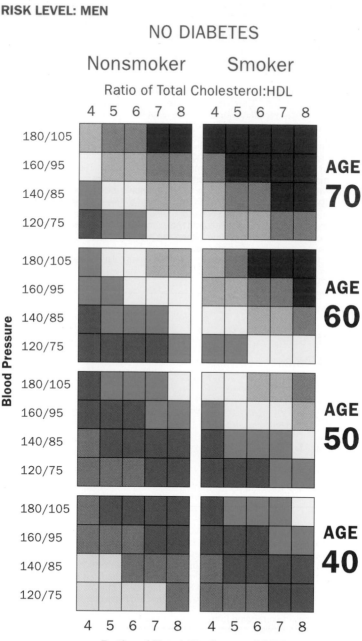

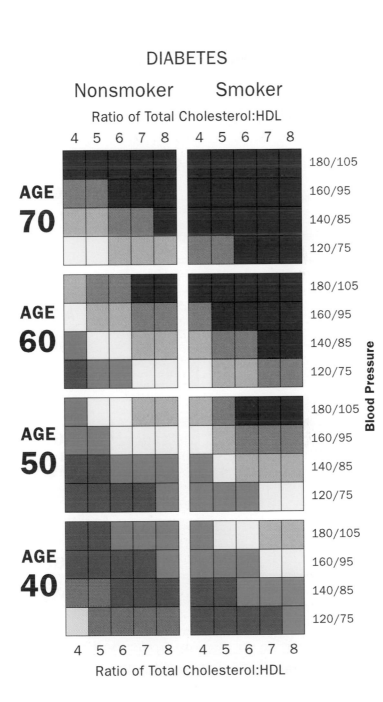

DIABETES

Estimating cardiovascular risk and treatment benefit

RISK LEVEL: WOMEN

NO DIABETES

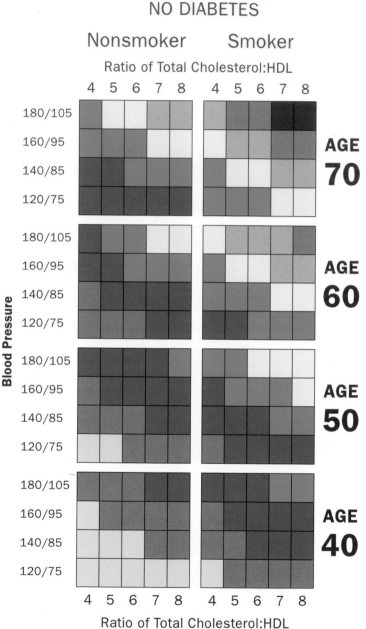

Estimating cardiovascular risk and treatment benefit

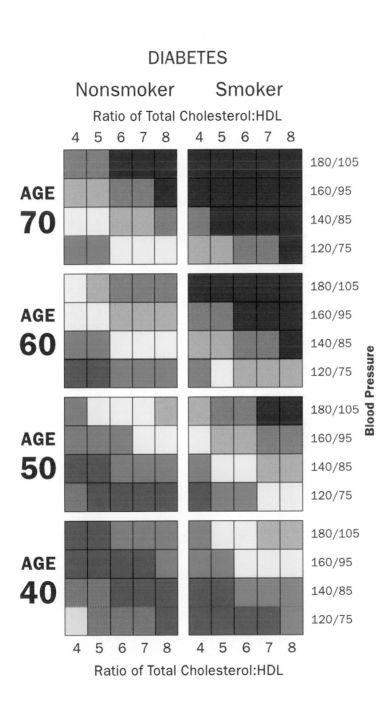

DIABETES

Nonsmoker   Smoker

Ratio of Total Cholesterol:HDL

Blood Pressure

Estimating cardiovascular risk and treatment benefit

Mid-range value	Benefit CVD events prevented per 100 treated over 5 years			Benefit NNT to prevent one event over 5 years		
	One intervention Estimated absolute risk reduction (ARR) 25%	Two interventions Estimated absolute risk reduction (ARR) 45%	Three interventions Estimated absolute risk reduction (ARR) 55%	One intervention 1/ARR	Two interventions 1/ARR	Three interventions 1/ARR
>30%	>8	>14	>17	<13	<7	<6
27.5	7	12	15	15	8	7
22.5	6	10	12	18	10	8
17.5	4	8	10	23	13	10
12.5	3	6	7	32	18	15
7.5	2	3	4	53	30	24
2.75	0.7	1.2	1.5	145	81	66
<2.5	<0.6	<1.1	<1.4	>160	>89	>73

Assumptions:
- A conservative estimate that each intervention: aspirin, blood pressure treatment (lowering systolic BP by 10 mm Hg) or lipid modification (lowering LDL-C by 20%) reduces cardiovascular risk by about 25% over 5 years;
- The relative risk of a CVD event over 5 years after one intervention compared to no treatment is 0.75, after two is 0.75 x 0.75, and after three is 0.75 x 0.75 x 0.75 (i.e. the risk is multiplicative).

The number needed to treat: adjusting for baseline risk

Adapted with permission from Chatellier et al, 1996[1]

BACKGROUND

The number needed to treat (NNT) to avoid a single additional adverse outcome is a meaningful way of expressing the benefit of an active treatment over a control. It can be used both to summarise the results of a therapeutic trial or series of trials and to help medical decision making about an individual patient.

If the absolute risk of adverse outcomes in a therapeutic trial is ARC in the control group and ART in the treatment group, then the absolute risk reduction (ARR) is defined as (ARC − ART). The NNT is defined as the inverse of the ARR:

$$NNT = 1/(ARC − ART)$$

Since the Relative Risk Reduction (RRR) is defined as (ARC − ART)/ARC, it follows that NNT, RRR, and ARC are related by their definitions in the following way:

$$NNT \times RRR \times ARC = 1$$

This relationship can be used to estimate the likely benefits of a treatment in populations with different levels of baseline risk (that is different levels of ARC). This allows extrapolation of the results of a trial or meta-analysis to people with different baseline risks. Ideally, there should be experimental evidence of the RRR in each population. However, in many trials, subgroup analyses show that the RRR is approximately constant in groups of patients with different characteristics. Cook and Sackett therefore proposed that decisions about individual patients could be made by using the NNT calculated from the RRR measured in trials and the baseline risk in the absence of treatment estimated for the individual patient.[2]

The method may not apply to periods of time different to that studied in the original trials.

USING THE NOMOGRAM

The nomogram shown on the next page allows the NNT to be found directly without any calculation: a straight line should be drawn from the point corresponding to the estimated absolute risk for the patient on the left hand scale to the point corresponding to the relative risk reduction stated in a trial or meta-analysis on the central scale. The intercept of this line with the right hand scale gives the NNT. By taking the upper and lower limits of the confidence interval of the RRR, the upper and lower limits of the NNT can be estimated.

REFERENCES

1. Chatellier G, Zapletal E, Lemaitre D, et al. The number needed to treat: a clinically useful nomogram in its proper context. *BMJ* 1996;321:426–429.
2. Cook RJ, Sackett DL. The number needed to treat: a clinically useful measure of treatment effect. *BMJ* 1995;310:452–454.

Number needed to treat

Appendix 2

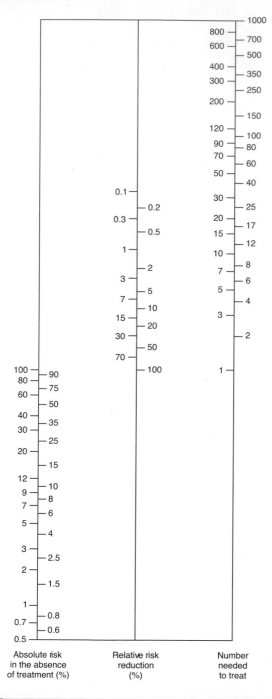

FIGURE Nomogram for calculating the number needed to treat. Published with permission.[1]